OXIDATIVE STRESS AND VASCULAR DISEASE

Developments in Cardiovascular Medicine

200. Walmor C. DeMello, Michiel J. Janse(eds.): *Heart Cell Communication in Health and Disease* ISBN 0-7923-8052-5
201. P.E. Vardas (ed.): *Cardiac Arrhythmias Pacing and Electrophysiology. The Expert View.* 1998 ISBN 0-7923-4908-3
202. E.E. van der Wall, P.K. Blanksma, M.G. Niemeyer, W. Vaalburg and H.J.G.M. Crijns (eds.) *Advanced Imaging in Coronary Artery Disease, PET, SPECT, MRI, IVUS, EBCT. 1998* ISBN 0-7923-5083-9
203. R.L. Wilensky (ed.) *Unstable Coronary Artery Syndromes, Pathophysiology, Diagnosis and Treatment. 1998.* ISBN 0-7923-8201-3
204. J.H.C. Reiber, E.E. van der Wall (eds.): *What's New in Cardiovascular Imaging?* 1998 ISBN 0-7923-5121-5
205. Juan Carlos Kaski, David W. Holt (eds.): *Myocardial Damage Early Detection by Novel Biochemical Markers. 1998.* ISBN 0-7923-5140-1
207. Gary F. Baxter, Derek M. Yellon, *Delayed Preconditioning and Adaptive Cardioprotection. 1998.* ISBN 0-7923-5259-9
208. Bernard Swynghedauw, *Molecular Cardiology for the Cardiologist, Second Edition* 1998. ISBN 0-7923-8323-0
209. Geoffrey Burnstock, James G.Dobson, Jr., Bruce T. Liang, Joel Linden (eds): *Cardiovascular Biology of Purines.* 1998. ISBN: 0-7923-8334-6
210. Brian D. Hoit, Richard A. Walsh (eds): *Cardiovascular Physiology in the Genetically Engineered Mouse.* 1998. ISBN: 0-7923-8356-7
211. Peter Whittaker, George S. Abela (eds.): *Direct Myocardial Revascularization: History, Methodology, Technology* 1998. ISBN: 0-7923-8398-2
212. C.A. Nienaber, R. Fattori (eds.): Diagnosis and Treatment of Aortic Diseases. 1999. ISBN: 0-7923-5517-2
213. Juan Carlos Kaski (ed.): *Chest Pain with Normal Coronary Angiograms: Pathogenesis, Diagnosis and Management.* 1999. ISBN: 0-7923-8421-0
214. P.A. Doevendans, R.S. Reneman and M. Van Bilsen (eds): *Cardiovascular Specific Gene Expression.* 1999 ISBN:0-7923-5633-0
215. G. Pons-Lladó, F. Carreras, X. Borrás, Subirana and L.J. Jiménez-Borreguero (eds.): *Atlas of Practical Cardiac Applications of MRI.* 1999 ISBN: 0-7923-5636-5
216. L.W. Klein, J.E. Calvin, *Resource Utilization in Cardiac Disease.* 1999. ISBN:0-7923-8509-8
217. R. Gorlin, G. Dangas, P. K. Toutouzas, M.M Konstadoulakis, *Contemporary Concepts in Cardiology, Pathophysiology and Clinical Management.*1999 ISBN:0-7923-8514-4
218. S. Gupta, J. Camm (eds.): *Chronic Infection, Chlamydia and Coronary Heart Disease.* 1999. ISBN:0-7923-5797-3
219. M. Rajskina: *Ventricular Fibrillation in Sudden Coronary Death.* 1999. ISBN:0-7923-8570-5
220. Z. Abedin, R. Conner: *Interpretation of Cardiac Arrhythmias: Self Assessment Approach.* 1999. ISBN:0-7923-8576-4
221. J. E. Lock, J.F. Keane, S. B. Perry: *Diagnostic and Interventional Catheterization In Congenital Heart Disease.* 2000. ISBN: 0-7923-8597-7
222. J.S. Steinberg: *Atrial Fibrillation after Cardiac Surgery.* 2000. ISBN: 0-7923-8655-8

Previous volumes are still available

KLUWER ACADEMIC PUBLISHERS - DORDRECHT/BOSTON/LONDON

OXIDATIVE STRESS AND VASCULAR DISEASE

Edited by:

John F. Keaney, Jr., M.D.
Associate Professor of Medicine and Pharmacology
Boston University School of Medicine
Boston, MA

KLUWER ACADEMIC PUBLISHERS

Boston/Dordrecht/London

Distributors for North, Central and South America:
Kluwer Academic Publishers
101 Philip Drive
Assinippi Park
Norwell, Massachusetts 02061 USA

Distributors for all other countries:
Kluwer Academic Publishers Group
Distribution Centre
Post Office Box 322
3300 AH Dordrecht, THE NETHERLANDS

Library of Congress Cataloging-in-Publication Data

Oxidative stress and vascular disease/edited by John F. Keaney, Jr.
    P. ; -- (Developments in cardiovascular medicine)
 Includes bibliographical references and index.
ISBN 0-7923-8678-7 (alk. Paper)
1. Blood-vessels--Pathophysiology. 2. Oxidation, Physiological 3. Stress
(Physiology) 4. Atherosclerosis--Pathophysiology. 5. Diabetic angiopathies--
Pathophysiology. 6. Hypertension--Pathophysiology. 7. Active oxygen in the body.
I. Keaney, John F. II. Series.
[DNLM: 1. Atherosclerosis--physiopathology. 2. Antioxidants. 3. Diabetes
Mellitus--physiopathology.   4.   Endothelium,   Vascular--metabolism.   5.
Hypertension--physiopathology. 6. Lipoproteins, LDL Cholesterol--metabolism. 7.
Oxidative Stress-physiology: WG 550 098 1999]
RC691.4.096 1999
616.1'307--dc21   99-046688

Printed on acid-free paper.

Printed in the United States of America

This book is dedicated to my parents, John and Rita, on the occasion of their fortieth wedding anniversary

Table of Contents

Contributors

John W. Baynes, Ph.D., Professor, Department of Chemistry and Biochemistry University of South Carolina, Columbia, SC 29208-0001

Bradford C. Berk, M.D., Ph.D., Professor of Cardiology, Chief, Cardiology Unit Director, Center for Cardiovascular Research, University of Rochester, 601 Elmwood Avenue, Box 679, Rochester, NY 14642

Judith A. Berliner, Ph.D., Professor, Department of Experimental Pathology and Laboratory Medicine, University of California, Los Angeles, 13-329 CHS, 650 Circle Drive South, Los Angeles, CA 90095-1732.

Elizabeth Biegelsen, M.D., Associate Physician, Boston Medical Center, 88 East Newton Street, Boston, MA 02118.

Richard Bucala, M.D., Ph.D., Professor and Head, Lab Medicine and Biochemistry, Picower Institute, 350 Community Drive, Manhasset, NY 11030

Sean Davies, BS., University of Utah, Eccles Institute of Human Genetics, Salt Lake City, UT 84112.

Elazer R. Edelman, M.D., Ph.D., Associate Professor of Medicine, Harvard-MIT Division of Health Science, MIT 16-343, Cambridge, MA 02139.

Jane Freedman, M.D., Assistant Professor of Medicine and Pharmacology, Georgetown University Medical Center, Med-Dent NE403, 3900 Reservoir Road NW, Washington, DC 20007

Balz Frei, Ph.D., Professor of Biochemistry and Biophysics, Director, Linus Pauling Institute at Oregon State University, 571 Weniger Hall, Corvallis, OR 97331.

J. Michael Gaziano, M.D., Assistant Professor of Medicine, Massachusetts Veterans Epidemiology Research Center, Brockton/West Roxbury Veterans Affairs Medical Center, 1300 VFW Parkway, West Roxbury, MA 02132

Kathy K. Griendling, Ph.D., Professor of Medicine, Emory University School of Medicine, Division of Cardiology, 1639 Pierce Dr., 319 WMB, Atlanta, GA 30322.

David G. Harrison, M.D., Professor of Medicine, Emory University School of Medicine, Division of Cardiology, 1639 Pierce Drive, WMB-319, Atlanta, GA 30322.

Jay W. Heinecke, M.D., Associate Professor of Medicine, Division of Atherosclerosis, Nutrition and Lipids, Washington University School of Medicine, Campus Box 8046, 660 S. Euclid Avenue, St. Louis, MO 63110-1093.

John F. Keaney, Jr., M.D., Associate Professor of Medicine and Pharmacology, Boston University School of Medicine, Whitaker Cardiovascular Institute, 715 Albany St. Room W507, Boston, MA 02118.

Charles Kunsch, Ph.D., Project Leader, Genomics, AtheroGenics, Inc., 8995 Westside Parkway, Alpharetta, GA 30004.

Norbert Leitinger, M.D., Department of Vascular Biology and Thrombosis Research, University of Vienna, Schwarzspanierstrasse 17, A-1090, Vienna, Austria.

Timothy Lyons, M.D., Associate Professor, Endocrinology Division, Medical University of South Carolina, 171 Ashley Ave., Charleston SC 29425.

Mark R. McCall, Ph.D., Linus Pauling Institute at Oregon State University, 571 Weniger Hall, Corvallis, OR 97331.

Thomas M. McIntyre, Ph.D., Professor, University of Utah, Eccles Institute of Human Genetics, Salt Lake City, UT 84112.

Russell Medford, M.D., Ph.D., CEO, AtheroGenics, Inc., 8995 Westside Parkway Alpharetta, GA 30004.

John Paolini, M.D., Cardiovascular Division, Brigham and Women's Hospital, 75 Francis St., Boston MA 02114.

Galen Pieper, Ph.D., Associate Professor, Department of Transplant Surgery, Medical College of Wisconsin, Froedfert East Clinic Building, 9200 West Wisconsin Avenue, Milwaukee, WI 53226.

Stephen M. Prescott, M.D., Professor of Medicine, Senior Research Director, Huntsman Cancer Institute, University of Utah, Bldg. 555, Rm. 540, Salt Lake City, Utah 84112.

Helmut Sies, M.D., Ph.D., Professor of Biochemistry, Institute of Physiol. Chem I Heinrich Heine University, Postfach 10 10 7, Dusseldorf, Germany D-40001 (2H, 88)

Mark Somers, M.D., Division of Cardiology, Emory University School of Medicine, 1639 Pierce Drive, WMB-319, Atlanta, GA 30322.

Daniel Steinberg, M.D., Ph.D., Professor of Medicine, University of California at San Diego, Department of Medicine 0682, 9500 Gilman Dr., La Jolla, CA 92093-0682.

Roland Stocker, Ph.D., Director, Biochemistry Group, The Heart Research Institute 145 Missenden Road, Camperdown, NSW, Sydney, Australia 2050

Suzanne R. Thorpe, Ph.D., Research Professor, Department of Chemistry and Biochemistry, University of South Carolina, Columbia, SC 29208-0001.

Sotirios Tsimikas, M.D., University of California at San Diego, Department of Medicine 0682, 9500 Gilman Drive, La Jolla, CA 92093-0682.

Joseph A. Vita, M.D., Associate Professor of Medicine, Boston Medical Center, Cardiology C-8, 88 E. Newton St., Boston, MA 02118.

Joseph Witztum, M.D., Professor of Medicine, University of California at San Diego, Department of Medicine 0682, 9500 Gilman Drive, La Jolla, CA 92093-0682.

Guy A. Zimmerman, M.D., Professor, Director, Program in Vascular Cell Biology, University of Utah, Eccles Institute of Human Genetics, Salt Lake City, UT 84112.

Foreword

One of the major biomedical triumphs of the post-World War II era was the definitive demonstration that hypercholesterolemia is a key causative factor in atherosclerosis; that hypercholesterolemia can be effectively treated; and that treatment significantly reduces not only coronary disease mortality but also all-cause mortality. Treatment to lower plasma levels of cholesterol – primarily low density lipoprotein (LDL) cholesterol – is now accepted as best medical practice and both physicians and patients are being educated to take aggressive measures to lower LDL. We can confidently look forward to important decreases in the toll of coronary artery disease over the coming decades. However, there is still uncertainty as to the exact mechanisms by which elevated plasma cholesterol and LDL levels initiate and favor the progression of lesions.

There is general consensus that one of the earliest responses to hypercholesterolemia is the adhesion of monocytes to aortic endothelial cells followed by their penetration into the subendothelial space, where they differentiate into macrophages. These cells, and also medial smooth muscle cells that have migrated into the subendothelial space, then become loaded with multiple, large droplets of cholesterol esters…the hallmark of the earliest visible atherosclerotic lesion, the so-called fatty streak. This lesion is the precursor of the more advanced lesions, both in animal models and in humans. Thus the centrality of hypercholesterolemia cannot be overstated. Still, the atherogenic process is complex and evolves over a long period of time. Factors initiating the lesion are not necessarily the same as those determining subsequent rate of progression. Undoubtedly many additional factors play important roles in the evolution of the lesion, *e.g.* the rate at which cells divide and deposit matrix, the remodeling of the stenotic lesion as it grows, the stabilization of the fibrous cap and so on. But in all animal models and in most humans with severe atherosclerosis some degree of dyslipidemia appears to be a necessary condition. New hypotheses should if possible be put into this context of established pathogenetic background.

This volume deals with one such hypothesis, namely, that oxidative modification of LDL and accompanying disturbances of oxidant/antioxidant balance may contribute importantly to the initiation and progression of lesions. The size of the volume testifies to the enormous amount of information that has been gathered…and in a relatively short time. A MEDLINE search shows that prior to 1989 there were a total of only 42 citations with the key word "oxidized LDL" (or "oxidised LDL", the latter being necessary to retrieve contributions from the United Kingdom). Between 1989 and the present time there have been an additional 1,773 articles so classified! The oxidation hypothesis has been heuristic and it continues to be viable. The intensity of interest in it undoubtedly stems in large part from the fact that several different antioxidant compounds have already been shown to be effective in slowing lesion progression in several different animal models. These effects have been independent of changes in plasma LDL or total cholesterol level. Thus, the effects to be expected from treatment with antioxidants should be additive to, or even synergistic with, the effects obtained by lowering plasma LDL levels.

The oxidative modification hypothesis was proposed in part because of the need to postulate some form of LDL that could account for the generation of foam cells----- uptake of native LDL could not induce foam cell formation. Oxidation of LDL, whether by cells in culture or by metal-catalyzed oxidation in the absence of cells, converted it to a form recognized by the scavenger receptors on macrophages, a form that could now induce foam cell formation. Another property of oxidized LDL that incriminated it early on was its cytotoxicity. Thus, incubation of cultured endothelial cells with LDL (in the absence of protective serum) led to cell death and this was shown to be due to oxidation of the LDL occurring during the incubation. These were the properties of oxidized LDL that initially led to its implication in atherogenesis. Subsequently, many additional biologic affects of oxidized LDL have been described that may also be highly relevant in atherogenesis. In addition, attention has been called to the changes in oxidant/antioxidant environment within the cells of animals or patients that are hypercholesterolemic. Actually, oxidation of LDL in the extracellular spaces and changes in the redox state of the cells probably occur simultaneously. Treatment with antioxidants would be expected to affect both.

The fatty streak lesion is clinically benign. Only when it has advanced to the state of a complex plaque that is either highly stenotic or that is unstable and predisposes to intravascular thrombosis does the atherosclerotic lesion become a clinical threat. The evolution of the fatty streak to the complex plaque has all the hallmarks of an inflammatory process and involves complex interactions among the cells in the developing lesion (monocyte/macrophages, T lymphocytes, smooth muscle cells and endothelial cells). Reactive oxygen and reactive nitrogen species play multiple complex roles in inflammation, affecting cell growth, cell viability, and gene expression. The precipitation of the fatal thrombosis in most instances is associated with an erosion of the cap of the lesion, with consequent exposure of the circulating blood to underlying pro-coagulant factors. Oxidized LDL and cellular redox state can regulate expression of metalloproteinases that could weaken the cap, for example. Exactly how oxidative processes impinge on other critical events in the evolution of the late lesion has yet to be elaborated and will undoubtedly be a major area of research in the coming decades.

It is still too early to say whether or not antioxidants will have the same effects in humans that they have in animal models. Speaking in favor, is the fact that the underlying pathology and pathogenesis of the disease in a variety of animal models (including the mouse, the rabbit, and the nonhuman primate) is fundamentally similar to that in humans. Moreover, there is a good deal of indirect evidence that oxidation of LDL does indeed occur in humans much as it does in animal models of atherosclerosis and that this can be affected by treatment with antioxidants. On the other hand, the rate of development of disease in humans is an order of magnitude slower than it is in animal models and thus interventions that work in the latter may not necessarily work in the former.

Only two large-scale double blind clinical intervention trials have been reported to date. One of these employed a rather low dose of vitamin E (50 mg/d) and there was no reduction in cardiovascular mortality. The other study utilized a much larger dose (400-800 mg/d) and observed a greater than 40% reduction in fatal and nonfatal myocardial infarctions. Fortunately, there are now in progress some 5 or 6 additional human intervention trials with various antioxidants and antioxidant combinations and we should have a definitive answer within the coming decade.

The papers in the present volume cover a broad spectrum of current research on oxidative stress and vascular disease. They are contributed by outstanding investigators at the forefront of their fields and cover everything from the most basic elements of free radical reactions to the potential clinical implications of oxidative stress in atherosclerosis. They provide a useful summary of the status of this rapidly growing field at the turn of the century.

Daniel Steinberg, M.D., Ph.D.
La Jolla, CA

Preface

The implication that oxidative stress and oxidative damage plays a major role in human disease is now well accepted. Although there has always been considerable interest in the role of oxidative stress in diseases such as cancer, inflammation, and neurodegenerative disorders, the role of oxidative stress in vascular disease is more recent. Since the late 1980s, it has become generally accepted that oxidative stress plays an important role in the development of atherosclerosis. This initial interest was a direct result of the "oxidative modification hypothesis" of atherosclerosis. However, as our knowledge base has increased, we have found evidence for involvement of oxidative stress in all manner of vascular diseases including diabetes, hypertension, and vascular remodeling.

The purpose of this book is to provide the reader with an overview of oxidative stress as it pertains to vascular diseases. The first part of the book is designed to help the reader grapple with important issues such as: Precisely what is oxidative stress?; What markers are available to assess oxidative stress?; and What are the precise sources of oxidative stress and antioxidant defenses in the vasculature? With this information as background, the book goes on to address the major vascular disease syndromes for which there is good evidence that oxidative stress may be involved. The greatest body of evidence exists for atherosclerosis and accordingly, this is the most extensive section. However, we have taken great care to try and provide the reader with objective evidence for the role of oxidative stress in other diseases such as diabetes, hypertension, and vascular remodeling. In each instance, the book is designed to provide a solid overview of the basic science data required to evaluate the role of oxidative stress. Animal data is then presented and finally, where applicable, the role of oxidative stress in human disease is discussed with the appropriate reference to epidemiologic data. The book is designed to appeal to both scientists and clinicians with an interest in vascular disease and its underlying pathophysiology.

No project occurs in a vacuum. I am deeply indebted to my contributors for without their help, this collection of work would not be possible.

John F. Keaney, Jr., M.D.
Boston, Massachusetts 1999

1 WHAT IS OXIDATIVE STRESS?

Helmut Sies

INTRODUCTION

Since the appearance in 1985 of the book, 'Oxidative Stress' (1), the biomedical area in particular has increasingly utilized this term in order to denote a challenge of the biological system by oxidants. The current cumulative number of Medline hits is 10,550, the 1,000/year mark having been passed in 1995, and the 3,000/year mark in 1997 (see Fig. 1). What precisely, does this term mean?

Let's start with a quote from the introductory chapter of a previous book (2): "As a biochemist, one may wonder whether Sclye's term should be stressed as it is in the present context. However, in recent years by something like a consensus in the biological-biomedical field 'oxidative stress' came to denote a disturbance in the pro-oxidant/antioxidant balance in favor of the former. Much experimental evidence now supports the thesis that the favorable aspects of aerobic life are also linked to potentially dangerous oxygen-linked oxidation processes. These are thought to form the basis of a number of physiological and pathophysiological phenomena and are participating in processes as diverse as inflammation, aging, carcinogenesis, drug action and drug toxicity, defense against protozoa and many others."

The *imbalance between oxidants and antioxidants in favor of the oxidants, potentially leading to damage*, forms the core of the definition of *'oxidative stress'*, as this author has discussed at various occasions before and after the 1985 book devoted to the term itself (2-8). Also two monographs have appeared (9, 10) and the first has stated: "In view of the proliferation of publications using the term [see Fig. 1], a few cautionary words might be appropriate. How can 'oxidative stress' be defined operationally? Considering the normal healthy state, oxidative challenge occurs in many cell types, but this alone does not constitute an oxidative stress. Likewise, a simple loss of antioxidants as resulting from limited nutritional supply is not sufficient. However, when there is an increased formation of pro-oxidants such as hydrogen peroxide, which is accompanied by a loss of glutathione and the formation of glutathione disulfide, we approach a definition. Even a severe loss of antioxidant may, however, still mean that there is no resulting damage." The second

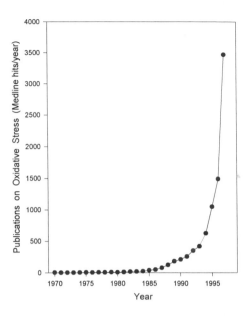

Figure 1. Hits for '*Oxidative Stress*' per year in Medline

monograph commented: "Novel roles of oxidants and antioxidants have been unraveled, as part of signaling cascades, and as mediators of an adaptive response, so that it is possible that the time course and even the final outcome of a variety of diseases can be critically modulated by strengthening the antioxidant side of the balance (10)."

The definition outlined above denotes a concept, in a nutshell. What does it encompass? As research has progressed, there have been ramifications and extensions, providing valuable further input to the scope of this term. Redox chemistry involves reduction-oxidation reactions, so obviously tipping the balance in favor of the reductants may also cause an imbalance (*i.e.*, 'reductive stress'). Further, the field of reactive species generated in biology has been extended, notably into the nitrogen-based reactants (which also contain oxygen), so there is a new term, 'nitrosative stress'. Without attempting a historical comprehensive digest of the field here, let's next look at some roots of these terms.

DEVELOPMENT OF CONCEPTS

The notion of oxidative challenge to biological systems most likely dates back to the early period of research on oxygen and its activation, *e.g.* to Otto Warburg, Leonor Michaelis, Britton Chance and other pioneers in this field. A hallmark in the development of the current topic is the work of Rebecca Gerschman in 1954 who viewed oxygen toxicity in common with X-irradiation (11). The body of knowledge that accumulated in the field was put together in a review on hydroperoxide metabolism in mammalian organs by Chance et al in 1979 (12). Searching available databases, one finds the following origins for the development of terms now synonymous with 'oxidative stress' were revealed:

Oxidative Stress. The study of hemolysis using exposure of red cells to conditions of oxidative challenge has been a very active field. In a study of glutathione in red cells in 1970, the effect of glutathione reductase deficiency on the stimulation of the hexose monophosphate shunt under oxidative stress was examined by Beutler's group (13); this may have been the first mention of the term, at least in a title of a publication readily retrievable. The next mention was only four years later, in work on a similar topic (14), and the research area was reviewed in 1975 (15). It took another decade until the book 'Oxidative Stress' (1) appeared.

Oxidant Stress. This term has been used much less frequently, but may be considered more or less synonymously, though sounding slightly ambiguous; the first mention again comes up in work on permeability properties in erythrocytes (16,17).

Pro-oxidant Stress Working on metal toxicity, again using red cells as a model, the effects of lead were described by Levander (18) employing this term. Cerutti (19) used the term 'pro-oxidant states' in his analysis of the role of oxidants in tumor promotion.

Dietary Oxidative Stress. The ability of dietary anti- and pro-oxidants to affect oxidative stress status has been widely discussed (see 20,21). Ames (22-24) has emphasized the importance of carcinogens and anti-carcinogens in food, and the term 'dietary oxidative stress' was coined by Levander (25,26). In particular, the relationship between oxidative stress and viral infections has been scrutinized in this regard (26,27). This area is receiving much attention in food science and in functional food considerations (28). In a recently proposed definition of dietary antioxidants, published by the Food and Nutrition Board of the National Academy of Sciences Institute of Medicine, (29), this term was described 'as a substance in foods that significantly decreases the adverse effects of reactive oxygen species, reactive nitrogen species, or both on normal physiological function in humans'.

Physiological Oxidative Stress. The fact that oxygen and its metabolites are not evenly distributed in organs and in subcellular organelles has led to the consideration that some sites are under what is called 'physiological' oxidative stress (30,31). Mitochondria are considered a site of physiological oxidative stress (32) and, in fact, one may consider that all cells, in the quasi-normal situation, are experiencing this form of challenge. In view of growing interest in *adaptive responses*, it is of interest to identify the need for and the extent of a physiological exposure to oxidative stress. The basal level of macrophage and neutrophil activation, for example, may fall into this category. Likewise, the physiological activity of glutamate (NMDA)- receptors could be included here. Thus, in specific locations in the physiological system there is a routine deployment of oxidants for normal functioning. A difficulty arises, of course, in defining the level at which the border to the pathological oxidative stress has been transcended. It may be that the accumulation of damage products, as part of the general definition of oxidative stress given above, could be a useful parameter in this regard. The adaptation to oxidative stress, initially studied predominantly with bacteria, *e.g.* in the oxyR-response (33-36), has also been demonstrated in eukaryotes (31,37,38), and may have interesting further functions in the mammalian organism. The responses of cell and tissues to oxidative stress in terms of gene expression in mammalian systems is developing rapidly (39).

The term 'exercised-induced oxidative stress' may also fall under the present heading (40). Spontaneous mutations and aging can be considered as being the result of exposure of the organism to oxidative stress, be it physiological or pathophysiological. The loss of the oxyR-regulon leads to an enormous increase in the number of spontaneous mutations (41,42). The relationship of oxidative stress to the aging process has been studied in many ways by Sohal (see 43). This pertains to Harman's (44-46) free radical theory of aging.

Oxidative Stress Status. The problem of assessing the biological status in intact systems has been tantalizing. Noninvasive methods are preferable, and stable endpoints are good candidates for useful applications (see 47-50). Our early work was on using GSSG efflux as an indicator (51-52). Many efforts continue to be directed to this topic, e.g. the use of 8-oxodG (53) or certain isoprostanes (50) in urinary samples. The topic of *biomarkers* would require a separate chapter.

Reductive Stress. In analogy to hyperoxia being linked to oxidative stress, hypoxia or anoxia may be linked to a reductive stress. The term 'reductive stress' was introduced by Wendel (54) to denote the metabolic initiation of iron redox cycling following overproduction of NADH (see also 55). Excessive redox cycling at the expense of reducing equivalents, either NADPH or NADH, is cytotoxic and is being utilized in chemotherapy, for example. Of course, the process of redox cycling ultimately involves oxidative stress, resulting from superoxide generation due to autoxidation of semiquinones serves as only one example (for review, see 56). From a toxicological point of view, therefore, NADPH (or NADH) can be considered as a 'detoxicant' and as a 'toxicant' (57). An oxidized compound, the disulfide lipoate, has been used to alleviate reductive stress (58) as has activation of the GSH exporter (59).

The effects caused by respiratory inhibition ('chemical hypoxia') which favors formation of toxic oxygen species have also been called 'reductive stress' (60,61). A role of VEGF in mediating vascular dysfunction induced by hypoxia-like cytosolic metabolic imbalances such as reductive stress and increased superoxide and nitric oxide production has been studied (62). As would be expected, reductive stress can be counteracted by pyruvate (63). A gene battery responsive to reductive stress has also been analyzed (64).

Nitrosative Stress. Working with nitrosothiols, Hausladen et al (65) observed a transcriptional activation of the *oxyR* regulon mentioned above, and these authors called this 'nitrosative stress'. It was also found that zinc release was mediated by nitrosative stress, and that this may be relevant in altering gene expression patterns (66). This area of particular interest to vascular physiology and pathophysiology has been evaluated in some detail recently (66-69).

SUMMARY

The developments sketched, in brief, in this introductory chapter focusing on vascular disease demonstrate the continuing need to assess and re-assess the concepts and terms used in ongoing research. It is obvious that the term 'oxidative stress' evokes different associations to researchers coming from different fields of interest. Thus, on some occasions it has been over used, and caution is advised when using this term in studies in which the molecular species causing "stress" are not specified.

The different concepts presented above may, in fact, not be at variance with each other. Rather, the different terms emphasize a common phenomenon. This has been pointed out by Kehrer and Lund (70) in their discussion of cellular reducing equivalents and oxidative stress. Likewise, there are many parallels between the reactions distinguished as nitrosative *vs.* oxidative. One chemical difference is, of course, the introduction of a nitroso group or a nitro group into a biological target (69).

Our own recent interest relates to protection against oxidative stress. Apart from analyzing the strategies in antioxidant defense in general (71), one area we have studied is the use of a seleno-organic compound, ebselen, as a glutathione peroxidase mimic (see review 72). Interestingly, this compound was shown to react very efficiently with peroxynitrite (73-74). An analogous function of selenocysteine in the selenoprotein, glutathione peroxidase, has recently been described, establishing its activity as a peroxynitrite reductase (75). This shows that protection can be afforded against oxidative stress as well as nitrosative stress simultaneously, and it underlines the close relationship between the two.

REFERENCES

1.   Sies H (ed.)*Oxidative Stress*, London, Academic Press, 1985, pp 1.
2.   Sies H: Oxidative Stress: Introductory remarks, in Sies H (ed): *Oxidative Stress*. London, Academic Press, 1985, pp 1.
3.   Cadenas E, Wefers H, Müller A, Brigelius R, Sies H. Active oxygen metabolites and their action in the hepatocyte. Studies on chemiluminescence responses and alkane production. *Agents Actions Suppl.* 1982;11:203.

4.   Sies H, Cadenas E: Oxidative stress: damage to intact cells and organs. *Philos Trans R Soc Lond B Biol Sci.* 1985;311:617.

5.   Cadenas E, Sies H. Oxidative stress: excited oxygen species and enzyme activity. *Adv Enzyme Regul.* 1985;23:217.

6.   Sies H: Biochemistry of Oxidative Stress. *Angew Chem Int Ed Engl.* 1986;25:1058.

7.   Sies H. Oxidative stress: from basic research to clinical application. *Am J Medi.* 1991;91:31S.

8.   Sies H. Oxidative stress: oxidants and antioxidants. *Exp Physiol.* 1997;82:291.

9.   Sies H (ed.)*Oxidative Stress: Oxidants and Antioxidants*, London, Academic Press, 1991, pp 1.

10.   Sies H (ed.)*Antioxidants in Disease Mechanisms and Therapy*, San Diego, Academic Press, 1997, pp 1.

11.   Gerschman R, Gilbert DL, Nye SW, Dwyer P, Fenn WO. Oxygen poisoning and X-irradiation: a mechanism in common. *Science.* 1954;119:623.

12.   Chance B, Sies H, Boveris A. Hydroperoxide metabolism in mammalian organs. *Physiol Rev.* 1979;59:527.

13.   Paniker NV, Srivastava SK, Beutler E. Glutathione metabolism of the red cells. Effect of glutathione reductase deficiency on the stimulation of hexose monophosphate shunt under oxidative stress. *Biochim Biophys Acta.* 1970;456.

14.   Gaetani GD, Parker JC, Kirkman HN. Intracellular restraint: A new basis for the limitation in response to oxidative stress in human erythrocytes containing low-activity variants of glucose-6-phosphate dehydrogenase. *Proc Natl Acad Sci USA.* 1974;71:3584.

15.   Benöhr HC, Waller HD. Glutathion (Bedeutung in Biologie und Medizin). *Klin Wschr.* 1975;53:789.

16.   Brownlee NR, Huttner JJ, Panganamala RV, Cornwell DG. Role of vitamin E in glutathione-induced oxidant stress: methemoglobin, lipid peroxidation, and hemolysis. *J Lipid Res.* 1977;18:635.

17.   Harm W, Deamer DW. Altered potassium permeability in vitamin E-deficient rat erythrocytes. *Physiol Chem & Physics.* 1977;9:501.

18.   Levander OA. Lead toxicity and nutritional deficiencies. *Environ Health Perspect.* 1979;29:1988.

19.   Cerutti PA. Prooxidant states and tumor promotion. *Science.* 1985;227:375.

20.   Halliwell B. How to characterize a biological antioxidant. *Free Radic Res Commun.* 1990;9:121.

21.   Halliwell B. Oxidative stress, nutrition and health. Experimental strategies for optimization of nutritional antioxidant intake in humans. *Free Radic Res.* 1996;25:57.

22.   Ames BN: Dietary carcinogens and anticarcinogens. Oxygen radicals and degenerative diseases. *Science.* 1983;221:1256.

23.   Ames BN, Shigenaga MK, Hagen TM. Oxidants, antioxidants, and the degenerative diseases of aging. *Proc Natl Acad Sci USA.* 1993;90:7915.

24.   Swirsky Gold L, Stern BR, Slone TH, Brown JP, Manley NB, Ames BN. Pesticide residues in food: investigation of disparities in cancer risk estimates. *Cancer Lett.* 1997;117:195.

25.   Levander OA, Fontela R, Morris VC, Ager AL, Jr. Protection against murine cerebral malaria by dietary-induced oxidative stress. *J Parasitol.* 1995;81:99.

26.   Beck MA, Levander OA. Dietary oxidative stress and the potentiation of viral infection. *Annu Rev Nutr.* 1998;18:93.

27.   Schwarz KB. Oxidative stress during viral infection: a review. *Free Radic Biol Med.* 1996;21:641.

28.   Diplock AT, Charleux JL, Crozier-Willi G, Kok FJ, Rice-Evans C, Roberfroid M, Stahl W, Vina-Ribes J: Functional food science and defence against reactive ocidative species. *Brit J Nutr.* 1998;77.

29.   Anonymous. Dietary reference intakes. Washington, Natl Acad Sci Press 1998;1-11

30.   Barja de Quiroga G. Brown fat thermogenesis and exercise: two examples of physiological oxidative stress? *Free Radic Biol Med.* 1992;13:325.

31.   Choi J, Liu RM, Forman HJ. Adaptation to oxidative stress: quinone-mediated protection of signaling in rat lung epithelial L2 cells. *Biochem Pharmacol.* 1997;53:987.

32. Kretzschmar M. Regulation of hepatic glutathione metabolism and its role in hepatotoxicity. *Exp Toxicol Pathol.* 1996;48:439.

33. Christman MF, Morgan RW, Jacobson FS, Ames BN. Positive control of a regulon for defenses against oxidative stress and some heat-shock proteins in Salmonella typhimurium. *Cell.* 1985;41:753.

34. Morgan RW, Christman MF, Jacobson FS, Storz G, Ames BN. Hydrogen peroxide-inducible proteins in Salmonella typhimurium overlap with heat shock and other stress proteins. *Proc Natl Acad Sci USA.* 1986;83:8059.

35. Imlay JA, Linn S. Mutagenesis and stress responses induced in Escherichia coli by hydrogen peroxide. *J Bacteriol.* 1987;169:296736.

36. Demple B, Amabile Cuevas CF. Redox redux: the control of oxidative stress responses. *Cell.* 1991;67:837.

37. Davies JM, Lowry CV, Davies KJ. Transient adaptation to oxidative stress in yeast. *Arch Biochem Biophys.* 1995;317:1.

38. Wiese AG, Pacifici RE, Davies KJ. Transient adaptation of oxidative stress in mammalian cells. *Arch Biochem Biophys.* 1995;318:231.

39. Janssen YM, Van Houten B, Borm PJ, Mossman BT. Cell and tissue responses to oxidative damage. *Lab Invest.* 1993;69:261.

40. Reddy KV, Anuradha D, Kumar TC, Reddanna P. Induction of Ya1 subunit of rat hepatic glutathione S-transferases by exercise-induced oxidative stress. *Arch Biochem Biophys.* 1995;323:6.

41. Storz G, Christman MF, Sies H, Ames BN. Spontaneous mutagenesis and oxidative damage to DNA in Salmonella typhimurium. *Proc Natl Acad Sci USA.* 1987;84:8917.

42. MacGregor JT, Wehr CM, Hiatt RA, Peters B, Tucker JD, Langlois RG, Jacob RA, Jensen RH, Yager JW, Shigenaga MK, Frei B, Eynon BP, Ames BN. 'Spontaneous' genetic damage in man: evaluation of interindividual variability, relationship among markers of damage, and influence of nutritional status. *Mutat Res.* 1997;377:125.

43. Sohal RS, Weindruch R. Oxidative stress, caloric restriction, and aging. *Science.* 1996,273.59.

44. Harman D, Piette LH. Free radical theory of aging: free radical reactions in serum. *J Gerontol.* 1966;21:560

45. Harman D. The aging process. *Proc Natl Acad Sci USA.* 1981;78:7124.

46. Harman D. The aging process: major risk factor for disease and death. *Proc Natl Acad Sci USA.* 1991;88:5360.

47. Pryor WA, Godber SS. Noninvasive measures of oxidative stress status in humans. *Free Radic Biol Med.* 1991,10:177.

48. Boveris A, Llesuy S, Azzalis LA, Giavarotti L, Simon KA, Junqueira VB, Porta EA, Videla LA, Lissi EA. In situ rat brain and liver spontaneous chemiluminescence after acute ethanol intake. *Toxicol Lett.* 1997;93:23.

49. Uppu RM, Cueto R, Squadrito GL, Salgo MG, Pryor WA. Competitive reactions of peroxynitrite with 2'-deoxyguanosine and 7,8-dihydro-8-oxo-2'-deoxyguanosine (8-oxodG): relevance to the formation of 8-oxodG in DNA exposed to peroxynitrite. *Free Radic Biol Med.* 1996;21:407.

50. Roberts LJ, 2d, Moore KP, Zackert WE, Oates JA, Morrow JD. Identification of the major urinary metabolite of the F2-isoprostane 8-iso-prostaglandin F2alpha in humans. *J Biol Chem.* 1996;271:20617.

51. Bartoli GM, Sies H. Reduced and oxidized glutathione efflux from liver. *FEBS Lett.* 1978;86:89.

52. Akerboom TP, Bilzer M, Sies H. The relationship of biliary glutathione disulfide efflux and intracellular glutathione disulfide content in perfused rat liver. *J Biol Chem.* 1982;257:4248.

53. Shigenaga MK, Aboujaoude EN, Chen Q, Ames BN. Assays of oxidative DNA damage biomarkers 8-oxo-2'-deoxyguanosine and 8-oxoguanine in nuclear DNA and biological fluids by high-performance liquid chromatography with electrochemical detection. *Methods Enzymol.* 1994;234:16.

54. Wendel A. Measurement of in vivo lipid peroxidation and toxicological significance. *Free Radic Biol Med.* 1987;3:355.

55.   Jaeschke H, Kleinwaechter C, Wendel A. NADH-dependent reductive stress and ferritin-bound iron in allyl alcohol-induced lipid peroxidation in vivo: the protective effect of vitamin E. *Chem Biol Interact.* 1992;81:57.

56.   Kappus H, Sies H. Toxic drug effects associated with oxygen metabolism: redox cycling and lipid peroxidation. *Experientia.* 1981;37:1233.

57.   Sies H, Brigelius R, Wefers H, Müller A, Cadenas E. Cellular redox changes and response to drugs and toxic agents. *Fundam Appl Toxicol.* 1983;3:200.

58.   Roy S, Sen CK, Tritschler HJ, Packer L. Modulation of cellular reducing equivalent homeostasis by alpha-lipoic acid - Mechanisms and implications for diabetes and ischemic injury. *Biochem Biophys Res Commun.* 1997;53:393

59.   Khan S, OBrien PJ. Rapid and specific efflux of glutathione before hepatocyte injury induced by hypoxia. *Bichem Biophys Res Commun.* 1997;238:320.

60.   Gores GJ, Flarsheim CE, Dawson TL, Nieminen AL, Herman B, Lemasters JJ. Swelling, reductive stress, and cell death during chemical hypoxia in hepatocytes. *Am J Physiol.* 1989;257:C347.

61.   Nishimura Y, Romer LH, Lemasters JJ. Mitochondrial dysfunction and cytoskeletal disruption during chemical hypoxia to cultured rat hepatic sinusoidal endothelial cells: The pH paradox and cytoprotection by glucose, acidotic pH, and glycine. *Hepatology.* 1998;27:1039.

62.   Tilton RG, Kawamura T, Chang KC, Ido Y, Bjercke RJ, Stephan CC, Brock TA, Williamson JR. Vascular dysfunction induced by elevated glucose levels in rats is mediated by vascular endothelial growth factor. *J Clin Invest.* 1997;99:2192.

63.   Kashiwagi A, Nishio Y, Asahina T, Ikebuchi M, Harada N, Tanaka Y, Takahara N, Taki H, Obata T, Hidaka H, Saeki Y, Kikkawa R. Pyruvate improves deleterious effects of high glucose on activation of pentose phosphate pathway and glutathione redox cycle in endothelial cells. *Diabetes.* 1997;46:2088.

64.   Halleck MM, Holbrook NJ, Skinner J, Liu H, Stevens JL. The molecular response to reductive stress in LLC-PK1 renal epithelial cells: Coordinate transcriptional regulation of gadd153 and grp78 genes by thiols. *Cell Stress Chaperones.* 1997;2:31.

65.   Hausladen A, Privalle CT, Keng T, DeAngelo J, Stamler JS. Nitrosative stress: activation of the transcription factor OxyR. *Cell.* 1996;86:719.

66.   Berendji D, Kolb-Bachofen V, Meyer KL, Grapenthin O, Weber H, Wahn V, Kröncke KD. Nitric oxide mediates intracytoplasmic and intranuclear zinc release. *FEBS Lett.* 1997;405:37.

67.   Szabo C, Dawson VL. Role of poly(ADP-ribose) synthetase in inflammation and ischaemia-reperfusion. *Trends Pharmacol Sci.* 1998;19:287.

68.   Wink DA, Cook JA, Kim SY, Vodovotz Y, Pacelli R, Krishna MC, Russo A, Mitchell JB, Jourd'heuil D, Miles AM, Grisham MB. Superoxide modulates the oxidation and nitrosation of thiols by nitric oxide-derived reactive intermediates. Chemical aspects involved in the balance between oxidative and nitrosative stress. *J Biol Chem.* 1997;272:11147.

69.   Wink DA, Mitchell JB. Chemical biology of nitric oxide: Insights into regulatory, cytotoxic and cytoprotective mechanisms of nitric oxide. *Free Radic Biol Med.* 1998;25:434(abstract).

70.   Kehrer JP, Lund LG. Cellular reducing equivalents and oxidative stress. *Free Radic Biol Med.* 1994;17:65.

71.   Sies H. Strategies of antioxidant defense. *Eur J Biochem.* 1993;215:213.

72.   Sies H. Ebselen, a selenoorganic compound as glutathione peroxidase mimic. *Free Radic Biol Med.* 1993;14:313.

73.   Masumoto H, Sies H. The reaction of ebselen with peroxynitrite. *Chem Res Toxicol.* 1996;9:262.

74.   Masumoto H, Kissner R, Koppenol WH, Sies H. Kinetic study of the reaction of ebselen with peroxynitrite. *FEBS Lett.* 1996;398:179.

75   Sies H, Sharov VS, Klotz LO, Briviba K. Glutathione peroxidase protects against peroxynitrite-mediated oxidations: a new function for selenoproteins as peroxynitrite reductase. *J Biol Chem.* 1997;272:27812.

2 SOURCES OF VASCULAR OXIDATIVE STRESS

Jay W. Heinecke

INTRODUCTION

Atherosclerotic vascular disease is the leading cause of death in industrialized society. One important risk factor for the onset of atherosclerosis is an elevated concentration of low density lipoprotein (LDL), the major carrier of blood cholesterol (1). It is thus paradoxical that LDL often fails to exert atherogenic effects *in vitro*. These observations led to the suggestion that LDL has to be modified to promote vascular disease (2,3). Subsequent studies indicate that cultured arterial cells modify LDL (4) and that the mechanism involves oxidative damage (5-7). Oxidized LDL, but not native LDL, exerts a multitude of potentially atherogenic effects *in vitro* and *in vivo* (8,9), suggesting that oxidation might be a physiologically relevant pathway for LDL modification in the artery wall.

Several lines of evidence implicate oxidatively damaged LDL as an atherogenic agent *in vivo* (reviewed in 8-10). First, oxidized LDL been isolated from atherosclerotic lesions (11,12). Second, chemical and immunohistochemical studies detect oxidized lipids in human and animal atherosclerotic lesions (13,14). Third, a number of structurally unrelated antioxidants retard lesion formation in hypercholesterolemic animals and non-human primates (15,16). Finally, therapy with vitamin E, a lipid-soluble antioxidant, dramatically reduces the risk for acute coronary events in patients with established coronary artery disease (17). Collectively, these observations suggest that oxidative stress may be one important factor in the genesis of atherosclerotic vascular disease.

The oxidation hypothesis of atherosclerosis raises a critical question: what are the pathways that oxidize LDL *in vivo*? In this review, we will evaluate studies that investigate mechanisms of lipoprotein oxidation, a topic that may be critical to choosing effective agents to block oxidation. Particular emphasis will be placed on recent results addressing the mechanisms for oxidative stress in the human artery wall.

MICROENVIRONMENTS AND MECHANISTIC ISSUES

Plasma contains high concentrations of antioxidants (18), which suggests that LDL oxidation takes place in another environment where antioxidants can become depleted. The artery wall potentially represents one such environment.

Consistent with this hypothesis, cultured arterial wall cells accelerate LDL oxidation (5-7), and these studies have resulted in a number of proposed mechanisms for LDL oxidation *in vivo*. However, there is considerable controversy over the relevant biochemical pathways. The discrepancies may stem in part from: (i) differing concentrations of free metal ions in tissue culture media, (ii) differing cell types, (iii) whether LDL contains preexisting hydroperoxides, (iv) differences in analytical methods, and (v) reliance on biological endpoints, which bear an uncertain relationship to the extent of lipid and protein oxidation.

PROPOSED PATHWAYS FOR VASCULAR OXIDATIVE STRESS

Extracellular Metal Ions

Redox active transition metal ions provide one important pathway for LDL oxidation *in vitro*. Cultured smooth muscle cells require either extracellular iron or copper to modify LDL (5). Metal chelators inhibit LDL oxidation by many other types of cells (5-7) and high concentrations of metal ions oxidize LDL in the absence of cells (5,7). Protein-bound metal ions in ceruloplasmin (19) and hemin (20) also promote LDL oxidation, though the mechanisms may differ from those of free metal ions.

Despite extensive study, the mechanisms by which metal ions stimulate LDL oxidation are poorly understood. Metal ions catalyze the decomposition of lipid peroxides into potent oxidizing species (21), but the relevance of this mechanism is uncertain because LDL isolated from plasma contains extremely low levels of hydroperoxides (22). However, it is important to note that a small fraction of LDL in plasma, termed LDL⁻, contains elevated levels of lipid oxidation products (23), suggesting that the conversion of preformed hydroperoxides into further lipid oxidation products might be physiologically relevant. The origin of LDL⁻ is uncertain, but it may be generated in blood or represent oxidized LDL generated in peripheral tissue that has reentered the circulation.

It has not yet been determined whether extracellular free metal ions (or low molecular weight chelates of metal ions) exist extracellularly *in vivo*. Redox active metal ions were found in tissue homogenates of atherosclerotic tissue, but results from normal aortic tissue subjected to the same homogenization procedure were not reported (24-26). Transferrin is the major carrier of iron in plasma, but its high-affinity binding sites for iron and copper are partially saturated in normal individuals (27). Moreover, low concentrations of albumin, the most abundant protein in plasma, inhibit metal ion-dependent LDL oxidation (28). This protein also avidly binds free copper (29), suggesting that extracellular free metal ions are unlikely to be present in normal arterial tissue.

Epidemiological studies examining the relationship between iron stores and risk for atherosclerosis have provided inconsistent results, which supports the notion that free iron is unlikely to be a major risk factor for atherosclerosis (reviewed in 30). Moreover, premature atherosclerosis is not a prominent feature of hemochromatosis (31,32), a common genetic disease that causes iron to accumulate in plasma and liver. Animal studies have also yielded inconsistent results regarding the effect of iron on atherosclerosis (33,34). Whether excess copper promotes LDL oxidation *in vivo* is less clear. Individuals with Wilson's disease appear not to be at increased risk for atherosclerosis, even though this disorder raises copper levels in liver, plasma and brain (35). However, it is important to note that levels of ceruloplasmin are low in this disorder (19,35).

Proteins that are oxidatively damaged by different reaction pathways *in vitro* exhibit distinct patterns of amino acid oxidation products (reviewed in 36). This suggests that the analysis of protein oxidation products in arterial tissue or in LDL, isolated from arterial tissue might provide insights into the mechanisms of oxidative damage *in vivo*. Proteins are particularly attractive candidates for such analysis because they are relatively difficult to oxidize. The spectrum of modified amino acids in an oxidized protein is thus likely to reflect the initial oxidative insult. In contrast, lipid peroxidation involves chain-propagating reactions that generate additional oxidizing intermediates and reaction products which may mask the initial oxidative insult.

Hydroxy radical is one important oxidant generated by metal ion-dependent reactions (37). One pathway for the *in vitro* generation of hydroxyl radical (HO$^\bullet$) involves the reaction of a reduced metal ion (such as Fe^{2+} or Cu^{1+}) with hydrogen peroxide (H_2O_2).

$$Fe^{2+} + H_2O_2 \rightarrow HO^\bullet + HO^- + Fe^{3+}$$

LDL and model proteins exposed to hydroxyl radical generated by metal ions exhibit a dramatic increase in ortho-tyrosine and meta-tyrosine (38,39). LDL oxidized by copper also demonstrates larger increases in ortho-tyrosine and meta-tyrosine (38). These observations suggest that these unusual tyrosine isomers might be useful markers of metal ion mediated damage *in vivo*.

We have used isotope dilution gas chromatography-mass spectrometry, a sensitive and specific analytical method, to quantify the levels of ortho-tyrosine and meta-tyrosine in plasma LDL and in LDL isolated from human atherosclerotic lesions (38). Lesion LDL did not contain higher levels of either oxidation product than plasma LDL. Moreover, the levels of ortho-tyrosine and meta-tyrosine were similar in normal aortic tissue and in fatty streaks, the earliest lesion of atherosclerosis. These observations suggest that metal ions are unlikely to play a role in oxidizing LDL early in the atherosclerotic process. In contrast, we did find a two- to three-fold increase in the levels of ortho-tyrosine and meta-tyrosine in advanced atherosclerotic lesions, though the increase was not statistically significant (38). This raises the possibility that redox active metal ions, perhaps released from necrotic or dystrophic cells, promote LDL oxidation late in the atherosclerotic process.

Superoxide

Superoxide, the one electron reduced form of molecular oxygen, is one well-characterized reactive oxygen species that promotes lipid peroxidation (40). Superoxide production by activated phagocytes plays a critical role in host defenses against invading microorganisms (41). The biochemical basis for superoxide production by neutrophils, monocytes and macrophages is a membrane-associated NADPH oxidase. The NADPH oxidase catalyzes the direct reduction of molecular oxygen to superoxide ($O_2^{\bullet-}$).

$$NADPH + 2\,O_2 \rightarrow 2\,O_2^{\bullet-} + NADP^+ + H^+$$

Monocyte activation promotes LDL oxidation (42,43) and the reaction is inhibited by superoxide dismutase, a scavenger of superoxide. Moreover, LDL oxidation is inhibited when phagocytes defective in superoxide production are substituted for normal phagocytes (42). These observations suggest that superoxide generated by phagocytes is one pathway for LDL oxidation *in vitro*.

Investigators have suggested that superoxide is involved in LDL oxidation by other types of cells because: (i) cell-mediated oxidation of LDL is inhibited by superoxide dismutase (44-46), (ii) levels of superoxide production correlate with cell-mediated oxidation of LDL (44-46), (iii) superoxide generated enzymatically (37) or radiolytically (47) promotes LDL oxidation when metal ions are present. However, the interpretation of these studies is complicated by several problems. First, superoxide dismutase can inhibit LDL oxidation by binding free metal ions rather than by scavenging superoxide (49). Second, superoxide dismutase does not uniformly inhibit LDL oxidation by cultured cells (48,49). However, free copper - which is widely used as a catalyst for LDL oxidation and is present at high concentrations in many tissue culture media (5) - also reacts with superoxide (50). The rate of reaction of superoxide with copper is near the diffusion controlled limit (50). When free copper is present at high concentrations in tissue culture medium, superoxide might react preferentially with free copper even when superoxide dismutase is present. This would make it difficult both to detect superoxide and to show that superoxide dismutase was inhibiting LDL oxidation.

It is unknown whether superoxide plays a role in oxidizing LDL *in vivo*. It is important to note that superoxide at neutral pH requires metal ions to promote LDL lipid peroxidation (37,40,44,47). In contrast, the protonated form of superoxide that forms under acidic conditions will directly stimulate lipid peroxidation (51). Superoxide might therefore promote LDL oxidation in the artery wall by several different mechanisms. Lipid-laden macrophages are the cellular hallmark of the early atherosclerotic lesion, and these cells are also prominent during latter stages of lesion development (8,9), suggesting that that superoxide generation might be one mechanism for oxidative damage in the artery wall. It would be of interest to determine whether atherosclerosis is inhibited in hypercholesterolemic mice that are deficient in phagocyte superoxide production.

Thiols

Early studies demonstrated that smooth muscle cells generate extracellular superoxide and that superoxide dismutase inhibits LDL oxidation, suggesting that the generation of reactive oxygen intermediates by cells might promote LDL oxidation *in vitro* (44,52). One mechanism for the generation of superoxide and other oxidizing species (such as sulfur centered radicals) involves thiols (51). We therefore investigated the role of autoxidizing thiols in lipid peroxidation. Incubating smooth muscle cells in medium free of L-cystine (the disulfide form of L-cysteine) inhibited both superoxide production and LDL oxidation (52). Both effects were reversed by adding L-cystine back to the medium. These results led us to propose that smooth muscle cells take up L-cystine and reduce it to a thiol, which leaves the cell. Autoxidation of the thiol then generates superoxide (51,52), which mediates LDL oxidation when metal ions are present . The ability of thiols to oxidize LDL in the absence of cells supports this proposal (53,54). Moreover, cultured macrophages and endothelial cells use an L-cystine-dependent pathway to generate extracellular thiol, which causes LDL oxidation in medium containing metal ions (55).

Thiols are also potent scavengers of certain reactive intermediates (51). Cells contain mM concentrations of glutathione, a thiol that plays a key role in protecting cells from oxidative stress. Whether thiols exert pro- or antioxidant effects *in vitro* depends critically on the reaction conditions. For example, thiols promote LDL oxidation when the reaction buffer contains free iron or low molecular weight chelates of copper, but inhibit LDL oxidation when free copper is used as the catalyst for oxidation (54,56). The effects of thiols on LDL oxidation *in vitro* is affected by a number of factors, including the chelators and metal ions in the medium.

Thiols may play a role in LDL oxidation *in vivo*. In persons with homocystinuria, a genetic disorder that results in massive elevations of plasma and urine homocystine, premature atherosclerosis and endothelial denudation are common (57). Elevated levels of homocysteine are an important risk factor for premature vascular disease in the general population (58). Moreover, infusing homocysteine into primates induces vascular injury (59). However, lipid peroxides are undetectable in the plasma of homocystinuric patients, arguing against the oxidation of circulating lipoproteins in plasma (60). The pathology of vascular damage in persons suffering from homocystinuria also differs morphologically from the usual forms of atherosclerosis (57), indicating that other mechanisms may mediate endothelial injury. It will be interesting to determine in animal studies whether elevated homocysteine promotes atherosclerosis.

Lipoxygenase

Lipoxygenases are intracellular enzymes that peroxidize polyunsaturated fatty acids into oxygenated lipids with potent biological effects (61). Lipoxygenases are present in macrophages, endothelial cells and smooth muscle cells - the major cellular elements of atherosclerotic lesions (8,9,61).

A combination of soybean lipoxygenase and phospholipase oxidized LDL *in vitro* (62), suggesting that lipoxygenases might be one pathway for LDL oxidation. Moreover, inhibitors of lipoxygenase blocked LDL oxidation by cultured cells (63). However, most of the inhibitors were non-specific, and they also blocked LDL oxidation by copper in the absence of cells (64,65). Both protein and mRNA for lipoxygenase have been found in atherosclerotic lesions (66). The patterns of immunostaining for 15-lipoxygenase, oxidation-specific epitopes and macrophages were similar. Moreover, transient overexpression of 15-lipoxygenase protein results in increased levels of oxidation specific epitopes in rabbit arteries (67). Taken together, these results indicate that lipoxygenase may be one pathway for LDL oxidation *in vivo*.

The mechanism by which an intracellular enzyme such as lipoxygenase could contribute to LDL oxidation has been the subject of much debate. One proposed pathway, the "seeding" mechanism, suggests that membrane phospholipids containing oxidized fatty acids are transferred from cells to LDL (63). Lipoxygenase might therefore promote LDL oxidation indirectly via "seeding" of LDL with products that promote subsequent oxidation reactions. Alternatively, oxygenated products generated by lipoxygenase might exert powerful biological effects on the artery wall without the direct involvement of LDL oxidation.

The stereospecific isomer 13S-hydroxy-9Z,11E-octadecadienoic acid (13S-HODE) is the major product of lipid peroxidation when LDL is incubated with 15-lipoxygenase (68). In contrast, LDL oxidized with copper yields a random mixture of 13S- and 13R-HODE isomers (68-70). LDL oxidized *in vitro* with 15-lipoxygenase exhibits an S/R ratio of 13-HODE products of approximately 2.5, whereas it is only about 1 when copper is the oxidant. Measuring the ratio of R to S isomers therefore might indicate whether lipoxygenase is active in a biological system.

Folcik et al. found an S/R ratio of 1.12 in total lipids extracted from advanced atherosclerotic lesions harvested at surgery (69). Kuhn et al found a ratio of 1.08 in HODEs extracted from early atherosclerotic lesions but no increased S/R ratio for lipids extracted from advanced atherosclerotic lesions (70). The detection of these small but statistically significant increases in 13S-HODE is consistent with the hypothesis that 15-lipoxygenase oxidizes lipids in the artery wall. It is important to note, however, that other enzymatic pathways also can produce stereospecific lipid peroxidation products (71).

Several groups have used the technique of homologous recombination to generate mice that are deficient in 12-lipoxygenase, the mouse analogue of human 15-lipoxygenase. A recent study has demonstrated that apo E-deficient mice lacking 12-lipoxygenase demonstrate less atherosclerosis than apo E-deficient mice with intact lipoxygenase activity (71a). Moreover, mice without 12-lopoxygenase also exhibit reduced IgG antibodies to oxidized LDL epitopes (71a). These data suggest that 12/15-lipoxygenase is involved in the process of atherosclerosis, presumably by contributing to the oxidation of LDL.

Glucose Autoxidation and Glycoxidation Reactions

Atherosclerotic vascular disease is greatly accelerated among persons with diabetes mellitus. Certain risk factors for atherosclerosis are frequently present in diabetics. They include hypertension, hyperlipidemia, central obesity and hyperinsulinemia (72). However, the increased risk associated with these factors does not appear adequate to explain the greatly increased incidence of atherosclerosis associated with diabetes.

Two factors have long been known to be powerful determinants of risk for the development of diabetic retinopathy and nephropathy: duration of disease and degree of glycemic control. The links between hyperglycemia and long-term diabetic complications have given rise to the "glucose hypothesis". The recent demonstration of a beneficial effect of intensive glucose-lowering therapy in Type I diabetics strongly supports the glucose hypothesis (73). The salutary effects of intensive glycemic control on the long-term complications of diabetes suggests that hyperglycemia plays a similar role in the pathogenesis of these complications. Therefore, glucose itself may constitute a toxin for the vasculature.

In its open chain form, glucose reacts non-enzymatically with the lysine residues of proteins (74). The resulting Schiff-base then undergoes an internal rearrangement reaction that results in the formation of fructoselysine, the stable Amadori product. Because of its reactive aldehyde group, the Amadori product can cross-link the protein to which it is attached to other proteins and lipoproteins, forming a variety of advanced glycated end products (AGEs)(74,75).

One important AGE is $^{\varepsilon}$N-(carboxymethyl)lysine (CML), formed by sequential glycation and oxidation reactions between reducing sugars and proteins (76). The formation of oxidants in glucose-dependent reactions with proteins and other biomolecules has been termed "glycoxidation." AGEs and glycoxidation have been proposed to promote vascular disease by a number of mechanisms (reviewed in 72,74,75 and Chapters 14 and 15), including the generation of oxidizing intermediates and dicarbonyl sugars, cross-linking of matrix-plasma components, and interactions with cell surface receptors.

Recent studies (77) have immunolocalized CML in skin, lung, heart, kidney and particularly in arteries. There was also an age-dependent increase in CML accumulation and acceleration of this process in diabetes (78). Several reactive oxygen species that could damage lipoproteins are also formed during glucose autoxidation and glycoxidation (72,74,75). These findings support the hypothesis that glycoxidation reactions and AGEs may contribute to oxidant damage occurring in atherosclerosis, aging and diabetes.

Nitric Oxide

Nitric oxide generated by endothelial cells is a major regulator of vascular tone in muscular arteries; it mediates a wide variety of biological effects that are potentially antiatherogenic (79,80). However, nitric oxide also is a relatively stable radical that may indirectly oxidize lipoproteins and promote atherosclerosis. This may be especially true for the much larger quantities of nitric oxide that are generated by inducible nitric oxide synthase as part of the inflammatory response.

When nitric oxide reacts with superoxide, it generates peroxynitrite (ONOO⁻), a powerful oxidizing intermediate (81).

$$NO + O_2^{\bullet-} \rightarrow ONOO^-$$

Peroxynitrite peroxidizes LDL lipids and converts the lipoprotein into a form that exerts pro-atherogenic effects on macrophages (82). Peroxynitrite also is a potent protein-nitrating reagent that produces high levels of 3-nitrotyrosine *in vitro* (83). Immunohistochemical studies have detected 3-nitrotyrosine in human atherosclerotic lesions, suggesting that reactive nitrogen species may promote LDL oxidation *in vivo* (84).

In contrast, other studies suggest that nitric oxide protects LDL from oxidation. LDL oxidation by murine macrophages was inhibited when the cellular production of nitric oxide was stimulated (85,86). LDL oxidation by copper is also inhibited by nitric oxide (87). Nitric oxide might suppress LDL oxidation by inhibiting heme-containing enzymes, scavenging superoxide, reacting with lipid radicals, or nitrosylating important cellular proteins (85-88). Recent studies in hypercholesterolemic rabbits and mice suggest that nitric oxide inhibits fatty streak formation (80,89), which supports the idea that nitric oxide is anti-atherogenic in these animal models.

To explore the possibility that reactive nitrogen species mediate LDL oxidation in the human artery wall, we used isotope dilution gas chromatography-mass spectrometry to quantify 3-nitrotyrosine levels in LDL isolated from atherosclerotic lesions (90). The level of 3-nitrotyrosine in lesion LDL was elevated 80-fold compared with circulating LDL. This observation raises the possibility that nitric oxide can render LDL atherogenic, counteracting in part nitric oxide's well established anti-atherogenic effects. Alternatively, the detection of elevated levels of 3-nitrotyrosine in lesion LDL may indicate that nitric oxide is one mechanism for inhibiting lipid peroxidation in the artery wall. The detection of nitrated lipids in atherosclerotic lesions would support this proposal.

Vitamin E

Vitamin E is a lipid-soluble compound that is a potent inhibitor of lipid peroxidation *in vitro* (51). The major isomer biologically active form of vitamin E is α-tocopherol. LDL is the major carrier of vitamin E in blood. Dietary supplementation with vitamin E increases the resistance of LDL to oxidation ex vivo with certain oxidants, suggesting that vitamin E might inhibit atherosclerosis (91,92). However, *in vitro* studies indicate that under certain conditions, oxidants convert α-tocopherol into α-tocopheroxyl radical that then initiates LDL lipid peroxidation (93-96). This reaction pathway, termed "tocopherol-mediated peroxidation," takes place with LDL exposed to many different oxidative insults (see chapter 3).

It is interesting to note that vitamin E at doses that fail to lower cholesterol levels has not exerted a consistent inhibitory effect on atherosclerosis in hypercholesterolemic animals (97-99). LDL isolated from the animals fed vitamin E was protected from oxidation ex vivo, documenting that vitamin E was incorporated into LDL and was able to inhibit lipid peroxidation induced by oxidative stress ex vivo.

In contrast to the animal studies, both epidemiological and clinical trials suggest that vitamin E is anti-atherogenic in humans (17,91,92). In the first prospective, randomized clinical trial that used atherosclerosis as the primary endpoint, vitamin E therapy reduced the risk of nonfatal myocardial infarction by 80% in patients with angiographically established coronary artery disease (17). This trial provides the first strong evidence that antioxidants can exert a powerful beneficial effect on human atherosclerosis. Remarkably, the effect appears to be greatest in patients with advanced atherosclerosis, whereas animal studies suggest that antioxidants are more likely to be beneficial early in the disease process (15). Collectively, these observations suggest that vitamin E might promote or inhibit LDL oxidation and atherosclerosis, depending in part on the species and the stage of disease.

Myeloperoxidase

Superoxide generated by phagocytes (or other biochemical reactions) dismutates to form hydrogen peroxide (40).

$$2\,O_2^{\bullet-} + 2\,H^+ \rightarrow H_2O_2 + O_2$$

Phagocytes also secrete the heme protein myeloperoxidase, which interacts with hydrogen peroxide to generate antimicrobial toxins (41,100). Because the active site of myeloperoxidase is buried deep in the center of the protein (101), it requires low molecular weight substrates to convey oxidizing equivalents from the enzyme's heme group to the target for damage. In contrast to most *in vitro* oxidation reactions, the reactions catalyzed by myeloperoxidase are independent of free metal ions.

Recent studies have shown that active myeloperoxidase is present in human atherosclerotic tissue (102). The enzyme co-localizes with macrophages in intermediate lesions. It is closely associated with cholesterol clefts in extracellular lipid deposits of advanced atherosclerotic lesions. A similar pattern of immunostaining for protein-bound lipid oxidation products has been reported for rabbit atherosclerotic lesions (14). The enzyme's ability to oxidize LDL *in vitro* by reactions that do not require free metal ions, together with its presence in atherosclerotic lesions, suggests that this heme protein may be one important agent for lipoprotein oxidation *in vivo*.

One reaction catalyzed by myeloperoxidase is the conversion of the phenolic amino acid L-tyrosine to tyrosyl radical (103). Tyrosyl radical generated by myeloperoxidase initiates LDL lipid peroxidation (104). This reaction bears remarkable biochemical similarities to the enzymatic peroxidation of polyunsaturated fatty acids by cyclooxygenase, which also is proposed to involve tyrosyl radical (105). Protein tyrosyl residues may also be a target because tyrosyl radical converts protein-bound tyrosines to dityrosine (106,107). Both the formation of o,o'-dityrosine and the initiation of LDL oxidation by myeloperoxidase are greatly enhanced by plasma concentrations of tyrosine (104,106,107). Dityrosine may serve as a marker for proteins that have been oxidatively damaged by activated phagocytes because it is an intensely fluorescent amino acid that is stable to acid hydrolysis.

LDL and model proteins exposed to tyrosine, hydrogen peroxide and myeloperoxidase exhibited a marked increase in dityrosine but little change in the level of ortho-tyrosine, a marker of protein oxidation by metal ions (38). To determine whether tyrosyl radical might play a role in oxidizing LDL *in vivo*, we quantified dityrosine levels using isotope dilution gas chromatography-mass spectrometry (38). LDL isolated from atherosclerotic lesions exhibited a dramatic 100-fold increase in dityrosine levels compared with circulating LDL. In striking contrast, there was no evidence of elevated ortho-tyrosine levels. Tissue dityrosine levels also increased markedly in fatty streaks (the earliest lesion of atherosclerosis) and in advanced atherosclerotic lesions. These results suggest that tyrosyl radical, perhaps generated in part by myeloperoxidase, contributes to LDL oxidation both early and late in the disease process.

The major reaction catalyzed by myeloperoxidase involves the conversion of chloride ion to hypochlorous acid (HOCl).

$$H_2O_2 + Cl^- + H^+ \rightarrow HOCl + H_2O$$

At plasma concentrations of halide ion, myeloperoxidase is the only human enzyme know to generate hypochlorous acid (108,109). Chlorinated biomolecules should therefore be specific markers of oxidative damage by activated phagocytes.

3-Chlorotyrosine is formed in the protein component of LDL oxidized by the myeloperoxidase-peroxide-chloride system (110,111). In contrast, 3-chlorotyrosine was undetectable in LDL oxidized by hydroxyl radical, copper, iron, horseradish peroxidase, hemin, glucose, or peroxynitrite, indicating that the chlorinated amino acid is a specific marker of oxidation by myeloperoxidase. We have recently used isotope dilution gas chromatography-mass spectrometry to show that 3-chlorotyrosine is dramatically elevated in LDL isolated from human atherosclerotic tissue and in atherosclerotic lesions harvested at surgery (111). These results provide strong evidence that oxidative damage to LDL - and perhaps to other macromolecules involved in plaque formation - can result from the action of myeloperoxidase in the human artery wall.

Immunohistochemical studies of atherosclerotic lesions suggest that oxidation specific epitopes are localized to phagolysosomal-like structures in macrophages (14). Phagocytosis is a potent stimulus for the secretion of both peroxide and myeloperoxidase into the phagolysosome, a cellular microenvironment where high concentrations of oxidants are generated that might overwhelm antioxidant defense mechanisms (41,101). These observations suggest that the phagolysosome might represent an ideal location for the promotion of LDL oxidation.

Recent studies indicate that myeloperoxidase also uses nitrite, a decomposition product of nitric oxide, to generate potent chlorinating and nitrating intermediates (112). Moreover, human neutrophils employ the myeloperoxidase system to both chlorinate and nitrate tyrosine residues (113). These observations, together with our demonstration that levels of 3-nitrotyrosine and 3-chlorotyrosine are elevated in human atherosclerotic tissue (90,111), raise the possibility that the myeloperoxidase pathway both nitrates and chlorinates host tissues *in vivo*.

SUMMARY AND FUTURE DIRECTIONS

These observations suggest a working model for the pathways that produce oxidative stress and LDL oxidation in the human artery wall. The detection of an excess of 13S-HODE in early and advanced atherosclerotic lesions suggests that 15-lipoxygenase may represent one pathway. Lipid oxidation products generated by lipoxygenase might promote LDL oxidation by the "seeding" mechanism or exert direct biological effects on the artery wall independent of lipoprotein oxidation.

Other pathways for vascular oxidative stress may involve myeloperoxidase, which is present and catalytically active in human atherosclerotic lesions and promotes

LDL oxidation *in vitro* by a variety of mechanisms. One mechanism may involve tyrosyl radical, which promotes dityrosine formation and peroxidation of LDL lipids. This hypothesis is supported by the detection of dramatically elevated levels of dityrosine in LDL isolated from human atherosclerotic lesions. Because 3-chlorotyrosine is a specific marker for oxidative damage by myeloperoxidase, the detection of elevated levels of 3-chlorotyrosine in lesion LDL provide even stronger evidence for the operation of this enzyme *in vivo*.

In striking contrast, there appears to be little evidence that free metal ions - the most widely studied *in vitro* model - play an important role in promoting LDL oxidation or tissue damage early in atherogenesis. However, the detection of elevated levels of ortho-tyrosine and meta-tyrosine - two markers for metal-catalyzed LDL oxidation - in advanced atherosclerotic lesions raises the possibility that metal ions contribute to the development of atherosclerosis latter in the disease process.

The detection of stable products of specific reaction pathways in atherosclerotic tissue and in LDL isolated from atherosclerotic lesions does not establish the biological significance of oxidative pathways. In future studies it will be important to study animal models that lack or overexpress oxidative enzymes, with the long-term goal of understanding the pathways that promote LDL oxidation and atherosclerosis. Such studies may ultimately led to the development of novel antioxidant therapies designed to interrupt atherogenesis.

REFERENCES

1.   Brown MS, Goldstein JL. Koch's postulates for cholesterol. *Cell.* 1992;71:187.
2.   Goldstein JL, Ho YK, Basu SK, Brown MS. Binding site on macrophages that mediates uptake and degradation of acetylated low density lipoprotein, producing massive cholesterol deposition. *Proc Natl Acad Sci USA.* 1979;76:333.
3.   Fogelman AM, Shechter I, Seager J, Hokom M, Child JS, Edwards PA. Malondialdehyde alteration of low density lipoproteins leads to cholesteryl ester accumulation in human monocyte-macrophages. *Proc Natl Acad Sci USA.* 1980;77:2214.
4.   Henriksen T, Mahoney EM, Steinberg D. Enhanced macrophage degradation of low density lipoprotein previously incubated with cultured endothelial cells: Recognition by receptors for acetylated low density lipoproteins. *Proc Natl Acad Sci USA.* 1981;78:6499.
5.   Heinecke JW, Rosen H, Chait A. Iron and copper promote modification of low density lipoprotein by human arterial smooth muscle cells in culture. *J Clin Invest.* 1984;74:1890.
6.   Morel DW, DiCorleto PE, Chisolm GM. Endothelial and smooth muscle cells alter low density lipoprotein *in vitro* by free radical oxidation. *Arteriosclerosis.* 1984;4:357.
7.   Steinbrecher UP, Parthasarathy S, Leake DS, Witztum JL, Steinberg D. Modification of low density lipoprotein by endothelial cells involves lipid peroxidation and degradation of low density lipoprotein phospholipids. *Proc Natl Acad Sci USA.* 1984;81:3883.
8.   Witztum JL, Steinberg D. Role of oxidized low density lipoprotein in atherogenesis. *J Clin Invest.* 1991;88:1785.
9.   Berliner JA, Heinecke JW. The role of oxidized lipoproteins in atherogenesis. *Free Rad Biol Med.* 1996;20:707.
10.   Esterbauer H, Gebicki J, Puhl H, Jurgens G. The role of lipid peroxidation and antioxidants in oxidative modification of LDL. *Free Rad Biol Med.* 1992;13:341.
11.   Daugherty A, Zweifel BS, Sobel BE, Schonfeld G. Isolation of low density lipoprotein from

atherosclerotic vascular tissue of Watanabe Heritable Hyperlipidemic rabbits. *Arteriosclerosis.* 1988;8:768.

12. Yla-Herttuala S, Palinski W, Rosenfeld ME, Parthasarathy S, Carew TE, Butler S, Witztum JL, Steinberg D. Evidence for the presence of oxidatively modified low density lipoprotein in atherosclerotic lesions of rabbit and man. *J Clin Invest.* 1989;84:1086.

13. Haberland ME, Cheng L, Fong D. Malondialdehyde-altered protein occurs in atheroma of Watanabe Heritable hyperlipidemic rabbits. *Science.* 1988;241:215.

14. Rosenfeld ME, Palinski W, Yla-Herttuala S, Butler S, Witztum JL. Distribution of oxidation specific lipid-protein adducts and apolipoprotein-B in atherosclerotic lesions of varying severity from WHHL rabbits. *Arteriosclerosis.* 1990;10:336.

15. Steinberg D. Clinical trials of antioxidants in atherosclerosis: Are we doing the right thing? *Lancet.* 1995;346:36.

16. Diaz MN, Frei B, Vita JA, Keaney JF. Antioxidants and atherosclerotic heart disease. *N Eng J Med.* 1997;337:408.

17. Stephens NG, Parsons A, Schofield PM, Kelly F, Cheeseman K, Mitchinson MJ, Brown MJ. Randomised controlled trial of vitamin E in patients with coronary disease: Cambridge Heart Antioxidant Study (CHAOS). *Lancet.* 1996;347:781.

18. Frei B, Stocker R, Ames, BN, Antioxidant defenses and lipid peroxidation in human blood plasma. *Proc Natl Acad Sci USA.* 1988;85.9748.

19. Ehrenwald E, Chisolm GM, Fox PL. Intact ceruloplasmin oxidatively modifies low density lipoprotein. *J Clin Invest.* 1994;93:1493.

20. Balla G, Eaton JW, Belcher JD, Vercellotti GM. Hemin: A possible physiological mediator of low density lipoprotein oxidation and endothelial injury. *Arterioscler Thromb.* 1991;11:1700.

21. Thomas JP, Kalyanaraman B, Girotti W. Involvement of preexisting lipid hydroperoxides in Cu^{2+} -stimulated oxidation of low-density lipoprotein. *Arch Biochem Biophysics.* 1994;315:244.

22. Bowry VW, Stanley KK, Stocker R. High density lipoprotein is the major carrier of lipid hydroperoxides in human blood plasma of fasting donors. *Proc Natl Acad Sci USA.* 1992;89:10316.

23. Hodis HN, Kramsch DM, Avogaro P, Bittolo-Bon G, Cazzolato G, Hwang J, peterson H, Sevanian A. Biochemical and cytotoxic characteristics of an *in vivo* circulating oxidized low density lipoprotein (LDL-). *J. Lipid Res.* 1994;35:669.

24. Smith C, Mitchinson MJ, Aruoma OI, Halliwell B. Stimulation of lipid peroxidation and hydroxyl radical generation by the contents of human atherosclerotic lesions. *Biochem J.* 1992;286:901.

25. Swain J, Gutteridge JMC. Prooxidant iron and copper, with ferroxidase and xanthine oxidase activity in human atherosclerotic material. *FEBS Let.* 1995;368:513.

26. Lamb D, Mitchinson MJ, Leake DS. Transition metals within human atherosclerotic lesions can catalyze the oxidation of low density lipoprotein by macrophages. *FEBS Let.* 1995;374:12.

27. Aasa R, Malmstrom BG, Saltman P, Vanngard T. The specific binding of iron (III) and copper (II) to transferrin and conalbumin. *Biochem Biophys Acta.* 1963;75:203.

28. Thomas CE. The influence of medium components on Cu-dependent oxidation of low density lipoproteins and its sensitivity to superoxide dismutase. *Biochim Biophys Acta.* 1992;1128:50.

29. Peters T Jr, Blumenstock FA. Copper-binding properties of bovine serum albumin and its amino-terminal peptide fragment. *J Biol Chem.* 1967;242:1574.

30. Ascherio A, Willett WC. Are body iron stores related to the risk of coronary heart disease? *N Eng J Med.* 1994;330:1152.

31. Bothwell TH, Charlton RW, Cook JD, Finch CA. Iron metabolism in man. 1979;Oxford:Blackwell Scientific Pub.

32. Miller M, Hutchins GM. Hemochromatosis, multiorgan hemosiderosis, and coronary artery disease. *JAMA.* 1994;272:231.

33. Dabbagh AJ, Shwaery GT, Keaney JF, Frei B. Effect of iron overload and iron deficiency on atherosclerosis in the hypercholesterolemic rabbit. *Arterioscler Thromb Vasc Biol.* 1997;17:2638.

34.   Araujo JA, Romano EL, Brito BE, Parthe V, Romano M, Bracho M, Montano RF, Cardier J. Iron overload augments the development of atherosclerotic lesions in rabbits. *Arterioscler Thromb Vasc Biol.* 1995;15:1172.

35.   Danks DM. Disorders of copper transport. In: Scriver, C.R., Beaudet, A.L. Sly, W.S., Valley, D. Eds. The metabolic basis of inherited disease. 6th ed. New York: McGraw-Hill, Inc. 1989:1411.

36.   Heinecke JW. Mechanisms of oxidative damage of low density lipoprotein in human atherosclerosis. *Cur Opin Lipid.* 1997;8:268.

37.   Lynch SM, Frei B. Mechanisms of copper-dependent and iron-dependent oxidative modification of human low density lipoprotein. *J Lipid Res.* 1993;34:1745.

38.   Leuwenburgh C, Rasmussen JE, Hsu FF, Mueller DM, Pennathur S, Heinecke JW. Mass spectrometric quantification of markers for protein oxidation by tyrosyl radical, copper, and hydroxyl radical in low density lipoprotein isolated from human atherosclerotic plaques. *J Biol Chem.* 1997;272:3520.

39.   Huggins TG, Wells-Knecht MC, Detorie NA, Baynes JW, Thorpe SR. Formation of o-tyrosine and dityrosine in proteins during radiolytic and metal-catalyzed oxidation. *J Biol Chem.* 1993;268:12341.

40.   Fridovich I. The biology of oxygen radicals. *Science.* 1978;201:875.

41.   Klebanoff SF. Oxygen metabolism and the toxic properties of phagocytes. *Ann Int Med.* 1980;93:480.

42.   Hiramatsu K, Rosen H, Heinecke J, Wolfbauer G, Chait A. Superoxide initiates oxidation of low density lipoprotein by human monocytes. *Arteriosclerosis.* 1987;7:55.

43.   Cathcart MK, McNally AK, Morel DW, Chisolm GM. Superoxide anion participation in human monocyte-mediated oxidation of LDL and conversion of LDL to a cytotoxin. *J Immunol.* 1989;142:1963.

44.   Heinecke JW, Baker L, Rosen H, Chait A. Superoxide-mediated modification of low density lipoprotein by arterial smooth muscle cells. *J Clin Invest.* 1986;77:757.

45.   Stenbrecher UP. Role of superoxide in endothelial cell modification of LDL. *Biochem Biophys Acta.* 1988;959:20.

46.   Mukhopadhyay CK, Ehrenwald E, Fox PL. Ceruloplasmin enhances smooth muscle cell-and endothelial cell-mediated low density lipoprotein oxidation by a superoxide-dependent mechanism. *J Biol Chem.* 1996;271:14773.

47.   Bedwell SR, Dean T, Jessup W. The action of defined oxygen-centered radicals on human low-density lipoprotein. *Biochem J.* 1989;262:707.

48.   Parthasarathy S, Weiland E, Steinberg D. A role for endothelial cell lipoxygenase in the oxidative modification of low density lipoprotein. *Proc Natl Acad Sci USA.* 1989;86:1046.

49.   Jessup W, Simpson JA, Dean RT. Does superoxide radical have a role in macrophage mediated oxidative modification of LDL? *Atherosclerosis.* 1993;99:107.

50.   Rabini J, Klug-Roth D, Lilie J. Pulse radiolytic investigations of the catalyzed disproportionation of peroxy radicals. Aqueous cupric ions. *J Phys Chem.* 1973;77:1169.

51.   Buettner GR. The pecking order of free radicals and antioxidants: Lipid peroxidation, alpha-tocopherol, and ascorbate. *Arch Biochem Biophys.* 1993;300:535.

52.   Heinecke JW, Suzuki L, Rosen H, Chait A. The role of sulfur containing amino acids in superoxide production and modification of low density lipoprotein by arterial smooth muscle cells. *J Biol Chem.* 1987;262:10098.

53.   Parthasarthy S. Oxidation of low density lipoprotein by thiol compounds leads to its recognition by the acetyl-LDL receptor. *Biochem Biophys Acta.* 1987;917:337.

54.   Heinecke JW, Kawamura M, Suzuki L, Chait A. Oxidation of low density lipoprotein by thiols: superoxide-dependent and -independent mechanisms. *J Lipid Res.* 1993;34:2051.

55.   Sparrow CP, Olszewski J. Cellular oxidation of low density lipoprotein is caused by thiol production in media containing transition metal ions. *J Lipid Res* 1993;34:1219.

56.   Lynch SM, Frei B. Physiological thiol compounds exert pro- and anti-oxidant effects, respectively, on iron- and copper-dependent oxidation of human low-density lipoprotein. *Biochem Biophys Acta.* 1997;1345:215.

57.   Mudd SH, Levy HL, Skovby F. Disorders of transsulfuration. In: Scriver, CR, Beaudet AL, Sly WS, Valley D., eds. *The metabolic basis of inherited disease.* New York:McGraw-Hill.

1989:793.
58. Mayer EL, Jacobsen DW, Robinson K. Homocysteine and coronary atherosclerosis. *J Amer College Card.* 1996;27:517.
59. Harker LA, Ross R, Slichter SJ, Scott CR. Homocystine-induced arteriosclerosis. *J Clin Invest.* 1976;58:731.
60. Dudman NPD, Wilcken DEL, Stocker R. Circulating lipid hydroperoxide levels in human homocysteinemia. *Arterioscler Thromb.* 1993;13:512.
61. Yamamoto S. Mammalian lipoxygenases: Molecular structures and functions. *Biochem Biophys Acta.* 1992;1128:117.
62. Sparrow CP, Parthasarathy S, Steinberg D. Enzymatic modification of LDL by purified lipoxygenase plus phospholipase A2 mimics cell-mediated oxidative modification. *J Lipid Res.* 1988;29:745.
63. Parthasarathy S, Weiland E, Steinberg D. A role for endothelial cell lipoxygenase in the oxidative modification of low density lipoprotein. *Proc Natl Acad Sci USA.* 1989;86:1046.
64. Jessup W, Darley-Usmar V, O'Leary V, Bedwell OS. 5-Lipoxygenase is not essential for macrophage mediated oxidation of LDL. *Biochem J.* 1991;278:163.
65. Sparrow CP, Olszewski J. Cellular oxidative modification of LDL does not require lipoxygenases. *Proc Natl Acad Sci USA.* 1991;89:128.
66. Yla-Herttuala S, Rosenfeld ME, Parthasarathy S, Sigal E, Sarkioia T, Witztum JL, Steinberg D. Colocalization of 15-lipoxygenase mRNA and protein with epitopes of oxidized low density lipoprotein in macrophage-rich areas of atherosclerotic lesions. *Proc Natl Acad Sci USA.* 1987;87:6959.
67. Yla-Herttuala S, Luoma J, Viita H, Hiltunen T, Sisto T, Nikkari T. Transfer of 15-lipoxygenase gene into rabbit iliac arteries results in the appearance of oxidation-specific lipid-protein adducts characteristic of oxidized low density lipoprotein. *J Clin Invest.* 1995;95:2692.
68. Belkner J, Wiesner R, Rathman J, Barnett J, Sigal E, Kuhn H. Oxygenation of lipoproteins by mammalian lipoxygenases. *Eur J Biochem.* 1993;213:251.
69. Folcik VA, Nivar-Aristy RA, Krajewski LP, Cathcart MK. Lipoxygenase contributes to the oxidation of lipids in human atherosclerotic plaques. *J Clin Invest.* 1995;96:504.
70. Kuhn H, Heydeck D, Hugou I, Gniwotta C. *In vivo* action of 15-lipoxygenase in early stages of human atherosclerosis. *J Clin Invest.* 1997;99:888.
71. Rao SI, Wilks A, Hamberg M, Ortiz de Montellano PR. The lipoxygenase activity of myoglobin. *J Biol Chem.* 1994;269:7210.
71a. Tillman C, Witztum JL, Rader DJ, Tangirala R, Fazio S, Linton MF, Funk CD. Disruption of the 12/15-lipoxygenase gene diminishes atherosclerosis in apo E-deficient mice. *J Clin Invest.* 1999;103:1597.
72. Semenkovich CF, Heinecke JW. The mystery of diabetes and atherosclerosis: time for a new plot. *Diabetes.* 1997;46:327.
73. The Diabetes Control and Complication Trial. *N Eng J Med.* 1993;329.683.
74. Baynes JW. Role of oxidative stress in development of complications in diabetes. *Diabetes.* 1991;40:405.
75. Bucala R, Cerami A. Advanced glycosylation: chemistry, biology, and implications for diabetes and aging. *Adv Pharm.* 1992;23:1.
76. Ahmed MU, Thorpe SR, Baynes JW. Identification of N-(carboxymethyl)-lysine as a degradation product of fructoselysine in glycated proteins. *J Biol Chem.* 1986;261:4889.
77. Dyer DG, Dunn JA, Thorpe SR, Bailie KE, Lyons TJ, McCance DR, Baynes JW. Accumulation of Mailard reaction products in skin collagen in diabetes and aging. *J Clin Invest.* 1993;91:2463.
78. Schleicher ED, Wagner E, Nerlich AG. Increased accumulation of the glycoxidation product N9epsilon)-(carboxymethyl) lysine in human tissues in diabetes and aging. *J Clin Invest.* 1997;99:457.
79. Moncada S, Palmer RM, Higgs EA. Nitric oxide: Physiology, pathophysiology and pharmacology. *Pharmacol Rev.* 1991;43:109.
80. Cooke JP, Tsao PS. Is NO an endogenous antiatherogenic molecule? *Arterioscler Thromb.* 1994;14:653.

81.   Beckman JS, Beckman TW, Chen J, Marshall PA, Freeman BA. Apparent hydroxyl radical production by peroxynitrite: Implications for endothelial injury from nitric oxide and superoxide. *Proc Natl Acad Sci USA.* 1990;87:1620.
82.   Graham AN, Hogg N, Kalyanaraman B, O'Leary V, Darley-Usmar V, Moncade S. Peroxynitrite modifications of LDL leads to recognition by the macrophage scavenger receptor. *FEBS.* 1993;330:181.
83.   Beckman JS, Chen J, Ischiropoulos H, Crow JP. Oxidative chemistry of peroxynitrite. *Meth Enzym.* 1994;233:229.
84.   Beckman JS, Ye YZ, Anderson PG, Chen J, Accavitti MA, Tarpey MM, White CR. Extensive nitration of protein tyrosines in human atherosclerosis detected by immunohistochemistry. *Biol Chem Hoppe-Seyler.* 1994;375:81.
85.   Jessup W, Mohr D, Gieseg SP, Dean RT, Stocker R. The participation of nitric oxide in cell free and its restriction of macrophage-mediated oxidation of low-density lipoprotein. *Biochim Biophys Acta.* 1992;1180:73.
86.   Yates MT, Lambert LE, Whitten JP, MacDonald I, Mano M, Ku G, Mao SJT. A protective role for nitric oxide in the oxidative modification of low density lipoprotein by mouse macrophages. *FEBS Lett.* 1992;309:135.
87.   Hogg N, Kalyanaraman B, Joseph J, Struck A, Parthasarathy S. Inhibition of low-density lipoprotein oxidation by nitric oxide: Potential role in atherogenesis. *FEBS Lett.* 1993;334:170.
88.   Rubbo H, Parthasarathy S, Barnes S, Kirk M, Kalyanaraman B, Freeman BA. Nitric oxide inhibition of lipoxygenase-dependent liposome and low-density lipoprotein oxidation: Termination of radical chain propagation reactions and formation of nitrogen-containing oxidized lipid derivatives. *Arch Biochem Biophys.* 1995;324:1.
89.   Aji W, Ravalli S, Szabolcs M, Jiang X-C, Sciacca RR, Michler RE, Canon PJ. L-arginine prevents xanthoma development and inhibits atherosclerosis in LDL receptor knockout mice. *Circulation.* 1997;95:430.
90.   Leeuwenburgh C, Hardy MM, Hazen SL, Wagner P, Oh-ishi S, Steinbrecher UP, Heinecke JW. Reactive nitrogen intermediates promote low density lipoprotein oxidation in human atherosclerosis. *J Biol Chem.* 1997;272:1433.
91.   Gaziano JM, Hennekens CH. Vitamin antioxidants and cardiovascular disease. *Cur Opin Lipidology.* 1992;3:91.
92.   Jha P, Flather M, Lonn E, Farkouh M, Yusuf S. The antioxidant vitamins and cardiovascular disease - a critical review of epidemiological and clinical trial data. *Ann Int Med.* 1995;123:860.
93.   Bowry VW, Stocker R. Tocopherol-mediated peroxidation: the prooxidant effect of vitamin E on the radical-initiated oxidation of human low-density lipoprotein. *J Am Chem Soc.* 1993;115:6029.
94.   Ingold KU, Bowry VW, Stocker R, Walling C. Autoxidation of lipids and antioxidation by alpha-tocopherol and ubiquinol in homogeneous solution and in aqueous dispersions of lipids - unrecognized consequences of lipid particle size as exemplified by oxidation of human low density lipoprotein. *Proc Natl Acad Sci USA.* 1993;90:45.
95.   Lynch SM, Frei B. Reduction of copper, but not iron, by human low density lipoprotein (LDL)-implications for metal ion-dependent oxidative modification of LDL. *J Biol Chem.* 1995;270:5158.
96.   Kontush A, Meyer S, Finckh B, Kohlschutter A, Beisiegel U. Alpha-tocopherol as a reductant for Cu(II) in human lipoproteins-triggering role in the initiation of lipoprotein oxidation. *J Biol Chem.* 1996;271:11106.
97.   Shaish A, Daugherty A, O'Sullivan F, Schonfeld G, Heinecke JW. Beta-carotene inhibits atherosclerosis in hypercholesterolemic rabbits. *J Clin Invest.* 1995;96:2075.
98.   Kleinveld HA, Demacker PNM, Stalenhoef AFH. Comparative study on the effect of low-dose vitamin E and probucol on the susceptibility of LDL to oxidation and the progression of atherosclerosis in Watanabe Heritable Hyperlipidemic rabbits. *Arterioscler and Thromb.* 1994;14:1386.
99.   Kleinveld HA, Hak-Lemmers HLM, Hectors MPC, de Fouw NJ, Demacker PNM, Stalenhoef AFH. Vitamin E and fatty acid intervention does not attenuate the progression of

atherosclerosis in Watanabe Heritable Hyperlipidemic rabbits. *Arterioscler Thromb Vasc Biol.* 1995;15:290.

100.   Hurst JK, Barette WC. Leukocytic oxygen activation and microbicidal oxidative toxins. *CRC Critical Reviews Biochem Mol Biol.* 1989;24:271.

101.   Zeng J, Fenna RE. X-ray crystal structure of canine myeloperoxidase at 3A resolution. *J Mol Biol.* 1992;226:185.

102.   Daugherty A, Rateri DL, Dunn JL, Heinecke JW. Myeloperoxidase, a catalyst for lipoprotein oxidation, is expressed in human atherosclerotic lesions. *J Clin Invest.* 1994;94:437.

103.   Heinecke JW, Li W, Daehnke HL, Goldstein JA. Dityrosine, a specific marker of oxidation, is synthesized by the myeloperoxidase-hydrogen peroxide system of human neutrophils and macrophages. *J Biol Chem.* 1993;268:4069.

104.   Savenkova MI, Mueller DM, Heinecke JW. Tyrosyl radical generated by myeloperoxidase is a physiological catalyst for initiation of lipid peroxidation in low density lipoprotein. *J Biol Chem.* 1994;269:20394.

105.   Karthein R, Dietz R, Nastainczyk W, Ruff H. Higher oxidation states of prostaglandin H synthase. *Eur J Biochem.* 1988;171:313.

106.   Heinecke JW, Li W, Francis GA, Goldstein JA. Tyrosyl radical generated by myeloperoxidase catalyzes the oxidative cross-linking of proteins. *J Clin Invest* 1993;91:2866.

107.   Francis GA, Mendez AJ, Bierman EL, Heinecke JW. Oxidative tyrosylation of high density lipoprotein by peroxidase enhances cholesterol removal from cultured fibroblasts and macrophage foam cells. *Proc Natl Acad Sci USA.* 1993;90:6631.

108.   Harrison JE, Schultz J. Studies on the chlorinating activity of myeloperoxidase. *J Biol Chem.* 1976;251:1371.

109.   Weiss SJ, Test ST, Eckmann CM, Ross D, Regiani S. Brominating oxidants generated by human eosinophils. *Science.* 1986;234:200.

110.   Hazen SL, Hsu FF, Mueller DM, Crowley JR, Heinecke JW. Human neutrophils employ chlorine gas as an oxidant during phagocytosis. *J Clin Invest.* 1996,98.1283.

111.   Hazen SL, Heinecke JW. 3 Chlorotyrosine, a specific marker of myeloperoxidase-catalyzed oxidation, is markedly elevated in low density lipoprotein isolated from human atherosclerotic intima. *J Clin Invest.* 1997;99:2075.

112.   Eiserich JP, Cross CE, Jones AD, Halliwell B, Van der Vliet A. Formation of nitrating and chlorinating species by reaction of nitrite with hypochlorous acid: A novel mechanism for nitric oxide-mediated protein modification. *J Biol Chem.* 1996;271:19199.

113.   Eiserich JP, Hristova M, Cross CE, Jones AD, Freeman BA, Halliwell B, Van der Vliet A. Formation of nitric oxide-derived inflammatory oxidants by myeloperoxidase in neutrophils. *Nature.* 1998;391:393.

3 ANTIOXIDANT DEFENSES IN THE VASCULAR WALL

Roland Stocker

INTRODUCTION

Oxidative stress, defined as a disturbance in the pro-oxidant to anti-oxidant balance in favor of the former (1), may lead to oxidative damage, depending on its extent and duration, and the type of oxidant(s) involved. Within the vascular wall both radicals (*i.e.*, one electron) and nucleophilic (two electron) oxidants are likely produced and contribute to oxidative stress (see Chapter 2). This chapter describes antioxidant defenses in the vascular wall in atherosclerosis.

An antioxidant may be usefully characterized as any substance that, when present at low concentrations compared to those of an oxidizable substrate, significantly delays or prevents oxidation of that substrate (2). It follows that vascular antioxidant defenses must be considered in light of the potential targets and oxidants involved. With regards to vascular disease, particularly atherosclerosis, lipoproteins and low density lipoprotein (LDL) have received the most attention as targets for oxidative modifications (3). It is generally accepted that 'oxidized LDL' has numerous biological activities of potential relevance to atherosclerosis (3, 4). Therefore, antioxidant defenses relevant to the oxidative modification of LDL and atherosclerosis-induced changes to the nature and pool size of oxidizable lipid particles within the vascular wall will be described. The reader is reminded that 'oxidized LDL' is a functional term that remains chemically undefined and likely refers to a heterogeneous population of apolipoprotein B-100-containing lipoproteins and possibly other lipid containing particles in the arterial wall. Importantly, and despite much support for the oxidation hypothesis (3), it remains largely untested and hence unknown whether 'oxidized LDL' actually causes atherosclerosis or represents an important consequence of the disease.

Most of the potential proatherogenic properties associated with 'oxidized LDL' require the modified lipoprotein particle to be present outside cells. For this reason and because extracellular antioxidant defenses are considered inferior to those present inside cells (see below), it is generally assumed that oxidative modification of LDL occurs predominantly outside cells. Therefore, antioxidant defenses associated with and surrounding LDL in the extracellular fluid are considered to represent the primary antioxidant defense shield that prevents oxidative LDL modification.

Recent studies of the early stages of LDL oxidation indicate that lipoprotein-containing extracellular fluids represent heterogeneous emulsions of 'lipid droplets', the radical-induced oxidation of which proceeds via known chemistry reminiscent of emulsion polymerization rather than homogeneous phase chemistry (5,6). As this has important consequences for antioxidant defense, its principles will be introduced briefly and then contrasted to antioxidant defenses against oxidative modification of LDL induced by nucleophilic oxidants.

Tocopherol-Mediated Peroxidation

Tocopherol-mediated peroxidation describes a general model for the early, α-tocopherol-containing period of radical-induced lipoprotein lipid peroxidation. Tocopherol-mediated peroxidation provides a unifying mechanism for controlled peroxidation (Fig. 1) and effective antioxidation (Fig. 2) of LDL lipids (5,7). In this process, the fate of α-tocopheroxyl radical, rather than α-tocopherol (α-tocopherol, biologically the most active form of vitamin E), governs whether significant lipid peroxidation occurs (5-10).

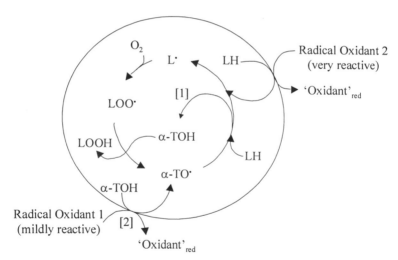

Figure 1. Tocopherol-mediated peroxidation of lipoprotein lipids. Tocopherol-mediated peroxidation describes the lipid peroxidation chain transfer (reaction [1]) and the phase transfer activity (reaction [2]) of α-tocopherol. Lipid peroxidation chain transfer is initiated by the rate-limiting reaction of α-tocopheroxyl radical with a lipid containing bisallylic hydrogen (LH). The resulting lipid-derived carbon centered radical (L˙) adds to molecular oxygen, giving rise to a lipid peroxyl radical (LOO˙) that is scavenged rapidly by α-TOH, thereby regenerating the chain-carrying α-TO˙ and producing a lipid hydroperoxide (LOOH). The phase transfer activity reflects the fact that as the most reactive molecule present on the surface of the lipoprotein particle, α-TOH preferentially reacts with relatively non-reactive aqueous radicals such as a peroxyl radical. This aids the transfer of radicals into the lipoprotein particle and can result in initiation of lipid peroxidation. Note that although more reactive aqueous radicals may not 'enter' the lipoprotein via reaction with α-TOH (top), they nevertheless give rise to α–TO˙ and hence can initiate tocopherol-mediated peroxidation.

Because α-tocopheroxyl radical is thermodynamically the most stable radical, it is formed independent of the chemical nature of the one electron oxidant LDL encounters (Fig. 1). Once formed, the single α-tocopheroxyl radical is 'trapped' within an oxidizing particle and physically segregated from other radicals present in the aqueous phase or within other oxidizing particles. The most effective protection of LDL lipids is obtained in the presence of both α-tocopherol and suitable reducing substances (termed co-antioxidants). The latter 'export' the radical character from an oxidizing particles into the aqueous phase where it is converted into non-radical product(s) (Fig. 2). In the absence of such co-antioxidants however, α-tocopheroxyl radical can initiate lipid peroxidation through abstraction of a bisallylic hydrogen atom from core or surface lipids of LDL (Fig. 1).

Hydrogen abstraction by α-tocopheroxyl radical is the rate limiting reaction in tocopherol-mediated peroxidation (TMP) of LDL's lipids. The rate of this reaction (*i.e.*, kTMP) is about three orders of magnitude lower than that of the lipid peroxidation chain propagation reaction catalyzed by lipid peroxyl radicals in homogeneous phase (*i.e.*, kLOO˙ + LH) (11). Tocopherol-mediated peroxidation thus represents retarded lipid peroxidation when compared to that of uninhibited lipid peroxidation taking place in the absence of α-tocopherol.

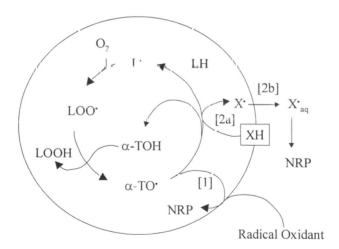

Figure 2. Inhibition of tocopherol-mediated peroxidation of lipoprotein lipids. Lipoprotein lipid peroxidation is inhibited by either radical-radical termination (reaction [1]) or co-antioxidation (reactions [2a] plus [2b]). Radical-radical termination requires the entry of a 'second' radical into the of α-tocopheroxyl radical containing lipoprotein particle. In this case, abstraction of bisallylic hydrogens and hence initiation of tocopherol-mediated peroxidation is prevented through formation of non-radical products (NRP), at the expense of α-tocopherol consumption. By contrast, co-antioxidation prevents tocopherol-mediated peroxidation without loss of α-TOH and formation of lipid hydroperoxides. It requires the presence of an agent (XH) capable of reducing of α-tocopheroxyl radical (reaction [2]) as well as 'exporting' the radical (present as co-antioxidant-derived radical, X˙) from the particle into the aqueous phase (reaction [2b]), where it decays to NRP. For a detailed description of co-antioxidation and natural and synthetic co-antioxidants see refs. 9, 13 and 15.

Tocopherol-mediated peroxidation is inhibited by either radical-radical termination and co-antioxidation (reactions [1] and [2], respectively in Fig. 2). The former is prominent under conditions of high frequency of radical encounter by the lipoprotein that increase the chance of a 'second' radical entering an α-tocopheroxyl radical containing particle. In this case, the second radical combines rapidly with α-tocopheroxyl radical resulting in both the elimination of the lipid peroxidation chain carrying vitamin E radical (and hence the prevention of tocopherol-mediated peroxidation) and the consumption of α-tocopherol (Fig. 2). The biological relevance of this pathway is unknown though not likely of major importance in developing human lesions. Thus, the content of aortic α-tocopherol remains largely intact (see below), and even at the most advanced stages of atherosclerosis, the concentration of α-tocopherol-adducts (produced as radical-radical termination reactions occur) account for 0.75 - 20% of the vitamin E present (A. Terentis, D. Liebler, R. Stocker, unpublished).

Co-antioxidation prevents tocopherol-mediated peroxidation without both the loss of α-tocopherol and formation of lipid hydroperoxides. Co-antioxidants are agents capable of reducing α-tocopheroxyl radical (reaction [2] in Fig. 2) and 'exporting' the radical (present as the resulting co-antioxidant-derived radical) from the particle into the aqueous phase (reaction [2b]). Different co-antioxidants achieve this in various ways (6, 9). A number of natural and synthetic co-antioxidants have been identified, including ascorbate, α-tocopheryl hydroquinone, ubiquinol-10, 3-hydroxyanthranilic acid and albumin-bound bilirubin (9, 12-15). As α-tocopheroxyl radical is formed independent of the initial radical oxidant, inhibition of tocopherol-mediated peroxidation by co-antioxidants represents a unifying antioxidant defense against LDL lipid peroxidation. Furthermore, co-antioxidation prevents the formation of lipid hydroperoxides more effectively than α-tocopherol in its classical mode of action as a chain-breaking antioxidant, during which lipid hydroperoxides are formed for each molecule of lipid peroxyl radical scavenged by the vitamin.

Table 1. Tocopherol-mediated peroxidation of lipoprotein lipids: Effect of particle size on apparent lipid peroxidation chain length.

Lipoprotein	Relative apparent chain length[†] $(LO(O)H/ROO^{\bullet})$
Human high density lipoprotein (HDL)	0.3
Human low density lipoprotein (LDL)	1.0
Human very low density lipoprotein (VLDL)	2.0
Rat chylomicron (rCM)	3.6

Results shown are taken from (5, 16, 17, 19, 54). [†]For comparative purpose, lipid peroxidation chain lengths are given relative to that in LDL. Values are calculated as the relative (to LDL) number of molecules of primary lipid oxidation products (hydroperoxides for LDL, VLDL and rCM; hydroxides and hydroperoxides for HDL; see reference 102) formed per molecule of peroxidation-initiating peroxyl radical (ROO$^{\bullet}$) under directly comparable oxidizing conditions.

Although described initially for LDL only, tocopherol-mediated peroxidation governs lipid peroxidation in all tocopherol-containing lipoproteins present in human plasma (16-19). However, the different classes of lipoproteins vary with respect to the oxidative damage α-tocopheroxyl radical inflicts. This damage, expressed as the relative number of molecules of primary oxidized lipids formed per initiating radical, increases with increasing particle size (Table 1).

ANTIOXIDANT DEFENSES IN THE VASCULAR WALL

The antioxidant defenses in the extracellular fluid present in the vascular wall have not been evaluated systematically since this fluid is difficult to obtain for experimentation. However, it is reasonable to assume that the antioxidant composition of the fluid surrounding cells, extracellular matrix and lipoprotein particles in the intima is comparable to that of human blood plasma (20) and suction blister fluid (21). The antioxidant defenses in human blood plasma have been reviewed previously (22, 23) and will only be summarized in the following, with special emphasis on events relevant to vascular lipoprotein lipid oxidation.

Extracellular Defenses

Plasma constituents are present in the artery wall (24). As the diffusion from the vasculature into the interstitium is inversely proportional to the size of the molecule, the concentration of small molecular weight aqueous antioxidants such as ascorbate and urate in interstitial fluids is similar to that in plasma. In contrast, the levels of lipoprotein-associated antioxidants (α tocopherol, ubiquinol-10) are lower (8-20%) and resemble the concentration of lipoprotein-associated lipids (13-23%) (21).

Enzymatic and proteinaceous antioxidants

Compared to cells, extracellular fluids are largely devoid of the classical antioxidant enzymes Cu,Zn- and Mn-superoxide dismutase, glutathione peroxidase (GSH peroxidase) and reductase (GSH reductase), glutathione transferase (GST), and catalase (Table 2) (22, 23). While effective against H_2O_2 and fatty acid hydroperoxides, glutathione peroxidase does not act on hydroperoxides of phospholipids, cholesteryl esters and triglycerides, although the latter are by far the predominant primary lipid oxidation products formed in lipoproteins undergoing oxidation. Extracellular fluids are also devoid of phospholipid glutathione-dependent peroxidase (PH-glutathione peroxidase) (25), the only enzyme known to reduce complex lipid hydroperoxides in oxidized lipoproteins to the corresponding hydroxides in a catalytic and stoichiometric fashion (26, 27). Despite this, hydroperoxides of phospholipids and cholesteryl esters in plasma are converted to the corresponding hydroxides (20). This appears to involve a chemical rather than enzymatic reaction (27). Recent evidence (28, 29) indicates that methionine residues in apolipoproteins A-I, A-II and, possibly to a lesser extent, apolipoprotein B-100 (30), reduce lipid hydroperoxides in lipoproteins while becoming oxidized to methionine sulfoxide:

Table 2. Enzymatic antioxidant levels in human plasma and homogenates of normal human arteries and atherosclerotic plaques.

Antioxidant	Plasma	Normal Artery	Plaque
GSH-related[†]			
GSH Peroxidase (mU/mg protein)	5	11.9 ± 3.8	3.55 ± 2.1*
GSH Reductase (mU/mg protein)	0.38	3.2 ± 1.2	1.07 ± 0.4*
GST-Peroxidase (mU/mg protein)	0	ND	1.37 ± 0.35*
Total GST (mU/mg protein)	0.06	22.5 ± 6.0	20.9 ± 5.3
SOD-related			
EC-SOD (U/mg protein)	$0.06 - 0.25$	104 ± 49	77 ± 55
Cu,Zn-SOD (U/mg protein)	ND	100 ± 50	90 ± 42
Mn-SOD (U/mg protein)	ND	2.5 ± 1.4	3.6 ± 1.9

Results shown (mean ± SD) are taken from (23 plasma), (70 glutathione-related enzymes), and (35 SODs). [†]Data obtained from 13 internal mammary arteries (Normal Artery) and 13 endarterectomy-derived carotid plaques (Plaque). [¶]Data obtained from post-mortem aortic samples classified by macroscopic examination into Normal Artery (n = 8) and Plaque (lesion types IV, V, and Vc; n = 8). For comparative purpose, the results shown here are adjusted to protein and presented without statistical analysis as this appears to have been carried out on non-adjusted values (see reference 35). Abbreviations: Cu, Zn-SOD, cytosolic SOD; EC-SOD, extracellular SOD; GSH peroxidase, selenium-dependent glutathione peroxidase; GSH reductase, glutathione disulfide reductase; GST, glutathione transferase; GST-Px, selenium-independent peroxidase; Mn-SOD, manganese SOD; ND, not detectable. *$P<0.05$ vs normal artery.

$$Met_{apolipoprotein} + LOOH_{lipoprotein} ------> Methionine\ sulfoxide_{apolipoprotein} + LOH_{lipoprotein}$$

As indicated, the above reaction is slow and *in vitro* occurs typically within hours, although it can be accelerated considerably by presently unknown factor(s) released by liver (31). While conversion of the hydroperoxides to hydroxides eliminates potential pro-oxidants, the physiological relevance of this reaction remains to be demonstrated. The average residence time of lipoproteins in the sub-endothelial space is longer than that in plasma, so that even a slow reduction may be important. On the other hand, it is presently not known whether formation of Methionine sulfoxide results in functional alteration of the apolipoproteins and thus may represent oxidative damage rather than antioxidant defense. Human plasma also contains low levels of thioredoxin and glutaredoxin (32) which can reduce lipid hydroperoxides (33), although it is not known whether, and if so, how effectively these proteins act on complex lipoprotein lipid hydroperoxides.

A striking exception to enzymatic antioxidants in interstitial fluids is the presence of large amounts of extracellular SOD (EC-SOD) within the artery wall, particularly the arteries (34, 35) (Table 2). In contrast, the levels of (extracellular) Cu,Zn- and Mn-SOD are low compared to other tissues (34). In normal human aorta, EC-SOD is produced by and surrounds smooth muscle cells beneath the endothelium and is localized throughout the connective tissue matrix of the vessel (36). The role of EC-SOD (37) and Cu,Zn-SOD (38) is likely to prevent inactivation of nitrogen mono oxide (nitric oxide, NO) by superoxide anion radical ($O2^{-\cdot}$), and hence to protect endothelium-dependent arterial relaxation. If so, the primary antioxidant function of EC-SOD related to oxidative modification of aortic lipoproteins may be to prevent the formation of the strongly oxidizing peroxynitrous acid (HONOO).

Transition metals and particularly copper are commonly used *in vitro* oxidants for LDL. Little is known about the amounts of intravascular proteins that bind metals or biological iron and copper complexes, such as ceruloplasmin, transferrin, haptoglobin and hemopexin. Despite this however, albumin even at a relative (to lipoproteins) low concentration present in the sub-endothelial space (24), is capable of preventing *in vitro* oxidation of LDL induced by transition metals (39) and ceruloplasmin (40). In support of the presence of effective antioxidation against such type of oxidation, the high-molecular weight fraction of human suction blister fluid completely prevents Cu(II)-induced LDL oxidation *in vitro* (21).

Compared to antioxidant defenses against radicals, relatively little is known about the antioxidant defenses against nucleophilic oxidants. Among the latter, hypochlorous acid (HOCl) is thought to be produced during atherogenesis (41, 42). Protein thiols provide the primary defense against HOCl (43, 44) and HOCl-derived chloramines (unpublished). Given the relative (to human plasma) low concentration of albumin (*i.e.*, likely the major extracellular thiol) in the artery wall (24), it appears possible that antioxidant defense of HOCL-related oxidations could become limited during the early stages of atherosclerosis (see below).

Non-enzymatic small molecular antioxidants

As indicated above, interstitial fluid (21) and lymph (19) contain ascorbate and urate at concentrations comparable to those present in human blood plasma. Among the water-soluble antioxidants, ascorbate has received most attention as a radical scavenger and inhibitor of LDL oxidation. It is now generally accepted that the reduced form of vitamin C represents a first line antioxidant defense against lipid peroxidation induced by radical oxidants (see Chapter 5). Briefly, in the presence of ascorbate substantial amounts of lipid hydroperoxides do not accumulate (20, 45). Ascorbate is a highly efficient scavenger of various radicals including α-tocopheroxyl radical (46) and it prevents tocopherol-mediated peroxidation (5). The one electron oxidation product of ascorbic acid, ascorbyl radical, is unreactive. It appears that at least in the case of aqueous alkyl peroxyl radicals, direct scavenging of these radicals, rather than reduction of α-tocopheroxyl radical is responsible for the extremely efficient antioxidant protection of lipoprotein lipids by ascorbate (10). In contrast to the situation with radicals however, ascorbate prevents oxidative damage induced by nucleophilic oxidants less effectively (44). Similarly, urate is unable to prevent tocopherol-mediated peroxidation of lipoprotein lipids (5) although it can directly scavenge aqueous (radical) oxidants (47).

A second line of extracellular aqueous co-antioxidant defense can be provided by 3-hydroxyanthranilic acid (14). This tryptophan-derived aminophenol is produced and released by activated human monocytes and macrophages. It is a highly efficient radical scavenger (48) responsible for the inhibition of LDL oxidation by interferon-γ-activated human macrophages (49), and capable of eliminating of α-tocopheroxyl radical in LDL (14). Bilirubin, produced during the breakdown of heme by heme oxygenase and biliverdin reductase, is a strong reducing agent and antioxidant (50). In extracellular fluids, the pigment is present predominantly complexed to albumin. Albumin-bound bilirubin retains antioxidant activity (51) and can inhibit LDL lipid peroxidation via reduction of α-tocopheroxyl radical (12).

Among the lipid-soluble antioxidants, α-tocopherol plays a central role as it controls radical-induced lipoprotein lipid peroxidation and its prevention (see above and Figure 1). Compared to α-tocopherol, γ-tocopherol is less reactive and hence less able to control radical-induced LDL lipid peroxidation (52). However, γ-tocopherol may be important in the detoxification of nitrogen dioxide (53), though the physiological significance of this remains unknown. Ubiquinol-10, the reduced and antioxidant active form of coenzyme Q_{10}, scavenges peroxyl radicals with slightly higher efficiency than α-tocopherol, although it is present in LDL at comparatively much lower concentration. The strong lipid peroxidation inhibitory activity of ubiquinol-10 observed *in vitro* (54-56) is likely due to the ability of the hydroquinone to interact with α-tocopherol (6, 56); ubiquinol-10 can reduce α-tocopheroxyl radical (57).

Table 3. Non-proteinaceous antioxidants in human blood plasma and homogenates of normal human arteries and atherosclerotic plaques.

Antioxidant	Plasma	Normal Artery[†]	Plaque[‡]
Water-soluble (nmol/mg protein)			
Ascorbate	0.11 – 1.88	0.12 ± 0.07	1.30 ± 0.87
Urate	2.0 – 5.6	0.11 ± 0.09	3.32 ± 2.26
Lipid-soluble (mmol/mol free cholesterol)			
α-Tocopherol	8.9 – 23.7	4.2 ± 1.7	6.3 ± 4.8
α-Tocopherol*	8.9 – 16.3	---	28.6 ± 21.8
γ-Tocopherol	0.5 – 1.1	ND	0.24 ± 0.18
Coenzyme Q_{10}	0.3 – 0.8	1.5 ± 1.5	1.5 ± 0.15
Lycopene	0.3 – 0.6	Traces	0.05 ± 0.06
Carotene	0.2 – 0.5	Traces	0.05 ± 0.04

Data (range or mean ± SD) are taken from (58). [†]Normal Iliac arteries, n=6. [‡]Advanced fibro-fatty lesions obtained from patients udergoing surgery of the femoral artery (n=7) or carotid endarterectomy (n=4). *Expressed as mmol/mol cholesterol linoleate.

Non-enzymatic antioxidants in the normal artery wall

To date, only a few reports have addressed the content of non-proteinaceous antioxidants in the interstitial fluid of normal human arteries and veins, and the available information is restricted to homogenates prepared from the vessels (58-60). Suarna et al. evaluated water- and lipid-soluble antioxidants in homogenates of normal and diseased human vessels. Table 3 compares the contents of non-proteinaceous antioxidants in these tissues vs human blood plasma. As can be seen, normal arteries overall contain about one third of plasma ascorbate, though substantially less urate. Unfortunately, it is not known whether the ascorbate detected (58) was derived from intra– and/or extracellular sites. However, in analogy to other interstitial fluids (21) and considering that plasma proteins are present in the sub-endothelial space (24), it seems reasonable to speculate that at least part of the ascorbate in healthy arteries is present within the extracellular space. On the other hand, most of the α-tocopherol (and coenzyme Q_{10}) is likely located within cells given the relatively (to albumin) low concentration of lipoproteins in healthy arteries (24).

ATHEROSCLEROSIS-INDUCED BIOCHEMICAL CHANGES IN THE ARTERIAL WALL RELEVANT TO OXIDATIVE STRESS AND ANTIOXIDANT DEFENSES

Changes in Pool Size of Lipoproteins and Lipid Targets for Oxidation

The concept of transition of normal arteries to fatty streaks, fibro-fatty plaques and complex plaques is now generally accepted (61). In normal human intima (of the descending thoracic and upper abdominal region of the aorta), the absolute amount of lipoproteins correlates highly with the subject's serum cholesterol. This correlation weakens however when the lipoprotein content is expressed in terms of the interstitial fluid volume of the subject from which the intimal lipoproteins are isolated (24). This suggests that in normal arteries lipoproteins from a constant amount of interstitial fluid are retained in the intima. This amount increases slightly with increasing age, and most of the incremental lipid is localized to the region of the (fragmentary) elastic laminae (24).

As fatty streaks develop, the concentration of lipoproteins initially decrease despite an increase in the tissue content of unesterified cholesterol. With further lesion development, the intimal content of lipoproteins, particularly LDL, increases to values several-fold higher than that in normal vessels (24). Compared to LDL, the increase in intimal content of high-density lipoprotein (HDL), quantified by the concentration of apolipoprotein A-I, is less pronounced, leading to marked decrease in the apolipoprotein A-I to apolipoprotein B-100 ratio (62). At the advanced stage of atherosclerosis, *i.e.*, the presence of a dense cap and an underlying amorphous 'atheroma', the lipoprotein concentration decreases again. Thus, with the exception of fatty streaks, lesions of all developmental stage contain higher concentrations of LDL than normal arteries.

Lipid-rich particles in the arterial wall during atherogenesis

Considering the concept of lesion transition (61) and the defenses against the 'oxidative modification' of LDL, a key question is how LDL is metabolized upon entry into the artery wall. As indicated above, lipid deposition in early human fatty streaks is characterized by a decreased extracellular content of lipoproteins. Instead, cholesteryl esters, mostly cholesteryl oleate, accumulate as large lipid droplets within cells (24, 61-63). It is thought that these cellular cholesteryl esters are derived mainly from LDL. Upon uptake, LDL cholesteryl linoleate (the major cholesteryl ester) undergoes hydrolysis, and the cholesterol is reesterified by acyl coenzyme A:cholesterol acyltransferase, primarily to cholesteryl oleate (see e.g. (64)).

LDL-derived lipoproteins that accumulate within the artery wall and that give rise to the intracellular accumulation of lipid droplets (*i.e.*, the formation of foam cells) are likely to at least initially contain several molecules of α–tocopherol per particle, and hence to oxidize via tocopherol-mediated peroxidation. Evidence for this is based in part on the work of Frank and co-workers (65, 66). They demonstrated that upon injection into rabbits, human LDL is initially deposited in the subendothelial-intimal space as lipid-like particles enmeshed in the filaments of the matrix. Although initially the size of the injected lipoprotein, these particles group together in clusters and in focal areas of the intima fuse to particles 7 to 8-times the size of normal LDL (65, 66). Mechanistic studies with model LDL aggregates (produced by physical means or by complexation with proteoglycans) indicate that also in aggregated form, LDL lipid peroxidation proceeds with typical tocopherol-mediated peroxidation kinetics (K. Morris, R. Stocker, unpublished). Each LDL particle entering the sub-endothelial space carries 6 to 10 molecules of α–tocopherol (7) and the size of the intimal particles, on average, is larger than that of LDL. It is therefore likely that each intimal LDL-derived particle contains several molecules of α–tocopherol. Because gross consumption of the vitamin does not appear to occur (see above and below), tocopherol-mediated peroxidation likely governs lipid peroxidation in these particles. If so, the prevention of tocopherol-mediated peroxidation may represent a key element of the antioxidant defense against oxidative modification of LDL during the early developmental stages of atherogenesis.

During the intermediate stages of atherogenesis, the extracellular accumulation of lipid particles becomes increasingly prominent (see above). Two types of such particles, esterified and unesterified cholesterol-rich, have been isolated from human lesions (24, 67-69). The esterified cholesterol-rich particles have a density of <1.01 g/mL and are composed of an esterified cholesterol core surrounded by a monolayer of phospholipids and unesterified cholesterol, *i.e.*, a structure similar to that of lipoproteins. By contrast, unesterified cholesterol-rich lipid particles are multilamellated, solid structures and vesicles comprised of single or multiple lamellas (69). The vast majority of both particles range in size between 40 to 200 nm, *i.e.*, up to 9-fold the size of plasma LDL (69). Linoleate is the major fatty acid in the cholesteryl ester fraction of both particles, whereas the sphingomyelin-rich phospholipid fraction contains largely palmitate and oleate. The accumulation of these particles in developing lesions may thus explain why overall there is a disease stage- and age-dependent increase in the relative content of linoleate in the artery wall (24), so that cholesteryl linoleate represents the single major readily oxidizable substrate in human atherosclerotic lesions. The origins and role of these two types of lipid particles in the artery wall are presently unknown. Similarly, the mechanism(s) of oxidation and antioxidation of the lipid components of these particles is unknown.

Changes in Antioxidant Defenses

It is clear from the discussion above that atherosclerosis is associated with complex changes to the content, structure, chemical composition and location of lipid/lipoprotein particles within the vascular wall, all of which are likely to affect the mechanism and efficacy of various types of antioxidant defenses. Compared to our knowledge of these changes, very little is known about the changes in the antioxidant defenses occurring during atherogenesis, even when information from various animal models of atherosclerosis is included. To date no systematic study on the disease stage-dependent changes in antioxidant defenses in the artery wall has been carried out. Also, the available literature on human tissue is restricted largely to the advanced stages of atherosclerosis. This represents a major limitation, given that a central component of the 'oxidation theory' is that oxidative LDL modification represents an early causative event of atherosclerosis. Furthermore, almost all of our knowledge on antioxidants in lesions is derived from experiments carried out with homogenates prepared from entire or large parts of vessels (mostly aortas). Given these severe limitations, the following can only serve as an indication of gross changes that may be occurring; it does not provide insight into putative events taking place in focal areas of the intima, such as those where intimal lipoprotein fusion (see above) and perhaps oxidative modification that precede cellular uptake may occur.

Enzymatic antioxidants in atherosclerosis

Table 2 summarizes the changes to the glutathione-related enzymatic antioxidants and superoxide dismutases occurring during atherogenesis. Compared to the normal artery, the activities of the selenium-dependent glutathione peroxidase and glutathione reductase, and EC-SOD are decreased in advanced human plaque (35, 70). By contrast, selenium-independent glutathione peroxidase activity (GST-Px) is increased in plaque vs control artery. Cucurullo and co-workers also examined changes in the aortic antioxidant defenses in cholesterol-fed rabbits: in this situation glutathione peroxidase increased with increasing disease, whereas glutathione reductase and glutathione s-transferase activities decreased (71). The inconsistency in the changes observed in human vs rabbit tissue illustrates some of the difficulties associated with the interpretation of such results in light of the 'oxidation theory' of atherosclerosis. In addition to the different location of intimal LDL/lipid particles vs cellular enzymes, and the questionable relevance of *e.g.* glutathione peroxidase as an antioxidant for complex lipids in LDL (see above), both an increase or decrease in enzyme activity may be seen as evidence of oxidative stress. However, evaluation of a causal relationship between these changes and atherogenesis is not possible using this experimental approach.

Godin et al. compared the antioxidant status and susceptibility to atherosclerosis in cholesterol-fed male vs female Japanese quails (72). When fed a cholesterol-enriched diet, male quails developed substantial aortic lesions, whereas aortas of females remained largely free of macroscopic lesions (Table 4). Comparison of the aortic activities of glutathione-dependent enzymes in the same animals with those of quails fed a normal diet showed little difference, with the exception of a small increase in glutathione peroxidase in male quails. More importantly, and despite the large difference in the extent of atherosclerotic lesions, aortas from male and female quails had comparable levels of antioxidant enzymes (Table 4). Thus, it appears that at least in this animal model, gross changes to the glutathione-dependent antioxidant enzyme activities are not required for differences in the extent of atherogenesis. The use of glutathione peroxidase gene knockout mice (73) may provide a useful tool to investigate whether a lack of this enzyme results in accelerated atherogenesis in

Table 4. Atherosclerosis and enzymatic antioxidant defenses in aortas of female and male Japanese quails[†].

Parameter	Control (0 weeks)	Control (9 weeks)	Cholesterol-fed (9 weeks)[‡]
GSH-Reductase (nmol/min/mg protein)			
Females	0.54 ± 0.02	0.52 ± 0.03	0.52 ± 0.04
Males	0.51 ± 0.02	0.54 ± 0.03	0.52 ± 0.04
GSH-Peroxidase (nmol/min/mg protein)			
Females	0.96 ± 0.05	0.83 ± 0.05	0.83 ± 0.06
Males	0.87 ± 0.06	0.70 ± 0.03	0.84 ± 0.04*
SOD (U/mg protein)			
Females	0.35 ± 0.02	0.30 ± 0.01	0.26 ± 0.01
Males	0.37 ± 0.02	0.29 ± 0.02	0.30 ± 0.01
Plaque score			
Females	0	0	0.1 ± 0.1
Males	0	0	2.7 ± 0.3*

[†]Data (mean ± SEM, n = 15) are taken from (72). Eight weeks old animals of a strain of Japanese quails (Coturnix Japanica) selected for susceptibility to cholesterol-induced atherosclerosis were used for the experiment. Plaque score was assessed blinded by microscopic examination of the aortas using a semi-quantitative scale of 0 (normal) to 4 (severe atherosclerosis). [‡]1% cholesterol by weight. GSH = glutathione. *Significantly different from 9 week controls.

these animals. In any case, the relevance of the above findings to human atherosclerosis remains to be examined.

The activity of EC-SOD is decreased in advanced human lesions compared to normal arteries (35). This together with an increased expression of inducible NO synthase (iNOS) may result in a disturbance in the balance of $O2^{-}$ and NO. This could lead to dysfunctional endothelium-dependent vasorelaxation (38) and an increase in the production of HONOO (35). Indeed, there is an increase in nitrated proteins in plaque (35, 74), including an LDL-fraction isolated from it (75). However, the interpretation and relevance of the above observations to atherogenesis are not clear. For example, the activities of EC- and Cu,Zn-SOD in plaque are comparable (Table 2) and their relative contribution to the elimination of $O2^{-}$ (to maintain adequate NO efficacy) and how this relates to oxidative stress in the artery wall and atherogenesis, are not known. Chronic inhibition of Cu,Zn-SOD in rats decreases the ex vivo response of aortic rings from such animals to endothelium-derived NO and increases non-enzymic lipid peroxidation (38). This appears to indicate a role of this form of SOD as a protective agent against atherosclerosis. In apparent contrast to this however, over-expression of Cu,Zn-SOD increases rather than decreases fatty streak formation in fat-fed C57BL/6 mice (76). Therefore, the role of SOD in intimal LDL oxidation and atherogenesis remains unknown. Again, experiments with EC-SOD gene knockout mice may provide useful information on a possible contribution of this antioxidant to atherosclerosis.

While increased aortic activity of iNOS in lesions is commonly considered to have adverse effects by altering endothelium-dependent vasorelaxation and/or increasing formation of HONOO, unambiguous evidence for both a causative link between atherosclerosis and endothelial dysfunction as well as the occurrence of HONOO-mediated oxidative damage remains unclear. In this context, it is worth considering that increased formation of NO may represent an antioxidant defense, thus, NO can inhibit lipid peroxidation (77, 78). Stimulation of iNOS in murine macrophages by interferon-γ and lipopolysaccharide inhibits rather than promotes the ability of these cells to oxidize LDL (79-81); this antioxidant activity is prevented by inhibition of NO formation, yet unaffected by the simultaneous production of $O2^{-}$ by these cells (82). The latter indicates that cellular production of $O2^{-}$ and NO may not necessarily lead to HONOO formation and hence a pro-oxidant environment for LDL, in contrast to the situation where these two radicals are produced chemically (79, 83).

As indicated above, developing atherosclerotic lesions are characterized by a decrease in the ratio of albumin and apolipoprotein A-I to LDL (24, 62). A relative decrease in albumin could affect the metal-binding capacity of the interstitial fluid so that redox active transition metals could become available; it also would be expected to lower the relative (to target LDL) concentration of thiols which are important scavengers of nucleophilic oxidants (see above). The implied relative decrease in intimal HDL vs LDL could overall favor oxidative modification of the latter. An antioxidant protective role of HDL for LDL has been proposed (84) and

HDL-associated paraoxonase is thought to be play a key role in this protective action (85-88). Indeed, paraoxonase is present in interstitial fluid where it appears to be associated with HDL (89) and hence active. Furthermore, female paraoxonase gene knockout mice fed a cholate-containing high fat diet develop larger atherosclerotic lesions in the proximal aortae than the corresponding control C57BL/6J mice (90). However, the molecular basis of the antioxidant activity of paraoxonase (an arylesterase) is obscure and studies documenting the proposed protective role of paraoxonase against LDL oxidation exclusively used indirect methods to assess lipid oxidation (85-88). Also, the difference in lesion size between control and paraoxonase knockout mice was small. Furthermore, paraoxonase deficient animals were produced using stem cells from 129/SvJ mice, and were subsequently back-crossed onto C57BL/6J strain mice for only three generations (90). Thus, genetic heterogeneity may have remained. Despite these uncertainties however, a decrease in the relative concentration of intimal HDL and associated proteins, including methionine residues of its apolipoproteins (see above), could overall increase the tendency of LDL to become oxidized as atherosclerosis develops.

Heme oxygenase-1 the heme-degrading enzyme induced under various conditions of oxidative stress (91), is expressed in endothelial cells and foam cells in human atherosclerotic lesions (92). While it remains to be demonstrated that increased expression of heme oxygenase-1 is associated with increased heme oxygenase activity, such induction could represent a local antioxidant response (93). This is particularly so if biliverdin reductase activity were present and if increased heme oxygenase-1 activity were associated with simultaneous induction of ferritin synthesis (91, 94, 95). Together, this would result in the removal of the potential pro-oxidant heme, the production of the co-antioxidant bilirubin (see above), and the sequestration of iron (94, 95). In this context it is interesting that *in vitro* oxidized LDL induces heme oxygenase-1 in macrophages (92). Also, circulating levels of bilirubin are inversely associated with the risk of cardiovascular disease (see e.g. refs. 96 and 97), though it is unclear whether, and if so how, this relates to the observed expression of heme oxygenase-1 in human atherosclerotic lesions.

There is evidence that interferon-γ is present in human atherosclerotic lesions (98). Also, preliminary studies indicate the expression in human lesions of indoleamine 2,3-dioxygenase, the rate-limiting enzyme in oxidative tryptophan metabolism leading to the formation of 3-hydroxyanthranilic acid (S.R. Thomas, R. Stocker, unpublished), raising the possibility that this co-antioxidant may be present in the extracellular fluid in diseased arteries.

Non-enzymic antioxidants in atherosclerosis

The above results demonstrate that atherosclerosis can be associated with changes in enzymatic antioxidants, though with the exception of EC-SOD and the formation and release of NO and possibly bilirubin, most of these changes are likely to be localized within cells. While a change in the cellular redox state and enzymatic antioxidants may also contribute to atherogenesis (see ref. 99 and Chapter 8), stronger evidence exists for a causative role of extracellular redox changes, particularly those related to oxidative modification of LDL (see ref. 3 and Chapter 4.).

Table 3 shows the levels of non-enzymatic antioxidants associated with and surrounding LDL, some of which are known to effectively inhibit LDL lipid peroxidation *in vitro*. An early study reported that ascorbate levels in human aortic diseased tissue to be similar to those in plasma (100). This was confirmed by a more recent study employing homogenized plaque samples, in which the levels of urate were also reported to be intact (Table 3). The observations that ascorbate is converted rapidly into dehydroascorbic acid during sample work-up, that in plaque and normal arteries only small and comparable amounts of vitamin C are present as dehydroascorbic acid, and that plaque contains several times more ascorbate than normal arteries, all argue against the redox status of vitamin C being deficient in any way in human plaque.

Similar to ascorbate, the concentrations of α-tocopherol in homogenates of advanced (Table 3), early and intermediate human atherosclerotic lesions (J. Upston and R. Stocker, unpublished) are comparable to those in plasma. This is particularly so when the results are expressed per cholesteryl linoleate, the major readily oxidizable lipids (see legend to Table 3). Considering this together with the fate of LDL entering the intimal space (see above), these findings suggest that the non-enzymatic, extracellular antioxidant defense in form of at least ascorbate and α-tocopherol appears to remain intact in the artery wall of a developing lesion. Thus, the argument used to suggest that oxidative damage to LDL must occur in the intima rather than plasma (*i.e.*, that plasma has an overwhelming antioxidant capacity) appears undermined by these observations.

A striking feature of advanced human lesions is that despite the presence of these co-antioxidants, some 5 - 10 % of plaque cholesteryl linoleate is oxidized (58). As indicated earlier, tocopherol-mediated peroxidation of lipids in human plasma (20) and isolated LDL (54) is effectively prevented as long as ascorbate and α-tocopherol are present. Thus, the question arises of how relatively large amounts of oxidized lipids can co-exist and perhaps be formed in human plaque in the presence of ascorbate and α-tocopherol. The above findings (58) were obtained using homogenates of plaques and aortic vessels. Thus, a local depletion of ascorbic acid, for example within the filaments of the extracellular matrix where LDL becomes enmeshed and lipoprotein particle fusion occurs (65, 66), cannot be excluded. Such a putative local exclusion is not likely valid for the co-antioxidant ubiquinol-10 which associates with LDL. Unfortunately, information on the concentrations of ubiquinol-10 in human lesions is not available at present. The study of Suarna et al. (58) did not allow distinction to be made between endogenous oxidation of ubiquinol-10 and that occurring during sample work-up.

SUMMARY

Atherogenesis is associated with complex quantitative and qualitative changes in the pools of lipid substrates potentially available for oxidative modification. Compared to the knowledge of these changes, and despite the overwhelming literature on and interest in the 'oxidative theory' of atherosclerosis, our understanding of the nature and location of the various antioxidant defenses within the artery wall, and how they change during atherogenesis, is at best rudimentary. While several changes in enzymatic antioxidants have been reported to occur, the relevance of these to aortic LDL oxidation and, even more so, to atherogenesis, remains largely obscure. The limited data available on non-enzymatic, non-proteinaceous antioxidants surprisingly suggests that substantial amounts of oxidized lipids are present in plaque despite the absence of a gross deficiency in the levels of ascorbate and α-tocopherol. Our present knowledge of the mechanism underlying lipoprotein lipid peroxidation cannot readily explain these latter findings, unless we introduce the concept of local sites where aqueous co-antioxidants become limited or excluded. What is clear is that substantial lipid oxidation occurs despite the presence of apparently normal levels of vitamin E. Preliminary results with synthetic antioxidants suggest that effective inhibition of aortic lipoprotein lipid peroxidation can be achieved by lipophilic co-antioxidants. If confirmed, these could have important implications for future intervention trials. Further studies are needed to resolve these issues.

Acknowledgements

This work was supported by The National Health & Medical Research Council of Australia and a Fellowship for Visiting Scientists by the International Atherosclerosis Society. I thank Dr. M.R. McCall for carefully reading the manuscript and stimulating discussions

REFERENCES

1. Sies H. Oxidative stress: introductory remarks. In: Sies H, ed. Oxidative Stress. New York: Academic, 1985:1.
2. Halliwell B. How to characterize a biological antioxidant. *Free Rad Res Comm.* 1990;9:1.
3. Steinberg D, Parthasarathy S, Carew TE, Khoo JC, Witztum JL. Beyond cholesterol: Modifications of low-density lipoprotein that increase its atherogenicity. *N Engl J Med.* 1989;320:915.
4. Berliner JA, Heinecke JW. The role of oxidized lipoproteins in atherogenesis. *Free Rad Biol Med.* 1996;20:707.
5. Bowry VW, Stocker R. Tocopherol-mediated peroxidation. The pro-oxidant effect of vitamin E on the radical-initiated oxidation of human low-density lipoprotein. *J Am Chem Soc.* 1993;115:6029.
6. Ingold KU, Bowry VW, Stocker R, Walling C. Autoxidation of lipids and antioxidation by α–tocopherol and ubiquinol in homogeneous solution and in aqueous dispersions of lipids. The unrecognized consequences of lipid particle size as exemplified by the oxidation of human low density lipoprotein. *Proc Natl Acad Sci USA.* 1993;90:45.
7. Witting PK, Upston JM, Stocker R. The molecular action of α–tocopherol in lipoprotein lipid peroxidation: pro- and antioxidant activity of vitamin E in complex heterogeneous lipid emulsions. In: Quinn P, Kagan V, eds. Subcellular Biochemistry: Fat-Soluble Vitamins. London: Plenum, 1998:345.
8. Bowry VW, Ingold KU, Stocker R. Vitamin E in human low-density lipoprotein. When and how this antioxidant becomes a pro-oxidant. *Biochem J.* 1992;288:341.

9.   Bowry VW, Mohr D, Cleary J, Stocker R. Prevention of tocopherol-mediated peroxidation of ubiquinol-10-free human low density lipoprotein. *J Biol Chem*. 1995;270:5756.
10.   Neuzil J, Thomas SR, Stocker R. Requirement for, promotion, or inhibition by α–tocopherol of radical-induced initiation of plasma lipoprotein lipid peroxidation. *Free Rad Biol Med* 1997;22:57.
11.   Mukai K, Sawada K, Kohno Y, Terao J. Kinetic study of the prooxidant effect of tocopherol. Hydrogen abstraction from lipid hydroperoxides by tocopheroxyls in solution. *Lipids*. 1993;28:747.
12.   Neuzil J, Stocker R. Free and albumin-bound bilirubin is an efficient co-antioxidant for α–tocopherol, inhibiting plasma and low density lipoprotein lipid peroxidation. *J Biol Chem*. 1994;269:16712.
13.   Witting PK, Westerlund C, Stocker R. A rapid and simple screening test for potential inhibitors of tocopherol-mediated peroxidation of LDL lipids. *J Lipid Res*. 1996;37:853.
14.   Thomas SR, Witting PK, Stocker R. 3-Hydroxyanthranilic acid is an efficient, cell-derived co-antioxidant for α–tocopherol, inhibiting human low density lipoprotein and plasma lipid peroxidation. *J Biol Chem*. 1996;271:32714.
15.   Neuzil J, Witting PK, Stocker R. α–Tocopheryl hydroquinone is an efficient multifunctional inhibitor of radical-initiated oxidation of low-density lipoprotein lipids. *Proc Natl Acad Sci USA*. 1997;94:7885.
16.   Bowry VW, Stanley KK, Stocker R. High density lipoprotein is the major carrier of lipid hydroperoxides in fasted human plasma. *Proc Natl Acad Sci USA*. 1992;89:10316.
17.   Mohr D, Stocker R. Radical-mediated oxidation of isolated human very low density lipoprotein. *Arterioscl Thromb*. 1994;14:1186.
18.   Thomas SR, Neuzil J, Mohr D, Stocker R. Co antioxidants make α–tocopherol an efficient antioxidant for LDL. *Am J Clin Nutr*. 1995;62:1357S.
19.   Mohr D, Umeda Y, Redgrave TG, Stocker R. Antioxidant defenses in rat intestine and mesenteric lymph. *Redox Report*. 1998;in press.
20.   Frei B, Stocker R, Ames BN. Antioxidant defenses and lipid peroxidation in human blood plasma. *Proc Natl Acad Sci USA*. 1988;85:9748.
21.   Dabbagh AJ, Frei B. Human suction blister interstitial fluid prevents metal ion-dependent oxidation of low density lipoprotein by macrophages and in cell-free systems. *J Clin Invest* 1995;96:1958.
22.   Halliwell B, Gutteridge JMC. The antioxidants of human extracellular fluids. *Arch Biochem Biophys*. 1990;280:1.
23.   Stocker R, Frei B. Endogenous antioxidant defenses in human blood plasma. In: Sies H, ed. Oxidative stress: Oxidants and antioxidants. London: Academic Press, 1991:213-243.
24.   Smith EB. The relationship between plasma and tissue lipids in human atherosclerosis. *Adv Lipid Res* 1974;12:1.
25.   Ursini F, Maiorino M, Valente M, Ferri L, Gregolin C. Purification from pig liver of a protein with protects liposomes and biomembranes from peroxidative degradation and exhibits glutathione peroxidase activity on phosphatidyl-choline liposomes. *Biochim Biophys Acta*. 1982;710:197.
26.   Thomas JP, Geiger PG, Maiorino M, Ursini F, Girotti AW. Enzymatic reduction of phospholipid and cholesterol hydroperoxides in artificial bilayers and lipoproteins. *Biochim Biophys Acta*. 1990;1045:252.
27.   Sattler W, Maiorino M, Stocker R. Reduction of HDL- and LDL-associated cholesterylester- and phospholipid hydroperoxides by phospholipid hydroperoxide glutathione peroxidase and Ebselen (PZ 51). *Arch Biochem Biophys*. 1994;309:214.
28.   Garner B, Waldeck AR, Witting PK, Rye K-A, Stocker R. Oxidation of high density lipoproteins. II. Evidence for direct reduction of HDL lipid hydroperoxides by methionine residues of apolipoproteins AI and AII. *J Biol Chem*. 1998;273:6088.
29.   Mashima R, Yamamoto Y, Yoshimura S. Reduction of phosphatidylcholine hydroperoxide by apolipoprotein A-I: purification of the hydroperoxide-reducing proteins from human blood plasma. *J Lipid Res*. 1998;39:1133.
30.   Sattler W, Christison JK, Stocker R. Cholesterylester hydroperoxide reducing activity associated with isolated high- and low-density lipoproteins. *Free Rad Biol Med*. 1995;18:421.
31.   Christison JK, Karjalainen A, Brauman J, Bygrave F, Stocker R. Rapid reduction and removal of HDL- but not LDL-associated cholesterylester hydroperoxides by in situ perfused rat liver. *Biochem J*. 1996;314:739.

32.   Nakamura H, Vaage J, Valne G, Padilla CA, Björnstedt M, Holmgren A. Measurement of plasma glutaredoxin and thioredoxin in healthy volunteers and during open-heart surgery. *Free Rad Biol Med.* 1998;24:1176.

33.   Björnstedt M, Hamberg M, Kumar S, Xue J, Holmgren A. Human thioredoxin reductase directly reduces lipid hydroperoxides by NADPH and selenocystine strongly stimulates the reaction via catalytically generated selenols. *J Biol Chem.* 1995;270:11761.

34.   Strålin P, Karlsson K, Johansson BO, Marklund SL. The interstitium of the human arterial wall contains very large amounts of extracellular superoxide dismutase. *Arterioscl Thromb Vasc Biol.* 1995;15:2032.

35.   Luoma JS, Strålin P, Marklund SL, Hiltunen TP, Sarkioja T, Ylä-Herttuala S. Expression of extracellular SOD and iNOS in macrophages and smooth muscle cells in human and rabbit atherosclerotic lesions: colocalization with epitopes characteristic of oxidized LDL and peroxynitrite-modified proteins. *Arterioscler Thromb Vasc Biol.* 1998;18:157.

36.   Oury TD, Day BJ, Crapo JD. Extracellular superoxide dismutase in vessels and airways of humans and baboons. *Free Rad Biol Med.* 1996;20:957.

37.   Abrahamsson T, Brandt U, Marklund SL, Sjoqvist PO. Vascular bound recombinant extracellular superoxide dismutase type C protects against the detrimental effects of superoxide radicals on endothelium-dependent arterial relaxation. *Circ Res.* 1992;70:264.

38.   Lynch SM, Frei B, Morrow JD, et al. Vascular superoxide dismutase deficiency impairs endothelial vasodilator function through direct inactivation of nitric oxide and increased lipid peroxidation. *Arterioscler Thromb Vasc Biol.* 1997; 17:2975.

39.   van Hinsburg VWM, Scheffer M, Havekes L, Kempen HJM. Role of endothelial cells and their products in the modification of low-density lipoproteins. *Biochim Biophys Acta.* 1986;878:49.

40.   Ehrenwald E, Chisolm GM, Fox PL. Intact human ceruloplasmin oxidatively modifies low density lipoprotein. *J Clin Invest.* 1994; 93:1493.

41.   Daugherty A, Dunn JL, Rateri DL, Heinecke JW. Myeloperoxidase, a catalyst for lipoprotein oxidation, is expressed in human atherosclerotic lesions. *J Clin Invest.* 1994;94:437.

42.   Hazell LJ, Arnold L, Flowers D, Waeg G, Malle E, Stocker R. Presence of hypochlorite-modified proteins in human atherosclerotic lesions. *J Clin Invest.* 1996;97:1535.

43.   Winterbourn CC. Comparative reactivities of various biological compounds with myeloperoxidase-hydrogen peroxide-chloride, and similarity of the oxidant to hypochlorite. *Biochim Biophys Acta.* 1985;840:204.

44.   Hu ML, Louie S, Cross CE, Motchnik P, Halliwell B. Antioxidant protection against hypochlorous acid in human plasma. *J Lab Clin Med.* 1993;121:257.

45.   Frei B, England L, Ames BN. Ascorbate is an outstanding antioxidant in human blood plasma. *Proc Natl Acad Sci USA.* 1989;86:6377.

46.   Packer JE, Slater TF, Willson RL. Direct observation of a free radical interaction between vitamin E and vitamin C. *Nature.* 1979;278:737.

47.   Ames BN, Cathcart R, Schwiers E, Hochstein P. Uric acidprovides an antioxidant defense in humans against oxidant- and radical-caused aging and cancer: a hypothesis. *Proc Natl Acad Sci USA.* 1981;78:6858.

48.   Christen S, Peterhans E, Stocker R. Antioxidant activities of some tryptophan metabolites: Possible implication for inflammatory diseases. *Proc Natl Acad Sci USA.* 1990;87:2506.

49.   Christen S, Thomas SR, Garner B, Stocker R. Inhibition by interferon-g of human mononuclear cell-mediated low density lipoprotein oxidation. Participation of tryptophan metabolism along the kynurenine pathway. *J Clin Invest.* 1994;93:2149.

50.   Stocker R, Yamamoto Y, McDonagh AF, Glazer AN, Ames BN. Bilirubin is an antioxidant of possible physiological importance. *Science.* 1987;235:1043.

51.   Stocker R, Glazer AN, Ames BN. Antioxidant activity of albumin bound bilirubin. *Proc Natl Acad Sci USA.* 1987;84:5918.

52.   Witting PK, Bowry VW, Stocker R. Inverse deuterium kinetic isotope effect for peroxidation in human low-density lipoprotein (LDL): a simple test for tocopherol-mediated peroxidation of LDL lipids. *FEBS Lett.* 1995;375:45.

53.   Cooney RV, Franke AA, Harwood PJ, Hatch-Pigott V, Custer LJ, Mordan LJ. g-Tocopherol detoxification of nitrogen dioxide: superiority to α–tocopherol. *Proc Natl Acad Sci USA.* 1993;90:1771.

54. Stocker R, Bowry VW, Frei B. Ubiquinol-10 protects human low density lipoprotein more efficiently against lipid peroxidation than does α–tocopherol. *Proc Natl Acad Sci USA.* 1991;88:1646.

55. Mohr D, Bowry VW, Stocker R. Dietary supplementation with coenzyme Q10 results in increased levels of ubiquinol-10 within circulating lipoproteins and increased resistance of human low density lipoprotein to the initiation of lipid peroxidation. *Biochim Biophys Acta.* 1992;1126:247.

56. Thomas SR, Neuzil J, Stocker R. Co-supplementation with coenzyme Q prevents the pro-oxidant effect of α–tocopherol and increases the resistance of low-density lipoprotein towards transition metal-dependent oxidation initiation. *Arterioscl Thromb Vasc Biol.* 1996;16:687.

57. Mukai K, Morimoto H, Kikuchi S, Nagaoka S. Kinetic study of free-radical-scavenging action of biological hydroquinones (reduced forms of ubiquinone, vitamin K and tocopherol quinone) in solution. *Biochim Biophys Acta.* 1993;1157:313.

58. Suarna C, Dean RT, May J, Stocker R. Human atherosclerotic plaque contains both oxidized lipids and relatively large amounts of α–tocopherol and ascorbate. *Arterioscler Thromb Vasc Biol.* 1995;15:1616.

59. Carpenter KL, Cheeseman KH, van der Veen C, Taylor SE, Walker MK, Mitchinson MJ. Depletion of alpha–tocopherol in human atherosclerotic lesions. *Free Rad Res.* 1995;23:549.

60. Killion SL, Hunter GC, Eskelson CD, et al. Vitamin E levels in human atherosclerotic plaque: the influence of risk factors. *Atherosclerosis.* 1996;126:289.

61. Guyton JR, Klemp KF. Development of the atherosclerotic core region. Chemical and ultrastructural analysis of microdissected atherosclerotic lesions from human aorta. *Arterioscler Thromb.* 1994;14:1305.

62. Ylä-Herttuala S. Biochemistry of the arterial wall in developing atherosclerosis. *Ann NY Acad Sci.* 1991;623:40.

63. Lundberg B. Chemical composition and physical state of lipid deposits in atherosclerosis. *Atherosclerosis.* 1985;1985:93.

64. Cignarella A, Brennhausen B, von Eckardstein A, Assmann G, Cullen P. Differential effects of lovastatin on the trafficking of endogenous and lipoprotein derived cholesterol in human monocyte-derived macrophages. *Arterioscl Thromb Vasc Biol.* 1998;18:1322.

65. Frank JS, Fogelman AM. Ultrastructure of the intima in WHHL and cholesterol-fed rabbit aortas prepared by ultra rapid freezing and freeze etching. *J Lipid Res.* 1989;30:967.

66. Nievelstein PFEM, Fogelman AM, Mottino G, Frank JS. Lipid accumulation in rabbit aortic intima 2 hours after bolus infusion of low density lipoprotein. A deep-etch and immunolocalization study of ultrarapidly frozen tissue. *Arterioscl Thromb.* 1991;11:1795.

67. Simionescu N, Vasile E, Lupu F, Popescu G, Simionescu M. Prelesion events in atherogenesis. Accumulation of extracellular cholesterol-rich liposomes in the arterial intima and cardiac valves of the hyperlipidemic rabbit. *Am J Pathol.* 1986;123:109.

68. Chao F-F, Amende LM, Blanchette-Mackie EJ, et al. Unesterified cholesterol-rich lipid particles in atherosclerotic lesions of human and rabbit aortas. *Am J Pathol.* 1988;131:73.

69. Chao F-F, Blanchette-Mackie EJ, Chen Y-J, et al. Characterization of two unique cholesterol-rich lipid particles isolated from human atherosclerotic lesions. *Am J Pathol.* 1990;136:169.

70. Lapenna D, de Gioia S, Ciofani G, et al. Glutathione-related antioxidant defenses in human atherosclerotic plaques. *Circulation.* 1998;97:1930.

71. Del Boccio G, Lapenna D, Porreca E, et al. Aortic antioxidant defense mechanisms: time-related changes in cholesterol-fed rabbits. *Atherosclerosis.* 1990;81:127.

72. Godin DV, Garnett ME, Cheng KM, Nichols CR. Sex-related alterations in antioxidant status and susceptibility to atherosclerosis in Japanese quail. *Can J Cardiol.* 1995;11:945.

73. de Haan JB, Bladier C, Griffiths P, et al. Mice with a homozygous null mutation for the most abundant glutathione peroxidase, Gpx1, show increased susceptibility to the oxidative stress-induced agents paraquat and hydrogen peroxide. *J Biol Chem.* 1998;273:22528.

74. Beckman JS, Ye YZ, Anderson PG, et al. Extensive nitration of protein tyrosine in human atherosclerosis detected by immunohistochemistry. *Biol Chem Hoppe Seyler.* 1994;375:81.

75. Leeuwenburgh C, Hardy MM, Hazen SL, et al. Reactive nitrogen intermediates promote low density lipoprotein oxidation in human atherosclerotic intima. *J Biol Chem.* 1997;272:1433.

76. Tribble DL, Gong EL, Leeuwenburgh C, et al. Fatty streak formation in fat-fed mice expressing human copper-zinc superoxide dismutase. *Arterioscler Thromb Vasc Biol.* 1997;17:1734.

77.   Kanner J, Harel S, Granit R. Nitric oxide as an antioxidant. *Arch Biochem Biophys.* 1991;289:130.
78.   Kanner J, Harel S, Granit R. Nitric oxide, an inhibitor of lipid oxidation by lipoxygenase, cyclooxygenase and hemoglobin. *Lipids.* 1992;27:46.
79.   Jessup W, Mohr D, Gieseg SP, Dean RT, Stocker R. The participation of nitric oxide in cell free- and its restriction of macrophage-mediated oxidation of low-density lipoprotein. *Biochim Biophys Acta.* 1992;1180:73.
80.   Yates MT, Lambert LE, Whitten JP, et al. A protective role for nitric oxide in the oxidative modification of low density lipoproteins by mouse macrophages. *FEBS Lett.* 1992;309:135.
81.   Jessup W, Dean RT. Autoinhibition of murine macrophage-mediated oxidation of low-density lipoprotein by nitric oxide synthesis. *Atherosclerosis.* 1993;101:145.
82.   Jessup W. Cellular modification of low-density lipoproteins. *Biochem Soc Trans.* 1993;21:321.
83.   Darley-Usmar VM, Hogg N, O'Leary VJ, Wilson MT, Moncada S. The simultaneous generation of superoxide and nitric oxide can initiate lipid peroxidation in human low density lipoprotein. *Free Rad Res Comm.* 1992;17:9.
84.   Mackness MI, Abbott C, Arrol S, Durrington PN. The role of high-density lipoprotein and lipid-soluble antioxidant vitamins in inhibiting low-density lipoprotein oxidation. *Biochem J.* 1993;294:829.
85.   Mackness MI, Arrol S, Durrington PN. Paraoxonase prevents accumulation of lipoperoxides in low-density lipoprotein [published erratum appears in FEBS Lett 1991 Nov 4;292(1-2):307]. *FEBS Lett.* 1991;286:152.
86.   Mackness MI, Arrol S, Abbott C, Durrington PN. Protection of low-density lipoprotein against oxidative modification by high-density lipoprotein associated paraoxonase. *Atherosclerosis.* 1993;104:129.
87.   Watson AD, Berliner JA, Hama SY, et al. Protective effect of high density lipoprotein associated paraoxonase. Inhibition of the biological activity of minimally oxidized low density lipoprotein. *J Clin Invest.* 1995;96:2882.
88.   Van Lenten BJ, Hama SY, de Beer FC, et al. Anti-inflammatory HDL becomes pro-inflammatory during the acute phase response. Loss of protective effect of HDL against LDL oxidation in aortic wall cell cocultures. *J Clin Invest.* 1995;96:2758.
89.   Mackness MI, Mackness B, Arrol S, Wood G, Bhatnagar D, Durrington PN. Presence of paraoxonase in human interstitial fluid. *FEBS Lett.* 1997;416:377.
90.   Shih DM, Gu L, Xia Y-R, et al. Mice lacking serum paraoxonase are susceptible to organophosphate toxicity and atherosclerosis. *Nature.* 1998;394:284.
91.   Vile GF, Basu-Modak S, Waltner C, Tyrrell RM. Heme oxygenase 1 mediates an adaptive response to oxidative stress in human skin fibroblasts. *Proc Natl Acad Sci USA.* 1994;91:2607.
92.   Wang JJ, Lee TS, Lee FY, Pai RC, Chau LY. Expression of heme oxygenase-1 in atherosclerotic lesions. *Am J Pathol.* 1998;152:711.
93.   Stocker R. Induction of haem oxygenase as a defense against oxidative stress. *Free Rad Res Comm.* 1990;9:101.
94.   Balla G, Jacob HS, Balla J, et al. Ferritin: a cytoprotective antioxidant strategem of endothelium. *J Biol Chem.* 1992;267:18148.
95.   Vile GF, Tyrrell RM. Oxidative stress resulting from ultraviolet A irradiation of human skin fibroblasts leads to a heme oxygenase-dependent increase in ferritin. *J Biol Chem.* 1993;268:14678.
96.   Schwertner HA, Jackson WG, Tolan G. Association of low serum concentration of bilirubin with increased risk of coronary artery disease. *Clin Chem.* 1994;40:18.
97.   Hopkins PN, Wu LL, Hunt SC, James BC, Vincent GM, Williams RR. Higher serum bilirubin is associated with decreased risk for early familial coronary artery disease. *Arterioscler Thromb Vasc Biol.* 1996;16:250.
98.   Hansson GK, Holm J, Jonasson L. Detection of activated T lymphocytes in the human atherosclerotic plaque. *Am J Pathol.* 1989;135:169.
99.   Offermann MK, Medford RM. Antioxidants and atherosclerosis: a molecular perspective. *Heart Disease and Stroke.* 1994;3:52.
100.   Willis GC, Fishman S. Ascorbic acid content of human arterial tissue. *Can M A J.* 1955;72:500.

101.   Upston JM, Neuzil J, Witting PK, Alleva R, Stocker R. 15-Lipoxygenase-induced enzymic oxidation of low density lipoprotein associated free fatty acids stimulates nonenzymic, α–tocopherol-mediated peroxidation of cholesteryl esters. *J Biol Chem.* 1997;272:30067.
102.   Garner B, Witting PK, Waldeck AR, Christison JK, Raftery M, Stocker R. Oxidation of high density lipoproteins. I. Formation of methionine sulfoxide in apolipoproteins AI and AII is an early event that correlates with with lipid peroxidation and can be enhanced by α–tocopherol. *J Biol Chem.* 1998;273:6080.

4 THE OXIDATIVE MODIFICATION HYPOTHESIS OF ATHEROGENESIS

Sotirios Tsimikas and Joseph L. Witztum

INTRODUCTION

Atherosclerosis, and its clinical sequelae continue to be the leading cause of mortality and morbidity in the western world. It is a complex and chronic disease that is influenced by a wide variety of genetic, environmental and behavioral activities. Yet, there can be little doubt now that hypercholesterolemia is a dominant risk factor for atherosclerosis. Indeed, at any plasma cholesterol level above ~ 160 mg/dl it is likely that the risk of developing clinical coronary artery disease (CAD) increases proportionately. Many clinical trials have now demonstrated convincingly that lowering plasma cholesterol levels can dramatically reduce both morbidity and mortality due to coronary and cerebrovascular disease, and even reduce total mortality.

Nevertheless, at any given concentration of plasma cholesterol there is great variability in the expression of clinical disease, undoubtedly due to the fact that many other risk factors are also involved in atherogenesis. Indeed, the mechanisms by which elevated levels of lipoproteins, chiefly the apolipoprotein (apo) B-containing lipoproteins, such as LDL, cause atherogenesis are only incompletely understood. However, there is now a large body of evidence to support the hypothesis that the atherogenicity of LDL derives in large part from the fact that it becomes modified in one or more ways once it enters the arterial wall (1,2). In particular, it is widely believed that the oxidation of LDL is one such modification that is involved in the atherogenic process. Indeed **the oxidative modification hypothesis of atherogenesis states that oxidation of lipids and lipoproteins, such as LDL, is important, if not obligatory for the atherogenic process.**(3-5) This hypothesis has not only been of great heuristic value in guiding research into the pathophysiology of atherogenesis, but attracted considerable attention because if clinically relevant it predicts that inhibition of such lipid peroxidation could ameliorate, and in conjunction with effective hypolipidemic therapy, might even prevent atherosclerosis and its clinical sequelae. While this chapter will focus on the oxidative modification hypothesis of atherogenesis, it is clearly recognized that this is but one component of a complex interplay of circulating blood elements, activated endothelial cells, chemo-attractants, cytokines, growth factors, T-cells, macrophages and smooth muscle cells that profoundly influence the atherogenic process. However, the purpose of this chapter will be to summarize the potential role that oxidation of lipoproteins, and LDL in particular, could play in this process.

The earliest atherosclerotic lesion that is morphologically visible is the fatty streak, a lesion that occurs under an intact endothelium. Fatty streaks are found even in early fetal life (6) and progressively increase from infancy to adulthood (7). Fatty streaks are composed primarily of cholesteryl ester-laden foam-cells, which in large part consist of monocyte-derived macrophages that have penetrated through the endothelial layer, as well as modified smooth muscle cells that have presumably migrated from the media (8,9). The fatty streak is widely accepted to be the precursor of the more advanced and complicated plaques, which cause symptoms both by compromising the lumen diameter, as well as by altering normal vasomotor activity. In addition, advanced lesions, particularly those enriched in macrophages and lipid, are the sites of plaque rupture, which results in intravascular thrombosis leading to acute clinical events (10-12). Understanding the precise mechanisms responsible for fatty streak formation should provide insights into novel approaches to prevent early lesion formation, which in turn should result in reduced clinical sequelae.

OXIDIZED LDL, BUT NOT NATIVE LDL, LEADS TO FOAM CELL FORMATION

The appreciation that macrophages were the chief cell within the artery wall giving rise to foam cells led to an intensive effort in understanding the mechanisms by which elevations of LDL caused foam cell formation. It was initially anticipated that LDL uptake via the LDL receptor would cause foam cell formation, several observations suggested this was not correct. First, patients with homozygous familial hypercholesterolemia, who genetically lack LDL receptors, nevertheless develop the most severe forms of atherosclerosis, even during the first decade of life. Second, incubation of LDL with normal macrophages that contain a full complement of LDL receptors, did not lead to accumulation of cholesterol and foam cell formation. In this setting, the high concentrations of LDL in the medium led to a down-regulation of LDL receptors. Thus, uptake of native LDL could not explain foam cell formation.

The answer to this paradox was provided by Goldstein and associates (13) who demonstrated that chemical modification of LDL, produced by acetylation of lysine residues, modified LDL such that it was taken up in an unregulated manner and greatly enhanced rate, leading to true foam cell formation. This process was mediated by a specific saturable receptor which was termed the "acetyl LDL receptor"(14). It is now known to be a member of an ever growing family of so-called "scavenger receptors" present on macrophages and other cell types (15). Several other chemical modifications of LDL such as aceto-acetylation, or reaction with malondialdehyde (MDA) also modified LDL in a manner that supported enhanced uptake via the acetyl LDL receptor.(16) However, there appeared little evidence that any of these modifications occurred to a significant extent *in vivo*.

Subsequent studies by Steinberg and colleagues (17) showed that incubation of LDL with cultured endothelial or smooth muscle cells converted it into a modified form that was rapidly taken up by macrophages via the scavenger receptor and caused foam cell formation. Steinbrecher *et al.* (18) then showed that the modification induced by cells was the initiation of lipid peroxidation in LDL, a finding confirmed for smooth muscle cell modification as well (19). In parallel studies, LDL was shown to be cytotoxic to endothelial cells and smooth muscle cells and this was due to oxidation of LDL lipids occurring during the incubation (20). It is now well established that oxidation of LDL can be induced by incubation under appropriate conditions with a variety of cells including endothelial cells, smooth muscle cells, macrophages, or even fibroblasts.

While the acetyl LDL receptor was identified as the original "scavenger" receptor, it is now well established that there are a family of different scavenger receptors present not only on macrophages but other cells as well (21). The acetyl LDL receptor was cloned and shown to exist in two forms, termed the scavenger receptor A (SRA types I and II) (14). In addition, a number of other putative scavenger receptors have also been identified, including CD36, SR-B1, LOX-1, and CD68 (macrosialin) (4,22). The relative importance of each of these receptors in mediating the binding and internalization of oxidized LDL (oxLDL) remains to be established. However, SRA knockout mice have been generated and crossed into apo E-deficient mice. Macrophages from such animals bind and degrade oxLDL approximately 40% less than macrophages from wild type animals. Furthermore these mice develop less atherosclerosis than apo E deficient mice with a normal complement of SRA receptors (23,23). Monocyte/macrophages from humans with CD36 deficiency also have a reduced ability to bind and degrade oxLDL (24). Recently, CD36 knockout animals have been generated and macrophages from these animals also demonstrate about a 40% reduction in binding of oxLDL, implying a major role for this receptor as well (25).

Many of these receptors appear to recognize a wide variety of ligands, including components of certain bacterial cell walls, suggesting an evolutionary role in the recognition and removal of a variety of modified structures (26). For example, *both* the modified lipid and the modified apo B of oxLDL are ligands for macrophage scavenger receptors (27,28). Furthermore, scavenger receptors appear to mediate the binding and internalization of oxidized cells and cells undergoing apoptosis as well (29). Indeed, apoptotic cells and oxLDL express common "oxidation-specific" epitopes recognized by monoclonal antibodies which bind to certain oxidized phospholipids and other oxidation-specific epitopes (30). These data suggest that such scavenger receptors play an important evolutionarily conserved role in maintenance of homeostasis and urge caution in any attempt to interfere with their normal function. For example, the SRA knockout mice are more susceptible to certain bacterial infections than wild type controls(23).

MECHANISMS OF LDL OXIDATION *IN VITRO*

It has been estimated that the average LDL particle contains 700 molecules of phospholipids, 600 molecules of free cholesterol, 1600 molecules of cholesterol ester, 185 triglyceride molecules and 1 molecule of apo B, which consists of 4536 amino acids including 270 lysines. Both these lipids and apo B are subject to oxidative modification, and the complex chemistry that results can lead to a large spectrum of oxidation byproducts ranging from so-called minimally modified-LDL, (MM-LDL, see also Chapter 7) (31) to heavily oxidized LDL (oxLDL) (32). MM-LDL demonstrates oxidative changes in its lipids, but minimal changes to apo B. Because the LDL receptor binding site of apo B is dependent on intact lysine residues, MM-LDL is still recognized by the LDL receptor but not by the scavenger receptor. In contrast, heavily oxidized LDL ceases to be a ligand for the LDL receptor as its lysine residues are altered, but is recognized by one or more scavenger receptors on macrophages.

When polyunsaturated fatty acids (PUFAs) undergo lipid peroxidation, free radical-mediated reactions are propagated and result in widespread modification and decomposition of PUFAs (33, see also Chapter 5). This results in the generation of many highly reactive breakdown products including ketones and aldehydes such as malondialdehyde (MDA), which can modify amino groups such as apo B lysine residues or phospholipids such as phosphatidylethanolamine. Blocking lysine residues of apo B decreases LDL binding to the LDL receptor and generates a change in apo B protein charge and configuration that creates new ligands for macrophage scavenger receptor recognition. In addition, the residual phospholipid remaining after degradation of the *sn*2 PUFA may also retain a reactive group and the intact oxidized phospholipid may then covalently attach to apo B, creating a phospholipid-apo B adduct, which also appears to be a ligand for macrophage scavenger receptors (27). For example, 1-palmitoyl-2-(5-oxovaleroyl)-3-phosphatidylcholine (POVPC), resulting from the degradation of the arachidonic acid in 1-palmitoyl-2-arachidonoyl-3 phosphatidylcholine (PAPC), appears to be a potent ligand mediating binding of both oxLDL and apoptotic cells to macrophages (27,30). In addition to POVPC, other oxidatively modified phospholipids have important biological effects as well (see Chapters 6 and 7).

The biologic activity of oxLDL is not restricted to phospholipid oxidation. The oxidation of cholesterol molecules also occurs, leading to a variety of oxysterols, as well as oxidized cholesteryl esters (34). Undoubtedly, many of these products are sufficiently polar to leave the modified LDL particle and cause a myriad of biological effects. In addition, apo B is subject to direct oxidative modification as a consequence of free radical attack (35). LDL oxidized *in vitro* displays extensive fragmentation of its apo B moiety and LDL isolated from atherosclerotic plaques shows similar fragmentation (36,37). Other covalent modifications of apo B amino acid have also been described such as generation of dityrosine, parahydroxyphenylacetaldehyde, and chlorinated tyrosines, in part, as a result of myeloperoxidase activity (38).

The extraordinarily complex chemistry involved in LDL oxidative modification and the number of species generated provides a rationale for the multiple biologic effects that have been ascribed to oxLDL. It is of the utmost importance to recognize that the term "oxLDL" denotes a highly heterogeneous series of particles and modified molecules. This is likely to be true for LDL particles modified *in vitro*, as well as *in vivo*. Furthermore, the same oxidized LDL particle may contain different modified lipids that have opposing effects on a given biological parameter. It is likely that this heterogeneity not only accounts for the many different biologic effects noted, but also explains, in part, the often discordant reports of oxLDL bioactivity. In this context it should be appreciated that it is difficult to reproducibly generate any given form of "oxLDL" and this problem complicates interpretation of research results. The isolation of components responsible for a given biologic effect should greatly strengthen our ability to understand the pathologic effects of oxLDL and hasten our ability to design specific and effective therapies.

MECHANISMS OF LDL OXIDATION *IN VIVO*

As detailed below, there is considerable evidence that LDL undergoes oxidation *in vivo* and oxLDL can be found in abundance in the atherosclerotic arterial wall. Because plasma and even extracellular fluid contain abundant antioxidant defenses (39) it is not clear how such oxidation can occur. *In vitro*, oxidation of LDL can be readily accomplished by exposure to transition metal ions such as copper. Indeed, such *in vitro* oxidative modification can be completely inhibited by heavy metal chelators such as EDTA (40). In addition, free radicals generated by azo compounds or ionizing radiation can also generate forms of oxLDL that have biologic properties similar to oxLDL generated by exposure to cells in culture (41). As noted above, the co-incubation of LDL with a wide variety of cells in culture can lead to its oxidation, particularly when the medium contains trace amounts of free metals. The original studies which revealed the ability of endothelial cells to oxidatively modify LDL were conducted in F-10 medium and oxidation could be abolished by the presence of EDTA. In contrast, incubation in DMEM which contains few free metals prevented oxidative modification.

Studies in cell culture have identified a number of enzyme systems that could potentially mediate the ability of cells to oxidize LDL. These enzyme systems produce reactive oxygen species, such as superoxide anion and hydrogen peroxide which can be released into the extracellular space. As a result the LDL particle can be "seeded" with lipid hydroperoxides (2). These can decompose in the presence of transition metals generating free radicals which lead to propagation reactions that amplify the number of lipid hydroperoxides and the formation of both "conjugated dienes" and the generation of reactive aldehyde molecules. Enzyme systems that could play a role in this process include NADPH oxidase (42), the mitochondrial electron transport system, myeloperoxidase (43), and 15-lipoxygenase. In particular, substantial evidence has been accumulated to support a role for 15-lipoxygenase. Inhibitors of 15-lipoxygenase can decrease the ability of several cell types to modify LDL *in vitro* (44,45), and fibroblasts constitutively lacking lipoxygenase expression demonstrate an enhanced ability to modify LDL when transfected with human 15-lipoxygenase (46,47). Treatment of hypercholesterolemic rabbits with inhibitors of 15-lipoxygenase decreases the extent of atherosclerosis (48,49). Recently, a definitive study by Cyrus *et al.*(50) has shown that homozygous disruption of the 12/15-lipoxygenase gene in an apo E-deficient background dramatically reduced the progression of atherosclerosis even though marked hypercholesterolemia persisted. Furthermore, this was accompanied by decreased autoantibody titers to epitopes of oxLDL, providing strong, though indirect, evidence that oxidation of LDL had been greatly diminished. The fact that disruption of 15-lipoxygenase so profoundly inhibited atherosclerosis, even in the presence of massive hypercholesterolemia, strongly supports the hypothesis that many, if not most, of the adverse effects of hypercholesterolemia on the artery wall are mediated via altered oxidative processes. Recent data suggest that hypercholesterolemia itself is associated with an enhanced rate of lipid peroxidation (51). There is no data yet on the importance of the 15-lipoxygenase enzyme in atherogenesis in man, but 15-lipoxygenase mRNA and protein are abundantly present in human lesions (52,53) as are stereospecific products of 15-lipoxygenase activity (54,55), supporting an important role in human lesions as well.

It is likely that other processes are also involved in human lesion formation. It is of greatest importance to understand the mechanisms by which LDL is oxidized *in vitro*, and the mechanisms that regulate the redox state in the artery wall in general, since it so profoundly affects many other functions such as vasomotor tone and endothelial cell adhesion molecule expression (see Chapters 8 and 9). Because such processes have broad biological implications, the more detailed knowledge we have of the mechanisms responsible for the control of the redox state in the artery, the more accurately and specifically can we design effective therapies that will target pathological processes, but not interfere with beneficial ones.

ATHEROGENICITY OF OXIDIZED LDL

The original interest in oxLDL stemmed from observations that the unregulated uptake of oxLDL by macrophage scavenger receptors generated foam cells, the earliest morphologic lesion of atherosclerosis. However, it is now clear that oxLDL, and/or its many oxidatively modified molecules have a wide variety of biological effects that could influence the atherogenic process. Many of these potential mechanisms are summarized in Table 1, but it is likely that these are many other mechanisms as well. Many of the identified mechanisms are discussed in detail in other chapters of this book and only a brief overview will be given here. In nearly all experimental animal models hypercholesterolemia is needed to initiate the atherosclerotic process. Although endothelial cell activation appears to be an early event that occurs soon after the initiation of hypercholesterolemia in experimental animals(56), the signals that result from hypercholesterolemia that alter endothelial cell function have not yet been defined, but are likely to be due to products of oxLDL(57,58). When hypercholesterolemia is produced experimentally there is an increased rate of entry of circulating LDL into the artery wall and a decreased rate of exit, particularly at sites that are lesion prone(59,60). Presumably once within the artery wall, there is enhanced binding of LDL by extracellular matrix, which prolongs its half life within the intima, rendering it more susceptible to various modifications, including oxidation. For example, after undergoing mild degrees of oxidation, it becomes an excellent substrate for sphingomyelinase, which can aggregate LDL and enhance macrophage uptake (61). The rapidity with which LDL can be oxidized once it enters the artery wall was demonstrated in experiments by Calara *et al.* (62) in which the intravenous injection of normal human LDL into a rat aorta resulted in the appearance of the human LDL in the aorta approximately 6 hours after injection as detected by an anti human LDL antibody. After 12 hours there was the co-localization of oxidation-specific epitopes of oxLDL. Furthermore, injection of LDL enriched with probucol prevented the appearance of the oxidation specific epitopes in the artery wall, even though the human LDL was still detected there. In human fetal arteries, lipid-filled lesions are readily observed and in many of these lesions, the presence of oxLDL can be seen without any accompanying monocyte/macrophages(63). Thus, the generation of oxLDL within the artery wall appears to be among the earliest events that occur as a result of hypercholesterolemia. As discussed above, the mechanisms by which LDL becomes oxidized are unclear, but even the earliest form of oxLDL, MM-LDL, is directly chemotactic for monocytes. In addition, it can alter gene expression of neighboring arterial cells to cause increased expression of a variety of chemotactic molecules including MCP-1, colony stimulating factors, IL-1 as well as increasing endothelial cell expression of adhesive molecules such as VCAM-1, P-selection and others (64). Some of the biologic effects of oxLDL reside in the lipid components and in particular POVPC has recently been demonstrated to be capable of inducing expression of endothelial cell adhesive molecules (65-67). Lysophosphatidylcholine, a product of more extensively oxLDL, can also induce the expression of adhesion molecules and contribute to monocyte recruitment (68). These combined events result in the migration of monocytes into the subendothelial space and their conversion to macrophages. oxLDL inhibits the motility of macrophages and prevents their egress from the lesions. Macrophages in turn can effectively further modify the LDL to maximally oxLDL(69), which is now readily taken up by scavenger receptors resulting in foam cell formation.

A very important and increasingly recognized property of products of oxLDL is their ability to influence gene expression, probably through the wide variety of modified lipids generated. For example, a number of pro-inflammatory genes and their products, such as heme oxygenase, SAA and ceruloplasmin are induced by oxLDL(70). MM-LDL or oxLDL can induce enhanced expression of macrophage scavenger receptors thereby leading to its own enhanced uptake(71). oxLDL can also enhance macrophage expression of PPARg and products of oxLDL can activate PPARg (72-74). The latter in turn can affect the expression of a wide variety of macrophage genes potentially involved in atherogenesis and inflammation. For example PPARg activation in macrophages can induce CD36 expression, but inhibit pro-inflammatory genes such as NO synthase and B-gelatinase.

A potential important property of oxLDL is its cytotoxicity to various cells including endothelial cells. This could result in functional or even overt damage to endothelium or other cells. Cytotoxicity has been shown to be due in part to Oxysterols(34). Ironically, cytotoxicity could also be induced in the very macrophages that have taken up oxLDL, leading to necrosis and release of undigested pro-inflammatory oxidized lipids in the developing atheroma. Furthermore, oxLDL may also promote apoptosis as well (75,76).

oxLDL is immunogenic and induces a profound humoral and cellular response(77), the consequences of which are complex but likely to be important, especially in the more slowly evolving lesions seen in human subjects. As discussed in detail elsewhere in this book, oxLDL, or its products, either directly or indirectly decrease the generation and/or delivery of nitric oxide to smooth muscle cells, thereby blunting or even producing paradoxical vasoconstriction in response to stimuli such as acetylcholine. This has been shown both *in vitro* and *in vivo* in animal and human studies. Moreover, this may occur even in patients who have only modest degrees of hypercholesterolemia but do not have obvious atherosclerotic lesions. Pretreatment with antioxidants has been shown to partially restore the normal response.

Table 1. Potential mechanisms by which oxidized forms of LDL (oxLDL) may influence atherogenesis

OxLDL has enhanced uptake by macrophages leading to foam cell formation.

Products of oxLDL are chemotactic for monocytes and T-cells and inhibit the motility of tissue macrophages.

Products of oxLDL are cytotoxic, in part due to oxidized sterols, and can induce apoptosis.

OxLDL, or products, are mitogenic for smooth muscle cells and macrophages.

OxLDL, or products, can alter gene expression of vascular cells, e.g. induction of MCP-1, colony-stimulating factors, IL-1 and expression of adhesion molecules.

OxLDL, or products, can increase expression of macrophage scavenger receptors, thereby enhancing its own uptake.

OxLDL, or products, can induce pro-inflammatory genes, e.g. heme oxygenase, SAA and ceruloplasmin.

OxLDL can induce expression and activate PPARg, thereby influencing many gene functions.

OxLDL is immunogenic and elicits autoantibody formation and activated T-cells.

Oxidation renders LDL more susceptible to aggregation, which independently leads to enhanced uptake. Similarly, oxLDL is a better substrate for sphingomyelinase, which also aggregates LDL.

OxLDL may enhance procoagulant pathways, e.g. by induction of tissue factor and platelet aggregation.

Products of oxLDL can aversely impact arterial vasomotor properties.

Modified from Steinberg, D and Witztum, JL: Lipoproteins, Lipoprotein Oxidation and Atherogenesis in Molecular Basis of Heart Disease. Chien, K.R. ed. W.B. Saunders Co., Philadelphia, 1999.

In summary, as shown in Table 1, there are many potential mechanisms by which oxLDL and its various products can both initiate atherogenesis and, through various pro-inflammatory and immunologic mechanisms, participate in the conversion of the early foam-cell lesion into intermediate and late complicated atheromas that are rich in oxidized lipids and prone to rupture. The rather striking decrease in formation of early and even late atherosclerotic lesions observed in animal models treated with a wide variety of antioxidants, (as described below) or by deletion of pro-oxidant enzymes such as 15-lipoxygenase, strongly support a critical role for many of these mechanisms in the atherogenic process.

EVIDENCE THAT OXIDATION OF LDL TAKES PLACE *IN VIVO*

When LDL is incubated *in vitro* with cultured cells, or with transition metal such as copper, it undergoes rapid lipid peroxidation after its endogenous content of antioxidants is depleted (78). However, if the LDL or medium is enriched with antioxidants, such as probucol or vitamin E, or with 5% serum or even albumin, oxidation can be completely inhibited. Because of the ubiquitous presence of proteins and/or aqueous antioxidants in plasma and because the concentrations of these appear to be sufficient even in the extracellular fluid to confer antioxidant protection under ordinary circumstances (79) there was initially much skepticism about the possibility that oxidation of LDL could occur *in vivo*. However, as summarized below there are now many lines of evidence to support the hypothesis that this does occur and furthermore that it is quantitatively important. How then does one account for oxidation of LDL *in vivo*? Although the mechanisms responsible for such oxidation are not known with certainty, it does occur. Because plasma has such a large content of antioxidants it does not seem likely that any significant degree of oxidation can occur in the circulation. Therefore, oxidation of LDL most likely occurs in sequestered microenvironments within the arterial intima, either adjacent to the arterial cells and/or bound to extracellular matrix. In the same way that neutrophils create a localized microenvironment in which a sufficient concentration of ROS are generated to kill bacteria, or in which monocyte/macrophages create "black holes" (80), so might microdomains be generated adjacent to vascular cells. The evidence that oxidation of LDL takes place *in vivo* can be summarized as follows:

1.   *There is now extensive evidence for the presence of epitopes of oxLDL in atherosclerotic lesions.* When LDL undergoes oxidative modifications a variety of structural changes occur as noted above. In particular, a variety of breakdown products from oxidized PUFAs are generated which, in turn, can form adducts with adjacent epsilon-amino groups of lysine, for example MDA-lysine, or 4-hydroxynonenal-lysine. Antibodies have been generated that recognize such lipid-protein adducts, which we have termed "oxidation-specific epitopes". To develop antibodies that would recognize these epitopes, model compounds, such as MDA-LDL and 4-hydroxynonenal LDL were prepared from homologous LDL and used to immunize donor animals. Such oxidation-specific antibodies have been used by us and others to immunostain atherosclerotic lesions in rabbits, mice, nonhuman primates and humans. No staining is seen with normal arterial tissue.(36,81-85)

2.   *OxLDL can be isolated from atherosclerotic lesions.* Because the oxidation-specific antibodies are specific for the adduct itself e.g., MDA-lysine, and would recognize this epitope to some degree even when present on other similarly modified proteins other than apo B, it was necessary to demonstrate that oxLDL itself was oxidatively modified. To accomplish this, LDL was gently extracted from atherosclerotic tissue of rabbits and humans and shown to posses all of the

physical, biological, and immunologic properties observed with LDL oxidized *in vitro*. In particular, LDL isolated from fatty streak lesions had enhanced uptake by macrophage scavenger receptors and this uptake could be competed for by LDL that had been oxidized *in vitro* (37).

3.   *Lipid peroxidation is specific for diseased tissue.*   Oxidized lipids, including oxidized sterols are demonstrable in atherosclerotic tissue but not in normal aortic tissue (86).   Certain F_2-isoprostanes, which are non-enzymatic breakdown products of arachidonic acid that has undergone lipid peroxidation, have been demonstrated in atherosclerotic tissue by immunohistology and chemical techniques (87,88). As described above, 15-lipoxygenase mRNA and protein have been demonstrated in atherosclerotic tissue and the presence of the 15-lipoxygenase products demonstrates 15-lipoxygenase activity in the artery wall and suggests at least one mechanism by which macrophages mediate the oxidation of LDL *in vivo*. The observation that deletion of 12/15-lipoxygenase in mice dramatically reduced the progression of atherosclerosis also suggests that oxidation is a quantitatively important pathway.

4.   *Small quantities of modified LDL have been detected in the circulation.* As noted above, abundant antioxidant defenses exist in plasma and extracellular fluid that makes it highly unlikely that LDL could be oxidized to any major extent in the circulation. Furthermore the presence of high concentrations of scavenger receptors in hepatic sinusoidal cells would rapidly remove any heavily modified forms of LDL. Nevertheless, MM-LDL forms of oxLDL could be present and indeed both immunological and physical techniques have demonstrated that a small fraction of circulating LDL displays indices of early stages of oxidation (89-91). As originally described by Schwenke and Carew, (59) LDL circulates through a variety of tissues, including the artery wall itself and could well undergo minimal or early degrees of modification during such tissue passages. In particular, oxidation of LDL could occur in tissues other than the artery, such as at sites of inflammation, where the concentration of LDL in the inflammatory fluid might be higher than in normal extracellular fluid because of changes in permeability. For example, during diet induced hypercholesterolemia in mice, a number of pro-inflammatory genes were induced in the liver, and this was accompanied by enhanced indices of lipid peroxidation (70).   Under these circumstances, LDL seeded with lipid hydroperoxides could be generated in the liver, but would not have enhanced clearance from plasma. Consequently, upon entering the artery wall, being partially oxidized, it would require little further modification to produce proatherogenic oxLDL forms.

5.   *Even minimal modifications of autologous LDL render it immunogenic.* Because oxLDL is present *in vivo* in atherosclerotic tissues, it should follow that autoantibodies to a variety of oxidation-specific epitopes of LDL should exist and indeed this has been demonstrated (92). In a prospective study of LDL receptor negative mice, the titer of autoantibodies rose progressively with the progression of atherosclerosis, and at the end of the study, correlated significantly with the extent of lesion formation (93). Apolipoprotein E-deficient mice, which have exceedingly

high plasma cholesterol levels and marked atherosclerosis, have extraordinarily high titers of such autoantibodies, making it possible to clone out monoclonal autoantibodies by using their spleens to generate hybridomas, even without exogenous immunization (90). Antibody titers to epitopes of oxidized LDL are also found in humans. In our original report, titers to MDA-LDL were shown to be a highly significant predictor of the progression of carotid intimal-medial thickness in a group of middle age Finnish males (94). Since that initial report a large number of studies in humans suggest that the titers of autoantibodies to oxLDL, or model epitopes, is associated with manifestations of atherosclerosis or with traditional risk factors for atherosclerosis such as hypertension, diabetes and smoking. This has been reviewed elsewhere (77,95). Not only are autoantibodies to epitopes of oxidized LDL found in the circulation but they are also found in atherosclerotic lesions of animals and humans as part of immune complexes with oxLDL (96).

6.   *OxLDL epitopes in vivo can be quantified.* There is an old saying that seeing is believing. In order to demonstrate that oxidation specific epitopes are present *in vivo*, and in order to visualize and quantitate the extent of these lesions in the entire aorta, we have radiolabeled and directly injected intravenously monoclonal antibodies specific for oxidation-specific epitopes, such as MDA-LDL (97). This allows one to visualize at a whole body level the extent of oxidized LDL present in an atherosclerotic lesion (Fig 1).

7.   *Animal studies suggest reducing LDL oxidation limits atherosclerosis.* All of these data prove conclusively that oxidation of LDL exists *in vivo*. However, these data do not directly address the issue of whether oxidation of LDL is causally related to atherogenesis and whether it is quantitatively important If oxidation results in promotion of atherogenesis, then inhibition by the use of appropriate antioxidants, or other techniques to reduce the prooxidant status of the artery wall, should effectively reduce atherogenesis. As originally shown by Carew and colleagues (98) and Kita and colleagues (99) the use of the potent lipophilic antioxidant, probucol, which is transported within the LDL particle itself, profoundly inhibits atherogenesis, independent of any effects on plasma cholesterol levels. In fact, in several rabbit studies probucol inhibited atherosclerosis by 40-80% despite the fact that it lowered HDL levels. By now there are a large series of studies demonstrating that a variety of antioxidants can inhibit atherosclerosis in animal models independent of lowering plasma cholesterol levels. These studies are summarized in Table 2.

Although there are major questions about the mechanisms by which these compounds work, there is considerable evidence that supports the hypothesis that antioxidant mechanisms are responsible for their protective effect. First, antioxidants of widely differing structure have proved effective and are unlikely to share other biological properties other than their antioxidant effect. Second, those compounds that have conferred the most potent antioxidant protection to LDL such as probucol and probucol analogs almost universally inhibit the progression of atherosclerosis (except for mice as discussed below) whereas those compounds that are weaker have often failed. Indeed in a study of the effects of probucol in nonhuman primates, a significant correlation was found between the extent of antioxidant protection of plasma LDL and the extent of inhibition of aortic atherosclerosis (100). However, not all studies in animals have shown a positive

Table 2. Effects of antioxidants in animal models of atherosclerosis

Type of Study	Reference	Result
Probucol in LDLR$^{-/-}$ rabbits	Carew et al (128)	+
	Kita et al (99)	+
	Mao et al (129)	+
	Daugherty et al (130)	±
	Fruebis et al (101)	+
	Morel et al (131)	+
	Witting et al (132)	+
Probucol analogs in LDLR-/- rabbits	Mao et al (133)	+
	Fruebis et al (101)	-
	Witting et al (132)	-
Probucol in cholesterol-fed rabbits	Stein et al (134)	-
	Daugherty et al (135)	+
	Prasad et al (136)	+
Other antioxidants in rabbits		
DPPD	Sparrow et al (137)	+
BHT	Bjorkhem et al (138)	+
Vitamin E	Mantha et al (139)	+
	Morel et al (131)	-
	Kleinveld et al (140)	-
	Shaish et al (141)	-
	Fruebis et al (142)	-
Antioxidants in rodents		
Probucol in hamsters	Parker et al (129)	+
Vitamin E in hamsters	Parker et al (133)	+
DPPD in apoE-/- mice	Tangirala et al (143)	+
Probucol in apoE-/- mice	Zhang et al (104)	-*
Probucol in LDLR-/- mice	Bird et al (105)	-*
Probucol in LDLR-/- mice	Cynshi et al (106)	-*
Probucol analog in LDLR-/-	Cynshi et al (106)	+
Probucol metabolite in LDLR-/-/apoE-/-	Witting et al (108)	+
Vitamin E in apoE-/-	Pratico et al (88)	+
Dietary antioxidants in LDLR-/-	Crawford et al (109)	+
Antioxidants in nonhuman primates		
Probucol	Sasahara et al (100)	+
Vitamin E	Verlangieri and Bush (144)	±

Modified from Steinberg, D and Witztum JL: Lipoproteins, Lipoprotein Oxidation and Atherogenesis. In: Molecular Basis of Heart Disease. Chien, K.R. and W.B. Saunders Co, Philadelphia 1999. + = positive study (Atherosclerosis decreased); - = negative study (atherosclerosis unchanged); + = atherosclerosis equivocal; -* = atherosclerosis enhanced

benefit of antioxidant therapy. For example, Fruebis and colleagues tested probucol and a probucol analog in WHHL rabbits. Probucol provided potent protection to the LDL from oxidation, prolonging the lag time for conjugated-diene formation of the LDL over 8-fold, whereas the probucol analog prolonged the lag time only 4-fold. Although probucol strongly inhibited atherosclerosis, the probucol analog did not

(101). This finding suggests that for any given degree of pro-oxidant stress, a certain threshold of antioxidant protection may be needed. For example, mild degrees of antioxidant protection may be sufficient under mild degrees of hypercholesterolemia, but insufficient in the face of marked hypercholesterolemia. Support for this hypothesis can be found in the studies of Parker and associates (102) who examined the ability of probucol and vitamin E to protect against atherosclerosis in a cholesterol-fed hamster model. When the hamsters were fed sufficient cholesterol to result in marked hyperlipidemia, neither probucol nor vitamin E was protective, but at lower levels of plasma cholesterol, both vitamin E and probucol were effective. Determining the validity of this concept is of particular relevance to humans because it might suggest that the antioxidant protection required for a non-smoking, mildly hypercholesterolemic individual may be quite different than that required for an individual with increased oxidative stress as would occur with severe hypercholesterolemia, smoking and hypertension.

Other experiments strongly suggest that under some circumstances the degree of *ex vivo* protection observed in circulating LDL may not necessarily be a reflection of the antiatherogenic potential of the compound (103). For example, the site of important antioxidant protection is likely to be in the artery itself, and the intracellular concentration may be the most important variable. This could differ significantly between differing antioxidants, even though the degree of protection conferred on circulating LDL might be similar.

Genetically engineered murine models of atherosclerosis have been of great value in the study of atherosclerosis. Considerable evidence supported the hypothesis that oxidation of LDL was as important in these animals as in other animal models studied. However, treatment of both LDL receptor negative and apo E-deficient mice with probucol resulted in *enhanced* atherosclerosis, not protection, calling into question the relevance of oxidation in these models (104-106). However, five studies have now shown that antioxidants slow the development of atherosclerosis in murine models. One study used Diphenylphenylenediamine in the apo E-deficient mouse (107); one used a synthetic analog of probucol in LDL receptor-deficient mice (106); one used vitamin E in apo E-deficient mice (88), one used a metabolite of probucol in apo E, LDL receptor double knockout mice (108), and one used a combination of different dietary antioxidants in LDL receptor-negative mice (109).

The study by Pratico *et al.* (88) warrants particular consideration. That study nicely demonstrated a direct correlation between the concentration of administered vitamin E and both the progression and regression of atherosclerosis in apo E-deficient mice. In that study, a rise in $iPF_2\alpha$-V1 (a specific isoprostane) levels in plasma, urine, and arterial tissue was observed over time that paralleled the ongoing progression of atherosclerotic lesions. Vitamin E administration led to a reduction in isoprostane excretion and inhibition of lesion formation without affecting plasma cholesterol levels. Plasma vitamin E levels correlated inversely with plasma, urinary, and lesion isoprostanes levels as well as with the extent of aortic lesions. These data provide definitive evidence for a direct relationship between atherogenesis and *in vivo* lipid peroxidation. Finally, a recent report by Cyrus *et al.* (50) demonstrated that absence of 12/15-lipoxygenase dramatically protected against lesion formation despite marked hypercholesterolemia and provides compelling evidence that oxidation plays a crucial role in atherogenesis. The fact that autoantibodies to oxLDL were greatly diminished in the lipoxygenase knockout animals strongly supports the hypothesis that the mechanism by which lipoxygenase inhibition worked was by inhibition of oxidation of the LDL. In aggregate, these data argue strongly in favor of the hypothesis that oxidation of LDL is *quantitatively* important, if not obligatory, in the progression of atherosclerosis in murine models, as in other animal models. It is likely that worsening of atherosclerosis observed in probucol-treated mice reflects some other biologic property of probucol, or one of its metabolites that is particular to the mouse.

In summary these data suggest that not only does oxLDL occur *in vivo* with the resultant generation of foam cells and a large variety of oxidatively modified lipids and proteins, but that this process is quantitatively important, if not obligatory in a wide variety of experimental models of atherosclerosis. The relevance of these observations to humans remains to be determined.

INHIBITING OXIDATION OF LDL *IN VIVO*

In considering modifiable factors that might facilitate inhibition of LDL oxidation, it is useful to contrast factors *intrinsic* to the LDL particle, with those factors *extrinsic* to LDL such as tissue conditions or the cellular environment where LDL oxidation likely occurs. With regard to factors intrinsic to LDL, a major determinant of lipid peroxidation is the fatty acid composition. Because PUFAs are more susceptible to oxidation than their unsaturated counterparts, one would anticipate that LDL enriched in PUFAs is more susceptible to oxidation than LDLs with highly saturated fatty acids. This is indeed the case (110,111). Substitution of monounsaturated fatty acids, as opposed to PUFAs, for saturated fatty acids not only leads to lower plasma cholesterol levels but also, theoretically produces LDL with a reduced susceptibility to oxidation. Again, this has been demonstrated experimentally (112), as well as with LDL obtained from free living subjects consuming so-called "Mediterranean" diets (113).

A second major determinant of LDL susceptibility to oxidation is the endogenous content of antioxidants including natural substances such as vitamin E, ubiquinol-10, beta carotene and other poorly characterized compounds such as flavonoids, and at least in women, estrogen esters (114). Studies from many laboratories have shown that increasing the dietary content of vitamin E can produce ~1.5-fold increase in the per particle LDL vitamin E content that confers a 40-50% increase in the resistance of LDL to copper-mediated oxidation, as measured by various *in vitro* assays (115-117). Contrary to expectations, supplementation with beta carotene, despite increasing LDL content up to 20-fold, does not lead to an increase in the resistance of LDL to oxidation (115). Treatment with potent lipophilic antioxidants such as probucol, is a highly effective method of protecting LDL from oxidation since these compounds are strategically located within the LDL particle. Probucol can nearly completely protect LDL from *in vitro* oxidation mediated by transition metals, although it appears not to be as effective against free radical-mediated oxidation from azo compounds. One might speculate that a variety of other analogs of probucol, or other similar compounds, could be developed that will share this property of probucol. From a practical point of view, supplementation of LDL with lipophilic antioxidants would seem to be a major therapeutic target to inhibit its oxidation.

There are also many other properties of LDL that may influence its susceptibility to oxidation, including its endogenous content of phospholipase A_2 activity which appears attributable, in large part, to platelet activating factor (PAF) acetylhydrolase activity. It appears that this activity degrades some of the oxidized phospholipids that may have adverse biological activities (118). Another property that influences the susceptibility to oxidation of LDL is the size of the particle. Small, dense LDL particles appear to be more susceptible to oxidation (119) and in turn, the density of such particles appears to be inversely related to the degree of hypertriglyceridemia. Thus, plasma triglyceride reduction, which in general shifts the distribution of LDL size to more buoyant particles, might indirectly affect the susceptibility of LDL to oxidation. LDL from diabetic patients has significant degrees of nonenzymatic glycation, as well as the presence of advanced glycosylation end productions (AGEs), each of which enhances the susceptibility of LDL to oxidation. Theoretically achieving normoglycemia should help reduce this modification of LDL. Finally, variations in the primary sequence of apo B could affect the ability of LDL to bind to the extracellular matrix, thereby affecting its half-life within the artery wall (120). Much evidence indicates that the binding of LDL to extracellular matrix may be an important determinant of its residence time in the extracellular space of the intima, which in turn renders it more susceptible to oxidation. The identification of crucial residues, either on LDL, or in the extracellular matrix responsible for such interactions could well lead to the development of novel small molecules that could prevent LDL binding and thereby indirectly inhibit LDL accumulation and its subsequent modification.

There are also a large number of factors extrinsic to the LDL that may influence the ability of tissues, such as the artery, to modify LDL. Among these factors is the strong evidence to support a role for 15-lipoxygenase as described above. The use of 15-lipoxygenase inhibitors has been shown in several animal models to significantly reduce the extent of atherosclerosis and this would seem to be an excellent target for investigation. Other cellular enzymes affecting redox state such as NADPH oxidase, phospholipid glutathione peroxidase, catalase and myeloperoxidase also need to be considered. The secretory form of PLA_2 may also modify oxLDL (121). Similarly, paraoxonase, an enzyme that is capable of hydrolyzing oxidized short-chain fatty acids in the *sn*2 position of phospholipids, and is carried on HDL, also seems to play a significant role in mediating the so-called antioxidant-activity of HDL (122,123). Since such oxidized phospholipids appear to mediate numerous pro-inflammatory properties of MM-LDL, paraoxonase (as well as PAF acetylhydrolase) may play an important regulatory role in the degradation of oxidized compounds.

There is a well known inverse correlation between HDL levels and the extent of atherosclerosis. Using *in vitro* assays, HDL has been shown to protect LDL from oxidation and to inhibit the release from MM-LDL of many bioactive molecules. Thus, attempts to raise HDL are likely to be associated with increased paraoxonase levels as well, since this is the exclusive carrier of paraoxonase in plasma. These enzymatic activities may represent attractive targets for pharmacologic manipulation. However, since many such activities are involved in important biological processes such as in warding off infections, one will need to be extremely cautious in attempts to intervene at this level.

It should be emphasized once again that the most effective way to reduce the number of oxidized LDL particles in the artery wall is to reduce the concentration of LDL in the circulation. Similarly, assuming that the protective role of HDL is, in part, related to its antioxidant activities, then enhancement of HDL levels would be expected to be of benefit. Thus, even from the perspective of the oxidative modification hypothesis, lowering LDL levels and raising HDL levels are important goals for therapy of patients at risk for atherosclerosis.

RELEVANCE OF THE OXIDATIVE MODIFICATION HYPOTHESIS FOR HUMAN DISEASE

The oxidative modification hypothesis of atherogenesis is strongly supported by a large body of experimental evidence. What is the evidence that it is relevant to man? With the exception of prospective intervention trials in animals, much of the evidence listed in the sections above applies to human disease as well. Immunocytochemical studies demonstrate the presence of oxidation-specific epitopes in human atherosclerotic tissues. LDL extracted from atherosclerotic tissue of humans has all of the physical, immunologic, and biologic properties of LDL oxidized *in vitro*. Immunochemical and physical techniques can demonstrate early forms of oxLDL in plasma, and improvement in endothelium-dependent vasodilation in hypercholesterolemic human subjects following LDL apheresis best correlates with a decrease in the presence of oxidation-specific epitopes on LDL particles (124). A variety of oxidized lipids, including products of the lipoxygenase pathway, isoprostanes, and oxidized sterols, are found in human atherosclerotic tissue. Oxidized LDL is immunogenic and autoantibodies to epitopes of oxLDL are found in human subjects and correlate with a variety of indices of atherosclerosis. Finally, autoantibodies to oxLDL are present in atherosclerotic lesions as part of immune complexes.

All of these data demonstrate unequivocally the presence of oxLDL in humans, as in experimental animals, but do not demonstrate a causal relationship. This latter evidence can only come from prospective interventional trials, which are thus far lacking in human subjects. While there is epidemiological support of a relation between increased antioxidant vitamin intake and reduced risk for coronary heart disease (see Chapter 13), the number of prospective intervention trials demonstrating a clinical benefit with a variety of antioxidants is not yet sufficient to assess the importance of this pathway in man.

Of those studies available, most have been performed with either vitamin E or beta carotene and were planned and initiated before the implications for LDL antioxidant protection were appreciated. For example, dietary substitution with beta carotene, even though it substantially increases LDL carotene concentrations, fails to significantly protect LDL against oxidation *ex vivo*. Not surprisingly, in the three large-scale trials of beta carotene that have been reported none demonstrated any beneficial effect with respect to cardiovascular disease, or even cancer.

Supplementation with vitamin E, on the other hand, both increases plasma and LDL vitamin E levels and confers significant protection of LDL against *ex vivo* oxidation. In the Finnish α-tocopherol, beta carotene study (125), male smokers were treated with either 20 mg/day of beta carotene, 50 mg/day of vitamin E, both or neither. There was no significant effect of vitamin E on cardiovascular end points, however, the dose of vitamin E used was unlikely to confer any significant antioxidant protection. Indeed, prolongation of diene conjugation lag time becomes significant at vitamin E doses of about 150 mg/day and maximal at 800 to 1200 mg/day. A dramatic benefit of vitamin E was reported from a randomized trial in England known as the Cambridge Heart Antioxidant Study (CHAOS) (126). In that study, vitamin E supplementation of 400 or 800 IU/D vs placebo was administered to 2,002 patients with angiographic evidence of CAD. After a mean of follow-up of only 510 days, vitamin E supplementation significantly reduced the primary end point of nonfatal myocardial infarction and cardiovascular death by 47% and produced an overall 74% decrease in nonfatal myocardial infarction. The rather dramatic results of this study need to be confirmed. In the only clinical study of probucol reported, the Probucol Quantitative Regression Swedish Trial (PQRST) (127) examined the effects of probucol superimposed on cholestyramine and diet therapy using angiographic assessment of femoral atherosclerosis as an endpoint. No impact was seen with probucol therapy. It should be noted that disease in the femoral arteries is generally more advanced and the lesions tend to be rather fibrotic and thus, would be unlikely to respond to antioxidant therapy. In addition, the 24% reduction in HDL cholesterol levels seen with probucol treatment may have masked any beneficial effect of the antioxidant.

Thus, while there is strong epidemiologic data to support the antioxidant hypothesis in humans, we must await the results of prospective clinical trials to determine if there is indeed a causal relationship between oxidation of LDL and atherogenesis.

SUMMARY

The oxidative modification hypothesis of atherogenesis is strongly supported by a large body of experimental evidence, both in experimental animals and in man. In animal studies a variety of antioxidants inhibit atherosclerosis providing strong support that oxidative modification of LDL is a quantitatively important, if not obligatory, event in atherogenesis. Although epidemiologic data in humans support a role for antioxidants in the prevention of clinical events, intervention trials thus far have given mixed results. In part, this may be due to the fact that techniques to adequately provide an index of *in vivo* lipid peroxidation have only recently become available to design and monitor effective antioxidant intervention trials. We lack sufficient measures to identify high-risk groups that would theoretically benefit most from antioxidant intervention and we have lacked reliable measures to determine the *in vivo* effectiveness of antioxidant intervention. In the absence of such information, current (and some future) clinical trials may give incorrect conclusions regarding the use of these agents. This could occur because of the inclusion of populations that would not be expected to benefit from antioxidant supplementation and/or because the dose or agent yielded insufficient antioxidant protection. Not only do we need to understand in a mechanistic way the factors responsible for oxidation of LDL, we also need techniques to measure *in vivo* lipid peroxidation, and ideally, measures that would reflect events occurring in the artery wall. The recent development of measurements for specific isoprostanes in plasma and in urine, the measurement of autoantibodies to epitopes of oxLDL, and the measurement of "oxidation-specific" epitopes on LDL in plasma are potential methods that might yield such information. In addition, it may be possible to utilize

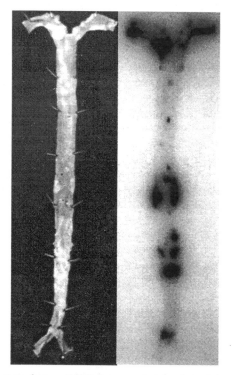

Figure 1. Shown is an aorta from a LDLR-/- mouse that has been injected with the radiolabeled antibody MDA2, which is specific for MDA-LDL (MDA-lysine residues). After the aorta was harvested it was pinned out and stained for the presence of neutral fat (shown in bright grayscale on the left) and an autoradiograph performed (shown on the right) to demonstrate the uptake of MDA2 by the lesion, as described in reference 97. Note that the uptake exactly reflects the lipid staining.

antibodies directed against oxidation-specific epitopes to image the burden of oxidation in the arterial wall *in vivo* as shown in Figure 1 and potentially quantitate lesion burden. It is of great importance to determine the relevance of the oxidative modification hypothesis to humans. If the oxidation hypothesis of atherosclerosis is relevant to humans, then measures to inhibit such LDL oxidation, when combined with effective hypolipidemic therapy, might lead to the amelioration or even the ability to prevent atherosclerosis.

Reference List

1. Steinberg D, Parthasarathy S, Carew TE, Khoo JC, Witztum JL. Beyond cholesterol. Modifications of low-density lipoprotein that increase its atherogenicity]. *N Engl J Med* 1989; 320:915-924.
2. Witztum JL, Steinberg D. Role of oxidized low density lipoprotein in atherogenesis. *J Clin Invest* 1991; 88:1785-1792.
3. Witztum JL. The oxidation hypothesis of atherosclerosis. *Lancet* 1994; 344:793-795.
4. Steinberg D. Low density lipoprotein oxidation and its pathobiological significance. *J Biol Chem* 1997; 272:20963-20966.
5. Steinberg D, Witztum JL. Lipoproteins, Lipoprotein Oxidation, and Atherogenesis. Chien KR, editor. 458-475. 1999. Philadelphia, W. B. Saunders Co. *Molecular Basis of Cardiovascular Disease.*
6. Napoli C, D'Armiento FP, Mancini FP, Postiglione A, Witztum JL, Palumbo G, Palinski W. Fatty streak formation occurs in human fetal aortas and is greatly enhanced by maternal hypercholesterolemia. Intimal accumulation of low density lipoprotein and its oxidation precede monocyte recruitment into early atherosclerotic lesions. *J Clin Invest* 1997, 100(11):2680-2690.
7. Strong JP, Malcom GT, McMahan CA, Tracy RE, Newman WP, Herderick EE, Cornhill JF. Prevalence and extent of atherosclerosis in adolescents and young adults: implications for prevention from the Pathobiological Determinants of Atherosclerosis in Youth Study. *JAMA* 1999; 281(8):727-735.
8. Steinberg D, Witztum JL. Lipoproteins and atherogenesis. Current concepts. *JAMA* 1990; 264:3047-3052.
9. Ross R. Atherosclerosis--an inflammatory disease. *N Engl J Med* 1999; 340(2):115-126.
10. Davies MJ. Anatomic features in victims of sudden coronary death. Coronary artery pathology. *Circulation* 1992; 85:I19-24.
11. Libby P. Molecular bases of the acute coronary syndromes. Circulation 1995; 91:2844-2850.
12. Newby AC, Libby P, van der Wal AC. Plaque instability--the real challenge for atherosclerosis research in the next decade? *Cardiovasc Res* 1999; 41(2):321-322.
13. Goldstein JL, Ho YK, Basu SK, Brown MS. Binding site on macrophages that mediates uptake and degradation of acetylated low density lipoprotein, producing massive cholesterol deposition. *Proc Natl Acad Sci U S A* 1979; 76:333-337.
14. Kodama T, Freeman M, Rohrer L, Zabrecky J, Matsudaira P, Krieger M. Type I macrophage scavenger receptor contains alpha-helical and collagen-like coiled coils. *Nature* 1990; 343:531-535.
15. Krieger M, Acton S, Ashkenas J, Pearson A, Penman M, Resnick D. Molecular flypaper, host defense, and atherosclerosis. Structure, binding properties, and functions of macrophage scavenger receptors. *J Biol Chem* 1993; 268:4569-4572.
16. Fogelman AM, Shechter I, Seager J, Hokom M, Child JS, Edwards PA. Malondialdehyde alteration of low density lipoproteins leads to cholesteryl ester accumulation in human monocyte-macrophages. *Proc Natl Acad Sci U S A* 1980; 77:2214-2218.
17. Henriksen T, Mahoney EM, Steinberg D. Enhanced macrophage degradation of low density lipoprotein previously incubated with cultured endothelial cells: recognition by receptors for acetylated low density lipoproteins. *Proc Natl Acad Sci U S A* 1981; 78:6499-6503.

18.   Steinbrecher UP, Parthasarathy S, Leake DS, Witztum JL, Steinberg D. Modification of low density lipoprotein by endothelial cells involves lipid peroxidation and degradation of low density lipoprotein phospholipids. *Proc Natl Acad Sci U S A* 1984; 81:3883-3887.

19.   Heinecke JW, Rosen H, Chait A. Iron and copper promote modification of low density lipoprotein by human arterial smooth muscle cells in culture. *J Clin Invest* 1984; 74:1890-1894.

20.   Morel DW, Hessler JR, Chisolm GM. Low density lipoprotein cytotoxicity induced by free radical peroxidation of lipid. *J Lipid Res* 1983; 24:1070-1076.

21.   Acton S, Rigotti A, Landschulz KT, Xu S, Hobbs HH, Krieger M. Identification of scavenger receptor SR-BI as a high density lipoprotein receptor . *Science* 1996; 271:518-520.

22.   Krieger M. The other side of scavenger receptors: pattern recognition for host defense. *Curr Opin Lipidol* 1997; 8(5):275-280.

23.   Suzuki H, Kurihara Y, Takeya M, Kamada N, Kataoka M, Jishage K, Ueda O, Sakaguchi H, Higashi T, Suzuki T, Takashima Y, Kawabe Y, Cynshi O, Wada Y, Honda M, Kurihara H, Aburatani H, Doi T, Matsumoto A, Azuma S, Noda T, Toyoda Y, Itakura H, Yazaki Y, Kodama T. A role for macrophage scavenger receptors in atherosclerosis and susceptibility to infection. *Nature* 1997; 386(6622):292-296.

24.   Nozaki S, Kashiwagi H, Yamashita S, Nakagawa T, Kostner B, Tomiyama Y, Nakata A, Ishigami M, Miyagawa J, Kameda-Takemura K. Reduced uptake of oxidized low density lipoproteins in monocyte- derived macrophages from CD36-deficient subjects. *J Clin Invest* 1995; 96:1859-1865.

25.   Febbraio M, Abumrad NA, Hajjar DP, Sharma K, Cheng W, Pearce SF, Silverstein RL. A null mutation in murine CD36 reveals an important role in fatty acid and lipoprotein metabolism. *J Biol Chem* 1999; 274(27):19055-19062.

26.   Krieger M, Acton S, Ashkenas J, Pearson A, Penman M, Resnick D. Molecular flypaper, host defense, and atherosclerosis. Structure, binding properties, and functions of macrophage scavenger receptors. *J Biol Chem* 1993; 268:4569-4572.

27.   Hörkkö S, Bird DA, Miller E, Itabe H, Leitinger N, Subbanagounder G, Berliner JA, Friedman P, Dennis EA, Curtiss LK, Palinski W, Witztum JL. Monoclonal autoantibodies specific for oxidized phospholipids or oxidized phospholipid-protein adducts inhibit macrophage uptake of oxidized low-density lipoproteins. *J Clin Invest* 1999; 103(1):117-128.

28.   Bird DA, Gillotte KL, Hörkkö S, Friedman P, Dennis EA, Witztum JL, Steinberg D. Receptors for oxidized low-density lipoprotein on elicited mouse peritoneal macrophages can recognize both the modified lipid moieties and the modified protein moieties: Implications with respect to macrophage recognition of apoptotic cells. *Proc Natl Acad Sci U S A* 1999; 96:6347-6352.

29.   Sambrano GR, Steinberg D. Recognition of oxidatively damaged and apoptotic cells by an oxidized low density lipoprotein receptor on mouse peritoneal macrophages: role of membrane phosphatidylserine. *Proc Natl Acad Sci U S A* 1995; 92:1396-1400.

30.   Chang MK, Bergmark C, Laurila A, Hörkkö S, Han KH, Friedman P, Dennis EA, Witztum JL. Monoclonal antibodies against oxidized low-density lipoprotein bind to apoptotic cells and inhibit their phagocytosis by elicited macrophages: evidence that oxidation-specific epitopes mediate macrophage recognition. *Proc Natl Acad Sci U S A* 1999; 96(11):6353-6358.

31.   Berliner JA, Territo MC, Sevanian A, Ramin S, Kim JA, Bamshad B, Esterson M, Fogelman AM. Minimally modified low density lipoprotein stimulates monocyte endothelial interactions. *J Clin Invest* 1990; 85:1260-1266.

32.   Witztum JL. Role of oxidised low density lipoprotein in atherogenesis. *Br Heart J* 1993; 69:S12-8.

33.   Esterbauer H, Dieber-Rotheneder M, Waeg G, Striegl G, Jurgens G. Biochemical, structural, and functional properties of oxidized low-density lipoprotein. *Chem Res Toxicol* 1990; 3:77-92.

34.   Chisolm GM, Ma G, Irwin KC, Martin LL, Gunderson KG, Linberg LF, Morel DW, DiCorleto PE. 7 beta-hydroperoxycholest-5-en-3 beta-ol, a component of human atherosclerotic lesions, is the primary cytotoxin of oxidized human low density lipoprotein. *Proc Natl Acad Sci U S A* 1994; 91:11452-11456.

35.   Uchida K, Toyokuni S, Nishikawa K, Kawakishi S, Oda H, Hiai H, Stadtman ER. Michael addition-type 4-hydroxy-2-nonenal adducts in modified low-density lipoproteins: markers for atherosclerosis. *Biochemistry* 1994; 33:12487-12494.

36.   Palinski W, Rosenfeld ME, Yla-Herttuala S, Gurtner GC, Socher SS, Butler SW, Parthasarathy S, Carew TE, Steinberg D, Witztum JL. Low density lipoprotein undergoes oxidative modification *in vivo*. *Proc Natl Acad Sci U S A* 1989; 86:1372-1376.

37.   Ylä-Herttuala S, Palinski W, Rosenfeld ME, Parthasarathy S, Carew TE, Butler S, Witztum JL, Steinberg D. Evidence for the presence of oxidatively modified low density lipoprotein in atherosclerotic lesions of rabbit and man. *J Clin Invest* 1989; 84:1086-1095.

38.   Heinecke JW. Mass spectrometric quantification of amino acid oxidation products in proteins: insights into pathways that promote LDL oxidation in the human artery wall. *FASEB J* 1999; 13(10):1113-1120.

39.   Stocker R, Yamamoto Y, McDonagh AF, Glazer AN, Ames BN. Bilirubin is an antioxidant of possible physiological importance. *Science* 1987; 235:1043-1046.

40.   Steinbrecher UP, Parthasarathy S, Leake DS, Witztum JL, Steinberg D. Modification of low density lipoprotein by endothelial cells involves lipid peroxidation and degradation of low density lipoprotein phospholipids. *Proc Natl Acad Sci U S A* 1984; 81:3883-3887.

41.   Khouw AS, Parthasarathy S, Witztum JL. Radioiodination of low density lipoprotein initiates lipid peroxidation: protection by use of antioxidants. *J Lipid Res* 1993; 34:1483-1496.

42.   McNally AK, Chisolm GM, Morel DW, Cathcart MK. Activated human monocytes oxidize low-density lipoprotein by a lipoxygenase-dependent pathway. *J Immunol* 1990; 145(1):254-259.

43.   Daugherty A, Dunn JL, Rateri DL, Heinecke JW. Myeloperoxidase, a catalyst for lipoprotein oxidation, is expressed in human atherosclerotic lesions. *J Clin Invest* 1994; 94:437-444.

44.   Parthasarathy S, Wieland E, Steinberg D. A role for endothelial cell lipoxygenase in the oxidative modification of low density lipoprotein. *Proc Natl Acad Sci U S A* 1989; 86:1046-1050.

45.   Scheidegger KJ, Butler S, Witztum JL. Angiotensin II increases macrophage-mediated modification of low density lipoprotein via a lipoxygenase-dependent pathway. *J Biol Chem* 1997; 272(34):21609-21615.

46.   Benz DJ, Mol M, Ezaki M, Mori-Ito N, Zelaan I, Miyanohara A, Friedmann T, Parthasarathy S, Steinberg D, Witztum JL. Enhanced levels of lipoperoxides in low density lipoprotein incubated with murine fibroblast expressing high levels of human 15-lipoxygenase. *J Biol Chem* 1995; 270(10):5191-5197.

47.   Ezaki M, Witztum JL, Steinberg D. Lipoperoxides in LDL incubated with fibroblasts that overexpress 15-lipoxygenase. *J Lipid Res* 1995; 369):1996-2001.

48.   Bocan TM, Rosebury WS, Mueller SB, Kuchera S, Welch K, Daugherty A, Cornicelli JA. A specific 15-lipoxygenase inhibitor limits the progression and monocyte-macrophage enrichment of hypercholesterolemia-induced atherosclerosis in the rabbit. *Atherosclerosis* 1998; 136(2):203-216.

49.   Sendobry SM, Cornicelli JA, Welch K, Bocan T, Tait B, Trivedi BK, Colbry N, Dyer RD, Feinmark SJ, Daugherty A. Attenuation of diet-induced atherosclerosis in rabbits with a highly selective 15-lipoxygenase inhibitor lacking significant antioxidant properties. *Br J Pharmacol* 1997; 120(7):1199-1206.

50.   Tillman C, Witztum JL, Rader DJ, Tangirala R, Fazio S, Linton MF, Funk CD. Disruption of the 12/15-lipoxygenase gene diminishes atherosclerosis in apo E-deficient mice. *J Clin Invest.* 1999;103:1597.

51.   Reilly MP, Praticao D, Delanty N, DiMinno G, Tremoli E, Rader D, Kapoor S, Rokach J, Lawson J, FitzGerald GA. Increased formation of distinct F2 isoprostanes in hypercholesterolemia. *Circulation* 1998; 98(25):2822-2828.

52.   Ylä-Herttuala S, Rosenfeld ME, Parthasarathy S, Glass CK, Sigal E, Witztum JL, Steinberg D. Colocalization of 15-lipoxygenase mRNA and protein with epitopes of oxidized low density lipoprotein in macrophage-rich areas of atherosclerotic lesions. *Proc Natl Acad Sci U S A* 1990; 87:6959-6963.

53.   Ylä-Herttuala S, Rosenfeld ME, Parthasarathy S, Sigal E, Sarkioja T, Witztum JL, Steinberg D. Gene expression in macrophage-rich human atherosclerotic lesions. 15-lipoxygenase and acetyl low density lipoprotein receptor messenger RNA colocalize with oxidation specific lipid- protein adducts. *J Clin Invest* 1991; 87:1146-1152.

54.   Kuhn H, Belkner J, Zaiss S, Feahrenklemper T, Wohlfeil S. Involvement of 15-lipoxygenase in early stages of atherogenesis. *J Exp Med* 1994; 179(6):1903-1911.

55.   Folcik VA, Nivar-Aristy RA, Krajewski LP, Cathcart MK. Lipoxygenase contributes to the oxidation of lipids in human atherosclerotic plaques. *J Clin Invest* 1995; 96:504-510.

56.   Li H, Cybulsky MI, Gimbrone MA, Jr., Libby P. An atherogenic diet rapidly induces VCAM-1, a cytokine- regulatable mononuclear leukocyte adhesion molecule, in rabbit aortic endothelium. *Arteriosclerosis and Thrombosis* 1993; 13:197-204.

57.   Kume N, Gimbrone MJ. Lysophosphatidylcholine transcriptionally induces growth factor gene expression in cultured human endothelial cells. *J Clin Invest* 1994; 93(2):907-911.

58.   Khan BV, Parthasarathy SS, Alexander RW, Medford RM. Modified low density lipoprotein and its constituents augment cytokine-activated vascular cell adhesion molecule-1 gene expression in human vascular endothelial cells. *J Clin Invest* 1995; 95(3):1262-1270.

59.   Schwenke DC, Carew TE. Initiation of atherosclerotic lesions in cholesterol-fed rabbits. I. Focal increases in arterial LDL concentration precede development of fatty streak lesions. *Arteriosclerosis* 1989; 9(6):895-907.

60.   Schwenke DC, Carew TE. Initiation of atherosclerotic lesions in cholesterol-fed rabbits. II. Selective retention of LDL vs. selective increases in LDL permeability in susceptible sites of arteries. *Arteriosclerosis* 1989; 9(6):908-918.

61.   Williams KJ, Tabas I. The response-to-retention hypothesis of atherogenesis reinforced. *Curr Opin Lipidol* 1998; 9(5):471-474.

62.   Calara F, Dimayuga P, Niemann A, Thyberg J, Diczfalusy U, Witztum JL, Palinski W, Shah PK, Cercek B, Nilsson J, Regnstreom J. An animal model to study local oxidation of LDL and its biological effects in the arterial wall. *Arterioscl Thromb Vasc Biol* 1998; 18(6):884-893.

63.   Napoli C, D'Armiento FP, Mancini FP, Postiglione A, Witztum JL, Palumbo G, Palinski W. Fatty streak formation occurs in human fetal aortas and is greatly enhanced by maternal hypercholesterolemia. Intimal accumulation of low density lipoprotein and its oxidation precede monocyte recruitment into early atherosclerotic lesions. *J Clin Invest* 1997; 100(11):2680-2690.

64.   Navab M, Berliner JA, Watson AD, Hama SY, Territo MC, Lusis AJ, Shih DM, Van Lenten BJ, Frank JS, Demer LL, Edwards PA, Fogelman AM. The Yin and Yang of oxidation in the development of the fatty streak. A review based on the 1994 George Lyman Duff Memorial Lecture. *Arterioscler Thromb Vasc Biol* 1996; 16:831-842.

65.   Watson AD, Leitinger N, Navab M, Faull KF, Heorkkeo S, Witztum JL, Palinski W, Schwenke D, Salomon RG, Sha W, Subbanagounder G, Fogelman AM, Berliner JA. Structural identification by mass spectrometry of oxidized phospholipids in minimally oxidized low density lipoprotein that induce monocyte/endothelial interactions and evidence for their presence *in vivo*. *J Biol Chem* 1997; 272(21):13597-13607.

66.   Witztum JL, Berliner JA. Oxidized phospholipids and isoprostanes in atherosclerosis. *Curr Opin Lipidol* 1998; 9(5):441-448.

67.   Shih PT, Elices MJ, Fang ZT, Ugarova TP, Strahl D, Territo MC, Frank JS, Kovach NL, Cabanas C, Berliner JA, Vora DK. Minimally modified low-density lipoprotein induces monocyte adhesion to endothelial connecting segment-1 by activating beta1 integrin. *J Clin Invest* 1999; 103(5):613-625.

68.   Kume N, Cybulsky MI, Gimbrone MJ. Lysophosphatidylcholine, a component of atherogenic lipoproteins, induces mononuclear leukocyte adhesion molecules in cultured human and rabbit arterial endothelial cells. *J Clin Invest* 1992; 90(3):1138-1144.

69.   Rankin SM, Parthasarathy S, Steinberg D. Evidence for a dominant role of lipoxygenase(s. in the oxidation of LDL by mouse peritoneal macrophages. *J Lipid Res* 1991; 32:449-456.

70.   Liao F, Andalibi A, deBeer FC, Fogelman AM, Lusis AJ. Genetic control of inflammatory gene induction and NF-kappa B- like transcription factor activation in response to an atherogenic diet in mice. *J Clin Invest* 1993; 91:2572-2579.

71.   Yoshida H, Quehenberger O, Kondratenko N, Green S, Steinberg D. Minimally oxidized low-density lipoprotein increases expression of scavenger receptor A, CD36, and macrosialin in resident mouse peritoneal macrophages. *Arterioscler Thromb Vasc Biol* 1998; 18(5):794-802.

72.   Ricote M, Huang J, Fajas L, Li A, Welch J, Najib J, Witztum JL, Auwerx J, Palinski W, Glass CK. Expression of the peroxisome proliferator-activated receptor gamma (PPARgamma. in human atherosclerosis and regulation in macrophages by colony stimulating factors and oxidized low density lipoprotein. *Proc Natl Acad Sci U S A* 1998; 95(13):7614-7619.

73.   Ricote M, Li AC, Willson TM, Kelly CJ, Glass CK. The peroxisome proliferator-activated receptor-gamma is a negative regulator of macrophage activation. *Nature* 1998; 391(6662):79-82.

74.   Nagy L, Tontonoz P, Alvarez JG, Chen H, Evans RM. Oxidized LDL regulates macrophage gene expression through ligand activation of PPARgamma. *Cell* 1998; 93(2):229-240.

75. Bjorkerud B, Bjeorkerud S. Contrary effects of lightly and strongly oxidized LDL with potent promotion of growth versus apoptosis on arterial smooth muscle cells, macrophages, and fibroblasts. *Arterioscler Thromb Vasc Bio* 1996; 16(3):416-424.

76. Mitchinson MJ, Hardwick SJ, Bennett MR. Cell death in atherosclerotic plaques. *Curr Opin Lipidol* 1996; 7(5):324-329.

77. Witztum JL, Palinski W. Are immunological mechanisms relevant for the development of atherosclerosis?. *Clin Immunol* 1999; 90(2):153-156.

78. Esterbauer H, Gebicki J, Puhl H, Jurgens G. The role of lipid peroxidation and antioxidants in oxidative modification of LDL. *Free Radic Biol Med* 1992; 13:341-390.

79. Dabbagh AJ, Frei B. Human suction blister interstitial fluid prevents metal ion-dependent oxidation of low density lipoprotein by macrophages and in cell-free systems. *J Clin Invest* 1995; 96(4):1958-1966.

80. Heiple JM, Wright SD, Allen NS, Silverstein SC. Macrophages form circular zones of very close apposition to IgG- coated surfaces. *Cell Motil Cytoskeleton* 1990; 15:260-270.

81. Haberland ME, Fong D, Cheng L. Malondialdehyde-altered protein occurs in atheroma of Watanabe heritable hyperlipidemic rabbits. *Science* 1988; 241:215-218.

82. Palinski W, Yla-Herttuala S, Rosenfeld ME, Butler SW, Socher SA, Parthasarathy S, Curtiss LK, Witztum JL. Antisera and monoclonal antibodies specific for epitopes generated during oxidative modification of low density lipoprotein. *Arteriosclerosis* 1990; 10:325-335.

83. Rosenfeld ME, Palinski W, Yla-Herttuala S, Butler S, Witztum JL. Distribution of oxidation specific lipid-protein adducts and apolipoprotein B in atherosclerotic lesions of varying severity from WHHL rabbits. *Arteriosclerosis* 1990; 10:336-349.

84. Boyd HC, Gown AM, Wolfbauer G, Chait A. Direct evidence for a protein recognized by a monoclonal antibody against oxidatively modified LDL in atherosclerotic lesions from a Watanabe heritable hyperlipidemic rabbit. *Am J Path* 1989; 135(5):815-825.

85. Palinski W, Ord VA, Plump AS, Breslow JL, Steinberg D, Witztum JL. ApoE-deficient mice are a model of lipoprotein oxidation in atherogenesis. Demonstration of oxidation-specific epitopes in lesions and high titers of autoantibodies to malondialdehyde- lysine in serum. *Arterioscler Thromb* 1994; 14:605-616.

86. Hulten LM, Lindmark H, Diczfalusy U, Bjorkhem I, Öttosson M, Liu Y, Bondjers G, Wiklund O. Oxysterols present in atherosclerotic tissue decrease the expression of lipoprotein lipase messenger RNA in human monocyte-derived macrophages. *J Clin Invest* 1996; 97(2):461-468.

87. Pratico D, Iuliano L, Mauriello A, Spagnoli L, Lawson JA, Maclouf J, Violi F, FitzGerald GA. Localization of distinct F2-isoprostanes in human atherosclerotic lesions. *J Clin Invest* 1997; 100:2028-2034.

88. Pratico D, Tangirala RK, Rader DJ, Rokach J, FitzGerald GA. Vitamin E suppresses isoprostane generation *in vivo* and reduces atherosclerosis in ApoE-deficient mice. *Nat Med* 1998; 4(10):1189-1192.

89. Sevanian A, Hwang J, Hodis H, Cazzolato G, Avogaro P, Bittolo-Bon G. Contribution of an *in vivo* oxidized LDL to LDL oxidation and its association with dense LDL subpopulations. *Arterioscler Thromb Vasc Biol* 1996; 16(6):784-793.

90. Palinski W, Hörkkö S, Miller E, Steinbrecher UP, Powell HC, Curtiss LK, Witztum JL. Cloning of monoclonal autoantibodies to epitopes of oxidized lipoproteins from apolipoprotein E-deficient mice. Demonstration of epitopes of oxidized low density lipoprotein in human plasma. *J Clin Invest* 1996; 98(3):800-814.

91. Holvoet P, Perez G, Zhao Z, Brouwers E, Bernar H, Collen D. Malondialdehyde-modified low density lipoproteins in patients with atherosclerotic disease. *J Clin Invest* 1995; 95(6):2611-2619.

92. Palinski W, Rosenfeld ME, Ylä-Herttuala S, Gurtner GC, Socher SS, Butler SW, Parthasarathy S, Carew TE, Steinberg D, Witztum JL. Low density lipoprotein undergoes oxidative modification *in vivo. Proc Natl Acad Sci U S A* 1989; 86(4):1372-1376.

93. Palinski W, Tangirala RK, Miller E, Young SG, Witztum JL. Increased autoantibody titers against epitopes of oxidized LDL in LDL receptor-deficient mice with increased atherosclerosis. *Arterioscl Thromb Vasc Biol* 1995; 15(10):1569-1576.

94. Salonen JT, Ylä-Herttuala S, Yamamoto R, Butler S, Korpela H, Salonen R, Nyyssonen K, Palinski W, Witztum JL. Autoantibody against oxidised LDL and progression of carotid atherosclerosis. *Lancet* 1992; 339:883-887.

95.   Ylä-Herttuala S. Is oxidized low-density lipoprotein present *in vivo? Curr Opin Lipidol* 1998;
        9(4):337-344.
96.   Ylä-Herttuala S, Palinski W, Butler SW, Picard S, Steinberg D, Witztum JL. Rabbit and
        human atherosclerotic lesions contain IgG that recognizes epitopes of oxidized LDL.
        Arterioscler Thromb 1994; 14:32-40.
97.   Tsimikas S, Palinski W, Halpern SE, Yeung DW, Curtiss LK, Witztum JL. Radiolabeled
        MDA2, an oxidation-specific, monoclonal antibody, identifies native atherosclerotic lesions
        in vivo. J Nucl Cardiol 1999; 61 Pt 1):41-53.
98.   Carew TE, Schwenke DC, Steinberg D. Antiatherogenic effect of probucol unrelated to its
        hypocholesterolemic effect: evidence that antioxidants *in vivo* can selectively inhibit low
        density lipoprotein degradation in macrophage-rich fatty streaks and slow the progression of
        atherosclerosis in the Watanabe heritable hyperlipidemic rabbit. *Proc Natl Acad Sci U S A*
        1987; 84:7725-7729.
99.   Kita T, Nagano Y, Yokode M, Ishi K, Kume N, Ooshima A, Yoshida H, Kawai C. Probucol
        prevents the progression of atherosclerosis in Watanabe heritable hyperlipidemic rabbit, an
        animal model for familial hypercholesterolemia. *Proc Natl Acad Sci USA* 1987; 84:5928-
        5931.
100.   Sasahara M, Raines EW, Chait A, Carew TE, Steinberg D, Wahl PW, Ross R. Inhibition of
        hypercholesterolemia-induced atherosclerosis in the nonhuman primate by probucol. I. Is the
        extent of atherosclerosis related to resistance of LDL to oxidation? *J Clin Invest* 1994;
        94:155-164.
101.   Fruebis J, Steinberg D, Dresel HA, Carew TE. A comparison of the antiatherogenic effects of
        probucol and of a structural analogue of probucol in low density lipoprotein receptor-deficient
        rabbits. *J Clin Invest* 1994; 94:392-398.
102.   Parker RA, Sabrah T, Cap M, Gill BT. Relation of vascular oxidative stress, alpha-tocopherol,
        and hypercholesterolemia to early atherosclerosis in hamsters. *Arterioscler Thromb Vasc Biol*
        1995; 15:349-358.
103.   Fruebis J, Bird DA, Pattison J, Palinski W. Extent of antioxidant protection of plasma LDL is
        not a predictor of the antiatherogenic effect of antioxidants. *J Lipid Res* 1997; 38(12):2455-
        2464.
104.   Zhang SH, Reddick RL, Avdievich E, Surles LK, Jones RG, Reynolds JB, Quarfordt SH,
        Maeda N. Paradoxical enhancement of atherosclerosis by probucol treatment in
        apolipoprotein E-deficient mice. *J Clin Invest* 1997; 99(12):2858-2866.
105.   Bird DA, Tangirala RK, Fruebis J, Steinberg D, Witztum JL, Palinski W. Effect of probucol
        on LDL oxidation and atherosclerosis in LDL receptor-deficient mice. *J Lipid Res* 1998;
        39(5):1079-1090.
106.   Cynshi O, Kawabe Y, Suzuki T, Takashima Y, Kaise H, Nakamura M, Ohba Y, Kato Y,
        Tamura K, Hayasaka A, Higashida A, Sakaguchi H, Takeya M, Takahashi K, Inoue K,
        Noguchi N, Niki E, Kodama T. Antiatherogenic effects of the antioxidant BO-653 in three
        different animal models. *Proc Natl Acad Sci U S A* 1998; 95(17):10123-10128.
107.   Tangirala RK, Casanada F, Miller E, Witztum JL, Steinberg D, Palinski W. Effect of the
        antioxidant N,N'-diphenyl 1,4-phenylenediamine (DPPD. on atherosclerosis in apoE-deficient
        mice. *Arterioscl Thromb Vasc Biol* 1995; 15(10):1625-1630.
108.   Witting PK, Pettersson K, Ostlund-Lindqvist AM, Westerlund C, Eriksson AW, Stocker R.
        Inhibition by a coantioxidant of aortic lipoprotein lipid peroxidation and atherosclerosis in
        apolipoprotein E and low density lipoprotein receptor gene double knockout mice. *FASEB J*
        1999; 13(6):667-675.
109.   Crawford RS, Kirk EA, Rosenfeld ME, LeBoeuf RC, Chait A. Dietary antioxidants inhibit
        development of fatty streak lesions in the LDL receptor-deficient mouse. *Arterioscl Thromb
        Vasc Biol* 1998; 18(9):1506-1513.
110.   Reaven PD, Witztum JL. Oxidized LDL in atherogenesis: role of dietary modification. In:
        McCormack D, editor. *Annual Review of Nutrition. Palo Alto*: Annual Reviews Inc., 1996:
        51-71.
111.   Tsimikas S, Reaven PD. The role of dietary fatty acids in lipoprotein oxidation and
        atherosclerosis. *Curr Opin Lipidol* 1998; 94):301-307.
112.   Reaven P, Parthasarathy S, Grasse BJ, Miller E, Steinberg D, Witztum JL. Effects of oleate-
        rich and linoleate-rich diets on the susceptibility of low density lipoprotein to oxidative
        modification in mildly hypercholesterolemic subjects. *J Clin Invest* 1993; 91:668-676.

113. Tsimikas S, Philis-Tsimikas A, Alexopoulos S, Sigari F, Lee C, Reaven PD. LDL isolated from Greek subjects on a typical diet or from American subjects on an oleate-supplemented diet induces less monocyte chemotaxis and adhesion when exposed to oxidative stress. *Arteriscl Thromb Vasc Biol* 1999; 19(1):122-130.
114. Shwaery GT, Vita JA, Keaney JJ. Antioxidant protection of LDL by physiologic concentrations of estrogens is specific for 17-beta-estradiol. *Atherosclerosis* 1998; 138(2):255-262.
115. Reaven PD, Khouw A, Beltz WF, Parthasarathy S, Witztum JL. Effect of dietary antioxidant combinations in humans. Protection of LDL by vitamin E but not by beta-carotene. *Arterioscler Thromb* 1993; 13:590-600.
116. Reaven PD, Witztum JL. Comparison of supplementation of RRR-alpha-tocopherol and racemic alpha-tocopherol in humans. Effects on lipid levels and lipoprotein susceptibility to oxidation. *Arterioscler Thromb* 1993; 13:601-608.
117. Keaney JFJ, Vita JA. Atherosclerosis, oxidative stress, and antioxidant protection in endothelium-derived relaxing factor action. *Prog Cardiovasc Dis* 1995; 38:129-154.
118. Watson AD, Navab M, Hama SY, Sevanian A, Prescott SM, Stafforini DM, McIntyre TM, Du BN, Fogelman AM, Berliner JA. Effect of platelet activating factor-acetylhydrolase on the formation and action of minimally oxidized low density lipoprotein. *J Clin Invest* 1995; 95:774-782.
119. Lee C, Sigari F, Segrado T, Hcorkkeo S, Hama S, Subbaiah PV, Miwa M, Navab M, Witztum JL, Reaven PD. All ApoB-containing lipoproteins induce monocyte chemotaxis and adhesion when minimally modified. Modulation of lipoprotein bioactivity by platelet-activating factor acetylhydrolase. *Arterioscl Thromb Vasc Biol* 1999; 19(6):1437-1446.
120. Boraen J, Olin K, Lee I, Chait A, Wight TN, Innerarity TL. Identification of the principal proteoglycan-binding site in LDL. A single-point mutation in apo-B100 severely affects proteoglycan interaction without affecting LDL receptor binding. *J Clin Invest* 1998; 101(12):2658-2664.
121. Romano M, Romano E, Bjeorkerud S, Hurt-Camejo E. Ultrastructural localization of secretory type II phospholipase A2 in atherosclerotic and nonatherosclerotic regions of human arteries. *Arterioscl Thromb Vasc Biol* 1998; 18(4):519-525.
122. Mackness MI, Mackness B, Durrington PN, Fogelman AM, Berliner J, Lusis AJ, Navab M, Shih D, Fonarow GC. Paraoxonase and coronary heart disease. *Curr Opin Lipidol* 1998; 9(4):319-324.
123. Shih DM, Gu L, Xia YR, Navab M, Li WF, Hama S, Castellani LW, Furlong CE, Costa LG, Fogelman AM, Lusis AJ. Mice lacking serum paraoxonase are susceptible to organophosphate toxicity and atherosclerosis. *Nature* 1998; 394(6690):284-287.
124. Tamai O, Matsuoka H, Itabe H, Wada Y, Kohno K, Imaizumi T. Single LDL apheresis improves endothelium-dependent vasodilatation in hypercholesterolemic humans. *Circulation* 1997; 95(1):76-82.
125. The effect of vitamin E and beta carotene on the incidence of lung cancer and other cancers in male smokers. The Alpha-Tocopherol, Beta Carotene Cancer Prevention Study Group. *N Engl J Med* 1994; 330(15):1029-1035.
126. Stephens NG, Parsons A, Schofield PM, Kelly F, Cheeseman K, Mitchinson MJ, Brown MJ. Randomised controlled trial of vitamin E in patients with coronary disease: Cambridge Heart Antioxidant Study (CHAOS). *Lancet* 1996; 347:781-785.
127. Walldius G, Erikson U, Olsson AG, Bergstrand L, Hadell K, Johansson J, Kaijser L, Lassvik C. The effect of probucol on femoral atherosclerosis: the probucol quantitative regression Swedish trial (PQRST). *Am J Card* 1994; 74:875-883.
128. Carew TE, Schwenke DC, Steinberg D. Antiatherogenic effect of probucol unrelated to its hypocholesterolemic effect: evidence that antioxidants *in vivo* can selectively inhibit low density lipoprotein degradation in macrophage-rich fatty streaks and slow the progression of atherosclerosis in the Watanabe heritable hyperlipidemic rabbit. *Proc Natl Acad Sci U S A* 1987; 84:7725-7729.
129. Mao S, Yates M, Parker R, Chi E, Jackson R. Attenuation of atherosclerosis in a modified strain of hypercholesterolemic watanabe rabbits with use of a probucol analogue (MDL 29,311. that does not lower serum cholesterol. *Arterio and Thromb* 1991; 11:1266-1275.
130. Daugherty A, Zweifel BS, Schonfeld G. The effects of probucol on the progression of atherosclerosis in mature Watanabe heritable hyperlipidaemic rabbits. *Br J Pharmacol* 1991; 103:1013-1018.

74

Oxidative Modification Hypothesis

131.   Morel DW, de la Llera-Moya M, Friday K. Treatment of cholesterol-fed rabbits with dietary vitamins E and C inhibits lipoprotien oxidation but not development of atherosclerosis. *Am Inst Nutri* 1994;2123-2130.
132.   Witting P, Pettersson K, Ostlund-Lindqvist AM, Westerlund C, Wagberg M, Stocker R. Dissociation of atherogenesis from aortic accumulation of lipid hydro(pero)xides in Watanabe heritable hyperlipidemic rabbits. *J Clin. Invest* 1999; 104, 213-220.
133.   Mao SJ, Yates MT, Parker RA, Chi EM, Jackson RL. Attenuation of atherosclerosis in a modified strain of hypercholesterolemic Watanabe rabbits with use of a probucol analogue (MDL 29,311). that does not lower serum cholesterol. *Arterioscler Thromb* 1991; 11:1266-1275.
134.   Stein Y, Stein O, Delplanque B, Fesmire JD, Lee DM, Alaupovic P. Lack of effect of probucol on atheroma formation in cholesterol- fed rabbits kept at comparable plasma cholesterol levels. *Atherosclerosis* 1989; 75:145-155.
135.   Daugherty A, Zweifel BS, Schonfeld G. Probucol attenuates the development of aortic atherosclerosis in cholesterol-fed rabbits. *Br J Pharmacol* 1989; 98:612-618.
136.   Prasad K, Kalra J, Lee P. Oxygen free radicals as a mechanism of hypercholesterolemic atherosclerosis: effects of probucol. *International J Angio* 1994; 3:100-112.
137.   Sparrow CP, Doebber TW, Olszewski J, Wu MS, Ventre J, Stevens KA, Chao YS. Low density lipoprotein is protected from oxidation and the progression of atherosclerosis is slowed in cholesterol-fed rabbits by the antioxidant N,N'-diphenyl-phenylenediamine. *J Clin Invest* 1992; 89:1885-1891.
138.   Bjorkhem I, Henriksson-Freyschuss A, Breuer O, Diczfalusy U, Berglund L, Henriksson P. The antioxidant butylated hydroxytoluene protects against atherosclerosis. *Arterio and Thromb* 1991; 11:15-22.
139.   Mantha SV, Prasad M, Kalra J, Prasad K. Antioxidant enzymes in hypercholesterolemia and effects of vitamin E in rabbits. *Atherosclerosis* 1993; 101:135-144.
140.   Kleinveld HA, Hak-Lemmers H, Hectors M, de Fouw NJ, Demacker P, Stalenhoef A. Vitamin E and fatty acid intervention does not attenuate the progression of atherosclerosis in watanabe heritable hyperlipidemic rabbits. *Aterio Thromb and Vasc Biol* 1995; 15:290-297.
141.   Shaish A, Daugherty A, O'Sullivan F, Schonfeld G, Heinecke JW. Beta-carotene inhibits atherosclerosis in hypercholesterolemic rabbits. *J Clin Invest* 1995; 96:2075-2082.
142.   Fruebis J, Carew TE, Palinski W. Effect of vitamin E on atherogenesis in LDL receptor-deficient rabbitsl. *Atherosclerosis* 1996; 117:217-224.
143.   Tangirala RK, Casanada F, Miller E, Witztum JL, Steinberg D, Palinski W. Effect of the antioxidant N,N'-diphenyl 1,4-phenylenediamine (DPPD). on atherosclerosis in apoE-deficient mice. *Arterioscler Thromb Vasc Biol* 1995; 15:1625-1630.
144.   Verlangieri AJ, Bush MJ. Effects of d-α-tocopherol supplementation on experimentally induced primate atherosclerosis. *J Am Coll Nutri* 1992; 11:131-138.

5 MECHANISMS OF LDL OXIDATION

Mark R. McCall and Balz Frei

INTRODUCTION

Oxidative stress is generally thought to play an important contributory role in the pathogenesis of atherosclerosis. Although there are many determinants in the development of this disease, substantial *in vitro* evidence links the production of oxidized forms of LDL to molecular processes involved in atherogenesis (1-7). Depending on how LDL oxidation is initiated and the level of damage produced, a spectrum of damaged particles and biological effects are observed. Thus, LDL possessing low levels of oxidative damage induces the expression of chemo-attractants and adhesion molecules, thereby facilitating tethering, activation and attachment of monocytes to endothelial cells (8-12). In addition, low level oxidative damage to LDL results in the formation of oxidized lipids that can impair the function of key elements of the anti-atherogenic reverse cholesterol transport pathway (13). More pronounced oxidative damage to LDL increases its atherogenicity by inhibiting endothelium-derived relaxing factor (14,15) and exerting cytotoxic effects (16,17). Moreover, oxidized LDL can induce foam cell formation, since after sufficient oxidative modification LDL is taken up by the poorly-regulated scavenger receptor pathway bypassing the cells normal cholesterol homeostatic mechanisms (18,19).

In vivo studies support these *in vitro* observations, since LDL isolated from atherosclerotic lesions shares some functional and biological properties with LDL oxidized *in vitro* (20). Immunohistochemical studies with antibodies that specifically recognize LDL oxidation products also provide direct evidence that oxidized LDL is present within arterial lesions (21,22). What is presently unknown and a topic of much research and speculation is the mechanism of initiation and progression of LDL oxidation *in vivo*.

The lack of stable and mechanism-specific biomarkers of oxidative damage, coupled with LDL's large size and chemical complexity, have limited characterization of the precise pathway(s) involved in LDL oxidation *in vivo*. Structurally, LDL is a spheroid particle with a hydrophobic core of neutral lipids (*i.e.*, cholesteryl esters and triacylglycerols) and a surface of polar lipids (*i.e.*, unesterified cholesterol and phospholipids) and amphipathic apolipoproteins (predominantly the glycoprotein apo B) (23). Human LDL has a molecular weight in the range of 2-3 x 10^6 and the following chemical composition, as a percent of weight: cholesteryl esters, 28-30%; triacylglycerols, 7-11%; phospholipids, 24-30%; unesterified cholesterol, 9-12%; and protein, 20-22% (24). Approximately half of the fatty acids in LDL are polyunsaturated. In addition, monoenoic lipids (e.g., cholesterol and monounsaturated fatty acids) represent a significant proportion of LDL lipid molecules. Both lipid and protein constituents of LDL are potential targets for oxidative insult. However, with the exception of cysteine and methionine residues, protein amino acids and monoenoic lipids are not as susceptible to free radical-mediated oxidation as polyunsaturated fatty acids (PUFAs) possessing bisallylic hydrogens that are readily abstracted (25).

Thus, oxidative modification of LDL has generally been thought to be initiated by radical mediated hydrogen abstraction from a methylene carbon on a PUFA side chain (4,26). The resulting carbon-centered radical then undergoes molecular rearrangement followed by an interaction with molecular oxygen to form a peroxyl radical. Among possible fates of the nascent peroxyl radical is the abstraction of a hydrogen atom from an adjacent PUFA side chain, thereby producing a lipid hydroperoxide and another radical capable of propagating the oxidative injury (4,26). The lipid hydroperoxides produced by this process are fairly stable, however, in the presence of transition metal ions such as copper or iron, these molecules decompose into a variety of breakdown products (4,28). Some of these products can initiate new rounds of lipid peroxidation (e.g., lipid alkoxyl radicals, LO•) while others are cytotoxic (e.g., 4-hydroxynonenal, HNE (28)) or promote inflammation (platelet-activating factor-like oxidized phospholipids (27), see Chapter 6). In addition, it has been reported that aldehydic PUFA breakdown products promote foam cell formation by modifying specific LDL apo B amino acid residues, thereby targeting these LDL particles for uptake via the macrophage scavenger receptor pathway (18,28,29).

METAL ION-DEPENDENT OXIDATION OF LDL

In Vitro Findings

Free radical-mediated lipid peroxidation appears to be a plausible *in vivo* mechanism to account for many of oxidized LDL's atherogenic properties. Much scientific effort has been focused on identifying the radical species involved in this process and the reaction mechanisms by which they are produced. Reactions involving redox-active metal ions, such as iron and copper, constitute one important pathway for the initiation of LDL oxidation *in vitro* (2,4,5,26,30). It is noteworthy, however, that even in the simplest of systems, containing either copper or iron ions and isolated LDL in phosphate-buffered saline, the mechanistic details of LDL oxidation are still not well defined. Clearly, preformed lipid hydroperoxides, if present in isolated LDL, are potential targets for the initiation of LDL peroxidation by copper or iron ions (28,30) (Fig. 1).

Recent studies have demonstrated that classical ultracentrifugation methods for LDL isolation are likely to artifactually introduce lipid hydroperoxides during the two to three day LDL isolation procedure, subsequent dialysis, and storage (32,33). Thus,

Reductant (α-tocopherol, [protein] thiol, superoxide radical, etc.)

$$\text{LOOH} + \text{Me}^{(N)} \rightarrow \text{LO}\bullet + \text{OH}^- + \text{Me}^{(N+1)}$$

"Re-initiation" of lipid peroxidation

Figure 1. Redox-active metal ion-catalyzed lipid peroxidation. The oxidized metal ion ($\text{Me}^{(N+1)}$) is reduced by a reductant; the reduced metal ion (Me^N) reacts with a lipid hydroperoxide (LOOH) to form a lipid alkoxyl radical (LO•), which can re-initiate lipid peroxidation. This reaction scheme is thermodynamically favored over the reaction of $\text{Me}^{(N+1)}$ with LOOH to produce lipid peroxyl radicals. It should be noted, however, that it has recently been suggested that the reduction of Cu^{2+} by LOOH may overcome the thermodynamic barriers to the reaction in lipid environments such as those found in LDL (31).

much of the literature in this field is marred by this uncontrolled *ex vivo* artifact and may require re-analysis. It should also be noted that classical non-specific indices of LDL lipid peroxidation (*i.e.*, thiobarbituric acid-reactive substances, TBARS) do not always correlate with more direct and sensitive methods of assessing LDL oxidation (34).

Stocker and co-workers, using methods designed to reduce the artifactual peroxidation of LDL during isolation, have shown that lipid hydroperoxides, if present in freshly isolated LDL, are generally below the detection limit (< 1 cholesteryl ester hydroperoxide molecule per 2000 LDL particles) of a highly sensitive HPLC assay utilizing postcolumn chemiluminescence (35,36). Thus, it has been possible to examine metal ion-catalyzed LDL peroxidation in a system essentially free of preformed lipid hydroperoxides (37). Although some studies suggest the reductive chemistry associated with copper ion-catalyzed LDL peroxidation involves specific amino acid residues in apo B (e.g., thiols or histidine (38,39)), it is now apparent that the major reductant involved in copper ion-catalyzed LDL peroxidation is α-tocopherol (37,40,41). Paradoxically, α-tocopherol is considered the major lipid-soluble chain-breaking antioxidant associated with LDL. It is likely that in cell-free systems ceruloplasmin, a putative endogenous source of redox-active copper (42), exerts its pro-oxidant effects through this mechanism.

α-Tocopherol-mediated peroxidation (TMP) was covered in chapter 3 and therefore will be discussed only briefly here. Stocker and others have shown that tocopherol can reduce copper ions during copper-dependent oxidation of LDL (37,40,41).

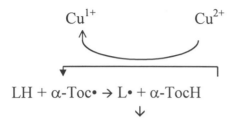

$$Cu^{1+} \qquad\qquad Cu^{2+}$$

$$LH + \alpha\text{-Toc}\bullet \to L\bullet + \alpha\text{-TocH}$$

Initiation of lipid peroxidation

Figure 2. Copper-mediated TMP. The reduction of copper by α-tocopherol (α-TocH) results in the formation of the α-tocopheroxyl radical (α-Toc•). LDL lipid peroxidation ensues if appropriate co-antioxidants are not available to scavenge the α-tocopheroxyl radical (see text).

According to the TMP model, the α-tocopheroxyl radical (α-Toc•) produced by this reaction abstracts a bisallylic hydrogen from an unsaturated surface or core lipid in LDL, thereby initiating LDL lipid peroxidation (Fig. 2). Since α-tocopherol in TMP not only mediates the entry of radicals into LDL from the aqueous phase, but also participates in the lipid peroxidation cascade, α-tocopherol has been described as both a "phase-transfer" and a "chain-transfer" agent (37). This important *in vitro* LDL peroxidation pathway proceeds only in the absence of compounds capable of eliminating the α-tocopheroxyl radical from the peroxidizing LDL particle. Thus, when ubiquinol-10 is depleted, and the aqueous phase "co-antioxidants" ascorbate and albumin-bound bilirubin are absent (as is the situation when isolated LDL is incubated in a buffer system with copper ions), TMP appears to be the most relevant LDL peroxidation pathway (37).

Although iron and copper are both used *in vitro* to oxidize LDL, the mechanism(s) by which these redox-active metals exert their pro-oxidant effects appear dissimilar (43,44). Copper binds to specific amino acid residues on apo B (38,39) and, as discussed above, appears to initiate LDL lipid peroxidation by directly interacting with LDL-associated α-tocopherol (37,40,41). Thus, the reduction of Cu^{2+} to Cu^{1+} by α-tocopherol with the concomitant generation of the α-tocopheroxyl radical is thought to result in the initiation of LDL lipid peroxidation (Fig. 2). Iron, like copper, requires reduction to initiate LDL oxidation. In contrast to copper, however, Fe^{3+} can not initiate LDL oxidation without an external reductant such as superoxide radicals or free thiols (44). Thus, it is currently not clear if TMP plays a role in iron-induced LDL oxidation.   Moreover, unless preformed lipid hydroperoxides are present in LDL (Fig. 1), the precise mechanism by which Fe^{2+} induces LDL oxidation remains speculative.

It has been demonstrated in cell culture experiments that many of the cell types present in developing atherosclerotic lesions (*i.e.*, endothelial cells, monocytes, macrophages and smooth muscle cells) can peroxidize LDL through reactions requiring copper or iron ions (45-48). Considering the metabolic complexity of these cell culture systems (compared to cell-free incubations) and the difficulties associated with identifying the nature and source of specific radical species and oxidation products, it is not surprising that the precise mechanisms of cell-mediated LDL oxidation are unclear.   Moreover, many of the problems discussed above related to LDL isolation practices and the fact that frequently used analytical methods such as TBARS do not always correlate with more direct and sensitive methods of assessing LDL oxidation (*i.e.*, HPLC separation followed by chemiluminescence detection) have further complicated the identification of the relevant peroxidation pathways.

It is generally thought that metal ions require cell-derived reductants in order to oxidize LDL in cell culture systems. Superoxide radicals may play such a role in a variety of cell types (49-51). The proposed mechanism by which superoxide produces this effect is by reducing copper or iron ions, which in turn catalyze the decomposition of hydrogen peroxide or preformed lipid hydroperoxides (Figure 1) into hydroxyl radicals and lipid alkoxyl radicals, respectively. These radical species are capable of initiating (hydroxyl radical) or re-initiating (lipid alkoxyl radical) lipid peroxidation.   Thus, endothelial cells, smooth muscle cells, and monocytes have all been shown to produce and release superoxide, which in turn stimulates LDL oxidation in the presence of (media-contained) redox-active metal ions (49-51). Recently, Mukhopadhyay and Fox have provided evidence that the acute phase copper-containing protein ceruloplasmin induces LDL oxidation by a redox process, whereby one ceruloplasmin-bound copper is reduced by cell-derived superoxide (52,53).   It is important to note, however, that a causal role for superoxide in the initiation of LDL oxidation has only been inferred and not conclusively demonstrated. Thus, not all investigators have been able to demonstrate an increase in LDL peroxidation in response to enhanced cellular superoxide production (34).

Metal ion-dependent oxidation of LDL by cultured vascular cells may also proceed by a mechanism requiring the reductive capacity of free thiols (54-57).   This reaction is thought to proceed by an L-cystine-dependent pathway that involves the intracellular reduction of L-cystine and subsequent release of a thiol (presumably L-cysteine) into the culture medium (54). In the presence of metal ions in the culture medium the thiol autooxidizes with the production of superoxide; LDL oxidation then proceeds as described above for superoxide.   Alternatively, it has been suggested that metal ions can be directly reduced by the free thiol, thereby facilitating metal ion-catalyzed decomposition of preformed lipid hydroperoxides in

LDL or hydrogen peroxide produced by the cells (58). It is currently not clear if these thiol-dependent pathways proceed only in the presence of peroxides, or if sulfur-centered radicals capable of abstracting a hydrogen atom from PUFAs can also participate (55). Wood and co-workers, however, have recently argued that although sulfur-centered radicals can initiate lipid peroxidation under certain *in vitro* conditions, it is unlikely that these conditions exist in the cell culture systems used for LDL oxidation (58).

Interestingly, Garner and co-workers have provided evidence for a pathway by which macrophages can directly reduce transition metals (59). These investigators showed that a trans-plasma membrane electron transport mechanism may account for much of the thiol-independent copper reduction and cell-mediated LDL oxidation observed with macrophages in culture. Thus, although alternative explanations have been suggested (5), it appears that cells in culture enhance metal ion-induced LDL oxidation by providing a means of reducing metal ions, so that they can facilitate the decomposition of peroxides.

In Vivo Evidence

The physiological relevance of transition metal ion-catalyzed LDL oxidation is controversial, since plasma as well as the interstitial fluid in the subendothelial space of the arterial wall possesses considerable capacity for metal ion chelation and antioxidation (60-62). Plasma and a fluid similar to subendothelial interstitial fluid (*i.e.*, suction blister fluid) prevent metal ion-dependent oxidation of LDL at very low concentrations. There are, however, a number of plausible mechanisms by which metal ions and redox-active metal complexes can be released from enzymes and transport proteins (63). Most of these mechanisms require the participation of reactive oxygen species (ROS) or reactive nitrogen species (RNS) and therefore, are likely to occur only at sites of injury or inflammation, where normal protective mechanisms have been overwhelmed and where plausible mechanisms for the generation of hydrogen peroxide and "seeding" lipid hydroperoxides exist. Thus, in atherosclerosis, LDL oxidation is thought to occur predominately, if not exclusively, in sequestered spaces or "microenvironments" within the arterial intima, where LDLs are retained (64,65) and antioxidant defense mechanisms have been overwhelmed (66).

Compelling evidence for a role of metal ions in atherogenesis, however, has not been obtained. Although it has been shown that tissue homogenates prepared from atherosclerotic lesions contain detectable levels of redox-active metal ions, it has not been determined whether this reflects the situation *in vivo* or if this redox-active material was artifactually generated during homogenization (67,68). In addition, genetic disorders resulting in the accumulation of iron or copper in tissues and plasma are generally not associated with premature atherosclerosis (5). Finally, damage to specific LDL-associated amino acid residues (e.g., oxidative damage to phenylalanine resulting in the formation of o- and m-tyrosine) isolated from fatty streaks, and intermediate lesions resected from human vascular tissue at necropsy, are not consistent with a mechanism involving metal-catalyzed oxidation in early lesion development (see below, Table 1) (69).

Cellular necrosis is thought to be a prominent feature of advanced atherosclerotic lesions. Dying cells may release redox-active metal ions, thereby facilitating LDL oxidation. Evidence in support of metal-catalyzed oxidation within advanced fibro-fatty lesions has been recently provided by Fu and co-workers (70). These investigators determined the levels of specific oxidation products of six different amino acids in proteins isolated from normal human intima and carotid artery plaque. Relative increases in hydroxy-valine, hydroxy-leucine, o-tyrosine, m-tyrosine and 3,4-dihydroxy-phenylalanine (Dopa) in the carotid samples were interpreted as evidence for hydroxyl radical-mediated damage in advanced atherosclerosis. It is important to note, however, that the specificity and validity of specific amino acid oxidation products as an index of type of oxidative insult are still under investigation. Thus, an *in vivo* role for transition metal-catalyzed LDL oxidation is still quite speculative, and seems unlikely in the initial stages of atherosclerosis.

LIPOXYGENASE-DEPENDENT OXIDATION OF LDL

In Vitro Findings

Non-heme iron-containing lipoxygenases have been proposed as initiators of LDL lipid peroxidation (71-74). Based on the positional specificity of oxygen insertion into arachidonic acid, four mammalian lipoxygenases have been identified: 5-, 8-,12- and 15-lipoxygenase (75). These lipoxygenases stereospecifically incorporate molecular oxygen into PUFAs, and in some instances PUFA side chains, generating PUFA hydroperoxides with specific positional (depending on the lipoxygenase) and optical (S enantiomer) properties (75). As a result of this enzymatic specificity, the reaction products from lipoxygenase reactions can be distinguished from those generated by the non-enzymatic metal ion-catalyzed reactions discussed above (71-73). Non-enzymatic processes result in the formation of PUFA hydroperoxides positionally the same as those catalyzed by lipoxygenases, but with equal quantities of the S and R stereoisomers at the peroxidized position (71-73). Thus, stereochemical evidence consistent with lipoxygenases participating in LDL peroxidation has been presented (71,76-79). However, as will be discussed below, the *in vivo* importance of these observations is still an area of considerable speculation and controversy.

In vitro studies have, in general, supported the hypothesis that lipoxygenase enzymes can oxidize LDL, thereby potentially facilitating atherogenesis. Studies in cell-free systems as well as with cells have provided support for a role of 15-lipoxygenase in LDL oxidation (71-73). Unlike other lipoxygenases, this enzyme is capable of oxygenating not only free fatty acids, but also fatty acid esters, including the major neutral lipid component of LDL, cholesterol linoleate (71,77,79). Thus, in cell-free systems LDL peroxidation mediated by 15-lipoxygenase can proceed in the presence or absence of lipid-hydrolyzing enzymes (e.g., phospholipase A_2) (78,79). When lipid-hydrolyzing enzymes are absent, and incubation times are short and LDL concentrations low (LDL to lipoxygenase molar ratio = 1:10), the primary products are cholesteryl ester hydroperoxides. The S/R ratio of 13-hydroxy-9Z,11E-octadecadienoic acid (13-HODE (Z,E)) in this instance (77/23) is consistent with the enzymatic activity of 15-lipoxygenase (79). Interestingly, longer incubation times or higher LDL concentrations (LDL to lipoxygenase molar ratio = 1:1) also result in cholesteryl ester hydroperoxides being the predominant peroxidized lipid species formed, however, the S/R ratio of 13-HODE (Z,E) in this case approximates 1 (79). This observation suggests that free radical-mediated secondary reactions predominate *in vitro* at higher enzyme concentrations or during longer incubation periods. Neuzil and co-workers have provided convincing evidence that the non-enzymatic secondary reactions responsible for LDL peroxidation with 15-lipoxygenase *in vitro* are the result of TMP (78). This appears to be especially true when lipases (e.g., secretory phospholipase A_2) are present in the reaction mixture. These investigators speculated that some fraction of free fatty acid peroxyl radicals (or cholesteryl ester peroxyl radicals) generated by 15-lipoxygenase are released from the enzyme's active site, leading to the co-oxidation of α-tocopherol and the formation of α-tocopheroxyl radicals (78); LDL peroxidation then proceeds as described above for metal ion-catalyzed TMP (Fig. 2). This observation is consistent with earlier observations that 15-lipoxygenase-catalyzed LDL oxidation proceeds in the presence of endogenous α-tocopherol (76,77,80).

15-lipoxygenase is an intracellular enzyme and therefore an unlikely candidate for the initiation of extracellular LDL peroxidation (71-74). Recent studies, however, provide limited evidence that the cellular expression of this enzyme can result in enhanced LDL peroxidation. Interleukin-4 and interleukin-13, cytokines that induce the expression of 15-lipoxygenase, enhance the ability of activated monocytes to peroxidize LDL (81). In addition, macrophages isolated from mice lacking the rodent homologue of human 15-lipoxygenase (12/15-lipoxygenase) have a reduced capacity for LDL oxidation when stimulated with opsonized zymosan, compared to similarly stimulated macrophages from wild-type control mice (82). Moreover, stably transfected murine fibroblasts that overexpress 15-lipoxygenase have an increased ability to peroxidize LDL compared to cells transfected with β-galactosidase (control) (83,84). Even when the degree of LDL oxidation is similar (as assessed by TBARS or change in percent distribution of LDL fatty acids), LDL isolated from the medium of fibroblasts overexpressing 15-lipoxygenase possess an enhanced ability to stimulate monocyte adhesion to endothelial cells (84). This observation indicates that specific products of the lipoxygenase reaction exert bioactivity similar to that of lipids isolated from minimally modified LDL.

Although these studies with cells demonstrate that the cellular expression of 15-lipoxygenase can result in enhanced LDL peroxidation, they represent very specialized experimental systems. These results, therefore, can not be unambiguously interpreted. For example, due to some similarity in sequence and positional specificity, mouse 12/15-lipoxygenase is thought to be a homologue of human 15-lipoxygenase. This assumption may prove to be incorrect, as human 15-lipoxygenase and mouse 12/15-lipoxygenase differ in how they are regulated and in some of the cell types in which they are expressed (75). Furthermore, studies with transfected murine fibroblasts overexpressing 15-lipoxygenase failed to examine cell-conditioned medium for 15-lipoxygenase activity (83,84); thus, it remains possible that the intracellular enzyme was released and induced LDL peroxidation extracellularly. It should also be noted that these recent cell culture studies have not provided any direct evidence for the accumulation of stereochemically specific 15-lipoxygenase reaction products.

In Vivo Evidence

Although there are no data concerning the accumulation of stereospecific 15-lipoxygenase lipid oxidation products in LDL *in vivo*, there are studies that have analyzed oxidized lipids extracted from atherosclerotic lesions (85-88). These studies have provided limited evidence for the presence of 15-lipoxygenase-modified lipids in lesions. Human studies using carotid endarterectomy samples or post mortem resected aortic lesion material have shown S/R ratios that are racemic or very close to 1 (85-88). A single study using the cholesterol fed rabbit as a model of human atherosclerosis has provided data consistent with 15-lipoxygenase being of pathophysiological importance during the early stages of atherogenesis. This study documented that in rabbits consuming a cholesterol-rich diet for 12 weeks, 74% of the 13-HODE isolated from atherosclerotic aortas was in the S-form (85). Considering the difficulties encountered in detecting elevated S/R ratios *in vitro* with purified LDL, the findings of this study with lesion lipids are quite remarkable.

Immunohistochemical studies have demonstrated the presence of 15-lipoxygenase in macrophage-rich regions of atherosclerotic lesions in both humans and rabbits (89,90). Moreover, epitopes of oxidized LDL co-localize with these regions of 15-lipoxygenase expression (89). Normal intima does not appear to express this enzyme, however, hypercholesterolemia in rabbits resulting from either cholesterol feeding or an inherited lack of functional LDL receptors (*i.e.*, Watanabe rabbits) results in the induction of 15-lipoxygenase expression at sites of lesion development (91). A more recent study using a retrovirus to mediate the transfer of the 15-lipoxygenase gene into the iliac arteries of rabbits demonstrated that an increase in 15-lipoxygenase activity alone is not sufficient for the generation of oxidation-specific protein adducts, as assessed with antibodies to malondialdehyde (MDA)-modified LDL (92). Oxidation-specific protein adducts were observed only after the animals were fed a diet enriched in cholesterol. Taken together these data provide suggestive evidence that the expression of 15-lipoxygenase in the arterial wall requires permissive concentrations of lipoproteins to induce LDL peroxidation.

The recent development of transgenic animal models that overexpress the 15-lipoxygenase gene is of importance to address the question of whether 15-lipoxygenase expression in the arterial wall is causally related to LDL oxidation and atherogenesis (93,94). Interestingly, transgenic rabbits that overexpress the human 15-lipoxygenase gene in a macrophage-specific manner develop significantly less atherosclerosis when fed a high-cholesterol diet than their non-transgenic litter mates (94). In contrast, inhibition of 15-lipoxygenase by a selective inhibitor lacking antioxidant properties reduces the development of atherosclerosis in hypercholesterolemic rabbits (95,96). The lack of agreement between these studies is intriguing and has generated considerable discussion in several recent reviews (73,74). Whether these results can be explained by effects related to the abnormal sustained expression of 15-lipoxygenase activity in macrophages or by unknown *in vivo* effects of the lipoxygenase inhibitor requires further study. Cross-breeding studies in progress (73,74), using transgenic mice overexpressing human 15-lipoxygenase in vascular endothelial cells (93) should provide important new information on the role of 15-lipoxygenase in LDL oxidation and atherogenesis. In fact, a recent study has demonstrated that apo E-deficient mice lacking 12/15-lipoxygenase have less atherosclerosis than littermate controls (93a). These data support a role for 12/15-lipoxygenase in atherosclerosis, although the precise mechanism remains to be determined.

NITROGEN MONOXIDE (NITRIC OXIDE)-MEDIATED OXIDATION OF LDL

In Vitro Findings

The complex nature of nitrogen monoxide (NO) chemistry and biology has been the subject of several recent reviews (30,97-99). NO is a radical species generated endogenously from arginine by nitric oxide synthases. This radical, in addition to possessing numerous important regulatory functions *in vivo*, has also been linked to LDL oxidation (30). NO itself does not react with LDL at physiological pH. *In vitro* studies have shown that peroxynitrite [oxoperoxonitrate(1-)], the product of the facile reaction of NO with the superoxide radical, can undergo a variety of chemical reactions, some of which are capable of oxidizing LDL (100,101). Peroxynitrite can mediate both one- and two-electron oxidations, and it has been suggested that at low oxidant-to-lipoprotein ratios peroxynitrite is capable of oxidizing LDL via TMP, a one electron oxidation cascade (102). In addition, among other potentially damaging reactions, peroxynitrite oxidizes methionine residues and thiol groups in proteins, hydroxylates and nitrates aromatic amino acid residues, and oxidizes PUFAs (97). Thus, peroxynitrite has been shown to be capable of initiating LDL oxidation and converting this lipoprotein into a ligand for the scavenger receptors of macrophages (100,101).

Of some importance in understanding peroxynitrite chemistry in LDL oxidation is the observation that peroxynitrite reacts rapidly with carbon dioxide in the presence of physiological concentrations of bicarbonate, to generate an unstable nitrosoperoxy-carbonate anion adduct (103). The decomposition of this anion produces oxidizing, nitrating and nitrosating species that can subsequently react with LDL-associated proteins, lipids and carbohydrates (98,103). Recently, it has been shown that bicarbonate in the presence of the peroxynitrite generator 3-morpholinosydnonimine (SIN-1) enhances LDL oxidation, as assessed by either the loss of tryptophan residues (an index of protein oxidation) or an increase in cholesteryl ester hydroperoxides (an index of lipid oxidation) (102).

The cellular mechanisms involved in NO and superoxide radical generation are complex, as are the conditions *in vivo* which favor peroxynitrite formation (97,99). Studies with cultured cells have shown that stimulated endothelial cells, neutrophils and macrophages are capable of simultaneously generating both peroxynitrite precursors, superoxide and NO (104-106). Based on kinetic considerations (the rate of reaction of superoxide with NO exceeds the rate of superoxide dismutation by superoxide dismutase) it appears that even in the presence of superoxide dismutase peroxynitrite can be produced by stimulated phagocytic cells (97). In addition, it has recently been shown that inducible nitric oxide synthase in macrophages is capable of generating both superoxide and peroxynitrite when arginine availability is low (106). Thus, studies with cells in suspension have provided data consistent with the hypothesis that peroxynitrite mediates LDL oxidation *in vivo*.

In contrast to the pro-oxidant role described above, NO has also been shown to prevent or limit LDL oxidation (107-109). One mechanism by which NO is thought to inhibit LDL lipid peroxidation is through the scavenging of lipid alkoxyl and peroxyl radicals involved in propagating the peroxidative injury (99,107). As might be expected, considering the radical-radical nature of these reactions, the relative rates of NO and peroxyl or alkoxyl radical formation are critical in determining the efficacy of NO as an antioxidant. Thus, high fluxes of peroxyl radical production require high fluxes of NO production to limit oxidative damage (99,108). Interestingly, the product of this radical-radical reaction (an organic peroxynitrite) has been suggested to be an oxidant; however, this has not been demonstrated experimentally (99). Another mechanism by which NO is thought to inhibit LDL peroxidation is through its reaction with peroxynitrite (30,99). Thus, when NO is produced in excess of that required for the formation of peroxynitrite, lipid peroxidation actually decreases and reaction products other than lipid hydroperoxides are formed. This antioxidant effect is thought to be the result of peroxynitrite reacting with NO to form nitrogen dioxide, thereby preventing peroxynitrite or its homolysis products from initiating lipid peroxidation in LDL. Nitrogen dioxide (a radical) and dinitrogen trioxide (a non-radical) formed following the interaction of NO with peroxynitrite and nitrogen dioxide, respectively, are RNS thought to be involved in nitration and nitrosation reactions.

These RNS products are not as clearly deleterious as lipid peroxidation breakdown products. In fact, some nitrosation products are thought to be beneficial, acting as a reservoir of endothelium-derived relaxing factor activity (97).

In Vivo Evidence

Whether NO acts as a pro-oxidant or antioxidant *in vivo* is dependent on the balance between NO generation and the availability of superoxide radicals. Luoma and co-workers have recently reported that despite abundant expression of extracellular superoxide dismutase, epitopes characteristic of oxidized lipoproteins can be detected in both human and rabbit atherosclerotic lesions (110). These epitopes for both lipid oxidation products (MDA- and HNE-lysine) and peroxynitrite-modified proteins (*i.e.*, nitrotyrosine; see Fig. 3) were detected in inducible nitric oxide synthase-positive, macrophage-rich lesions. Simultaneous *in situ* hybridization and immunocytochemical analysis localized the inducible nitric oxide synthase and extracellular superoxide dismutase expression to both macrophages and smooth muscle cells (110). These observations are consistent with an earlier study by Buttery and co-workers (111) and imply that peroxynitrite formation and lipid peroxidation occur in atherosclerotic lesions even in the presence of extracellular superoxide dismutase. Moreover, the observation that very low levels of LDL-associated nitrotyrosine are detected in human plasma (69,112) and many fold higher levels in LDL isolated from human atherosclerotic lesions (see Table 1) (69) provides additional support for the *in vivo* importance of peroxynitrite in LDL oxidation in the arterial wall.

Table 1. Biomarkers of LDL oxidation isolated from plasma and atherosclerotic lesion LDL (69)

Protein oxidation products	Plasma LDL (mmol/mol apo B)	Lesion LDL (mmol/mol apo B)
m- and o-tyrosine	90	90
3-nitrotyrosine	1	120
3-chlorotyrosine	2	45
o,o' -dityrosine	<1	45

It is necessary to point out, however, that the use of nitrotyrosine as a specific marker of peroxynitrite-mediated protein oxidation has been questioned (113-116). It now appears that nitrotyrosine can be generated by mechanisms that are independent of the generation of superoxide. These superoxide-independent mechanisms require nitrite and either hypochlorous acid (HOCl) or myeloperoxidase (both potentially present in atherosclerotic lesions, see below) (113-115). The relative *in vivo* importance of these nitrotyrosine-generating pathways are currently unknown, and thus the role of peroxynitrite in LDL oxidation in the arterial wall remains uncertain.

MYELOPEROXIDASE-DEPENDENT OXIDATION OF LDL

In Vitro Findings

In vitro evidence has linked myeloperoxidase (MPO) to the oxidative conversion of LDL to an atherogenic form (5,117). MPO is a heme containing protein, released from activated neutrophils and monocytes that catalyzes the production of strong oxidants (5,117):

$$H_2O_2 + Cl^- + H^+ \xrightarrow{\text{MPO}} HOCl + H_2O$$

The predominant product of this enzyme at physiological chloride ion concentrations is HOCl, an oxidant that readily reacts with a variety of biomolecules (e.g. thiols, ascorbate and a variety of amines including amino acids) (118). Because of the high reactivity of HOCl, its reactions are dependent on the relative concentration and reactivities of compounds in the immediate vicinity of where it is produced. Thiols and methionine residues are many fold more reactive with HOCl than other amino acids and amines (118). At neutral pH, reagent or MPO-generated HOCl preferentially oxidizes LDL apo B (119-121). Neither LDL-associated lipids nor antioxidants (e.g., α-tocopherol or β-carotene) appear to represent major targets of HOCl. Of the various amino acid residues in apo B modified by HOCl, lysine residues appear to quantitatively represent the major target (119,120):

(a) $R\text{-}CH_2\text{-}NH_2 + HOCl \rightarrow R\text{-}CH_2\text{-}NHCl + H_2O$

(b) $R\text{-}CH_2\text{-}NHCl + H_2O \rightarrow R\text{-}CH{=}O + NH_4^+ + Cl^-$

The reaction of HOCl with the ε-amino group of lysine residues results in the formation of chloramines (reaction a), some of which subsequently decompose to form aldehydes (reaction b) (119,120). It is thought that once formed these aldehydes participate in the observed HOCl-induced crosslinking of apo B and aggregation of LDL (120). These physicochemical changes in LDL induced by HOCl treatment result in the conversion of LDL to a ligand for the scavenger receptors of macrophages (120). Thus, unlike lipoxygenase- or metal ion-dependent modification of LDL, which require the derivatization of lysine residues by lipid hydroperoxide breakdown products, HOCl directly modifies apo B lysine residues to enhance the atherogenicity of LDL.

The reaction of HOCl with amino acids or proteins generates additional products that may be relevant to LDL oxidation and atherogenesis. Anderson and co-workers have demonstrated that the MPO-H_2O_2-chloride system of polymorphonuclear neutrophils (PMNs) converts the hydroxy-amino acids L-serine and L-threonine into α-hydroxy aldehydes (122). In addition, the α,β-unsaturated aldehyde acrolein can be formed from L-threonine (122). These reactive aldehydic species can induce crosslinking of apo B (26). Other potentially relevant endproducts of reactions involving HOCl are: 3-chlorotyrosine (Fig. 3), a specific marker of MPO-catalyzed oxidation and therefore a potential *in vivo* biomarker of MPO activity (123); and nitrotyrosine (Fig. 3), a tyrosine derivative once thought to be a specific biomarker for peroxynitrite-mediated oxidation (see above) (113-115).

Although quantitatively not as important a target as apo B, LDL-associated lipids can also be oxidized by reagent HOCl or HOCl generated by the MPO-H_2O_2-chloride system (121). The mechanism of HOCl-induced lipid oxidation has recently been reviewed (124). It is thought that HOCl can react with unsaturated lipids generating a family of chlorohydrins (125). This reaction, however, does not generate lipid hydroperoxides and appears to be a favored reaction in LDL only at high HOCl concentrations and low pH. Alternatively, it has been suggested that HOCl can react with preformed LDL-associated lipid hydroperoxides to generate alkoxyl radicals, thereby re-initiating lipid peroxidation (124). This pathway is of some interest in that it does not depend on reduced metal ions for the decomposition of lipid hydroperoxides. The most recent proposed mechanism for HOCl-initiated lipid peroxidation involves secondary radical species produced by decomposition of HOCl-derived chloramines and chloramides (126). It is thought that some of the radicals produced by this process can initiate lipid peroxidation.

In vitro studies with PMNs suffer from many of the problems previously discussed concerning the use of culture media containing transition metal ions and the use of relatively insensitive and non-specific indices of LDL oxidation that do not distinguish between LDL and cell-derived lipid oxidation products. Moreover, the majority of these studies with cells in culture have focused on lipid rather than protein modifications (127-131). Studies using non-stimulated PMNs have suggested that increases in lipid peroxidation, as assessed by TBARS formation, are critically dependent on the presence of metal ions in the culture medium (127-128). In the absence of metal ions, it has been suggested that stimulated PMNs increase LDL lipid peroxidation by a superoxide-dependent, rather than HOCl-dependent, pathway (131). This conclusion likely reflects the fact that lipid oxidation rather than protein oxidation endpoints were measured. Considering that proteins rather than lipids appear to be the preferred targets of HOCl, it is surprising that the majority of *in vitro* LDL oxidation studies using PMNs have focused on lipid rather than protein oxidation products.

Heinecke and colleagues have suggested that L-tyrosine is another important physiological substrate for MPO. These investigators have provided convincing *in vitro* evidence that under specific experimental conditions purified MPO or stimulated neutrophils can generate tyrosyl radicals, which then initiate LDL lipid peroxidation either by directly abstracting a hydrogen atom from bis-allylic methylene groups of PUFAs or via TMP (117,132). Moreover, tyrosyl radicals can generate multiple protein-bound tyrosine oxidation products (133). The physiological relevance of these observations has come into question, however, since the same group of investigators has shown that o,o'-dityrosine (Fig. 3), a major reaction product under the experimental conditions used, is the major product formed by MPO only in the absence of chloride ion; at neutral pH and in the presence of physiological chloride ion concentrations, MPO converts L-tyrosine into p-hydroxyphenylacetaldehyde (134). The latter product is thought to result from the breakdown of HOCl-generated tyrosine-chlorine. Interestingly, this aldehydic product of L-tyrosine oxidation by the MPO-H_2O_2-chloride system covalently modifies ε-amino groups of protein lysine residues (135), potentially impacting LDL charge characteristics and affinity for the scavenger receptors of macrophages.

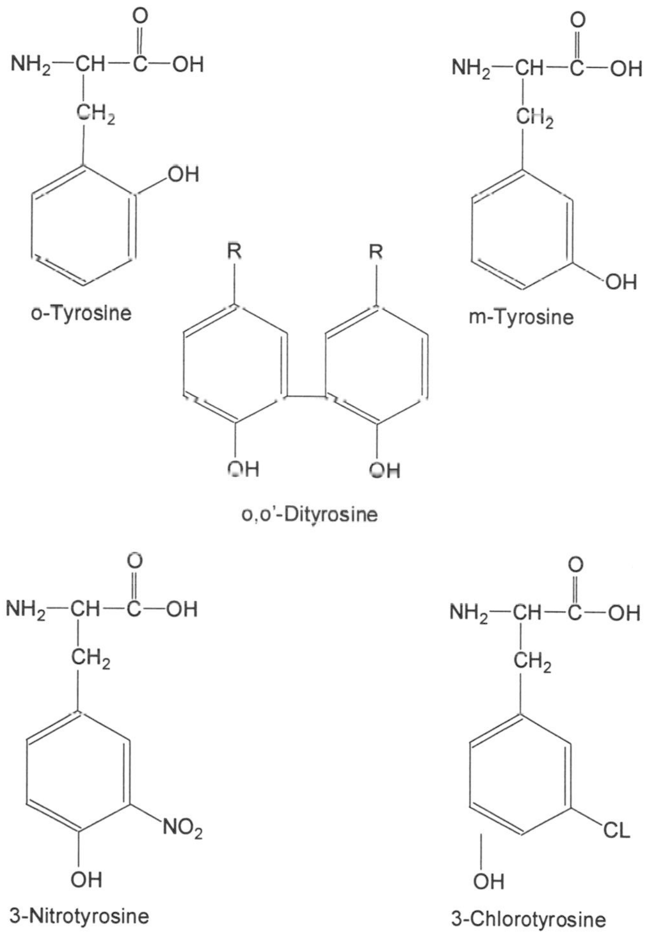

Figure 3. Structures of protein oxidation biomarkers that have been quantified for LDL isolated from atherosclerotic lesions.

In Vivo Evidence

The presence of immunoreactive and catalytically active MPO has been demonstrated in human atherosclerotic lesions (136). The enzyme appears to be localized both intra- and extra-cellularly and colocalizes with macrophages (136). Polyclonal antibodies against HOCl-modified LDL cross react with copper-oxidized LDL and LDL derivatized with either MDA or HNE. Conversely, polyclonal antibodies to copper- or aldehyde-modified LDL cross-react with HOCl-modified LDL, suggesting that these differing LDL preparations share common epitopes (137). These observations are of importance, since they indicate that early studies with polyclonal antibodies to copper- or aldehyde-modified LDL may have recognized epitopes generated by HOCl. More recent investigations with monoclonal antibodies specific for HOCl-modified proteins have demonstrated the presence of these proteins in both early and advanced lesions (138). Moreover, apo B-containing fractions obtained from atherosclerotic lesions were recognized by this antibody (138). Hazen and Heinecke recently demonstrated that 3-chlorotyrosine (Fig. 3), a specific marker of MPO-catalyzed oxidation, is elevated 30-fold in LDL isolated from human atherosclerotic lesions compared to plasma LDL (139).

It is also of interest to note that dityrosine (Fig. 3), generated by reaction of L-tyrosine with either HOCl or hydroxyl radicals, and nitrotyrosine (Fig. 3), generated by reaction of L-tyrosine with peroxynitrite and HOCl, are both elevated (100-fold and 90-fold, respectively) in lesion derived LDL compared to plasma LDL (Table 1) (69).

SUMMARY

In vitro and *in vivo* studies have discovered multiple oxidative pathways capable of altering LDL structure and, presumably, atherogenicity. Understanding the specific pathway or pathways involved in LDL oxidation *in vivo* is essential for evaluating whether a causal link exists between LDL oxidation and atherosclerotic lesion development. Moreover, if such a link exists, knowledge of these pathways is necessary to design strategies to inhibit LDL oxidation and its clinical sequelae. Considering the efficacy of plasma and interstitial fluid to sequester redox-active metal ions and to quench ROS and RNS, it appears that localized microenvironments in which antioxidant defenses have been overwhelmed underlie the focal nature of atherosclerosis. Defining this intimal microenvironment has proven difficult. The recent observation by Suarna and co-workers (140) that advanced fibro-fatty lesions from endarterectomy specimens, compared with healthy human arteries, possess elevated levels of lipid peroxidation products, and yet are not deficient in the antioxidant vitamins C and E illustrates the complexity of this problem. Further complicating the identification of relevant LDL oxidation pathways are a number of other conceptual and methodological problems including:

the ubiquitous nature of *in vitro* transition metal contamination; the continued use of relatively insensitive and non-specific indices of LDL oxidation, e.g., TBARS; LDL heterogeneity; artifactual *ex vivo* formation of lipid hydroperoxides during LDL isolation and storage; and the inadequate characterization of the various forms of oxidized LDLs experimentally generated. Clearly, the terms "minimally modified," "minimally oxidized" and "oxidized" LDL are inadequate to describe the spectrum of oxidized particles produced by the various pathways discussed in this chapter. Thus, the elucidation of the relevant *in vivo* pathways involved in LDL oxidation is still very much a work in progress.

The most relevant information to date concerning the potential mechanisms of LDL oxidation *in vivo* has come from immunohistochemical and biochemical analyses of animal and human atherosclerotic lesions and lipoproteins extracted from these lesions (Table 1). Ceruloplasmin, 15-lipoxygenase, myeloperoxidase and the enzymes essential for peroxynitrite production (nitric oxide synthase and NAD(P)H oxidase) are present in both animal and human lesions and could contribute to LDL oxidation. However, ceruloplasmin as well as other sources of redox-active metal ions are unlikely to participate in early lesion development, since specific markers for metal ion-catalyzed protein damage could not be found in early and intermediate atherosclerotic lesions. In contrast, lipid or protein oxidation products have been identified that are consistent with 15-lipoxygenase, myeloperoxidase and the enzymes essential for peroxynitrite production all participating in early lesion development.

The roles of 15-lipoxygenase and peroxynitrite in LDL oxidation and atherogenesis, however, are quite controversial. The fact that the mechanism by which the intracellular enzyme 15-lipoxygenase "seeds" extracellular LDL with hydroperoxides is unknown, and the observation that products of the 15-lipoxygenase pathway may be antiatherogenic have cast doubt on the importance of this enzyme to promote LDL oxidation and atherogenesis. Similarly, the fact that NO, an essential reactant in the generation of peroxynitrite, can also function as an antioxidant, and that nitrotyrosine appears not to be a specific marker for peroxynitrite damage has brought into question the relative importance of this pathway. The most compelling and consistent *in vivo* evidence for a specific LDL oxidation pathway is that involving myeloperoxidase-generated HOCl. Studies with myeloperoxidase knockout mice, now underway, should help elucidate the role of this enzyme in atherosclerotic lesion development.

REFERENCES

1.   Steinberg D, Witztum JL. Lipoproteins and atherogenesis: current concepts. *JAMA.* 1990;264:3047.
2.   Haberland ME, Steinbrecher UP. "Modified Low-Density Lipoproteins: Diversity and Biological Relevance in Atherogenesis." In *Molecular Genetics of Coronary Artery Disease*, Lusis AJ, Rotter JI, Sparkes RS, eds. Basel: Karger, 1992.

3.   Navab M, Berliner JA, Watson AD, Hama SY, Territo MC, Lusis AJ, Shih DM, Van Lenten BJ, Frank JS, Demer LL, Edwards PA, Fogelman AM. The yin and yang of oxidation in the development of the fatty streak: a review based on the 1994 George Lyman Duff memorial lecture. *Arterioscler Thromb Vasc Biol.* 1996;16:831.

4.   Jialal I, Devaraj S. Low-density lipoprotein oxidation, antioxidants, and atherosclerosis: a clinical biochemistry perspective. *Clin Chem.* 1996;42:498.

5.   Berliner JA, Heinecke JW. The role of oxidized lipoproteins in atherogenesis. *Free Rad Biol Med.* 1996;20:707.

6.   Hajjar DP, Haberland ME. Lipoprotein trafficking in vascular cells: molecular Trojan horses and cellular saboteurs. *J Biol Chem.* 1997;272:22975.

7.   Diaz MN, Frei B, Vita JA, Keaney JF Jr. Antioxidants and atherosclerotic heart disease. *New Engl J Med.* 1997;337:408.

8.   Cushing SD, Berliner JA, Valente AJ, Territo MC, Navab M, Parhami F, Gerrity R, Schwartz CJ, Fogelman AM. Minimally modified low density lipoprotein induces monocyte chemotactic protein 1 in human endothelial cells and smooth muscle cells. *Proc Natl Acad Sci USA.* 1990;87:5134.

9.   Rajavashisth TB, Andalibi A, Territo MC, Berliner JA, Navab M, Fogelman AM, Lusis AJ. Induction of endothelial cell expression of granulocyte and macrophage colony-stimulating factors by modified low-density lipoproteins. *Nature.* 1990;344:254.

10.   Navab M, Imes SS, Hama SY, Hough GP, Ross LA, Bork RW, Valente AJ, Berliner JA, Drinkwater DC, Laks H, Fogelman AM. Monocyte transmigration induced by modification of low density lipoprotein in cocultures of human aortic wall cells is due to induction of monocyte chemotactic protein 1 synthesis and is abolished by high density lipoprotein. *J Clin Invest.* 1991;88:2039.

11.   Frostegård J, Haegerstrand A, Gidlund M, Nilsson J. Biologically modified LDL increases the adhesive properties of endothelial cells. *Atherosclerosis.* 1991;90:119.

12.   Schwartz D, Andalibi A, Chaverri-Almada L, Berliner JA, Kirchgessner T, Fang Z-T, Tekamp-Olson P, Lusis AJ, Gallegos C, Fogelman AM, Territo MC. Role of the GRO family of chemokines in monocyte adhesion to MM-LDL-stimulated endothelium. *J Clin Invest.* 1994;94:1968.

13.   Bielicki JK, Forte TM, McCall MR. Minimally oxidized LDL is a potent inhibitor of lecithin:cholesterol acyltransferase activity. *J Lipid Res.* 1996;37:1012.

14.   Kugiyama K, Kerns SA, Morrisett JD, Roberts R, Henry PD. Impairment of endothelium-dependent arterial relaxation by lysolecithin in modified low-density lipoproteins. *Nature.* 1990;344:160.

15.   Chin JH, Azhar S, Hoffman BB. Inactivation of endothelial derived relaxing factor by oxidized lipoproteins. *J Clin Invest.* 1992;89:10.

16.   Hessler JR, Morel DW, Lewis LJ, Chisolm GM. Lipoprotein oxidation and lipoprotein-induced cytotoxicity. *Arteriosclerosis.* 1983;3:215.

17.   Kosugi K, Morel DW, DiCorleto PE, Chisolm GM. Toxicity of oxidized low-density lipoprotein to cultured fibroblasts is selective for S phase of the cell cycle. *J Cell Physiol.* 1987;130:311.

18.   Steinbrecher UP. Oxidation of human low density lipoprotein results in derivatization of lysine residues of apolipoprotein B by lipid peroxide decomposition products. *J Biol Chem.* 1987;262:3603.

19.   Steinbrecher UP, Lougheed M, Kwan W-C, Dirks M. Recognition of oxidized low density lipoprotein by the scavenger receptor of macrophages results from derivatization of apolipoprotein B by products of fatty acid peroxidation. *J Biol Chem.* 1989;264:15216.

20.   Hoff HF, O'Neil J. Lesion-derived low density lipoprotein and oxidized low density lipoprotein share a lability for aggregation, leading to enhanced macrophage degradation. *Arterioscler Thromb.* 1991;11:1209.

21.   Haberland ME, Fong D, Cheng L. Malondialdehyde-altered protein occurs in athero of Watanabe heritable hyperlipidemic rabbits. *Science.* 1988;241:215.

22.   Ylä-Herttuala S, Palinski W, Rosenfeld ME, Parthasarathy S, Carew TE, Butler S, Witztum JL, Steinberg D. Evidence for the presence of oxidatively modified low density lipoprotein in atherosclerotic lesions of rabbit and man. *J Clin Invest.* 1989;84:1086.

23. Yang C-Y, Pownall HJ. Structure and function of apolipoprotein B. In: Structure and Function of Apolipoproteins (ed. Rosseneu M). Boca Raton: CRC Press, Inc., 1992 pp. 64.

24. Edelstein C. General properties of plasma lipoproteins and apolipoproteins. In: Biochemistry and Biology of Plasma Lipoproteins (eds. Scanu AM, Spector AA). New York: Marcel Dekker, Inc., 1986 pp. 495.

25. Dean RT, Fu S, Stocker R, Davies MJ. Biochemistry and pathology of radical-mediated protein oxidation. *Biochem J.* 1997;324:1.

26. Esterbauer H, Gebicki J, Puhl H, Jürgens G. The role of lipid peroxidation and antioxidants in oxidative modification of LDL. *Free Rad Biol Med.* 1992;13:341.

27. Heery JM, Kozak M, Stafforini DM, Jones DA, Zimmerman GA, McIntyre TM, Prescott SM. Oxidatively modified LDL contains phospholipids with platelet-activating factor-like activity and stimulates the growth of smooth muscle cells. *J Clin Invest.* 1995;96:2322.

28. Fogelman AM, Shechter I, Seager J, Hokom M, Child JS, Edwards, PA. Malondialdehyde alteration of low density lipoproteins leads to cholesteryl ester accumulation in human monocyte-macrophages. *Proc Natl Acad Sci USA.* 1980;77:2214.

29. Haberland ME, Fogelman AM, Edwards PA. Specificity of receptor-mediated recognition of malondialdehyde-modified low density lipoproteins. *Proc Natl Acad Sci USA.* 1982;79:1712.

30. Darley-Usmar V, Halliwell B. Blood radicals: reactive nitrogen species, reactive oxygen species, transition metal ions, and the vascular system. *Pharm Res.* 1996;13:649.

31. Patel RP, Svistunenko D, Wilson MT, Darley-Usmar VM. Reduction of Cu(II) by lipid hydroperoxides: implications for the copper-dependent oxidation of low-density lipoprotein. *Biochem J.* 1997;322:425.

32. Sattler W, Mohr D, Stocker R. Rapid isolation of lipoproteins and assessment of their peroxidation by high-performance liquid chromatography postcolumn chemiluminescence. *Meth Enzymol.* 1994;233:469.

33. Shwaery GT, Mowri H, Keaney JF Jr, Frei B. Preparation of lipid hydroperoxide-free low-density lipoproteins. *Meth Enzymol.* 1999;300:17.

34. Garner B, Dean RT, Jessup W. Human macrophage-mediated oxidation of low-density lipoprotein is delayed and independent of superoxide production. *Biochem J.* 1994;301:421.

35. Stocker R, Bowry VW, Frei B. Ubiquinol-10 protects human low density lipoprotein more efficiently against lipid peroxidation than does α-tocopherol. *Proc Natl Acad Sci USA.* 1991;88:1646.

36. Bowry VW, Stanley KK, Stocker R. High density lipoprotein is the major carrier of lipid hydroperoxides in human blood plasma from fasting donors. *Proc Natl Acad Sci USA.* 1992;89:10316.

37. Neuzil J, Thomas SR, Stocker R. Requirement for, promotion, or inhibition by α-tocopherol of radical-induced initiation of plasma lipoprotein lipid peroxidation. *Free Rad Biol Med.* 1997;22:57.

38. Chen K, Frei B. The effect of histidine modification on copper-dependent lipid peroxidation in human low-density lipoprotein. *Redox Report.* 1997;3:175.

39. Wagner P, Heinecke JW. Copper ions promote peroxidation of low density lipoprotein lipid by binding to histidine residues of apolipoprotein B100, but they are reduced at other sites on LDL. *Arterioscler Thromb Vasc Biol.* 1997;17:3338.

40. Proudfoot JM, Croft KD, Puddey IB, Beilin LJ. The role of copper reduction by α-tocopherol in low-density lipoprotein oxidation. *Free Rad Biol Med.* 1997;23:720.

41. Perugini C, Seccia M, Bagnati M, Cau C, Albano E, Bellomo G. Different mechanisms are progressively recruited to promote Cu(II) reduction by isolated human low-density lipoprotein undergoing oxidation. *Free Rad Biol Med.* 1998;25:519.

42. Ehrenwald E, Chisolm GM, Fox PL. Intact human ceruloplasmin oxidatively modifies low density lipoprotein. *J Clin Invest.* 1994;93:1493.

43. Kuzuya M, Yamada K, Hayashi T, Funaki C, Naito M, Asai K, Kuzuya F. Oxidation of low-density lipoprotein by copper and iron in phosphate buffer. *Biochim Biophys Acta.* 1991;1084:198.

44. Lynch SM, Frei B. Reduction of copper, but not iron, by human low density lipoprotein (LDL). *J Biol Chem.* 1995;270:5158.

45. Heinecke JW, Rosen H, Chait A. Iron and copper promote modification of low density lipoprotein by human arterial smooth muscle cells in culture. *J Clin Invest.* 1984;4:1890.

46.   Steinbrecher UP, Parthasarathy S, Leake DS, Witztum JL, Steinberg D. Modification of low density lipoprotein by endothelial cells involves lipid peroxidation and degradation of low density lipoprotein phospholipids. *Proc Natl Acad Sci USA*. 1984;81:3883.

47.   Morel DW, DiCorleto PE, Chisolm GM. Endothelial and smooth muscle cells alter low density lipoprotein in vitro by free radical oxidation. *Arteriosclerosis*. 1984;4:357.

48.   Jessup W, Rankin SM, DeWhalley CV, Hoult JRS, Scott J, Leake DS. α-Tocopherol consumption during low-density-lipoprotein oxidation. *Biochem J*. 1990;265:399.

49.   Heinecke JW, Baker L, Rosen H, Chait A. Superoxide-mediated modification of low density lipoprotein by arterial smooth muscle cells. *J Clin Invest*. 1986;77:757.

50.   Hiramatsu K, Rosen H, Heinecke JW, Wolfbauer G, Chait A. Superoxide initiates oxidation of low density lipoprotein by human monocytes. *Arteriosclerosis*. 1987;7:55.

51.   Steinbrecher UP. Role of superoxide in endothelial-cell modification of low-density lipoproteins. *Biochim Biophys Acta*. 1988;959:20.

52.   Mukhopadhyay CK, Ehrenwald E, Fox PL. Ceruloplasmin enhances smooth muscle cell-and endothelial cell-mediated low density lipoprotein oxidation by a superoxide-dependent mechanism. *J Biol Chem*. 1996;271:14773.

53.   Mukhopadhyay CK, Fox PL. Ceruloplasmin copper induces oxidant damage by a redox process utilizing cell-derived superoxide as reductant. *Biochemistry*. 1998;37:14222.

54.   Heinecke JW, Rosen H, Suzuki LA, Chait A. The role of sulfur-containing amino acids in superoxide production and modification of low density lipoprotein by arterial smooth muscle cells. *J Biol Chem*. 1987;262:10098.

55.   Heinecke JW, Kawamura M, Suzuki L, Chait A. Oxidation of low density lipoprotein by thiols: superoxide-dependent and -independent mechanisms. *J Lipid Res*. 1993;34:2051.

56.   Sparrow CP, Olszewski J. Cellular oxidation of low density lipoprotein is caused by thiol production in media containing transition metal ions. *J Lipid Res*. 1993;34:1219.

57.   Graham A, Wood JL, O'Leary VJ, Stone D. Human (THP-1) macrophages oxidize LDL by a thiol-dependent mechanism. *Free Rad Res*. 1996;25:181.

58.   Wood JL, Graham A. Structural requirements for oxidation of low-density lipoprotein by thiols. *FEBS Lett*. 1995;366:75.

59.   Garner B, van Reyk D, Dean RT, Jessup W. Direct copper reduction by macrophages. Its role in low density lipoprotein oxidation. *J Biol Chem*. 1997;272:6927.

60.   Frei B, Stocker R, Ames B. Antioxidant defenses and lipid peroxidation in human blood plasma. *Proc Natl Acad Sci USA*. 1988;85:9748.

61.   Dabbagh AJ, Frei B. Human suction blister interstitial fluid prevents metal ion-dependent oxidation of low density lipoprotein by macrophages and in cell-free systems. *J Clin Invest*. 1995;96:1958.

62.   Stocker R, Frei B. Endogenous antioxidant defenses in human blood plasma. In: Oxidative Stress: Oxidants and Antioxidants (ed. Sies H). London: Academic Press Limited, 1991 pp. 213.

63.   Darley-Usmar V, Halliwell B. Blood radicals: reactive nitrogen species, reactive oxygen species, transition metal ions, and the vascular system. *Pharm Res*. 1996;13:649.

64.   Williams KJ, Tabas I. The response-to-retention hypothesis of early atherogenesis. *Arterioscler Thromb Vasc Biol*. 1995;15:551.

65.   Hurt-Camejo E, Olsson U, Wiklund O, Gondjers G, Camejo G. Cellular consequences of the association of apoB lipoproteins with proteoglycans. *Arterioscler Thromb Vasc Biol*. 1997;17:1011.

66.   Quinn MT, Parthasarathy S, Fong LG, Steinberg D. Oxidatively modified low density lipoproteins: a potential role in recruitment and retention of monocyte/macrophages during atherogenesis. *Proc Natl Acad Sci USA*. 1987;84:2995.

67.   Evans PJ, Smith C, Mitchinson MJ, Halliwell B. Metal ion release from mechanically-disrupted human arterial wall. Implications for the development of atherosclerosis. *Free Rad Res*. 1995;23:465.

68.   Lamb DJ, Mitchinson MJ, Leake DS. Transition metal ions within human atherosclerotic lesions can catalyse the oxidation of low density lipoprotein by macrophages. *FEBS Lett*. 1995;374:12.

69.   Leeuwenburgh C, Rasmussen JE, Hsu FF, Mueller DM, Pennathur S, Heinecke JW. Mass spectrometric quantification of markers for protein oxidation by tyrosyl radical, copper, and

hydroxyl radical in low density lipoprotein isolated from human atherosclerotic plaques. *J Biol Chem.* 1997;272:3520.

70. Fu S, Davies MJ, Stocker R, Dean RT. Evidence for roles of radicals in protein oxidation in advanced human atherosclerotic plaque. *Biochem J.* 1998;333:519.
71. Belkner J, Wiesner R, Rathman J, Barnett J, Sigal E, Kühn H. Oxygenation of lipoproteins by mammalian lipoxygenases. *Eur J Biochem.* 1993;213:251.
72. Wetterholm A, Samuelsson B. "The Lipoxygenase System." In *Oxidative Processes and Antioxidants,* R Paoletti et al., eds. New York: Raven Press, Ltd., 1994.
73. Feinmark SJ, Cornicelli JA. Is there a role for 15-lipoxygenase in atherogenesis? *Biochem Pharm.* 1997;54:953.
74. Kühn H, Chan L. The role of 15-lipoxygenase in atherogenesis: pro- and antiatherogenic actions. *Curr Opin Lipidol.* 1997;8:111.
75. Funk CD. The molecular biology of mammalian lipoxygenases and the quest for eicosanoid functions using lipoxygenase-deficient mice. *Biochim Biophys Acta.* 1996;1304:65.
76. Lass A, Belkner J, Esterbauer H, Kühn H. Lipoxygenase treatment renders low-density lipoprotein susceptible to Cu^{2+}-catalysed oxidation. *Biochem J.* 1996;314:577.
77. Upston JM, Neuzil J, Witting PK, Alleva R, Stocker R. Oxidation of free fatty acids in low density lipoprotein by 15-lipoxygenase stimulates nonenzymic, α-tocopherol-mediated peroxidation of cholesteryl esters. *J Biol Chem.* 1997;272:30067.
78. Neuzil J, Upston JM, Witting PK, Scott KF, Stocker R. Secretory phospholipase A_2 and lipoprotein lipase enhance 15-lipoxygenase-induced enzymic and nonenzymic lipid peroxidation in low-density lipoproteins. *Biochemistry.* 1998;37:9203.
79. Belkner J, Stender H, Kühn H. The rabbit 15-lipoxygenase preferentially oxygenates LDL cholesterol esters, and this reaction does not require vitamin E. *J Biol Chem.* 1998;273:23225.
80. Upston JM, Neuzil J, Stocker R. Oxidation of LDL by recombinant human 15-lipoxygenase: evidence for α-tocopherol-dependent oxidation of esterified core and surface lipids. *J Lipid Res.* 1996;37:2650.
81. Folcik VA, Aamir R, Cathcart MK. Cytokine modulation of LDL oxidation by activated human monocytes. *Arterioscler Thromb Vasc Biol.* 1997;17:1954.
82. Sun D, Funk CD. Disruption of 12/15-lipoxygenase expression in peritoneal macrophages: enhanced utilization of the 5-lipoxygenase pathway and diminished oxidation of low density lipoprotein. *J Biol Chem.* 1996;271:24055.
83. Benz DJ, Mol M, Ezaki M, Mori-Ito N, Zelán I, Miyanohara A, Friedmann T, Parthasarathy S, Steinberg D, Witztum JL. Enhanced levels of lipoperoxides in low density lipoprotein incubated with murine fibroblasts expressing high levels of human 15-lipoxygenase. *J Biol Chem.* 1995;270:5191.
84. Sigari F, Lee C, Witztum JL, Reaven PD. Fibroblasts that overexpress 15-lipoxygenase generate bioactive and minimally modified LDL. *Arterioscler Thromb Vasc Biol.* 1997;17:3639.
85. Kühn H, Belkner J, Zaiss S, Fährenklemper T, Wohlfeil S. Involvement of 15-lipoxygenase in early stages of atherogenesis. *J Exp Med.* 1994;179:1903.
86. Folcik VA, Nivar-Aristy RA, Krajewski LP, Cathcart MK. Lipoxygenase contributes to the oxidation of lipids in human atherosclerotic plaques. *J Clin Invest.* 1995;96:504.
87. Kühn H, Heydeck D, Hugou I, Gniwotta C. In vivo action of 15-lipoxygenase in early stages of human atherogenesis. *J Clin Invest.* 1997;99:8883.
88. Gniwotta C, Morrow JD, Roberts LJ II, Kühn H. Prostaglandin F_2-like compounds, F_2-isoprostanes, are present in increased amounts in human atherosclerotic lesions. *Arterioscler Thromb Vasc Biol.* 1997;17:3236.
89. Ylä-Herttuala S, Rosenfeld ME, Parthasarathy S, Glass CK, Sigal E, Witztum JL, Steinberg D. Colocalization of 15-lipoxygenase mRNA and protein with epitopes of oxidized low density lipoprotein in macrophage-rich areas of atherosclerotic lesions. *Proc Natl Acad Sci USA.* 1990;87:6959.
90. Ylä-Herttuala S, Rosenfeld ME, Parthasarathy S, Sigal E, Särkioja T, Witztum JL, Steinberg D. Gene expression in macrophage-rich human atherosclerotic lesions: 15-lipoxygenase and acetyl low density lipoprotein receptor messenger RNA colocalize with oxidation specific lipid-protein adducts. *J Clin Invest.* 1991;87:1146.

91.   Hiltunen T, Luoma J, Nikkari T, Ylä-Herttuala S. Induction of 15-lipoxygenase mRNA and protein in early atherosclerotic lesions. *Circulation*. 1995;92:3297.

92.   Ylä -Herttuala S, Luoma J, Viita H, Hiltunen T, Sisto T, Nikkari T. Transfer of 15-lipoxygenase gene into rabbit iliac arteries results in the appearance of oxidation-specific lipid-protein adducts characteristic of oxidized low density lipoprotein. *J Clin Invest*. 1995;95:2692.

93.   Harats D, Kurihara H, Belloni P, Oakley H, Ziober A, Ackley D, Cain G, Kurihara Y, Lawn R, Sigal E. Targeting gene expression to the vascular wall in transgenic mice using the murine preproendothelin-1 promoter. *J Clin Invest*. 1995;95:1335.

93a.   Tillman C, Witztum JL, Rader DJ, Tangirala R, Fazio S, Linton MF, Funk CD. Disruption of the 12/15-lipoxygenase gene diminishes atherosclerosis in apo E-deficient mice. *J Clin Invest*. 1999;103:1597.

94.   Shen J, Herderick E, Cornhill JF, Zsigmond E, Kim H-S, Kühn H, Guevara, NV, Chan L. Macrophage-mediated 15-lipoxygenase expression protects against atherosclerosis development. *J Clin Invest*. 1996;98:2201.

95.   Sendobry SM, Cornicelli JA, Welch K, Bocan T, Tait B, Trivedi BK, Colbry N, Dyer RD, Feinmark SJ, Daugherty A. Attenuation of diet-induced atherosclerosis in rabbits with a highly selective 15-lipoxygenase inhibitor lacking significant antioxidant properties. *Brit J Pharm*. 1997;120:1199.

96.   Bocan TMA, Rosebury WS, Mueller SB, Kuchera S, Welch K, Daugherty A, Cornicelli JA. A specific 15-lipoxygenase inhibitor limits the progression and monocyte-macrophage enrichment of hypercholesterolemia-induced atherosclerosis in the rabbit. *Atherosclerosis*. 1998;136:203.

97.   Koppenol WH. The basic chemistry of nitrogen monoxide and peroxynitrite. *Free Rad Biol Med*. 1998;25:385.

98.   Squadrito GL, Pryor WA. Oxidative ch emistry of nitric oxide: the roles of superoxide, peroxynitrite, and carbon dioxide. *Free Rad Biol Med*. 1998;25:392.

99.   Wink DA, Mitchell JB. Chemical biology of nitric oxide: insights into regulatory, cytotoxic, and cytoprotective mechanism of nitric oxide. *Free Rad Biol Med*. 1998;25:434.

100.   Graham A, Hogg N, Kalyanaraman B, O'Leary V, Darley-Usmar V, Moncada S. Peroxynitrite modification of low-density lipoprotein leads to recognition by the macrophage scavenger receptor. *FEBS Lett*. 1993;330:181.

101.   Moore KP, Darley-Usmar V, Morrow J, Roberts LJ II. Formation of F_2-isoprostanes during oxidation of human low-density lipoprotein and plasma by peroxynitrite. *Circ Res*. 1995;77:335.

102.   Thomas SR, Davies MJ, Stocker R. Oxidation and antioxidation of human low-density lipoprotein and plasma exposed to 3-morpholinosydnonimine and reagent peroxynitrite. *Chem Res Toxicol*. 1998;1:484.

103.   Uppu RM, Squadrito GL, Pryor WA. Acceleration of peroxynitrite oxidations by carbon dioxide. *Arch Biochem Biophys*. 1996;327:335.

104.   Kooy NW, Royall JA. Agonist-induced peroxynitrite production from endothelial cells. *Arch Biochem Biophys*. 1994;310:352.

105.   Carreras MC, Pargament GA, Catz SD, Poderoso JJ, Boveris A. Kinetics of nitric oxide and hydrogen peroxide production and formation of peroxynitrite during the respiratory burst of human neutrophils. *FEBS Lett*. 1994;341:65.

106.   Xia Y, Zweier JL. Superoxide and peroxynitrite generation from inducible nitric oxide synthase in macrophages. *Proc Natl Acad Sci USA*. 1997;94:6954.

107.   Hogg N, Kalyanaraman B, Joseph J, Struck A, Parthasarathy S. Inhibition of low-density lipoprotein oxidation by nitric oxide: potential role in atherogenesis. *FEBS Lett*. 1993;334:170.

108.   Goss, SPA, Hogg N, Kalyanaraman B. The effect of nitric oxide release rates on the oxidation of human low density lipoprotein. *J Biol Chem*. 1997;272:21647.

109.   Jessup W, Mohr D, Gieseg SP, Dean RT, Stocker R. The participation of nitric oxide in cell free- and its restriction of macrophage-mediated oxidation of low-density lipoprotein. *Biochim Biophys Acta*. 1992;1180:73.

110.   Luoma JS, Strålin P, Marklund SL, Hiltunen TP, Särkioja T, Ylä-Herttuala. Expression of extracellular SOD and iNOS in macrophages and smooth muscle cells in human and rabbit atherosclerotic lesions: colocalization with epitopes characteristic of oxidized LDL and peroxynitrite-modified proteins. *Arterioscler Thromb Vasc Biol*. 1998;18:157.

111. Buttery LD, Springall DR, Chester AH, Evans TJ, Standfield EN, Parums DV, Yacoub MH, Polak JM. Inducible nitric oxide synthase is present within human atherosclerotic lesions and promotes the formation and activity of peroxynitrite. *Lab Invest.* 1996;75:77.

112. Khan J, Brennan DM, Bradley N, Gao B, Bruckdorfer R, Jacobs M. 3-Nitrotyrosine in the proteins of human plasma determined by an ELISA method. *Biochem J.* 1998;330:795.

113. Halliwell B. What nitrates tyrosine? Is nitrotyrosine specific as a biomarker of peroxynitrite formation in vivo? *FEBS Lett.* 1997;411:157.

114. Kettle AJ, van Dalen CJ, Winterbourn CC. Peroxynitrite and myeloperoxidase leave the same footprint in protein nitration. *Redox Rep.* 1997;3:257.

115. Eiserich JP, Hristova M, Cross CE, Jones AD, Freeman BA, Halliwell B, van der Vliet A. Formation of nitric oxide-derived inflammatory oxidants by myeloperoxidase in neutrophils. *Nature.* 1998;391:393.

116. Sampson JB, Ye YZ, Rosen H, Beckman JS. Myeloperoxidase and horseradish peroxidase catalyze tyrosine nitration in proteins from nitrite and hydrogen peroxide. *Arch Biochem Biophys.* 1998;356:207.

117. Heinecke JW. Pathways for oxidation of low density lipoprotein by myeloperoxidase: tyrosyl radical, reactive aldehydes, hypochlorous acid and molecular chlorine. *BioFactors.*1997;6:145.

118. Winterbourn CC. Neutrophil oxidants: production and reactions. In: Oxygen Radicals: Systemic Events and Disease Processes (eds. Das DK, Essman WB). Basel: S Karger AG, pp. 32-70, 1990.

119. Hazell LJ, Stocker R. Oxidation of low-density lipoprotein with hypochlorite causes transformation of the lipoprotein into a high-uptake form for macrophages. *Biochem J.* 1993;290:165.

120. Hazell LJ, van den Berg JJM, Stocker R. Oxidation of low-density lipoprotein by hypochlorite causes aggregation that is mediated by modification of lysine residues rather than lipid oxidation. *Biochem J.* 1994;302:297.

121. Jerlich A, Fabjan JS, Tschabuschnig S, Smirnova AV, Horakova L, Hayn M, Auer H, Guttenberger H, Leis H-J, Tatzber F, Waeg G, Schaur RJ. Human low density lipoprotein as a target of hypochlorite generated by myeloperoxidase. *Free Rad Biol Med.* 1998;24:1139.

122. Anderson MM, Hazen SL, Hsu FF, Heinecke JW. Human neutrophils employ the myeloperoxidase-hydrogen peroxide-chloride system to convert hydroxy-amino acids into glycolaldehyde, 2-hydroxypropanal, and acrolein. a mechanism for the generation of highly reactive α-hydroxy and α,β-unsaturated aldehydes by phagocytes at sites of inflammation. *J Clin Invest.* 1997;99:424.

123. Hazen SL, Crowley JR, Mueller DM, Heinecke JW. Mass spectrometric quantification of 3-chlorotyrosine in human tissues with attomole sensitivity: a sensitive and specific marker for myeloperoxidase-catalyzed chlorination at sites of inflammation. *Free Rad Biol Med.* 1997;23:909.

124. Panasenko OM. The mechanism of the hypochlorite-induced lipid peroxidation. *BioFactors.* 1997;6:181.

125. Hazen SL, Hsu FF, Duffin K, Heinecke JW. Molecular chlorine generated by the myeloperoxidase-hydrogen peroxide-chloride system of phagocytes converts low density lipoprotein cholesterol into a family of chlorinated sterols. *J Biol Chem.* 1996;271:23080.

126. Hawkins CL, Davies MJ. Degradation of hyaluronic acid, poly- and mono-saccharides, and model compounds by hypochlorite: evidence for radical intermediates and fragmentation. *Free Rad Biol Med.* 1998;24:1396.

127. Wieland E, Brandes A, Armstrong VW, Oellerich M. Oxidative modification of low density lipoproteins by human polymorphonuclear leukocytes. *Eur J Clin Chem Clin Biochem.* 1993;31:725.

128. Katsura M, Forster LA, Ferns GAA, Änggård EE. Oxidative modification of low-density lipoprotein by human polymorphonuclear leucocytes to a form recognised by the lipoprotein scavenger pathway. *Biochim Biophys Acta.* 1994;1213:231.

129. Cathcart MK, Morel DW, Chisolm GM III. Monocytes and neutrophils oxidize low density lipoprotein making it cytotoxic. J Leukoc Biol 1985;38:341-350.

130. Tanabe F, Sato A, Ito M, Ishida E, Ogata M, Shigeta S. Low-density lipoprotein oxidized by polymorphonuclear leukocytes inhibits natural killer cell activity. *J Leukoc Biol.* 1988;43:204.

131.   Scaccini C, Jialal I.   LDL modification by activated polymorphonuclear leukocytes: a cellular model of mild oxidative stress. *Free Rad Biol Med.* 1994;16:49.

132.   Savenkova MI, Mueller DM, Heinecke JW. Tyrosyl radical generated by myeloperoxidase is a physiological catalyst for the initiation of lipid peroxidation in low density lipoprotein. *J Biol Chem.* 1994;269:20394.

133.   Jacob JS, Cistola DP, Hsu FF, Muzaffar S, Mueller DM, Hazen SL, Heinecke JW. Human phagocytes employ the myeloperoxidase-hydrogen peroxide system to synthesize dityrosine, trityrosine, pulcherosine, and isodityrosine by a tyrosyl radical-dependent pathway. *J Biol Chem.* 1996;271:19950.

134.   Hazen SL, Hsu FF, Heinecke JW. *p*-Hydroxyphenylacetaldehyde is the major product of L-tyrosine oxidation by activated human phagocytes: a chloride-dependent mechanism for the conversion of free amino acids into reactive aldehydes by myeloperoxidase. *J Biol Chem.* 1996;271:1861.

135.   Hazen SL, Gaut JP, Hsu FF, Crowley JR, d'Avignon A, Heinecke JW.   *p*-Hydroxyphenylacetaldehyde, the major product of L-tyrosine oxidation by the myeloperoxidase-H_2O_2-chloride system of phagocytes, covalently modifies ε-amino groups of protein lysine residues. *J Biol Chem.* 1997;272;16990.

136.   Daugherty A, Dunn JL, Rateri DL, Heinecke JW. Myeloperoxidase, a catalyst for lipoprotein oxidation, is expressed in human atherosclerotic lesions. *J Clin Invest.* 1994;94:437.

137.   Malle E, Hazell L, Stocker R, Sattler W, Esterbauer H, Waeg G. Immunologic detection and measurement of hypochlorite-modified LDL with specific monoclonal antibodies. *Arterioscler Thromb Vasc Biol.* 1995;15:982.

138.   Hazell LJ, Arnold L, Flowers D, Waeg G, Malle E, Stocker R. Presence of hypochlorite-modified proteins in human atherosclerotic lesions. *J Clin Invest.* 1996;97:1535.

139   Hazen SL, Heinecke JW. 3-Chlorotyrosine, a specific marker of myeloperoxidase-catalyzed oxidation, is markedly elevated in low density lipoprotein isolated from human atherosclerotic intima. *J Clin Invest.* 1997;99:2075.

140.   Suarna C, Dean RT, May J, Stocker R. Human atherosclerotic plaque contains both oxidized lipids and relatively large amounts of α-tocopherol and ascorbate. *Arterioscler Thromb Vasc Biol.* 1995;15:1616.

6 OXIDIZED PHOSPHOLIPIDS AS MEDIATORS OF VASCULAR DISEASE

Sean Davies, Thomas McIntyre, Stephen Prescott and Guy Zimmerman

INTRODUCTION

Atherosclerosis has been thought to be an inevitable consequence of aging, but progress in understanding the molecular and pathological basis of this vascular disease through the work of Brown and Goldstein (1) has made it clear that this need not be the case. Specific risk factors for this disease exist, and these elucidate general mechanisms underlying this disease. For example, failure to adequately remove plasma cholesterol in the form of low-density lipoprotein (LDL) from the bloodstream, due to mutations in the LDL receptor, leads to high concentration of plasma LDL that is sufficient to cause the disease. Other work (2) demonstrated that LDL underwent oxidative modification to generate particles that were more effective in causing pathological effects. Elevated levels of LDL promoted this pathologic change. Ross proposed a "response-to-injury" model of atherosclerosis (3), where damage to the vessel wall initiated the disease. A refined version of this model recognizes that the early steps in atherogenesis need not necessarily be initiated by the cytotoxicity of oxidized LDL, but rather by activation of an inflammatory response in vascular tissue. Oxidation inappropriately stimulates the normal inflammatory response of endothelial cells and leukocytes. Activation of this normally tightly regulated inflammatory response program, by factors which themselves are not well regulated, (i.e. oxidation of LDL by uncontrolled chemical reactions) leads to chronic, unregulated inflammation of the vascular wall. Such a chronic inflammatory process remodels the vessel wall, drives plaque formation, and destabilizes plaque structures, all key events in atherosclerosis.

To understand the basis of atherosclerosis, it is necessary to understand inflammation and in particular, the role of endothelial cells in determining the site, type, and magnitude of leukocyte activation. The field of inflammation has undergone tremendous advances in the last twenty years and a paradigm for the molecular basis of endothelial cell and leukocyte interaction is now well established. Extension of the paradigm from acute to chronic inflammation suggests the thesis summarized in this chapter: that oxidation of LDL produces modified phospholipids which are capable of activating leukocytes, endothelial cells, and smooth muscle cells.   Because the production of these oxidatively modified phospholipid occurs an unregulated manner, the acute inflammation produced is not rapidly turned off, generating chronic inflammation which leads to atherogenesis.

P-SELECTIN, PAF, AND INTEGRINS: A GENERAL PARADIGM FOR INFLAMMATION

The general paradigm for inflammation worked out over the last twenty years has identified adhesion proteins and paracrine molecules such as platelet-activating factor (PAF) which play a key role in the activation of endothelial cells and leukocytes.   Animal models where these molecules have been knocked-out or inhibited demonstrate that they also play a critical role in atherosclerosis. Oxidative stress can activate expression of these adhesion molecules and produce oxidatively modified phospholipids which mimic PAF, thereby producing the chronic inflammation which results in atherosclerosis.

Identification of Molecules Required for Acute Inflammatory Responses

Identification of the molecules and mechanisms that result in the coordinated activation of endothelial cells and leukocytes used an *ex vivo* model system of freshly isolated human umbilical vein endothelial cells (HUVEC), peripheral blood polymorphonuclear leukocytes (PMN) and monocytes. All of the elements defined in this system have now been validated in animal models of inflammation (4-8). These experiments demonstrated that regulated adhesion of leukocytes requires responses from both the endothelial cell and the leukocyte (Figure 1). Endothelial cells regulate the location, and identity of the responding cell type as well as magnitude of leukocyte activation.

Endothelial cells stimulated with rapidly acting agonists such as thrombin, histamine, or leukotriene C_4 acquire a surface that is adhesive for polymorphonuclear (PMN) leukocytes (9-12). This response begins within seconds, peaks between 5 to 15 minutes, and is resolved 30 to 60 minutes after exposure to the agonist.   The complete response requires the regulated expression of two molecules by the endothelial cell, and a subsequent response from the PMN leukocytes.   Stimulated endothelial cells translocate P-selectin, a member of the selectin family, from intracellular Weibel-Palade bodies (13) – endothelial cell-specific storage vesicles- to the plasma membrane, where it serves as a leukocyte tether by binding to P-selectin glycoprotein ligand-1 (PSGL-1) constitutively expressed on quiescent leukocytes (14-16).   This calcium-dependent lectin interaction with its sialylated target is characterized by rapid on and off interaction rates (17). In experiments using either purified P-selectin or Chinese hamster ovary (CHO) cells transfected with cDNA for P-selectin, we found that this interaction tethers the two cells together but is, by itself, insufficient to completely activate the PMN leukocytes (18). However, in response to the same stimuli and with the same time course, endothelial cells synthesize PAF (19).   This biologically active phospholipid has diverse actions (see below), but in this context induces leukocytes to activate their adhesive program. This includes activation of their own adhesion molecules (the β_2 integrins), development of the polarized morphology required for directed migration, and priming for enhanced responses to other stimuli. P-selectin and PAF are required for maximal adhesion of PMN leukocytes to endothelial cells, and the two molecules act cooperatively (19). The sum effect is a transfer of information from endothelial cell to circulating leukocytes and induction of an activated state.

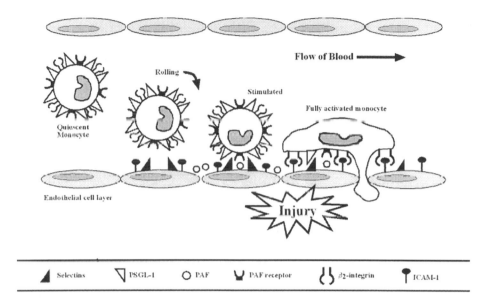

Figure 1. Stimulation of endothelial cells by vascular injury leads to display of P-selectin, E-selectin, and ICAM-1 on endothelial surface. Monocytes loosely adhere to P-selectin via P-selectin glycoprotein ligand (PSGL-1) and are juxtaposed to endothelial cell derived PAF. Activation of PAF receptor on monocyte leads to upregulation of integrins and tight adherence to intracellular adhesion molecule-1 (ICAM-1), allowing the monocyte to penetrate into the subendothelial space.

The General Paradigm For Inflammation Allows For Tight Regulation

This two-step adhesion and activation process has several advantages. First, the initiating signal is fixed in space so that leukocytes are recruited precisely where they are needed. Second, the initial tethering to the vessel wall without activation allows an editing step by the leukocyte. Leukocytes brought into close proximity to the vessel wall scan the endothelium for an activating signal. If one is present, the leukocytes are activated and their integrins dramatically augment the adhesive response. If no activator is present, the leukocyte can release from the tether due to the rapid off rate of selectin-ligand interactions, and re-enter the circulation without having undergone activation-dependent responses which would be detrimental should they occur in the circulation. This tethering is the molecular basis for the rolling of leukocytes on the endothelium that has been observed *in vivo* (20, 21). Third, the tethering effect of P-selectin provides specificity to the adhesive interaction because receptors for P-selectin are present on PMN leukocytes and monocytes but not on most lymphocytes or platelets (15,22). In contrast, platelets have PAF receptors and potentially could adhere to activated endothelium if there were no requirement for tethering by P-selectin. Finally, the P-selectin and β_2-integrin-dependent mechanisms of adhesion may operate to different extents under different conditions to fine-tune this cell-cell interaction. We have proposed that this two-step binding response is an example of juxtacrine activation, a term originally used to describe activation of target cells by membrane-anchored growth factors.

This two-step paradigm, defined through rapidly activated PMN leukocytes-endothelial cell responses, appears to be generally applicable to leukocyte-endothelial responses. Endothelial cells respond to more slowly activating agonists such as tumor necrosis factor (TNF) or interleukin-1 (IL-1) by synthesizing and expressing a number of leukocyte adhesion molecules such as E-selectin (23), ICAM-1, vascular cell adhesion molecule-1 (VCAM-1), and endothelial-leukocyte adhesion molecule-1 (ELAM-1). In each instance, a co-expressed activating signal also is required, and again the type of leukocyte recruited to its surface can be modulated by the agonist synthesized from the activated endothelial cell. Endothelial cells also release monocyte chemotactic protein-1 (MCP-1) after stimulation with the longer, more slowly acting agonists mentioned above (24). MCP-1 is chemotactic for monocytes and certain other inflammatory cells and thereby maximizes the response for these cells over other leukocytes.

Parallels between adhesion molecules important for acute inflammation those required for the chronic inflammation present in atherosclerosis are evident in experimental models of atherosclerosis. P-selectin expression increases in endothelium overlying atherosclerotic plaque (25). Antibodies to P-selectin attenuate ischemia/reperfusion injury in several animal models (26,27). In mouse models of atherosclerosis, the combined absence of P-selectin and E-selectin (28), of P-selectin and ICAM-1 (29), or of ICAM-1 and β_2-integrins, is associated with significantly less disease progression. Antibodies to both β_2-integrins and ICAM-1 significantly reduce lesion formation (30). Clearly then, expression of adhesion molecules is important for atherogenesis, and conditions which lead to inappropriate expression of these molecules are likely to contribute to atherosclerosis.

PLATELET-ACTIVATING FACTOR

Just as the adhesion molecules that participate in acute inflammation are also important in chronic inflammatory diseases, PAF and its receptor participate in both acute and chronic inflammation. Regulation of the inflammatory response is critical to protect against disease and platelet activating factor (PAF) plays a central role in the activation of granulocytes, monocytes, and platelets (Table 1). PAF synthesis, expression, release, and degradation are carefully regulated to prevent inappropriate stimulation of leukocytes, that can have pathological effects.

Table 1. *In vitro* effects of Platelet-Activating Factor (PAF)

RESPONSE	REFERENCES
MONOCYTE	
Aggregation	31
Complement-dependent phagocytosis	32
Tumor cell killing	33
TNF release	34
TNF release	35
Enhanced cytokine production by LPS-stimulated cells	36
Leukotriene synthesis	37
Fcε RII/CD23 expression	38
Adhesion to endothelial cells	39
MONOCYTE-DERIVED MACROPHAGE	
O_2 radical generation	40
PMN LEUKOCYTES	
Aggregation	41
Chemotaxis	41
Adhesion to endothelium	10
Degranulation	41-44
Priming of fMLP-dependent O_2 radical generation	45
PLATELET	
Histamine release	46
Aggregation	47
SMOOTH MUSCLE CELLS	
Enhancement of PDGF-induced proliferation	48
Proliferation	49

PAF is a potent inflammatory mediator, and was the first phospholipid identified to act in this role. PAF was originally described as a fluid-phase mediator (46) released from stimulated rabbit basophils that induced platelet activation; hence the origin of its trivial name. Independently, a polar lipid derived from kidney that lowered blood pressure was described (50) and these lines of investigation merged when the structure of the compound responsible for both responses was shown to be 1-*O*-alkyl-2-acetyl-*sn*-glycero-3-phosphocholine (51).

PAF is not stored, and is produced only when cells possessing the capability to synthesize it are appropriately stimulated (52). There are two known routes leading to PAF synthesis. The principal synthetic route in activated endothelial cells, PMN leukocytes, and monocytes is known as the remodeling pathway (53). The first step requires (54) a stimulated phospholipase A_2 that catalyzes the hydrolysis of the *sn-2* fatty acid from alkylcholinephosphoglycerides. This yields an intermediate, 1-*O*-alkyl-*sn*-glycero-3-phospholcholine (lysoPAF), and a free fatty acid. In the second step of the remodeling pathway, lysoPAF is converted to PAF by the addition of an acetyl residue, a reaction catalyzed by a specific acetylcoenzyme A:lysoPAF acetyltransferase that has yet to be molecularly identified. Both synthetic steps in the pathway are regulated by phosphorylation (55-57), a feature that implies tight control of the synthesis and accumulation of PAF in activated cells.

PAF acts via specific receptors expressed on the surface membranes of responsive cells. Receptors have been described on platelets, PMN leukocytes, monocytes, macrophages, eosinophils, basophils, and in brain and lung tissues (58). Honda *et al* (59) cloned a PAF receptor from guinea pig lung, and subsequently the human leukocyte PAF receptor was cloned (60-62). The 1.8 kb human PAF receptor cDNA encodes a 342 amino acid residue protein with a calculated Mr of 39,203. The human receptor shares 83% identity with its the guinea pig counterpart, and both possess seven putative membrane spanning domains. The human PAF receptor has two 5'-noncoding exons with distinct transcription initiation sites and promoters. These exons are alternatively spliced to a common splice acceptor site on exon 3 (58) with leukocytes solely expressing transcript 1. The PAF receptor is stereospecific, and binding studies with recombinant receptors demonstrate a K_d between 10^{-10} and 10^{-9} M that correlates well with PAF-stimulated functional responses in whole cells (61,63). The PAF receptor recognizes phospholipids other than 1-*O*-alkyl-2-acetyl-*sn*-glycero-3-phosphocholine, but for the most part with greatly reduced affinity. Analogs in which the *sn-1* ether linkage is replaced by an ester bond reduce binding affinity by 300-500-fold (64). Replacing the *sn-2* acetyl residue with acyl residues containing greater than five carbons essentially eliminates specific binding. Conversion of the choline headgroup to ethanolamine reduces binding by approximately 4000-fold.

Binding of PAF to its receptor can be blocked by numerous, chemically diverse (65) competitive antagonists, and these include many compounds without any discernable structural relationship to PAF. Nevertheless, several of these antagonists have proven to be remarkably specific: They do not interfere with other seven transmembrane spanning receptors, and this remains true for agents (*e.g.* WEB 2086) that were described over a decade ago (66). These first generation antagonists have not been effective in ameliorating human disease conditions in clinical trials (67-69). These antagonists are, however, considerably less efficient than PAF in binding to the receptor. As a consequence, the effective concentration of an antagonist in the fluid phase, or at the cell surface under conditions of juxtacrine activation by PAF, must be much higher than that of PAF itself to partially or completely inhibit biological responses. Thus, effective inhibition is not readily achieved with antagonists that possess only modest affinity for the PAF receptor. New agents with a high affinity for the PAF receptor do function well in animal models and asthmatic patients. (70,71)

PAF rapidly and potently induces alterations in the adhesive properties of leukocytes. It stimulates inside-out signaling of β_2-integrins (a qualitative alteration involving a change in affinity and clustering that makes the integrins competent to bind ligands) (72), and it causes a quantitative increase in the surface expression of β_2 heterodimers including $\alpha_M\beta_2$ (73,74). The integrins $\alpha_L\beta_2$ and $\alpha_M\beta_2$ on PAF-stimulated PMN leukocytes mediate adhesion to endothelial cells (75-77), and $\alpha_M\beta_2$ integrin also mediates PMN-PMN aggregation as well as adhesion to the subendothelial matrix (78).

PAF stimulates both degranulation and generation of active O_2 metabolites by human PMN leukocytes (41,43,44), two effector responses that are important in both physiologic and pathologic inflammation. The threshold concentrations of PAF required for degranulation are higher than those that induce adhesive responses, usually in the 100 nM range. Thus, PAF is most potent as an agonist for adhesion-dependent functions, inducing such responses at subnanomolar threshold concentrations. Conversely, it has intermediate potency as an agonist for degranulation depending on the marker used, and is a very weak agonist for oxygen radical generation (52).

PAF also induces the production of cytokines, such as TNF and MCP-1 by monocytes (35,79). It does so most effectively when the monocytes are adherent, for example to P-selectin expressed on platelets, transfected cells, or presented in purified immobilized form. This activity of PAF would be germane following PMN leukocyte adhesion to the P-selectin of activated endothelial cells, suggesting that while endothelial cells regulate the location of leukocyte activation, they could also regulate the inflammatory program of leukocytes as well. The net result of the integration of signals from the PAF receptor and from adhesion molecules is to convert transient signals and interactions into a sustained, well-directed inflammatory response (80).

OXIDATION OF CELLULAR AND CIRCULATING PHOSPHOLIPIDS GENERATE BIOLOGICALLY-ACTIVE MEDIATORS

In contrast to the regulated and directed inflammatory response outlined in the proceeding section, oxidative stress can generate dysregulated inflammation by inducing expression of adhesion molecules and by producing oxidized phospholipids which mimic PAF. The oxidative stress which produces such a response represents a failure to maintain homeostasis and therefore a failure in regulation. The products of this oxidative state are therefore themselves unregulated and can create pathological inflammation. An example of how oxidative stress can generate pathological inflammation is the role of LDL oxidation in atherosclerosis. Oxidation of LDL blocks its interaction with the LDL receptor, creates new binding motifs for scavenger receptors, and results in new bioactivities (Table 2). A number of the many new biologic effects of oxidized LDL are similar to those evoked by PAF, suggesting the thesis summarized here that oxidation of LDL produces oxidatively modified phospholipids that mimic the actions of PAF, and produce their effects through the PAF receptor.

Oxidation of phospholipid and cholesteryl ester unsaturated fatty acyl residues in either lipoprotein particles or cell membranes may generate compounds that activate several classes of lipid receptors and, as a consequence, trigger potentially deleterious inflammatory responses. Activation of the PAF receptor by oxidized phospholipids is among the best characterized of these pathologic responses and is closely allied with inflammation. However, other classes of oxidized lipids may also contribute to the overall response to phospholipid oxidation (81).

Table 2. Selected effects of oxidized LDL, including copper-, endothelial cell-, and minimally oxidized LDL on various cell types.

RESPONSE	REFERENCE
MONOCYTE	
Adhesion	82
Secretion of γIFN, IL-1	83,84
Tissue Factor expression	85
Increased thrombomodulin expression	86
Chemotaxis	87
Differentiation to macrophages	88
MACROPHAGES	
MCP-1 secretion	89
IL-1 secretion	90
PLATELET	
Aggregation	91, 92
T LYMPHOCYTES	
Chemotaxis	93
γIFN secretion, proliferation	94
ENDOTHELIAL CELLS	
ICAM-1 Expression	95
VCAM-1, ICAM-1, ELAM-1 expression	96,97
P-Selectin expression	98
MCP-1 secretion	99,100
SMOOTH MUSCLE CELLS	
Proliferation	101,102
PDGF production	103,104

Oxidation Of Phospholipids Generates PAF Receptor Agonists

Ozonelysis and reductive workup of 1-palmitoyl-2-arachidonyl-*sn*-glycero-3-phosphocholine (PAPC) results in 1-palmitoyl-2-(5-oxovaleroyl)-*sn*-glycero-3-phosphocholine (105). We tested this oxidation product, along with those produced by treatment of PAPC with soybean-lipoxygenase and subsequent exposure to air, for their ability to activate the PAF receptor on PMN leukocytes (106). At phosphate concentrations of 2.6-10 μM, these PAPC oxidation products induced PMN leukocytes adhesion to an immobilized ligand for β_2-integrins to an extent equivalent to that of 100 nM PAF. This adhesion was completely inhibited by preincubation of the PMN leukocytes with PAF receptor antagonists, and by preincubation of the oxidized PAPC with PAF acetylhydrolase (a phospholipase specific for PAF and oxidized phospholipids – see below). Thus the oxidation of phospholipids can produce compounds that mimic the actions of PAF because they are ligands for the PAF receptor. Oxidation of PAPC results in many fragmented and oxidized compounds (107) and results in phosphatidylcholines with short monocarboxylate, aldehydes, and dicarboxylate *sn-2* residues (Figure 2). Some of these fragmentation products have sufficiently short chains that they meet the stringent structural requirements of the PAF receptor, which requires short acyl chains at the sn-2 position for activity. The PAF receptor prefers alkylacyl phospholipids, but is promiscuous enough to accept diacyl phospholipids, although with a 300-500-fold lesser affinity.

Patel *et al* (108) demonstrated that the exposure of human umbilical vein endothelial cells (HUVEC) to H_2O_2, *t*-butyl hydroperoxide (*t*-BuOOH), or menadione induced 2-3 fold increase in PMN leukocytes adhesion. This was primarily due to P-selectin expression. Hydrogen peroxide induced the synthesis of PAF, although at levels less than that induced by thrombin and with a slower time course and the adhesion of PMN leukocytes to HUVEC could be blocked by a PAF receptor antagonist. In contrast to exposure to the water-soluble H_2O_2, exposure to the lipid soluble *t*-BuOOH did not induce PAF synthesis. However, similar concentrations of *t*-BuOOH did result in the formation of leukocyte agonists, and this activity (109) was blocked by a PAF receptor antagonist and by pretreatment with phospholipase C. As already noted, *t*-BuOOH treatment did not result in the synthesis of PAF, furthermore treatment with diisopropylfluorophosphate, which inhibits PAF synthesis, actually enhanced HUVEC secretion of the PMN leukocytes adhesion inducing factor (likely as a result of the inhibition of PAF acetylhydrolase). The adhesion-promoting activity from *t*-BuOOH treated endothelial cell supernatants migrates on TLC like PAF, but RP-HPLC produced two peaks, both of which eluted after authentic PAF. Together, these observations suggest that *t*-BuOOH exposed endothelial cells did not synthesize PAF, but rather produced a PAF-like lipid through the oxidation of endothelial cell lipids.

Diacyl phospholipids make up the overwhelming majority of cellular membrane and plasma phospholipids (110,111), and would therefore be expected to make up the majority of oxidized phospholipids created during exposure of membranes or lipoprotein particles to high levels of free radicals. For instance, Watson *et al* (112)

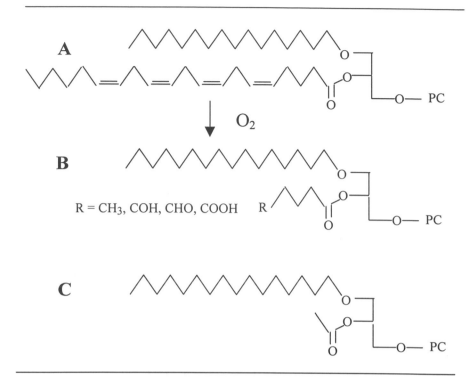

Figure 2 The oxidation of phosphatidylcholine generates compounds with structural similarities to Platelet-Activating Factor. **A.** 1-Hexadecyl -2-arachidonyl-*sn*-glycero-3-phosphocholine (HAPC). **B.** Oxidation of HAPC generates fragmented PC, typically with hydroxyl, aldehydic, or acid moieties. **C**. Authentic Platelet-Activating Factor.

have shown that the previously mentioned 1-palmitoyl-2-(5-oxovaleroyl)-*sn*-glycero-3-phosphocholine is one of the components of oxidized LDL that induces monocyte adherence to endothelial cells.

Although high micromolar concentrations were required for this activity, it was completely inhibited by the PAF receptor antagonist WEB 2086 (113). In contrast, oxidation of lipid extracts from bovine brain (114) and from krill (115), sources rich in alkylacyl phospholipids, creates oxidized phospholipids that activate the PAF receptor at much lower concentrations than required for oxidized diacyl lipids. Oxidation of alkylacyl phosphatidylcholines is not fundamentally different from that of diacyl phosphatidylcholines, and produce homologous oxidation products (116,117). Oxidation of semi-synthetic alkylacyl PC with unsaturated *sn*-2 residues showed that the oxidation products were about 1000-fold more potent than diacyl homologs (Authors' unpublished data).   While alkylacyl phosphatidylcholines typically constitute only about 1% of the total phospholipids present in most tissue, their potency suggests they may contribute to the PAF-like bioactivity produced during oxidation.

To test this directly, we determined whether the phospholipid fraction of oxidized LDL (oxLDL), which we had previously shown to contain PAF-like activity (49), would be degraded by PLA$_1$ treatment. Since only diacyl phospholipids would be destroyed during this process, the remaining PAF-like activity should be due to oxidized alkylacyl phospholipids. Incubation with phospholipase A$_1$ for 18 hours degraded nearly 99% of the phospholipid mass present in oxidized LDL, but did not significantly decrease the PAF-like activity present (Authors' unpublished data). Thus rare LDL phospholipids are precursors for the PAF-like lipids generated during LDL oxidation.

Biologically Active Oxidized Phospholipids Are Produced *In Vivo*

Together, the studies summarized above indicate that *in vitro* oxidation of LDL or intact cells generates phospholipid products with significant biological activity, but can such products ever be formed *in vivo* where intact antioxidant defenses protect against their formation? To examine this issue, we searched for a relevant pathophysiologic model where free radicals and oxidants are known to accumulate. An insult that fits this criteria is the oxidant stress caused by cigarette smoking where it is estimated that a single puff contains 5 nmoles of radicals (118). Furthermore, cigarette smoking is a major risk factor for atherogenesis (119). Hamsters exposed to cigarette smoke, like hamsters exposed to oxidized LDL (120), demonstrate a rapid, system-wide inflammatory response: there is rapid leukocyte adhesion to the systemic vascular wall and formation of intravascular leukocyte-platelet aggregates. These events use the components of physiologic inflammation; PAF receptor antagonists and anti-P-selectin antibody inhibit this effect. To determine if PAF or oxidized phospholipids were the mediators, lipid extracts from the plasma of hamsters exposed or unexposed to smoke were separated by HPLC where PAF-like bioactivity could be resolved from authentic PAF. This separation demonstrated that inflammatory mediators were present in the circulation of smoke-exposed animals, and that there were indeed PAF-like lipids. Importantly, dietary supplementation with vitamin C prevented the accumulation of PAF-like lipids in smoke-exposed animals. This not only shows the presence of PAF-like lipids is the direct result of oxidant stress, it suggests a way that antioxidants including dietary Vitamin C and E can inhibit atherogenesis (121,122). Further evidence that PAF-like oxidized phospholipids can be formed *in vivo* comes from the identification of 1-palmitoyl-2-(5-oxovaleroyl)-*sn*-glycero-3-phosphocholine and 1-palmitoyl-2-glutaryl-*sn*-glycero-3-phosphocholine in the atherosclerotic lesions of cholesterol fed rabbits (112). Oxidized phospholipid that activate the PAF receptor ligands may also play a role in ischemia/reperfusion injury because PAF receptor antagonists (123-128) inhibit the extent of injury in animal models.

In summary, the oxidation of cellular and lipoprotein phospholipids generate compounds which can activate the PAF receptor both *in vitro* and *in vivo*. Activation of the PAF receptor by these unregulated agonists stimulates monocytes and other leukocytes inappropriately, leading to pathological inflammation. The anti-atherogenic effects of anti-oxidants may be mediated by inhibiting the formation of these PAF-like compounds.

Lysophosphatidylcholine (lysoPC) is also generated during LDL oxidation

One of the major byproducts of phospholipid oxidation is lysoPC. LysoPC represents about 3.2% of the choline glycerophospholipids present in native LDL (110), but the oxidation of LDL increases this by 5 to 10 fold (129,130). LysoPC is also a product of the hydrolysis of oxidized phospholipid by PAF acetylhydrolase (49,107), an enzyme which associates with LDL (131). If this enzyme is not inhibited during mild oxidation of LDL, lysoPC is produced by virtue of the general increase in suitable substrates for the enzyme.

While no lysoPC receptor has been identified to date, lysoPC has been shown to have a number of specific effects including the chemotaxis of monocytes and T-lymphocytes (132), the induction of PDGF and FGF synthesis (133), the inhibition of nitric oxide synthesis and impairment of arterial relaxation (129), and the induction of smooth muscle cell proliferation (134). LysoPC has been reported to activate the PAF receptor (135), but a possible caveat to this result is that commercial preparation of lysoPC often contain trace amounts of PAF (authors' unpublished data). Whether the lysoPC produced by the oxidation of LDL plays a critical role in the effects of oxLDL is uncertain. Because about 150 µM lysoPC is already present in human plasma (136,137) and because 10-50 µM lysoPC typically induces *in vitro* responses, whether the relatively small increases in plasma lysoPC levels due to LDL oxidation generates significant biological activity seems doubtful.

PAF Acetylhydrolase Metabolizes Oxidized Phospholipids

PAF-acetylhydrolase is a substrate-specific phospholipase A_2 that converts the highly potent PAF to the considerably less active products lysoPAF and acetate. Stafforini *et al* (138) purified the LDL-associated PAF acetylhydrolase from human plasma and found plasma PAF acetylhydrolase has an apparent molecular weight of 43,000, does not require calcium, has preference for micellar versus monomeric substrate, and exhibits surface dilution kinetics (where substrate abundance at a surface, the phospholipid shell of lipoprotein particles for instance and not absolute concentration determine reaction rates.) The purified protein has an apparent K_m of 13.7 µM and a V_{max} of 568 µmol/h/mg with micellar PAF. It can act both on 1-O-alkyl and 1-acyl substrates and on ethanolamine analogs of PAF. However, the enzyme has a marked preference for the *sn-2* acetyl residue of PAF and can be considered as a specific PAF-acetylhydrolase as it can not hydrolyze long chain diacyl phosphatidylcholine.

Plasma PAF acetylhydrolase also degrades oxidized phospholipids. To identify potential substrates, we synthesized phosphatidylcholines with *sn-2* residues ranging from two to nine carbon atoms long, and found the V/k catalytic efficiency ratio rapidly decreased as the *sn-2* residue was lengthened: the C5 homologue was hydrolyzed 50%, the C6 20%, while the C9 homologue only 2% as efficiently as PAF. However, the presence of an omega-oxo function in the *sn-2* residue radically affected hydrolysis: the half-life of the *sn-2* 9-aldehydic homologue was identical to that of PAF (107). Hence PAF acetylhydrolase not only limits inflammation by degrading PAF, but can also protect against pathological inflammation by degrading oxidized phospholipids that are biologically-active, chemically reactive, or both.

Families with deficiencies in PAF acetylhydrolase activity have been identified in the Japanese population (139) at a high frequency—4% lack enzyme activity and 27% have only 50% of normal activity. This PAF acetylhydrolase deficiency is largely due to a Val279-Phe mutation near the active site of the enzyme (140). These families have a significantly higher risk for asthma, and the prevalence of the mutant gene is significantly higher in stroke patients (43.4%) compared to age/sex matched control patients (25.4%) (141). Mutation of glycine residue 994 of PAF acetylhydrolase to threonine has also been reported as an independent risk for coronary artery disease in Japanese men (142). It is therefore clear that the ability to eliminate PAF and oxidized phospholipid in a timely manner via PAF acetylhydrolase may be significant to the prevention of atherosclerosis.

SUMMARY

Advances in the understanding of atherosclerosis have led to a model that implicates chronic inflammation in the earliest as well as latter stages of the disease. The adhesion and activation of leukocytes by endothelial cell expression of PAF and P-selectin is a model of inflammation, which is relevant to atherosclerosis. Oxidative stress activates endothelial cells to express P-selectin on their surface, and results in the oxidation of LDL and cellular lipids. Oxidation of LDL leads to the formation of PAF-like lipids, which induce leukocyte adhesion, activation, and the secretion of inflammatory cytokines, thereby triggering a pathological response.

REFERENCES

1.   Brown MS, Goldstein JL. Lipoprotein metabolism in the macrophage: Implications for cholesterol deposition in atherosclerosis. *Ann Rev Biochem.* 1983;52:223.
2.   Steinberg D. Low density lipoprotein oxidation and its pathobiological significance. *J Biol Chem.* 1997;272:20963.
3.   Ross R. The pathogenesis of atherosclerosis – an update. *N Engl J Med.* 1986;314:488.
4.   Zimmerman GA, McIntyre TM, Prescott SM. Perspectives series: Cell adhesion in vascular biology. *J Clin Invest.* 1996;98:1699.
5.   McEver RP. Leukocyte-endothelial cell interactions. *Cur Opin Cell Biol.* 1992;4:840.
6.   McEver RP. Selectins. *Curr Opin Immunol.* 1994:6:75.
7.   Kubes P, Ibbotson G, Russell J, Wallace JL, Granger DN. Role of platelet-activating factor in ishemia/reperfusion-induced leukocyte adherence. *Am J Physiol.* 1990;259:G300.
8.   Shimizu Y, Newman W, Tanaka Y, Shaw S. Lymphocyte interactions with endothelial cells. *Immunology Today.* 1992;13:106.
9.   Zimmerman GA, McIntyre TM, Prescott SM. Thrombin stimulates the adherence of neutrophils to human endothelial cells *in vitro. J Clin Invest.* 1985;76:2235.
10.   Zimmerman GA, McIntyre TM, Mehra M, Prescott SM. Endothelial cell-associated platelet-activating factor: A novel mechanism for signaling intercellular adhesion. *J Cell Biol.* 1990;110:529.
11.   Geng J-G, Bevilacqua MP, Moore KL, McIntyre TM, Prescott SM, Kim JM, Bliss GA, Zimmerman GA, McEver RP. Rapid neutrophil adhesion to activated endothelium mediated by GMP-140. *Nature.* 1990;343:757.

12.   Sugama Y, Tiruppathi C, Offakidevi K, Andersen TT, Fenton JW, Malik AB. Thrombin-induced expression of endothelial P-selectin and intercellular adhesion molecule-1: a mechanism for stabilizing neutrophil adhesion. *J Cell Biol.* 1992;119:935.
13.   McEver RP. Beckstead JH, Moore KL, Marshall-Carlson L, Bainton DF. GMP-140, a platelet α-granule membrane protein, is also synthesized by vascular endothelial cells and is localized in Weibel-Palade bodies. *J Clin Invest.* 1989;84:92.
14.   Zhou Q, Moore KL, Smith DF, Varki A, McEver RP, Cummings RD. The selectin GMP-140 binds to sialylated, fucosylated lactosaminoglycans on both myeloid and nonmyeloid cells. *J Cell Biol.* 1991;115:557.
15.   Moore KL, Stults NL, Diaz S, Smith DF, Cummings RD, Varki A, McEver RP. Identification of a specific glycoprotein ligand for P-selectin (CD62) on myeloid cells. *J Cell Biol.* 1992;118:445.
16.   Norgard KE, Moore KL, Diaz S, Stults NL, Ushiyama S, McEver RP, Cummings RD, Varki A. Characterization of a specific ligand for P-selectin on myeloid cells. *J Biol Chem.* 1993;268:12764.
17.   Geng J-G, Moore KL, Johnson AE, McEver RP. Neutrophil recognition requires a Ca^{2+}-induced conformational change in the lectin domain of GMP-140. *J Biol Chem.* 1991;266:22313.
18.   Lorant DE, Tophan MK, Whatley RE, McEver RP, McIntyre TM, Prescott SM, Zimmerman GA. Inflammatory roles of P-selectin. *J Clin Invest.* 1993;92:559.
19.   Lorant DE, Patel KD, McIntyre TM, McEver RP, Prescott SM, Zimmerman GA. Coexpression of GMP-140 and PAF by endothelium stimulated by histamine or thrombin: a juxtacrine system for adhesion and activation of neutrophils. *J Cell Biol.* 1991;115:223.
20.   Allison F Jr., Smith MR, Wood WB Jr. The inflammatory reaction to thermal injury as observed in the rabbit ear chamber. *J Expl Med.* 1955;102:655.
21.   Moore KL, Patel KD, Bruehl RE, Fugang L, Johnson DA, Lichenstein HS, Cummings RD, Bainton DF, McEver RP. P-selectin glycoprotein ligand-1 mediates rolling of human neutrophils on P-selectin. *J Cell Biol.* 1995;128:661.
22.   Lenter M, Levinovitz A, Isenmann S, Vestweber D. Monospecific and common glycoprotein ligands for E- and P-selectin on myeloid cells. *J Cell Biol.* 1994;125:471.
23.   Bevilacqua MP, Johnston GI, Gimbrone MA Jr., McEver RP. Endothelial-leukocyte adhesion molecule-1 (ELAM-1) and granule membrane protein 140 (GMP-140) define a new family of inducible lectin-like receptors. *FASEB J.* 1989;3:A610.
24.   Rollins BJ, Pober JS. Interleukin-4 induces the synthesis and secretion of MCP-1/JE by human endothelial cells. *Am J Pathol.* 1991;138:1315.
25.   Johnson-Tidey RR, McGregor JL, Taylor PR, Poston RN. Increase in the adhesion molecule P-selectin in endothelial overlying atherosclerotic plaques. *Am J Pathol.* 1994;144:952.
26.   Winn RK, Vedder NB, Paulson JC, Harlan JM. Monoclonal antibodies to P-selectin are effective in preventing reperfusion injury to rabbit ears. *Circulation.* 1992;86:I-80.
27.   Weyrich AS, Ma X-L, Lefer DJ, Albertine KH, Lefer AM. *In vivo* neutralization of P-selectin protects feline heart and endothelium in myocardial ischemia and reperfusion injury. *J Clin Invest.* 1993;91:2620.
28.   Dong ZM, Chapman SM, Brown AA, Frenette PS, Hynes RO, Wagner DD. The combined role of P- and E-selectins in atherosclerosis. *J Clin Invest.* 1998;102:145.
29.   Nageh MF, Sandberg ET, Marotti KR, Lin AH, Melchoir EP, Bullard DC, Beaudet AL. Deficiency of inflammatory cell adhesion molecules protects against atherosclerosis in mice. *Arterioscler Thromb Vasc Biol.* 1997;17:1517.
30.   Russell PS, Chase CM, Colvin RB. Coronary atherosclerosis in transplanted mouse hearts. IV effects of treatment with omonclonal antibodies to intercellular adhesion molecule-1 and leukocyte function-associated antigen-1. *Transplantation.* 199;60:724.
31.   Yasaka T, Boxer LA, Baehner RL. Monocyte aggregation and superoxide anion release in response to formyl-methionyl-leucy-phylalanine (FMLP) and platelet-activating factor (PAF). *J Immunol.* 1982;128:1939.
32.   Bussolino F, Fischer E, Turrini F, Kazatchkine MD, Arese P. Platelet-activating factor enhances complement-dependent phagocytosis of diamide-treated erythrocytes by human monocytes through activation of protien kinase C and phosphorylation of complement receptor type one (CR1). *J Biol Chem.* 1989;264:21711.
33.   Valone FH, Philip R, Debs RJ. Enhanced human monocyte cytoxicity by platelet-activating factor. *Immunology.* 1988;64:715.

34.   Bonavida B, Mencia-Huerta J-M, Braquet P. Effect of platelet-activating factor on monocyte activation and production of tumor necrosis factor. *Internl Arch Allergy and Applied Immunol.* 1989;88:157.

35.   Weyrich AS, McIntyre TM, McEver RP, Prescott SM, Zimmerman GA. Monocyte tethering by P-selecting regulates monocyte chemotactic protein-1 and tumor necrosis factor-α secretion: Signal integration and NF-kB translocation. *J Clin Invest.* 1995;95:2297.

36.   Salem P, Deryckx S, Dulioust A, Vivier E, Denizot Y, Damais C, Dinarello CA, Thomas Y. immunoregulatory functions of paf-acether IV. Enhancement of IL-1 production by muramyl dipeptide-stimulated monocytes. *J Immunol.* 1990;144:1338.

37.   Fauler J, Sielhorst G, Frolich JC. Platelet-activating factor induces the production of leukotrienes by human monocytes. *Biochim Biophys Acta.* 1989:1013:80.

38.   Paul-Eugene N, Dugas B, Picquot S, Lagente V, Mencia-Huerta JM, Braquet P. Influence of interleukin-4 and platelet-activating factor on the Fc epsilon RII/CD23 expression on human monocytes. *J Lipid Mediat.* 1990;2:95.

39.   Kuijpers TW, Hakkert BC, van Mourik JA, Roos D. Distinct adhesive properties of granulocytes and monocytes to endothelial cells under statis and stirred conditions. *J Immunol.* 1990:145:2588.

40.   Rouis M, Nigon F, Chapman MJ. Platelet activating factor is a potent stimulant of the production of active oxygen species by human monocyte-derived macrophages. *Biochem Biophys Res Comm.* 1988;156:1293.

41.   Shaw JO, Pinckard RN, Ferrigni KS, McManus LM, Hanaha DJ. Activation of human neutrophils with 1-*O*-hexadecyl/octadecyl-2-acetyl-*sn*-glyceeryl-3-phosphorylcholine (platelet-activating factor). *J Immunol.* 1981;127:1250.

42.   Dewald B, Baggioline M. Platelet-activating factor as a stimulus of exocytosis in human neutrophils. *Biochimica et Biophysica Acta.* 1986;888:42.

43.   Wykle RL, Miller CH, Lewis JC, Schmitt JD, Smith JA, Surles JR, Piantadosi C, O'Flaherty JT. Sterospecific activity of 1-*O*-alkyl-2-*O*-acetyl-*sn*-glycero-3-phosphocholine and comparison of analogs in the degranulation of platelets and neutrophils. *Biochem Biophyisc Res Comm.* 1981;100:1651.

44.   O'Flaherty JT, Miller CH, Lewis JC, Wykle RL, Bass DA, McCall CE, Waite M, DeChatelet LR. Neutrophil responses to platclt-activating factor. *Inflammation.* 1981;5:193.

45.   Gay JC, Beckman JK, Zaboy KA, Lukens JN. Modulation of neutrophil oxidative responses to soluble stimuli by platelet-activating factor. *Blood.* 1986;67:931.

46.   Benveniste J, Henson PM, Cochrane C. Leukocyte-dependent histamine release from rabbit platelets: The role for IgE, basophils and a platelet-activating factor. *J Exper Med.* 1972:136:1356.

47.   Chignard M, Le Couedic JP, Tence M, Vargaftig BB, Benveniste J. The role of platelet-activating factor in platelet aggregation. *Nature.* 1979;279:799.

48.   Stoll LL, Spector AA. Interaction of platelet-activating factor with endothelial and vascular smooth muscle cells in coculture. *J Cell Physiol.* 1989;139:253.

49.   Heery JM, Kozak M, Stafforini DM, Jones DA, Zimmerman GA, McIntyre TM, Prescott SM. Oxidatively modified LDL contains phospholipids with PAF-like activity and stimulates the growth of smooth muscle cells. *J Clin Invest.* 1995;96:2322.

50.   Blank ML, Snyder F, Byers LW, Brooks B, Muirhead EE. Antihypertensive activity of an alkyl ether analog of phosphatidylcholine. *Biochem Biophysic Res Comm.* 1979;90:1194.

51.   Demopoulos CA, Pinckard RN, Hanahan DJ. Platelet-activating factor: Evidence for 1-*O*-alkyl-2-acetyl-*sn*-glyceryl-3-phosphorylcholine as the active component (a new class of lipid chemical mediators). *J Biol Chem.* 1979;254:9355.

52.   Zimmerman GA, Prescott SM, McIntyre TM. Platelet-activating factor: A fluid-phase and cell-mediator of inflammation. In: Gallin JI, Goldstein IM, Snyderman R, eds. *Inflammation: Basic principles and clinical correlates.* 2 ed. New York: Raven Press;1992:149.

53.   Snyder F. Enzymatic pathways for platelet-activating factor, related alkyl glycerolipids, and their precursors. In: Snyder F, ed. *Platelet-activating Factor and Related Lipids Mediators.* New York: Plenum Press;1987:89.

54.   Bonventre JV, Huange Z, Taheri MR, O'Leary E, Li E, Moskowitz MA, Sapirstein A. Reduced fertility and postischaemic brain injury in mice deficient in cystolic phospholipase A_{23}. *Nature.* 1997;390:622.

55.   Nieto ML, Velasco S, Crespo MS. Modulation of acetyl-CoA:1-alkyl-2-lyso-*sn*-glycero-3-phosphocholine (lyso-PAF) acetyltransferase in human polymorphonuclears: The role of

cyclic AMP-dependent and phospholipid sensitive, calcium-dependent protein kinases. *J Biol Chem.* 1988;263:4607.

56. Lenihan DJ, Lee T-C. Regulation of platelet-activating factor synthesis: Modulation of 1-alkyl-2-lyso-*sn*-glycero-3-pohophocholine: Acetyle-CoA acetyltransferease by phosphorylation and dephosphorylation in rat spleen microsomes. *Biochem Biophysic Res Comm.* 1984;120:834.

57. Holland MR, Whatley RE, Stroud ED, Zimmerman GA, McIntyre Tm, Prescott SM. Activation of the acetyl-CaA: LysoPAF acetyltransferase regulates platelet activating factor synthesis in endothelial cells. *Circulation.* 1990;82:III-372.

58. Shimizu T, Mutoh H, Kato S. Platelet-activating factor receptor. Gene structure and tissue-specific regulation. *Adv Exp Med Biol.* 1996;416:79.

59. Honda Z, Nakamura M, Miki I, Minami M, Watanabe T, Seyama Y, Okado H, Toh H, Ito K, Miyamoto T, Shimizu T. Cloning by functional expression of platelet-activating factor receptor from guinea-pig lung. *Nature.* 1991;349:342.

60. Nakamura M, Honda Z, Izumi T, Sakanaka C, Mutoh H, Minami M, Bito H, Seyama Y, Matsumoto T, Noma M, Shimizu T. Molecuar cloning and expression of platelet-activating factor receptor from human leukocytes. *J Biol Chem.* 1991;266:20400.

61. Kunz D, Gerard NP, Gerard C. The human leukocyte platelet-activating factor receptor. *J Biol Chem.* 1992;267:9101.

62. Seyfried CE, Schweickart VL, Godiska R, Gray PW. The human platelet activating factor receptor gene (PTAFR) contains no introns and maps to chromosome 1. *Genomics.* 1992;13:832.

63. Shen TY, Hwang S-B, Doebber TW, Robbins JC. The chemical and biological properties of PAF agaonists, antagonists, and biosynthetic inhbitors. In: Snyder F, ed. *Platelet-activating factor and related lipid mediators.* New York: Plenum Press;1987:153.

64. O'Flaherty JT, Tessner T, Greene D, Redman JR, Wykle RL. Comparison of 1-O-alkyl-, 1-O-alk-1'-enyl-, and 1-O-acyl-2-acetyl-sn-glycero-3-pohospoethanolamines and −3-phosphocholines as agonist of the platelet-activating factor family. *Biochim Biophys Acta.* 1994;1210:209.

65. Koltai M, Braquet PG. Involvment of PAF in atherogenesis. Brief Review. *Agents Actions Suppl.* 1992:37:333.

66. Casals-Stenzerl J, Muacevic G, Weber K-H. Pharmacologic actions of WEB 2086, a new specific antagonist of platelet activating factor. *J Pharmacol Exper Thera.* 1987;241:974.

67. Imaizumi T, Stafforni DM, Yamada Y, McIntyre TM, Prescott SM, Zimmerman GA. Platelet-activating factor: A mediator for clinicians. *J Intern Med.* 1995;238:5.

68. Kuitert LM, Angus RM, Barnes NC, Barnes PJ, Bone MF, Chung KF, Fairfax AJ, Higenbotham TW, O'Connor BJ, Piotrowska B, et al. Effect of a novel potent platelet-activating facotr antagonist, modipafant, in clinical asthma. *Am J Respir Crit Care Med.* 1995;151:1331.

69. Evans DJ, Barnes PJ, Cluzel M, O'Connor BJ. Effects of a potent platelet-activating factor antagonist, SR274174A, on allergen-induced asthmatic responses. *Am J Crit Care Med.* 1997;156:11.

70. Kagoshima M, Tomomatsu N, Iwahisa Y, Yamaguchi S, Matsuura M, Kawakami Y, Terasawa M. Suppressive effects of Y-24180, a receptor antagonist to platelet activating factor (PAF), on antigen-induced asthmatic responses in guinea pigs. *Inflamm Res.* 1997;46:147.

71. Hozawa S, Haruta Y, Ishioka S, Yamakido M. Effects of a PAF antagonist, Y-24180, on bronchial hyperresponsiveness in patients with asthma. *Am J Respir Crit Care Med.* 1995;152:1198.

72. Diamond MS, Springer TA. The dynamic regulation of integrin adhesiveness. *Curr Biol* 1994;4:506:

73. Shalit M, Von Allmen C, Atkins PC, Zweiman B. Platelet activating factor increases expression of complement receptors on human neutrophils. *J Leukocyte Biol.* 1988:44:212.

74. Dewald B, Thelen M, Baggiolini M. Two transduction sequences are necessary for neutrophil activation by receptor agonists. *J Biol Chem.* 1988:263:16179.

75. Anderson DC, Springer TA. Leukocyte adhesion deficiency: An inherited defect in the Mac-1, LFA-1, and p150,95 glycoproteins. *Ann Rev Med.* 1987;38:175.

76. Lo SK, van Seventer GA, Levin SM, Wright SD. Two leukocyte receptors (CD11a/CD18 and CD11b/CD18) mediate transient adhesion to endothelium by binding to different ligands. *J Immunol.* 1989:143:3325.

77. Schleiffenbaum B, Moser R, Patarroyo M, Fehr J. The cell surface glycoprotein Ma-1 (CD11b/CD18) mediated neutrophil adhesion and modulates degranulation independently of its quantitative cell surface expression. *J Immunol*. 1989:142:3537.

78. Kishimoto TK, Anderson DC. The role of integrins in inflammation. In: Gallin JI, Goldstein IM, Snyderman R, eds. *Inflammation: Basic Principles and Clinical Correlates*, 2nd edition. New York: Raven Press, Ltd. 1992 pp 353.

79. Weyrich AS, Elstad MR, McEver RP, McIntyre TM, Moore KL, Morrissey JH, Prescott SM, Zimmerman GA. Activated platlets signal chemokine synthesis by human monocytes. *J Clin Invest*. 1996;97:1525.

80. Zimmerman GA, Elstad MR, Lorant DE, McIntyre TM, Prescott SM, Topham MK, Weyrich AS, Whatley RE. Platelet-activating factor (PAF): signallying and adhesion in cell-cell interactions. *Adv Exp Med Biol*. 1996;416:297.

81. McIntyre TM, Zimmerman GA, Prescott SM. Biologically active oxidized phospholipids. *J Biol Chem*. 1998;in press.

82. Lehr HA, Krombach F, Munzing S, Bodlaj R, Glaubitt SI, Seiffge D, Hubner C, von Andrian UH, Messmer K. *In vitro* effects of oxidized low density lipoproteins on CD11b/CD18 and L-selectin presentation on neutrophils and monocytes with relevance for the *in vivo* situation. *Am J Pathol*. 1995;146:218.

83. Frotegard J, Huang YH, Ronnelid J, Schafer-Elinder L. Platelet-activating factor and oxidized LDL induce immune activation by a common mechanism. *Arterioscler Thromb Vasc Biol*. 1997;17:963.

84. Frostegard J, Wu R, Giscombe R, Holm G, Lefvert AK, Nilsson J. Induction of T-cell activation by oxidized low density lipoprotein. *Arterioscler Thromb*. 1992;12:461.

85. Lewis JC, Bennett-Cain AL, DeMars CS, Docllgast GJ, Grant KW, Jones NL, Gupta M. Procoagulant activity after exposure of monocyte-derived macrophages to minimally oxidized low density lipoprotein. Co-localization of tissue factor antigen and nascent fibrin fibers at the cell surface. *Am J Pathol*. 1995;147:1029.

86. Oida K, Tohda G, Ishii H, Horie S, Kohno M, Okada E, Suzuki J, Nakai T, Miyamori I. Effect of oxidized low density lipoprotein on thrombomodulin expression by THP-1 cells. *Thromb Haemost*. 1997;78.1228.

87. Muller K, Hardwick SJ, Marchant CE, Law NS, Waeg G, Esterbauer H, Carpenter KL, Mitchinson MJ. Cytotoxic and chemotactic potencies of several aldehydic components of oxidized low density lipoproteins for human monocyte-macrophages. *FEBS Lett*. 1996;388:165.

88. Frostegard J, Nilsson J, Haegerstrand A, Hamsten A, Wigzell H, Gidlund M. Oxidized low density lipoprotein induces differentiation and adhesion of human monocytes and the monocytic cell line U937. *Proc Natl Acad Sci USA*. 1990;87:904.

89. Wang GP, Deng ZD, Ni J, Qu ZL. Oxidized low density lipoproteins and very low density lipoprotein enhance expression of monocyte chemoattractant protein-1 in rabbit periotenal exudate macrophages. *Atherosclerosis*. 1997;133:31.

90. Ku G, Thomas CE, Akeson AL, Jackson RL. Induction of interleukin 1 beta expression from human peripheral blood monocyte-derived macrophages by 9-hydroxyoctadecadienoic acid. *J Biol Chem*. 1992;267:14183.

91. Ardlie NG, Selley ML, Simons LA. Platelet activation by oxidatively modified low density lipoproteins. *Atherosclerosis*. 1989;76:117.

92. Lehr HA, Frei B, Olofsson AM, Carew TE, Arfors KE. Protection from oxidized LDL-induced leukocyte adhesion to microvascular and macrovascular endothelium *in vivo* by vitamin C but not by vitamin E. *Circulation*. 1995;91:1525.

93. McMurray HF, Parthasarathy S, Steinberg D. Oxidatively modified low density liporotein is a chemoattractant for human T lymphocytes. *J Clin Invest*. 1993;92:1004.

94. Huang YH, Ronnelid J, Frostegard J. Oxidized LDL induces enhanced antibody formation and MHC class II-dependent IFN-gamma production in lymphocytes from healthy individuals. *Arterioscler Thromb Vasc Biol*. 1995;15:1577.

95. Jeng JR, Chang CH, Shieh SM, Chiu HC. Oxidized low-density lipoproteins enhances monocyte-endothelial cell binding against shear-stress induced detachment. *Biochim Biophys Acta*. 1993;1178:221.

96. Amberger A, Maczek C, Jurgens G, Michaelis D, Schett G, Trieb K, Ebert T, Jindal S, Xu Q, Wick G. Co-expression of ICAM-1, VCAM-1, ELAM-1 and Hsp60 in human arterial and venous endothelial cells in response to cytokines and oxidized low-density lipoproteins. *Cell Stress Chaperones*. 1997;2:94.

97.   Cominiacini L, Garbin U,Pasini AF, Davoli A, Campagnola M, Contessi GB, Pastorino AM, Lo Cascio V. Antioxidants inhibit the expression of intercellular cell adhesion molecule-1 and vascular cell adhesion molecule-1 induced by oxidized LDL on human umbilical vein endothelial cells. *Free Rad Biol Med.* 1997;22:117.

98.   Gebuhrer V, Murphy JF, Bordet JC, Reck MP, McGregor JL. Oxidized low-density lipoproteins induces the expression of P-selectin (GMP140/PADGEM/CD62) on human endothelial cells. *Biochem J.* 1995;306;293.

99.   Cushing SD, Berliner JA, Valente AJ, Territo MC, Navab M, Parhami F, Gerrity R, Schwartz CJ, Fogelman AM. Minimally modified low density lipoprotein induces monocyte chemotactic protein1 in human endothelial cells and smooth muscle cells. *Proc Natl Acad Sci USA.* 1990;87:5134.

100.   Takahara N, Kashiwagi A, Nishio Y, Harada N, Kojima H, Maegawa H, Hidaka H, Kikkawa R. Oxidized lipoprotins found in patients with NIDDM stimulate radical-induced monocyte chemoattractant protein-1 mRNA expression in cultured human endothelial cells. *Diabetologia.* 1997;40:662.

101.   Chatterjee S. Role of oxidized human plasma low density lipoproteins in atherosclerosis: effects on smooth muscle cell proliferation. *Mol Cell Biochem.* 1992;111:143.

102.   Heery JM, Kozak M, Stafforini DM, Jones DA, Zimmerman GA, McIntyre TM, Prescott SM. Oxidatively modified LDL contains phospholipids with platelet-activating factor-like activity and stimulates the growth of smooth muscle cells. *J Clin Invest.* 1995;96:2322.

103.   Zwijsen RM, Japenga SC, Heijen AM, van den Bos RC, Koeman JH. Induction of platelet-derived growth factor chain a gene expression in human smooth muscle cells by oxidized low density lipoproteins. *Biochem Biophys Res Comm.* 1992;186:1410.

104.   Stiko-Rahm A, Hultgardh-Nilsson A, Regnstrom J, Hamsten A, Nilsson J. Native and oxidized LDL enhances production of PDGF AA and the surface expression of PDGF receptors in cultured human smooth muscle cells. *Arterioscler Thromb.* 1992;12:1099.

105.   Stremler KE, Stafforini DM, Prescott SM, Zimmerman GA, McIntyre TM. An oxidized derivative of phosphatidylcholine is a substrate for the platelet-activating factor acetylhydrolase from human plasma. *J Biol Chem.* 1989;264:5331.

106.   Smiley PL, Stremler KE, Prescott SM, Zimmerman GA, McIntyre TM. Oxidatively fragmented phosphatidylcholines activate human neutrophils through the receptor for platelt-activating factor. *J Biol Chem.* 1991;266:11104.

107.   Stremler KE, Stafforini DM, Prescott SM, McIntyre TM. Human plasma platelet-activating factor acetylhydrolase: oxidatively-fragmented phospholipids as substratess. *J Biol Chem.* 1991;266:11095.

108.   Patel KD, Zimmerman GA, Prescott SM, McEver RP, McIntyre TM. Oxygen radicals induce human endothelial cells to express GMP-140 and bind neutrophils. *J Cell Biol.* 1991;112:749.

109.   Patel KD, Zimmerman GA, Prescott SM, McIntyre TM. Novel leukocyte agonists are released by endothelial cells exposed to peroxide. *J Biol Chem.* 1992;267:15168.

110.   Diagne A, Fauvel J, Record M, Chap H, Douste-Blazy L. Comparative composition of various tissues from human, rat and guinea pig. *Biochim Biophys Acta.* 1984;793:221.

111.   Sugiura T, Waku K. Composition of alkyl ether-linked phospholipids in mammalian tissues. In: Snyder F, ed. *Platelet-activating factor and related lipid mediators.* New York: Plenum Press. 1987 pp 55.

112.   Watson AD, Leitinger N, Navah M, Faull KF, Horkko S, Witztum JL, Palinski W, Schwenke D, Salomon RG, Sha W, Subbanagounder G, Fogelman AM, Berliner JA. Structural identification by mass spectrometry of oxidized phospholipids in minimally oxidized low density lipoprotein that induce monocyte/endothelial interactions and evidence for their presence *in vivo. J Biol Chem.* 1997;272:13597.

113.   Leitinger N, Watson AD, Faull KF, Fogelman AM, Berliner JA. Monocyte binding to endothelial cells induced by oxidized phospholipids present in minimally oxidized low density lipoprotein is inhbited by a platelet activating factor receptor antagonist. *Adv Exp Med Biol.* 1997;433:379.

114.   Yoshida J, Tokumura A, Fukuzawa K, Terao M, Takauchi K, Tsukatani H. A platelet-aggregating and hypotensive phospholipid isolated from bovine brain. *J Pharm Pharmacol.* 1986;38:878.

115.   Tanaka T, Tokumura A, Tsukatani H. Platelet-activating factor (PAF)-like phospholipids formed during peroxidation of phosphatidylcholines from different foodstuffs. *Biosci Biotechnol Biochem.* 1995;59:1389.

116. Tokumura A, Kamiyasu K, Takauchi K, Tsukatani H. Evidence for existence of various homologues and analogues of platelet activating factor in a lipid extract of bovine brain. *Biochem Biophys Res Comm*. 1987;145:415.

117. Tanaka T, Iimori M, Tsukatani H, Tokumura A. Platelet-aggregating effects of platelet-activating factor-like phospholipids formed by oxidation of phosphatidylcholines containing an sn-2-polyunsatuated fatty acyl group. *Biochim Biophys Act.*. 1994;1210:202.

118. Pryor WA, Stone K. Oxidants in cigarette smoke. *Ann NY Acad Sci*. 1993;686:12.

119. Stafford RS, Becker CG. Cigarette smoking and atherosclerosis. In: Fuster V, Ross R, Topol E, eds. *Atherosclerosis and coronary artery diseases*. Philadelpha, PA. Lippincott-Raven Publishers; 1996 pp. 303.

120. Lehr HA, Hubner C, Nolte D, Finckh B. Beisiegel U, Kohlschutter A, Mebmer K. Oxidatively modified human low-density lipoprotein stimulates leukocyte adherence to the microvascular endothelium *in vivo*. *Res Exper Med*. 1991;191:85.

121. Rimm E, Stampfer M. The role of antioxidants in preventive cardiology. *Curr Opin Cardiol*. 1997;12:188.

122. Chisolm G, Penn MS. Oxidized lipoproteins and atherosclerosis. In: Fuster V, Ross R, Topol E, eds. *Atherosclerosis and coronary artery diseases*. Philadelphia, PA: Lippincott-Raven Publishers; 1996 pp129.

123. Stahl GL, Terashita Z, Lefer AM. Role of platelet activating factor in propagation of cardiac damage during myocardial ischemia. *J Pharmacol Exp Ther*. 1988;244:898.

124. Montrucchio G, Alloatti G, Mariano F, de Paulis R, Comino A, Emanuelli G, Camussi G. Role of platelet-activating factor in the reperfusion injury of rabbit ischemic heart. *Am J Pathol*. 1990;137:71.

125. Kubes P, Ibbotson G, Russell J, Wallace JL, Granger DN. Role of platelet-activating factor in ischemia/reperfusion-induced leukocyte adherence. *Am J Physiol*. 1990;259:G300.

126. Alloatti G, Montrucchio G, Camussi G. Role of platelet-activating factor (PAF) in oxygen radical-induced cardiac dysfunction. *J Pharmacol Exp Ther*. 1994;269:766.

127. Matsuo Y, Kihara T, Ikeda M, Ninomiya M, Onodera H, Kogure K. Role of platelet-activating factor and thromboxane A2 in radical production during ischemia and reperfusion of the rat brain. *Brain Res.*. 1996;709:296.

128. Izuoka T, Takayama Y, Sugiura T, Taniguchi H, Tamura T, Kitashiro S, Jikuhara T, Iwasaka T. Role of platelet-activating factor on extravascular lung water after cornary reperfusion in dogs. *Jpn J Physiol*. 1998;48:157.

129. Kugiyama K, Kerns SA, Morrisett JD, Roberts R, Henry PD. Impairment of endothelium-dependent arterial relaxation by lysolecithin in modified low-density lipoproteins. *Nature*. 1990;344:160.

130. Chen L, Liang B, Froese DE, Liu S, Wong JT, Tran K, Hatch GM, Mymin D, Kroeger EA, Man RY, Choy PC. Oxidative Modification of low density lipoprotein in normal and hyperlipidemic patients: effect of lysophosphatidylcholine composition on vascular relaxation. *J Lipid Res*. 1997;38:546.

131. Stafforini DM, McIntyre TM, Carter ME, Prescott SM. Human plasma platelet-activating factor acetylhydrolase: association with lipoprotein particles and role in the degradation of platelet-activating factor. *J Biol Chem*. 1987;262:4215.

132. Quinn MT, Parthasarathy S, Steinberg D. Lysophosphatidylcholine: a chemotactic factor for human monocytes and its potential role in atherogenesis. *Proc Natl Acad Sci USA*. 1988;85:2805.

133. Kume N, Gimbrone MA Jr. Lysophosphatidylcholine transcriptionally induces growth factor gene expression in cultured human endothelial cells. *J Clin Invest*. 1994;93:907.

134. Tokumura A, Iimori M, Nishioka Y, Kitahara M, Sakashita M, Tanaka S. Lysophosphatidic acids induce proliferation of cultured vascular smooth muscle cells from rat aorta. *Am J Physiol*. 1994;267:C204.

135. Ogita T, Tanaka Y, Nakaoka T, Matsuoka R, Kira Y, Nakamura M, Shimizu T, Fujita T. Lysophosphatidylcholine transduces Ca^{2+} signaling via the platelet-activating factor receptor in macrophages. *Am J Physiol*. 1997;272:H17.

136. Subbaiah PV, Chen CH, Bagdade JD, Albers JJ. Substrate specificity of plasma lysolecithin acyltransferase and the molecular species of lecithin formed by the reaction. *J Biol Chem*. 1985;260:5308.

137. Rabini RA, Galassi R, Fumelli P, Dousset N, Solera ML, Valdiguie P, Curatola G, Ferretti G, Taus M, Mazzanti L. Reduced $NA^+ - K^+$ ATPase activity in diabetic patients. *Diabetes*. 1994;43:915.

138.   Stafforini DM, Prescott SM, McIntyre TM.   Human plasma platelet-activating factor acetylhydrolase: Purification and properties. *J Biol Chem.* 1987;262:4223.

139.   Miwa M, Miyake T, Yamanaka T, Sugatani J, Suzuki Y, Sakata S, Araki Y, Matsumoto M. Characterization of serum platelet-activating (PAF) acetylhydrolase: correlation between deficiency of serum PAF acetylhydrolase and respiratory symptoms in asthmatic children. *J Clin Invest.* 1988;82:1983.

140.   Stafforini DM, Satoh K, Atkinson DL, Tjoelker LW, Eberhardt C, Yoshida H, Imaizumi T-A, Takamatsu S, Zimmerman GA, McIntyre TM, Gray PW, Prescott SM.   Platelet-activating factor acetylhydrolase deficiency: a missense mutation near the active siet of an anti-inflammatory phospholipase. *J Clin Invest.* 1996;97:2784.

141.   Hiramoto M, Yoshida H, Imaizumi T, Yoshimizu N, Satoh K. A mutation in plasma platelet-activating factor acetylhydrolase (Val279→Phe) is a genetic risk factor for stroke. *Stroke.* 1997;28:2417.

142.   Yamada Y, Ichihara S, Fujimura T, Yokota M. Identification of the G994→T missense in exon 9 of the plasma platelet-activating factor acetylhydrolase gene as an independent risk factor for coronary artery disease in Japanese men. *Metabolism.* 1998;47:177.

7 MM-LDL AND ATHEROGENESIS – A MAJOR ROLE FOR PHOSPHOLIPID OXIDATION PRODUCTS

Norbert Leitinger and Judith A. Berliner

INTRODUCTION

Oxidative modification of low density lipoprotein (LDL) is thought to play a major role in atherogenesis (1,2,3). While unoxidized (native) LDL plays a physiologic role in lipid metabolism, oxidized LDL (oxLDL) is thought to cause pathologic changes in the vessel wall and oxidized lipids are likely to be involved in settings of general inflammation (4). Moreover, oxLDL has been isolated from atherosclerotic aorta and lipid oxidation products have been detected immunohistochemically in atherosclerotic lesions (5,6). In the development of chronic inflammatory diseases a role for oxidized lipids has been implicated and autoantibodies against lipid oxidation products in patients with atherosclerosis, diabetes, hypertension, rheumatoid arthritis and preeclampsia have been detected (7,8,9).

In 1990 Berliner and colleagues demonstrated that LDL which had been mildly oxidized by prolonged storage or using iron had unique properties different from those of native and oxLDL. This LDL was called minimally oxidized or minimally modified LDL (MM-LDL) and shown to induce monocyte-endothelial interactions, a key event in the formation of the atherosclerotic lesion (10). These findings showed the importance of distinguishing LDL which had been oxidized to different degrees, implicating that different oxidation products were responsible for the various effects seen with these different preparations. Here we summarize the unique biological properties of MM-LDL and the effects of oxidized phospholipids, present in MM-LDL, on atherogenesis.

CHEMICAL FEATURES OF MM-LDL: DIFFERENCES TO NATIVE AND HIGHLY OXIDIZED LDL

LDL is a heterogeneous particle, consisting of a variety of lipid components and a protein, apolipoprotein B100 (apo B). Both the lipid and the protein components are modified during oxidative modification of LDL (11). MM-LDL is LDL that has undergone depletion of antioxidants and oxidation of polyunsaturated fatty acids (much more arachidonic acid than linoleic acid), with little or no protein modification. MM-LDL can be produced by prolonged storage at 4°C (10), by oxidation with lipoxygenase (12) or iron (13), or by incubation with arterial wall cells (1). Although MM-LDL is primarily defined through its unique biological activity (i.e. it induces monocyte-endothelial interactions, as opposed to native and highly oxidized LDL), it also has unique chemical features by which it can be distinguished from native and highly oxidized LDL. These chemical features correspond to the various biological properties associated with MM-LDL (described below).

MM-LDL contains 2-5 nmoles of thiobarbituric acid-reactive substances (TBARS) as malondialdehyde (MDA) equivalents per mg cholesterol, that is only 1.5 - 2 fold higher than TBARS levels measured in freshly isolated (native) LDL (10). In contrast, oxLDL produced by copper oxidation contains 10-50 nmoles of TBARS (11). Hydroperoxide levels in MM-LDL as determined by a colorimetric assay using aluminum chloride as catalyst (15) were only 1.5 fold higher (10), while oxidation with copper caused up to 30 fold increases in peroxides (11). Cholesterol epoxide levels in MM-LDL were approximately 4 fold higher than in native LDL (10). Although levels of isoprostanes have not yet been determined in MM-LDL, there is considerable evidence for the presence of these biologically active compounds, as has been shown for oxLDL (16).

Free radical-induced oxidation of LDL can be divided into three stages: the lag phase, during which lipophilic antioxidants (vitamin E, β-carotene, ubiquinol) are depleted; the propagation phase, during which polyunsaturated fatty acids form lipid hydroperoxides and cholesterol gets oxidized to form oxycholesterol; and the decomposition phase, during which oxidized lipids undergo fragmentation, resulting in the formation of aldehydes capable of reacting with amino groups on the apo B and phospholipids. The reaction of these aldehydes with lysine groups on the apo B makes oxLDL a ligand for scavenger receptors (17). Extensive oxidation results in fragmentation of apo B. One important difference between native and oxidized LDL is the fact that native LDL is taken up by the LDL receptor in a highly regulated manner, while oxLDL is no longer recognized by the LDL receptor, but is taken up by scavenger receptors, a process which is no longer regulated by intracellular cholesterol content, leading to the formation of lipid laden foam cells, the hallmark of the atherosclerotic lesion. In contrast, MM-LDL is still recognized by the LDL receptor as demonstrated by degradation studies on endothelial cells (10). The rate of degradation of MM-LDL was comparable to that of native LDL, while degradation by endothelial cells of MDA-LDL (that is LDL where the lysine residues of the apo B had been modified with MDA, making it a ligand for the scavenger receptor, but unrecognizable for the LDL receptor) was about 3 times higher. In addition, native LDL, but not MDA-LDL suppressed uptake of MM-LDL and cross-competition studies confirmed that MM-LDL competed for native LDL uptake, but not for MDA-LDL (10). However, recent studies by Witztum and colleagues suggest that lipid components present in MM-LDL may bind to one or more macrophage scavenger receptors.

In terms of its atherogenicity, the probably most important feature of MM-LDL is its phospholipid modification. Watson *et al.* showed that the oxidized phospholipids in MM-LDL which are responsible for the induction of monocyte-endothelial interactions contain fragmented and oxygenated PUFAs at the *sn*-2 position (18). While in native LDL the PUFAs are still intact, in highly oxidized LDL the PUFAs at the sn-2 position of phospholipids have undergone extensive fragmentation leading to hydrolysis which results in the formation of lysophosphatidylcholine (lyso-PC). While the levels of biologically active "short-chain" phospholipids decreases, the lyso-PC content dramatically increases in oxLDL and is therefore an important measure for the degree of oxidation of LDL.

It is important to note that different MM-LDL preparations show a great degree of variation in biological activity due to the different lipid composition and oxidizability (antioxidant content, lipid composition) of LDL derived from different donors. Even MM-LDL preparations in which a small increase of TDARS had been measured sometimes lacked biological activity. Therefore, the optimum time for exposing native LDL to oxidants must be determined empirically for each LDL preparation in order to obtain biologically active MM-LDL. Additionally, exposing LDL to oxidants beyond the time required to produce biologically active oxidized phospholipids will result in the loss of its ability to induce monocyte-endothelial interactions. It has been shown that occasional isolates of endothelial cells are resistant to the effects of MM-LDL; therefore, several primary isolates should be screened (10).

BIOLOGICAL ACTIVITY OF MM-LDL

MM-LDL has unique biological properties that are not associated with native LDL or highly oxidized LDL. The effect of MM-LDL on vascular endothelial cells may be crucial for initiating the development of the atherosclerotic lesion. In atherosclerosis, similar to other chronic inflammatory diseases, mononuclear cells, but not polymorphonuclear cells, adhere to the vascular endothelium and transmigrate into the subendothelial space where they differentiate into macrophages (19). MM-LDL was shown to influence several steps involving monocytes during the development of the fatty streak in atherogenesis (Fig. 1). MM-LDL has been shown to stimulate endothelial cells *in vitro* to selectively bind monocytes, but not neutrophils (10). In contrast, the known inflammatory cytokines bacterial lipopolysaccharide (LPS), tumor necrosis factor (TNF), and interleukin-1 (IL-1) mediate both monocyte and neutrophil adhesion to the endothelium. The effects of MM-LDL related to vascular biology are summarized in Table 1.

MM-LDL And Monocyte Adhesion

A major goal was to identify the endothelial adhesion molecule induced by MM-LDL which led to the specific monocyte binding. The fact that MM-LDL induced specific adhesion of monocytes to endothelial cells without inducing expression of

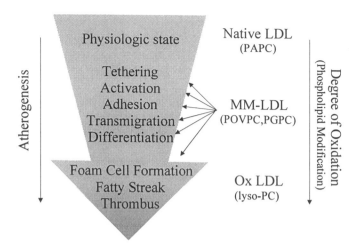

Figure 1. Influence of MM-LDL on various steps involving monocytes that consequently lead to clinical events of atherosclerosis.

E-selectin, VCAM-1 or ICAM-1 (20) suggested that another monocyte-specific adhesion molecule must be involved. Teng-Shih *et al.* found that MM-LDL-induced monocyte adhesion to endothelial cells is mediated by $\alpha_4\beta_1$ integrin, since antibodies to α_4 and β_1 significantly reduced monocyte binding induced by MM-LDL while antibodies to other integrins were ineffective (21). $\alpha_4\beta_1$ integrin is known to interact with VCAM-1 on endothelial cells, however, expression of VCAM-1 is not induced by MM-LDL and antibodies against VCAM-1 did not interfere with MM-LDL-induced monocyte adhesion. Interestingly, an alternatively spliced form of fibronectin, CS-1 fibronectin, was demonstrated to serve as the endothelial receptor for $\alpha_4\beta_1$ (21). Antibodies against the CS-1 region of fibronectin significantly decreased monocyte adhesion to MM-LDL-treated endothelial cells. CS-1 fibronectin was shown to be deposited on the surface of endothelial cells upon stimulation with MM-LDL. Confocal microscopy showed that CS-1 was located at perinuclear regions on the apical surface of endothelial cells (21).

Recently, a novel vascular monocyte adhesion-associated protein (VMAP-1) has been identified and shown to be induced by MM-LDL (23). VMAP-1, a 50 kD protein, was shown to play a role in adhesion of monocytes to activated endothelium since a specific antibody against VMAP-1 specifically blocked monocyte, but not neutrophil or lymphocyte, adhesion to endothelial cells stimulated with TNF, LPS or MM-LDL. Furthermore, VMAP-1 was expressed by mouse arterial and endocardial and rabbit aortic endothelial cells *in vivo*. This novel molecule is thought to function in conjunction with other adhesion molecules in regulating monocyte adhesion. Another adhesion molecule for monocytes, a 105 kD adhesion protein, was shown to be induced in endothelial cells by MM-LDL (24).

Table 1. Biological effects of MM-LDL related to vascular biology.

Effect	Cell type	Bioactive component	Ref.
Monocyte adhesion	HAEC, RAEC	POVPC, PGPC	10,20
β1-integrin activation	HAEC	OxPAPC	21
CS-1 fibronectin	HAEC	OxPAPC	21
VMAP-1	EC		22
Cell growth	EC		1
105 kD adhesion protein	EC		23
P-selectin	HAEC	OxPAPC	29
MCP-1	EC, SMC	OxPAPC	30,14
MCSF	EC		31
JE, KC, c-myc	Murine fibroblasts		35
Gro-chemokine	RAEC		36
IL 1α, IL 1β	monocytes		38
Scavenger receptor A, CD36, macrosialin	macrophages		39
Tissue factor	EC		41,42
Inhibits LCAT			43
Heme-oxygenase	HAEC	OxPAPC, PGPC	44
Calcification, proliferation	CVC	OxPAPC, 8-iso-PGE$_2$	45
Inhibits differentiation	preosteoblasts	OxPAPC, 8-iso-PGE$_2$	45
12-S-HETE	EC		49
Inhibits E-selectin, VCAM-1	HAEC		26
cAMP	EC, mesangial cells	OxPAPC	26,48
PDGF	Mesangial cells		48
calcium	EC, VSMC		49,50
NFκB	L-cells, RAEC		51,26
Stimulate Gs, inhibit Gi	EC	OxPAPC	47

This protein was recognized by mAb IG9 and shown to be expressed *in vivo* in inflamed human vessels and in atherosclerotic lesions in humans and rabbits.

Leukocyte recruitment and migration into the subendothelial space is a multistep process that involves rolling, activation, firm adhesion and transmigration (25). Rolling is mediated by a group of adhesion molecules, so called selectins, which, due to their presentation on the cell surface, permit weak interactions with leukocytes that, upon activation, then adhere firmly to the endothelium (26). Our group has shown that expression of E-selectin is not mediated by MM-LDL (20,27). Therefore, we tested the influence of MM-LDL on the expression and the release of P-selectin in endothelial cells. P-selectin is another molecule which brings about rolling of leukocytes on endothelial cells during inflammation. However, P-selectin is constitutively expressed in endothelial cells, stored in Weibel-Palade bodies (28) and mobilized to the surface of endothelial cells upon stimulation with agonists like histamin, phorbol esters, hydrogen peroxide, and thrombin (29). Vora *et al* found that MM-LDL induced intracellular accumulation of P-selectin, however, an additional stimulus was needed to release P-selectin to the surface (30).

Interestingly, highly oxidized LDL was capable of inducing P-selectin release, pointing to an interesting sequence of events during the oxidative modification of LDL. Again, the phospholipid component of MM-LDL was responsible for the effect on P-selectin expression and inhibition of cAMP formation abolished the effect. On the other hand, the fatty acid fraction of oxLDL was responsible for the mobilization of P-selectin to the cell surface. Furthermore, an increased expression of P-selectin in endothelial cells of human fatty streak lesions was demonstrated (29), suggesting a role for P-selectin in early monocyte recruitment during atherogenesis.

MM-LDL and Monocyte Transmigration and Differentiation

MM-LDL stimulates production of monocyte chemotactic protein-1 (MCP-1) in endothelial cells and smooth muscle cells (31) leading to monocyte transmigration into the subendothelial space, as determined by a transmigration assay using cocultures of vascular endothelial cells and smooth muscle cells (14). In addition, it was shown that MM-LDL had the potential to stimulate the maturation of monocytes into macrophages by inducing the synthesis of macrophage colony stimulating factor (MCSF) (32). MCSF (33, 34) and MCP-1 (35) were consequently found to be expressed in atherosclerotic lesions. In addition, it was shown that MM-LDL increased mRNA levels of the early response genes JE, KC and c-*myc* in murine fibroblasts (36). By expression screening of a cDNA library from rabbit aortic endothelial cells (RAEC) for molecules mediating monocyte adhesion, a cDNA homologous to growth-regulated oncogene (gro) was isolated. It was found that transcription of gro was induced by MM-LDL (37). In a study by Boisvert *et al.* it was demonstrated in LDL receptor deficient mice that expression of CXCR-2, the gro chemokine receptor, was important for macrophage accumulation in atherosclerotic lesions (38).

MM-LDL also stimulates monocytes by inducing transcription of inflammatory genes. When added to isolated human blood monocytes, MM-LDL induced gene expression of both interleukin 1α and 1β, however, expression of platelet-derived growth factor (PDGF) was inhibited (39). In addition to its atherogenic effects on endothelial cells and monocytes, Yoshida *et al.* showed that MM-LDL contributes to foam cell formation by directly acting on macrophages. MM-LDL induced the expression of receptors for internalization of highly oxidized LDL, namely scavenger receptor A, CD36, and macrosialin on mouse peritoneal macrophages (40). These results showed that MM-LDL, by inducing scavenger receptor expression, can prime macrophages for foam cell formation.

Consequently, it was tested whether MM-LDL was biologically active *in vivo*. Microgram quantities of MM-LDL were injected into mice and levels of colony stimulating factors (CSF) as well as JE (the mouse homologue of MCP-1), were determined. Both CSF in serum and JE in various tissues were markedly increased after 4 - 5 hours of injection with MM-LDL, but were not induced after injection of native LDL (41). These results indicated that MM-LDL indeed exerts biological activity *in vivo*.

Other Biological Activities of MM-LDL Related to Vascular Biology

It has been shown by Drake *et al.* that MM-LDL can also influence thrombus formation. These authors showed that MM-LDL induced tissue factor expression in endothelial cells (42) in a time and dose-dependent manner. Peak tissue factor coagulant activiy in cells treated with MM-LDL was observed at 4 to 6 hours, while mRNA levels peaked at 2-3 hours. Nuclear runoff transcription assays showed that regulation of tissue factor expression by MM-LDL in endothelial cells occured at the transciptional level (43).

Bielicki *et al.* showed that lipids from MM-LDL affect HDL function by inhibiting lecithin:cholesterol acyltransferase activity (44). Thus, MM-LDL may impair cholesteryl ester formation in HDL thereby limiting the beneficial effects of HDL in the antiatherogenic reverse cholesterol transport pathway.

Coculture modified LDL and oxidized phospholipids, but not native LDL, induced heme-oxygenase-1 (HO-1) mRNA in human aortic endothelial cells (HAEC). Induction of HO-1 subsequently inhibited monocyte transmigration induced by MM-LDL, pointing to an interesting protective mechanism by HO-1 (45) (Table 2).

When Parhami *et al.* investigated the effects of MM-LDL on arterial calcification, they found an interesting relationship between the effects of MM-LDL on calcifying vascular cells (CVC) and bone-derived preosteoblasts. MM-LDL, oxidized phospholipids, and another lipid peroxidation product which was also found to be present in oxLDL (8-iso-prostaglandin E_2), induced differentiation of CVCs and extensive areas of calcification, but inhibited differentiation of bone cells (46). On the other hand, cell proliferation was induced by these oxidized lipids in CVCs, but was inhibited in bone cells. These results suggest that oxidized lipids may be common factors underlying the pathogenesis of both atherosclerosis and osteoporosis and might help to explain the paradox of arterial calcification in osteoporotic patients.

Intracellular Signaling Induced by MM-LDL

The cellular mechanism by which MM-LDL induced monocyte endothelial interactions was not known until recently. There are several indications that the effects of MM-LDL on endothelial cells are receptor-mediated. However, the presence of a putative MM-LDL receptor remains speculative. From our studies with isolated and synthesized individual bioactive phospholipids, it seems that the effects of MM-LDL are mediated by receptors for bioactive phospholipids (described below). Studies from our laboratory showed that MM-LDL and OxPAPC act via a G-protein linked pathway, stimulating Gs and inhibiting Gi, thereby inducing the formation of cAMP (26,47). In a recent study performed with mesangial cells it was demonstrated that MM-LDL, but not oxLDL, induced mRNA expression for PDGF. This effect was shown to be mediated by protein kinase A (PKA) and elevation of cAMP levels (48). In addition, there are reports that MM-

LDL increases intracellular calcium in endothelial cells (49) and it was shown that MM-LDL evokes calcium-dependent retraction of vascular smooth muscle cells (50).

Moreover, the transcription factor NF-κB seems to play a major role in mediating transcription of several inflammatory genes induced by MM-LDL as shown in a study using L-cells (51). Using inbred mouse strains on an atherogenic diet, Liao *et al.* showed that atherosclerotic lesion formation and induction of inflammatory genes was associated with accumulation of lipid peroxidation products and activation of NFκB-like transcription factors (52). Furthermore, these authors showed that activation of NFκB-like transcription factors and induction of inflammatory genes cosegregated with aortic lesion formation in recombinant inbred strains derived from C57Bl/6J (susceptible to atherosclerotic lesion formation) and C3H/HeJ (resistant) mice (53). The same set of genes was activated after injection of MM-LDL into mice (52,54). Activation of NFκB by oxidized lipoproteins was shown by another study as well (55), however, one has to bear in mind that other inflammatory genes such as E-selectin and VCAM-1, which are also driven by NFκB, are inhibited by MM-LDL, most likely due to its ability to increase cAMP levels (56,57,58).

Recently, we showed that lipoxygenase metabolites play a major role in MM-LDL-induced monocyte binding to endothelial cells (49). Treatment of endothelial cells with inhibitors of lipoxygenase, 5,8,11,14-eicosatetraenoic acid (ETYA) or cinnamyl-3,4-dihydroxy-α-cyanocinnamate (CDC) blocked monocyte adhesion to MM-LDL-treated endothelial cells without reducing cAMP levels. In addition, arachidonate release and formation of 12-S-HETE were significantly increased in endothelial cells after MM-LDL treatment (49). Studies with the individual oxidized phospholipids will give more insight into the intracellular pathways leading to selective monocyte adhesion induced by MM-LDL.

BIOACTIVE OXIDIZED PHOSPHOLIPIDS IN MM-LDL

Separation and individual testing of the components in MM-LDL for bioactivity showed that only the lipid-soluble fraction of MM-LDL induced monocyte-endothelial interactions while the water-soluble fraction (containing apo B) was inactive (10). Further separation of the lipid fraction demonstrated that almost 100% of the bioactivity was associated with the polar lipid fraction, containing the phospholipids, whereas the neutral lipid fraction and fatty acids did not increase monocyte binding to endothelial cells (10). Since arachidonic acid-containing phospholipids in MM-LDL were especially prone to oxidation, 1-palmitoyl-2-archidonoyl-*sn*-glycero-3-phosphocholine (PAPC) was oxidized *in vitro* and tested for its ability to stimulate monocyte endothelial interactions. It turned out that oxidized PAPC (OxPAPC) could be used as a surrogate for MM-LDL in leukocyte adhesion experiments since it mimicked the effects of MM-LDL (18). Thus, OxPAPC stimulated endothelial cells to bind monocytes, but not neutrophils, in a concentration-dependent manner. However, the oxidation of PAPC results in the formation of numerous new phospholipids, due to either fragmentation of, or the

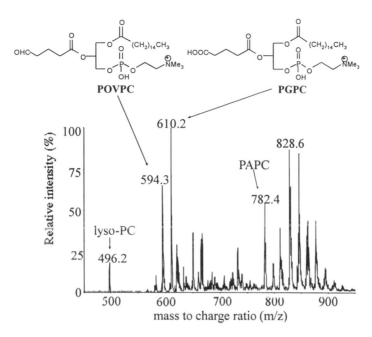

Figure 2. Electrospray-ionization mass spectrogram of oxidized PAPC. Chemical structures of biologically active oxidized phospholipids POVPC and PGPC.

addition of oxygen to the arachidonate moiety at the *sn*-2 position (Fig. 2). The molecular structures of biologically active oxidation products of PAPC were determined using liquid chromatography and electrospray ionization mass spectrometry in conjunction with chemical derivatization techniques. Two of three biologically active oxidized derivatives of PAPC were identified as 1-palmitoyl-2-(5-oxovaleryl)-*sn*-glycero-3-phosphocholine (POVPC) and 1-palmitoyl-2-glutaryl-*sn*-glycero-3-phosphocholine (PGPC) (Fig. 2), whereas the third molecule contained three oxygens added to the arachidonate moiety and had a mass of 828 Da (59). We found that oxidation of 1-stearoyl-2-archidonoyl-*sn*-glycero-3-phosphocholine (SAPC) followed exactly the same pattern as seen for PAPC, producing analoguous molecules with comparable bioactivity. These results indicated that the biological activity of oxidation products derived from arachidonoyl-containing phospholipids was not dependent on the lipid moiety at the *sn*-1 position. The two oxidized phospholipids present in MM-LDL and OxPAPC, POVPC and PGPC, were found to mediate monocyte-endothelial interactions (59). The effect of POVPC could be inhibited by a platelet activating factor (PAF) receptor antagonist, WEB 2086 (60). The action of PGPC, on the other hand, was not affected by WEB 2086, indicating different binding sites for POVPC and PGPC. PAF itself, however, did not induce monocyte-endothelial interactions (61). These results led us to hypothesize that specific receptors for POVPC and PGPC were present on endothelial cells. Although these experiments were performed with molecules either isolated from OxPAPC or produced by organic synthesis, POVPC and PGPC are likely to be active when embedded in the MM-LDL particle. The presentation of their

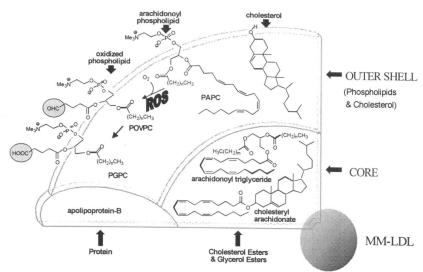

Figure 3. Hypothetical scheme of the arrangement of chemical components in MM-LDL. Phospholipids reside in the outer shell of the LDL particle and, upon oxidative modification of the PUFA moiety at the *sn*-2 position, present the functional group (aldehyde or carboxylic acid) on the outside. This way, in case of contact with cells, the functional groups can be recognized by respective receptors on the cell surface. ROS, reactive oxygen species. Figure was originally drawn by Dr. G.Subbanagounder.

functional groups on the surface of the MM-LDL particle makes POVPC and PGPC potential ligands for putative cell surface receptors (Fig. 3).

ENZYMES THAT REGULATE BIOACTIVITY OF MM-LDL

HDL was shown to prevent the formation of MM-LDL by cocultures of arterial wall cells (11,61), however, the molecular mechanisms for this protective effect were not known until recently. Watson *et al.* demonstrated that enzymes associated with HDL could destroy biologically active oxidized phospholipids in MM-LDL, thereby reducing its bioactivity. Due to their similar structures to PAF, oxidized "short chain" phospholipids are substrates for PAF-acetylhydrolase (PAF-AH), a serine esterase (62). Treatment of MM-LDL with PAF-AH eliminated the ability of MM-LDL to induce monocyte-endothelial interactions (63). When PAF-AH was inhibited with diisopropyl fluorophosphate, HDL was no longer protective and HPLC analysis revealed that the active oxidized phospholipid species in MM-LDL had been destroyed after PAF-AH treatment, increasing the amounts of lysophospholipids. Another enzyme associated with HDL is the ester hydrolase paraoxonase (64). Treatment of MM-LDL with purified paraoxonase significantly reduced the ability of MM-LDL to stimulate endothelial cells to bind monocytes. Furthermore, inactivation of paraoxonase in HDL by heat reduced the ability of HDL to protect against LDL modification (18). Isolated paraoxonase destroyed several oxygenated molecules in OxPAPC, rendering it inactive.

An enzyme which seems to contribute to the formation of bioactive oxidized phospholipids is secretory non-pancreatic phospholipase A_2 (group II $sPLA_2$). $sPLA_2$ is induced during inflammatory conditions, present in atherosclerotic lesions (65,66) and has been shown to act on lipoproteins (67). When transgenic mice expressing the group II $sPLA_2$ gene were fed a high fat diet, they developed severe atherosclerosis and marked inflammation in liver tissue (68). We investigated the mechanism by which group II $sPLA_2$ contributes to the development of inflammation and atherosclerotic lesions and showed that the biologically active oxidized phospholipids POVPC and PGPC, as well as the molecule with a mass of 828, but not lyso-PC, were increased in $sPLA_2$ transgenic mice. Analysis of the substrate specificity of human recombinant group II $sPLA_2$ by electrospray ionization-mass spectrometry revealed that the bioactive phospholipids were essentially resistant to hydrolysis by recombinant $sPLA_2$ whereas unoxidized PAPC was readily hydrolyzed by this enzyme. We showed that by liberating PUFAs, $sPLA_2$ may contribute to increased formation of oxidized phospholipids (69). Interestingly, HDL isolated from $sPLA_2$ transgenic animals had lost its ability to protect against LDL oxidation. This effect seemed to be correlated with reduced paraoxonase activity measured in the serum of these animals. Therefore, we hypothesize that $sPLA_2$ acts as an enhancer of inflammation by increasing the formation of biologically active oxidized phospholipids and abolishing the protective effects of HDL.

PRESENCE OF OXIDIZED PHOSPHOLIPIDS *IN VIVO*

We have shown that the biologically active oxidized phospholipids POVPC, PGPC and the molecule with a mass of 828 Da were present in atherosclerotic lesions of rabbits fed an atherogenic diet. The abundance of these molecules was significantly reduced when the diet had been supplemented with antioxidants such as vitamin E and probucol (59). Futhermore, the abundance of biologically active oxidized phospholipids in livers of recombinant inbred strains between mice which are highly susceptible to atherosclerosis when fed a high fat diet (C57/Bl6) and a resistant strain (C3H), correlated with aortic lesion size (70). POVPC, PGPC and the molecule with a mass of 828 Da were also increased in livers of group II $sPLA_2$ transgenic mice which were shown to develop atherosclerotic lesions, when compared to non-transgenic littermates (69).

MM-LDL is not the only source for biologically active oxidized phospholipids. It has been shown that vascular endothelial and smooth muscle cells, when subjected to oxidant stress, pinch off vesicles from their membranes (so called "blebs") which contain biologically active oxidized phospholipids (71). Therefore, it is very likely that at sites of inflammation, where increased oxidant stress has been reported, oxidized phospholipids are released from cells and contribute to the inflammatory process (72). (see Chapter 6).

Collectively, the data outlined above demonstrate that biologically active oxidized phospholipids are present in various tissues *in vivo* and suggest their contribution to the development of atherosclerosis and other inflammatory diseases.

SUMMARY

The current treatment of atherosclerosis is directed to altering lipoprotein levels. The finding that the molecules in MM-LDL responsible for induction of monocyte-endothelial interactions are oxidized phospholipids and the identification of their chemical structures leads to new possibilities for clinical intervention: (1) Cloning and identification of the individual receptors for these molecules as well as synthesis of specific receptor antagonists will help to inhibit the action of these lipid mediators at the receptor level. (2) More information is needed about the intracellular signalling pathways induced by the various bioactive lipids to devise strategies for pharmacological intervention at the cellular level. (3) Although bioactive oxidized phospholipids are generated through free radical-induced oxidation, identification of the most important enzymes that produce and destroy these radicals as well as enzymes that destroy bioactive phospholipids will lead to new strategies for clinical intervention.

References

1.   Berliner JA, Heinecke JW. The role of oxidized lipoproteins in atherogenesis. *Free Rad Biol Med.* 1996;20:707.
2.   Parthasarathy S, Rankin SM. The role of oxidized LDL in atherogenesis. *Prog Lipid Res.* 1992;31:127.
3.   Witztum JL, Steinberg D. Role of oxidized low density lipoprotein in atherogenesis. *J Clin Invest.* 1991;88:1785.
4.   Berliner JA, Navab M, Fogelman AM, Frank JS, Demer LL, Edwards PA, Watson AD, Lusis AJ. Atherosclerosis: Basic mechanisms: Oxidation, inflammation and genetics. *Circulation.* 1995;91:2488.
5.   Hoff HF, Gaubatz JW. Isolation, purification, and characterization of a lipoprotein containing Apo B from the human aorta. *Atherosclerosis.* 1982;42:243.
6.   Ylä-Herttuala S, Palinski W, Rosenfeld ME, Parthasarathy S, Carew TE, Butler S, Witztum JL, Steinberg D. Evidence for the presence of oxidatively modified low density lipoprotein in atherosclerotic lesions of rabbit and man. *J Clin Invest.* 1989;84:1086.
7.   Palinski W, Hörkkö S, Miller E, Steinbrecher UP, Powell HC, Curtiss LK, Witztum JL. Cloning of monoclonal autoantibodies to epitopes of oxidized lipoproteins from apolipoprotein E-deficient mice. *J Clin Invest.* 1996;98:800.
8.   Hörkkö S, Miller E, Dudl E, Reaven P, Curtiss LK, Zvaifler NJ, Terkeltaub R, Pierangeli SS, Branch DW, Palinski W, Witztum JL. Antiphospholipid antibodies are directed against epitopes of oxidized phospholipids. Recognition of cardiolipin by monoclonal antibodies to epitopes of oxidized low density lipoprotein. *J Clin Invest.* 1996;98:815.
9.   Hörkkö S, Miller E, Branch DW, Palinski W, Witztum JL. The epitopes of some antiphospholipid antibodies are adducts of oxidized phospholipid and beta2 glycoprotein 1 (and other proteins). *Proc Natl Acad Sci USA.* 1997;94:10356.
10.   Berliner JA, Territo MC, Sevanian A, Ramin,S, Kim JA, Bamshad B, Esterson M, Fogelman AM. Minimally modified low density lipoprotein stimulates monocyte endothelial interactions. *J Clin Invest.* 1990;85:1260.
11.   Esterbauer H, Dieber-Rotheneder M, Waeg G, Striegl G, Jürgens G. Biochemical, structural, and functional properties of oxidized low-density lipoprotein. *Chem Res Toxicol.* 1990;3:77.

12. Sparrow CP, Parathasarathy S, Steinberg D. Enzymatic modification of low density lipoprotein by purified lipoxygenase plus phospholipase A_2 mimics cell-mediated oxidative modification. *J Lipid Res.* 1988;29:745.

13. Kosugi K, Morel DW, Di Corleto PE,Chisholm GM. Toxicity of oxidized LDL to cultured fibroblasts is selective for S phase of the cell cycle. *J Cell Physiol.* 1987;130:311.

14. Navab M, Imes SS, Hama SY, Hough GP, Ross LA, Bork RW, Valente AJ, Berliner JA, Drinkwater DC, Laks H, Fogelman AM. Monocyte transmigration induced by modification of low density lipoprotein in co-cultures of human aortic wall cells is due to induction of monocyte chemotactic protein 1 synthesis and is abolished by high density lipoprotein. *J Clin Invest.* 1991;88:2039.

15. Asakawa T, Matsushita S. A colorimetric microdetermination of peroxide values utilizing aluminum chloride as the catalyst. *Lipids.* 1980;15:965.

16. Morrow JD, Roberts LJ. The isoprostanes: unique bioactive products of lipid peroxidation. *Prog Lipid Res.* 1997;36:1.

17. Steinbrecher UP. Oxidation of human LDL results in derivatization of lysine residues of apolipoprotein B by lipid peroxide decomposition products. *J Biol Chem.* 1987;262:3603.

18. Watson AD, Berliner JA, Hama SY, La Du BN, Faull KF, Fogelman AM, Navab M. Protective effect of high density lipoprotein associated paraoxonase. Inhibition of the biological activity of minimally oxidized low density lipoprotein. *J Clin Invest.* 1995;96:2882.

19. Berliner JA, Gerrity RG. Pathology of atherogenesis. In: Lusis AJ, Rotter JI, Sparkes RS, eds. *Molecular genetics of coronary artery disease.* 1992; 1.

20. Kim JA, Territo MC, Wayner E, Carlos TM, Parhami F, Smith CW, Haberland ME, Fogelman AM, Berliner JA. Partial characterization of leukocyte binding molecules on endothelial cells induced by minimally oxidized LDL. *Arterioscler Thromb.* 1994;14:427.

21. Teng P, Vora DK, Elices M, Frank J, Territo MC, Berliner JA. The role of alternatively spliced fibronectin in monocyte binding to endothelial cells treated with oxidized lipids. *FASEB J.* 1996;10:A1281.

22. Maier JAM, Barenghi L, Bradamante S, Pagani F. Induction of human endothelial cell growth by mildly oxidized low density lipoprotein. *Atherosclerosis.* 1996;123:115.

23. McEvoy LM, Sun H, Tsao PS, Cooke JP, Berliner JA, Butcher EC. Novel vascular molecule involved in monocyte adhesion to aortic endothelium in models of atherogenesis. *J Exp Med.* 1997;185:2069.

24. Calderon TM, Factor SM, Hatcher VB, Berliner JA, Berman JW. An endothelial cell adhesion protein for monocytes recognized by monoclonal antibody IG9. Expression in vivo in inflamed human vessels and atherosclerotic human and Watanabe rabbit vessels. *Lab Invest.* 1994;70:849.

25. Springer TA. Traffic signals for lymphocyte recirculation and leukocyte emigration: the multistep paradigm. *Cell.* 1994;76:311.

26. Lasky LA. Selectins: interpreters of cell-specific carbohydrate information during inflammation. *Science.* 1992;258:964.

27. Parhami F, Fang ZT, Fogelman AM, Andalibi A, Territo MC, Berliner JA. Minimally modified low density lipoprotein-induced inflammatory responses in endothelial cells are mediated by cyclic adenosine monophosphate. *J Clin Invest.* 1993;92:471.

28. McEver RP, Beckstead JH, Moore KL, Marshall-Carlson L, Bainton DF. GMP-140, a platelet alpha granule membrane protein is also synthesized by vascular endothelial cells and is localized in Weibel-Palade bodies. *J Clin Invest.* 1989;84:92.

29. Hattory R, Hamilton KK, Fugate RD, McEver RP, Sims PJ. Stimulation of secretion of endothelial von Willebrand factor is accompanied by rapid redistribution to the cell surface of the intracellular granule membrane protein GMP-140. *J Biol Chem.* 1989;264:7768.

30. Vora DK, Fang ZT, Liva SM, Tyner TR, Parhami F, Watson AD, Drake TA, Territo MC, Berliner JA. Induction of P-selectin by oxidized lipoproteins. Separate effects on synthesis and surface expression. *Circ Res.* 1997;80:810.

31. Cushing SD, Berliner JA, Valente AJ, Territo MC, Navab M, Parhami F, Gerrity R, Schwartz CJ, Fogelman AM. Minimally modified low density lipoprotein induces monocyte chemotactic protein 1 in human endothelial cells and smooth muscle cells. *Proc Natl Acad Sci USA.* 1990;87:5134.

32.   Rajavasisth TB, Andalibi A, Territo MC, Berliner JA, Navab M, Fogelman AM, Lusis AJ. Modified LDL induce endothelial cell expression of granulocyte and macrophage colony stimulating factors. *Nature*. 1990;344:254.

33.   Clinton SK, Underwood R, Hayes I, Sherman MI, Kufe DW, Libby P. Macrophage colony stimulating factor gene expression in vascular cells and in experimental and human atherosclerosis. *Am J Pathol*. 1992;140:301.

34.   Rosenfeld ME, Ylä-Herttuala S, Lipton BA, Ord VA, Witztum JL, Steinberg D. Macrophage colony-stimulating factor mRNA and protein in atherosclerotic lesions of rabbits and humans. *Am J Pathol*. 1992;140:291.

35.   Ylä-Herttuala S, Lipton BA, Rosenfeld ME, Sarkioja T, Yoshimura T, Leonard EJ, Witztum JL, Steinberg D. Macrophages express monocyte chemotactic protein (MCP-1) in human and rabbit atherosclerotic lesions. *Proc Natl Acad Sci USA*. 1991;88:5252.

36.   Bork RW, Svenson KL, Mehrabian M, Lusis AJ, Fogelman AM, Edwards PA. Mechanisms controlling competence gene expression in murine fibroblasts stimulated with minimally modified LDL. *Arterioscl Thromb*. 1992;12:800.

37.   Schwartz D, Chaverri-Almada L, Berliner JA, Kirchgessner T, Quismorio DC, Fang ZT, Tekamp-Olson P, Lusis AJ, Fogelman AM, Territo MC. The role of a gro homologue in monocyte adhesion to the endothelium. *J Clin Invest*. 1994;94:1068.

38.   Boisvert WA, Santiago R, Curtiss LK, Terkeltaub RA. Aleukocyte homologue of the IL-8 receptor CXCR-2 mediates the accumulation of macrophages in atherosclerotic lesions of LDL receptor-deficient mice. *J Clin Invest*. 1998;101:353.

39.   Li SR, Forster LA, Anggard EE, Ferns GA. RT-PCR study on the effects of minimally modified low-density lipoproteins and probucol treatment on gene expressions of interleukin-1 and platelet-derived growth factor B-chain in human peripheral blood mononuclear cells. *Biol Signals*. 1996;5:263.

40.   Yoshida H, Quehenberger O, Kondratenko N, Green S, Steinberg D. Minimally oxidized low-density lipoprotein increases expression of scavenger receptor A, CD 36, and macrosialin in resident mouse peritoneal macrophages. *Arterioscler Thromb Vasc Biol*. 1998;18:794.

41.   Liao F, Berliner JA, Mehrabian M, Navab M, Demer LL, Lusis AJ, Fogelman AM. Minimally modified low density lipoprotein is biologically active in vivo in mice. *J Clin Invest*. 1991;87:2253.

42.   Drake TA, Hannani K, Fei HH, Lavi S, Berliner JA. Minimally oxidized low density lipoprotein induces tissue factor expression in cultured human endothelial cells. *Am J Pathol*. 1991;138:601.

43.   Fei H, Berliner JA, Parhami F, Drake TA. Regulation of endothelial tissue factor expression by minimally oxidized LDL and lipopolysaccharide. *Arterioscler Thromb*. 1993;13:1711.

44.   Bielicki JK, Forte TM, McCall MR. Minimally oxidized LDL is a potent inhibitor of lecithin:cholesterol acyltransferase activity. *J Lipid Res*. 1996;37:1012.

45.   Ishikawa K, Navab M, Leitinger N, Fogelman AM, Lusis AJ. Induction of Heme Oxygenase-1 inhibits the monocyte transmigration induced by mildly oxidizd LDL. *J Clin Invest*. 1997;100:1209.

46.   Parhami F, Morrow AD, Balucan J, Leitinger N, Watson AD, Tintut Y, Berliner JA, Demer LL. Lipid oxidation products have opposite effects on calcifying vascular cell and bone cell differentiation. *Arterioscler Thromb Vasc Biol*. 1997;17:680.

47.   Parhami F, Fang ZT, Yang B, Fogelman AM, Berliner JA. Stimulation of Gs and inhibition of Gi protein functions by minimally oxidized LDL. *Arterioscl Thromb Vasc Biol*. 1995;15:2019.

48.   Ha H, Roh DD, Kirschenbaum MA, Kamanna VS. Atherogenic lipoproteins enhance mesangial cell expression of platelet-derived growth factor: role of protein tyrosine kinase and cyclic AMP-dependent protein kinase A. *J Lab Clin Med*. 1998;131:456.

49.   Honda HM, Leitinger N, Frankel M, Goldhaber JI, Natarajan R, Weiss JN, Nadler J, Berliner JA. Induction of monocyte binding to endothelial cells by MM-LDL: The role of lipoxygenase metabolites. *Arterioscl Thromb Vasc Biol*. in press.

50.   Auge N, Fitoussi G, Bascands JL, Pieraggi MT, Junquero D, Valet P, Girolami JP, Salvayre R, Negre-Salvayre A. Mildly oxidized LDL evokes a sustained Ca^{2+}-dependent retraction of vascular smooth muscle cells. *Circ Res*. 1996;79:871.

51.   Rajavashisth TB, Yamada H, Mishra NK. Transcriptional activation of the macrophage-colony stimulating factor gene by minimally modified LDL. Involvement of nuclear factor-kappa B. *Arterioscl Thromb Vasc Biol*. 1995;15:1591.

52. Liao F, Andalibi A, deBeer FC, Fogelman AM, Lusis AJ. Genetic control of inflammatory gene induction and NFkB-like transcription factor activation in response to an atherogenic diet in mice. *J Clin Invest.* 1993;91:2572.

53. Liao F, Andalibi A, Qiao JH, Allayee H, Fogelman AM, Lusis AJ. Genetic evidence for a common pathway mediating oxidative stress, inflammatory gene induction, and aortic fatty streak formation in mice. *J Clin Invest.* 1994;94:877.

54. Liao F, Lusis AJ, Berliner JA, Fogelman AM, Kindy M, deBeer MC, deBeer FC. Serum amyloid A protein family: differential induction by oxidized lipids in mouse strains. *Arterioscl Thromb.* 1994;14:1475.

55. Andalibi A, Liao F, Imes S, Fogelman AM, Lusis AJ. Oxidized lipoproteins influence gene expression by causing oxidative stress and activating the transcription factor NFkB. *Biochem Soc Trans.* 1993;21:651.

56. Collins T, Read MA, Neish AS, Whitley MZ, Thanos D, Maniatis T. Transcriptional regulation of endothelial cell adhesion molecules: NF-kappa B and cytokine-inducible enhancers. *FASEB J.* 1995;9:899.

57. Ghersa P, Hooft van Huijsduijnen R, Whelan J, Cambet Y, Pescini R, DeLamarter JF. Inhibition of E-selectin gene transcription through a cyclic AMP-dependent protein kinase pathway. *J Biol Chem.* 1994;269:29129.

58. Parry GCN, Mackman N. Role of cyclic AMP response element-binding protein in cyclic AMP inhibition of NF-κB-mediated transcription. *J Immunol.* 1997;159:5450.

59. Watson AD, Leitinger N, Navab M, Faull KF, Hörkkö S, Witztum JL, Palinski W, Schwenke D, Salomon RG, Sha W, Subbanagounder G, Fogelman AM, Berliner JA. Structural identification by mass spectrometry of oxidized phospholipids in minimally oxidized low density lipoprotein that induce monocyte/endothelial interactions and evidence for their presence in vivo. *J Biol Chem.* 1997;272:13597.

60. Leitinger N, Watson AD, Faull KF, Fogelman AM, Berliner JA. Monocyte binding to endothelial cells induced by oxidized phospholipids present in minimally oxidized low density lipoprotein is inhibited by a platelet activating factor receptor antagonist. In *Recent Advances in Prostaglandin, Thromboxane, and Leukotriene Research.* Sinzinger, H. et al., eds., Plenum Press, New York. 1998; pp 379.

61. Navab M, Berliner JA, Watson AD, Hama SY, Territo MC, Lusis AJ, Shih DM, Van Lenten BJ, Frank JS, Demer LL, Edwards PA, Fogelman AM. The Yin and Yang of oxidation in the development of the fatty streak. *Arterioscler Thromb Vasc Biol.* 1996;16:831.

62. Stafforini DM, Prescott SM, Zimmerman GA, McIntyre TM. Mammalian platelet-activating factor acetylhydrolases. *Biochim Biophys Acta.* 1996;1301:161.

63. Watson AD, Navab M, Hama SY, Sevanian A, Prescott SM, Stafforini DM, McIntyre TM, La Du BN, Fogelman AM, Berliner JA. Effect of platelet activating factor-acetylhydrolase on the formation and action of minimally oxidized low density lipoprotein. *J Clin Invest.* 1995;95:774.

64. Mackness MI, Mackness B, Durrington PN, Connelly PW, Hegele RA. Paraoxonase: biochemistry, genetics and relationship to plasma lipoproteins. *Curr Opin Lipidol.* 1996;7:69.

65. Menschikowski M, Kasper M, Lattke P, Schiering A, Schiefer S, Stockinger H, Jaross W. Secretory group II phospholipase A_2 in human atherosclerotic plaques. *Atherosclerosis.* 1995;118:173.

66. Hurt-Camejo E, Andersen S, Standal R, Rosengren B, Sartipy P, Stadberg E, Johansen B. Localization of nonpancreatic secretory phospholipase A_2 in normal and atherosclerotic arteries. *Arterioscler Thromb Vasc Biol.* 1997;17:300.

67. de Beer FC, de Beer MC, van der Westerhuyzen DR, Castellani LW, Lusis AJ, Swanson ME, Grass DS. Secretory non-pancreatic phospholipase A_2: influence on lipoprotein metabolism. *J Lipid Res.* 1997;38:2232.

68. Ivandic B, Castellani L, Wang XP, Qiao JH, Mehrabian M, Navab M, Fogelman AM, Grass DS, Swanson ME, de Beer MC, de Beer F, Lusis AJ. Role of group II secretory PLA_2 in atherosclerosis: 1. Increased atherogenesis and altered lipoproteins in transgenic mice expressing group II phospholipase A_2. *Arterioscl Thromb Vasc Biol.* in press.

69. Leitinger, N., Watson AD, Hama SY, Ivandic B, Qiao JH. Huber J, Faull KF, Grass DS, Navab M, Fogelman AM, de Beer FC, Lusis AJ, Berliner JA. Role of group II secretory PLA2 in atherosclerosis: 2. Potential involvement of biologically active oxidized phospholipids. *Arterioscl Thromb Vasc Biol.* in press.

70.   Berliner JA, Leitinger N, Watson AD, Huber J, Fogelman AM, Navab M. Oxidized lipids in atherogenesis: Formation, destruction and action. *Thromb Haemost.* 1997;78:195.
71.   Patel KD, Zimmerman GA, Prescott SM, McIntyre TM. Novel leukocyte agonists are released by endothelial cells exposed to peroxide. *J Biol Chem.* 1992;267:15168.
72.   Prescott SM, Patel KD, Smiley PL, Stafforini DM, Lorant DE, Zimmerman GA, McIntyre TM. Potential roles for oxidized phospholipids in inflammation and atherogenesis. *Atheroscl Rev.* 1993;25:59

8 OXIDATION-SENSITIVE TRANSCRIPTION AND GENE EXPRESSION IN ATHEROSCLEROSIS

Charles Kunsch and Russell M. Medford

INTRODUCTION

Historically, most research into the role of oxidative stress and reactive oxygen species (ROS) in inflammatory diseases such as rheumatoid arthritis, pulmonary emphysema, neurodegenerative disorders and atherosclerosis has focused on the putative role of ROS as cellular damaging agents through the potential toxic oxidative modification of macromolecules such as proteins, lipids and DNA and on the cytotoxicity of free radicals and their reaction products (1). In this context, ROS have been viewed as playing a destructive role in biology. Although this may be true for high concentrations of ROS, many cell types such as fibroblasts, endothelial cells and smooth muscle cells have been shown to produce ROS at relatively low levels where they play a role as intracellular messenger molecules. In this context, ROS serve as physiological second messengers to regulate signal transduction pathways that ultimately control gene expression and post-translational modifications of proteins.

ROS have been implicated in a variety of diseases including Alzheimer's, cancer, and vascular diseases such as restenosis and atherosclerosis. In the case of atherosclerosis, recent insights into the etiology and pathogenesis of this disease suggest that atherosclerosis may be viewed as an inflammatory disease linked to an abnormality in oxidation-mediated signals in the vasculature (2-4, see Chapter 4). The focus of this review is to summarize the current literature supporting the view of oxygen-mediated signals as physiological regulators of gene expression in the vasculature by modulating specific reduction-oxidation (redox)-sensitive signal transduction pathways and transcriptional regulatory events.

ATHEROSCLEROSIS, OXIDATIVE SIGNALS, AND VASCULAR
INFLAMMATORY GENE EXPRESSION

Although the precise cellular and molecular processes involved in atherogenesis are
unknown, atherosclerosis is generally viewed as a chronic inflammatory disease of
the arterial intima characterized by the formation of the atherosclerotic plaque – a
focal accumulation of foam cells, mononuclear leukocytes, smooth muscle cells,
lipids and extracellular matrix components (5, 6). One of the earliest detectable
events in the generation of atherosclerosis is the infiltration of inflammatory cells to
localized areas of the arterial wall and their subsequent transformation into lipid-
laden macrophages or foam cells. The initial recruitment of leukocytes into the
lesion is mediated by an increased gradient of chemotactic factors released from the
endothelium or smooth muscle cells and the expression of leukocyte adhesion
molecules by various inflammatory stimuli. Several lines of investigation suggest
that oxidative stress and the production of ROS play a key role in mediating the
pathologic manifestations of endothelial cell dysfunction associated with
atherosclerosis (see Chapter 4).

Hyperlipidemia, diabetes, hypertension and smoking are well-established risk
factors for the development of atherosclerosis. A current hypothesis suggests that
modulation of the expression of a selective set of vascular inflammatory genes by
intracellular oxidative signals may provide a molecular mechanism linking these
seemingly diverse risk factors with the early pathogenesis of atherosclerosis (5, 6).
This hypothesis suggests that various pro-inflammatory or pro-oxidant stimuli – *i.e.*
tumor necrosis factor–α (TNF–α), interleukin-1β (IL-1β), oxidatively modified low
density lipoprotein (oxLDL), angiotensin II, and hemodynamic forces – may directly
stimulate or sensitize vascular cells to generate ROS. Such ROS would then serve
as second messengers coupling these extracellular signals to the elevated expression
of atherogenic and pro-inflammatory gene products such as adhesion molecules and
cytokines, respectively. The induced expression of these gene products would thus
promote the infiltration of monocytes into the vessel wall and the release of
additional pro-inflammatory signals. Accordingly, this positive feedback loop
would serve to potentiate the local inflammatory response and endothelial cell
dysfunction. Conversely, chemical or cellular antioxidants would protect vascular
cells against oxidative stress by scavenging ROS generated from the inflammatory
stimuli and altering the oxidative milieu, or by directly modulating redox-sensitive
signaling pathways and blocking atherogenic gene expression (Figure 1).

Consistent with this hypothesis is the observation that the expression of vascular
inflammatory gene products such as vascular cell adhesion molecule-1 (VCAM-1)
and monocyte chemoattractant protein-1 (MCP-1) by diverse pro-inflammatory
stimuli occurs through a oxidation-sensitive mechanism involving the redox-
regulated transcription factor NF–κB (7-9). Thiol antioxidants such as pyrrolidine
dithiocarbamate (PDTC) and N-acetylcysteine (NAC) and other chemically distinct
antioxidants inhibit cytokine inducible expression of both VCAM-1 and MCP-1 in

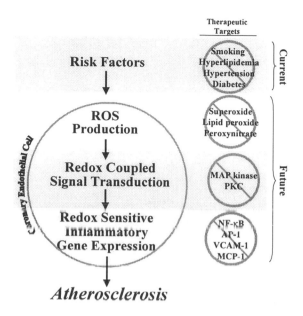

Atherosclerosis

Figure 1. Mechanism-based therapeutics for atherosclerosis. Various risk factors for atherosclerosis including smoking, hypertension, hyperlipidemia and diabetes result in the generation of intracellular oxidative stress in the endothelial cell. The mechanisms by which these risk factors generate oxidative stress are ill characterized and may act synergistically. The intracellular production of ROS in response to these risk factors act as second messagner coupling molecules in signal transduction pathways to modulate redox sensitive transcription factors and, ultimately, regulate redox-sensitive inflammatory gene expression. Current therapeutic strategies are aimed at the underlying risk factors associated with atherosclerosis. However, multiple molecular targets involved in redox-mediated signal transduction and gene expression could potentially serve as novel points of therapeutic intervention.

endothelial cells. Thus, ROS may act as specific regulators in the signal transduction network to relay environmental and physical signals generated at the cell membrane to nuclear regulatory signals resulting in modulation of inflammatory gene expression. In the following sections we will review the current literature with respect to understanding: i) physiological sources of oxidative stress in the vasculature, ii) specific transcriptional regulatory factors and signaling events modulated by an altered redox environment in the vasculature and iii) the functional implications of redox-sensitive modulation of gene expression in the vasculature with respect to the pathogenesis of atherosclerosis.

Sources of Oxidative Stress

A variety of processes associated with atherogenesis such as hyperglycemia, hypertension, oxidative modification of lipoproteins, and local hemodynamic stresses are known to mediate elevated expression of ROS in the vasculature (see Chapter 2). Potential cellular sources of ROS may include, but are not limited to, normal products of mitochondrial respiration, NADPH oxidase, nitric oxide synthases, cyclooxygenases, lipoxygenases and xanthine oxidase (12). Mammalian cells are protected from ROS by antioxidant defense mechanisms such as the enzymes catalase, superoxide dismutase (SOD) and glutathione peroxidase. When the normal redox homeostasis of the cell is upset and the rate of formation of ROS exceeds the capacity of the antioxidant defense system, a condition of oxidative stress exists (see Chapter 1). The role of various atherogenic risk factors and the cellular and enzymatic sources in cellular redox control has been extensively reviewed by others (13-15) and thus is only briefly discussed here with respect to their potential involvement in mediating redox-sensitive gene expression in the vasculature.

Hypertension and Angiotensin II

Hypertension is an important risk factor for the development of vascular disease and atherosclerosis (8). Hypertension due to the dysregulation of the renin-angiotensin may play a particularly important role in the pathogenesis of these diseases. Recent studies have suggested a role for Ang II in the generation of oxidative stress in the vasculature through induction of superoxide production via NADPH oxidase (16) (see Chapter 17). Angiotensin II has also been shown to stimulate both MCP-1 and VCAM-1 mRNA expression in rat aortas (17). In these experiments, NADPH oxidase inhibitors and catalase blocked angiotensin II-stimulated VCAM-1 and MCP-1 expression suggesting that NADPH oxidase may be contributing to oxidative stress and regulation of vascular inflammatory genes via the generation of hydrogen peroxide (H_2O_2). Thus, angiotensin II, via the formation of oxidative stress and increased levels of pro-inflammatory genes in the vessel wall, may serve as a molecular link between hypertension and a major form of atherosclerosis.

Hyperglycemia

Another established risk factor for the development of vascular disease is complications related to diabetes as a consequence of hyperglycemia (see Chapters 14 and 15). Diabetes-associated hyperglycemia produces an intracellular oxidative stress that leads to vascular dysfunction (13). High concentrations of serum glucose stimulate superoxide generation and enhance cell-mediated LDL peroxidation in endothelial cells (18-19). In addition, incubation of endothelial cells with high concentrations of glucose resulted in an increased activation of the transcription factor NF–κB (20) suggesting that hyperglycemia may activate endothelial gene expression via activation of NF–κB.

The hyperglycemia of diabetes generates advanced glycation end products (AGEs). AGEs are post-translational modifications of cellular proteins believed to play a role in the vascular complications associated with diabetes (21) (see Chapter 15). Chronic AGE accumulation in animals promotes VCAM-1 expression and formation of atherosclerotic lesions in the absence of hyperglycemia (22). Interaction of AGEs with cell surface receptors (RAGES) has been shown to generate ROS, decrease the levels of reduced glutathione and activate NF–κB (23, 24). In addition, AGE induced expression of VCAM-1 and monocyte/endothelial interactions can be blocked by antioxidants (22). These observations suggest that pathogenic processes associated with diabetes result in an oxidative stress and expression of redox-sensitive inflammatory genes in the vessel wall.

Modified LDL

One of the earliest events in atherosclerosis is the oxidative modification of lipoproteins (in particular, LDL) in the vessel wall to form oxidized LDL (oxLDL, see Chapter 4). oxLDL alters the intracellular redox-status of the cell in part through the generation of superoxide (25) and has been implicated as an important pro-oxidant signal in the pathogenesis of atherosclerosis (7, 26). Several studies suggest that oxLDL or fatty acid hydroperoxides (one of the more abundant components of oxLDL) act as pro-oxidant signals to regulate vascular gene expression such as ICAM-1 and VCAM-1 (27, 28) or redox-sensitive transcriptional factors such as c-Fos, c-Jun and NF–κB (29-31). Cellular lipoxygenases may mediate LDL oxidation and the formation of fatty acid hydroperoxides in several cell types. Increased levels of 15-lipoxygenase activity have been detected in atherosclerotic lesions in rabbit and human aorta compared to normal arteries (32, 33). Furthermore, transient over-expression of 15-lipoxygenase enhances TNF–α-induced VCAM-1 expression (34) and 5-lipoxygenase inhibitors blocked IL-1β-induced VCAM-1 expression in endothelial cells (35). Together, these studies suggest a role for oxLDL as a pro-oxidant signal that modulates the expression of redox-sensitive inflammatory gene products. As of yet, the exact nature of the cellular signals which lead to the generation of oxidized lipids are not known.

Hemodynamic Forces

Vascular endothelial cells are constantly subjected to the influence of hemodynamic forces including shear stress imposed by blood flow. The effects of fluid shear stress on endothelial biology and gene expression are the subject of extensive studies (36, 37). One of the biological effects of shear stress is alteration of endothelial cell/leukocyte interactions. This altered adhesivity of leukocytes for the endothelial cell is due, at least in part, to the regulation of the adhesion proteins ICAM-1 and VCAM-1. Recent evidence suggest that oxidative stress may contribute to shear-stress induced changes in endothelial gene expression.

Increased blood flow and fluid shear stresses alters the endothelial cell redox state and redox-sensitive gene expression (38-42). Laurindo *et al.* (38) provided both *ex vivo* and *in vivo* evidence that increases in blood flow lead to increased intracellular free radical release. In these studies, electron paramagnetic resonance spectroscopy was used to show that perfusion of isolated aortas led to increased levels of free radicals only in aortas containing an intact endothelium. This effect was completely blocked by addition of SOD, an antioxidant enzyme that accelerates the conversion of superoxide to H_2O_2. Similar effects were observed with *in vivo*-induced changes in blood flow. Hsieh and coworkers (40) demonstrated that exposure of endothelial cells to a steady laminar shear stress resulted in increased levels of intracellular ROS and expression of the redox-sensitive transcription factor c-Fos. These changes were abolished by treatment with the antioxidant NAC or catalase. Similar results were observed by Chiu *et al.* (41) who demonstrated that shear stress induced elevations of intracellular superoxide levels and ICAM-1 mRNA and promoter activities all of which could by blocked by NAC or SOD.

De Keulenaer and coworkers (39) recently showed that oscillatory shear stress induced the expression of NADH oxidase, superoxide, and the redox-sensitive gene heme oxygenase-1 in cultured endothelial cells. These effects could be blocked by pretreatment with the antioxidant NAC. In contrast, application of steady laminar shear induced only a transient increase in NADH oxidase and lower levels of superoxide. The authors suggest that steady laminar shear may induce compensatory antioxidant defense mechanisms by the observed increased expression of SOD an antioxidant defense enzyme whose level of expression adapts to changes in oxidative stress. Similar increases in SOD expression by shear stress were observed in human arterial endothelial cells (43) and human umbilical vein endothelial cells (44). The notion that steady laminar shear stress may play an protective role in vasculature is supported by the observation that steady unidirectional shear stress decreases the basal and cytokine-induced expression of VCAM-1 in human endothelial cells (45, 46).

In addition to the generation of ROS, shear stress is a potent stimulus for endothelial synthesis of nitric oxide (NO) (47, 48). This may be due, in part, to an increase in steady-state mRNA levels for the endothelial isoform of nitric oxide synthase (eNOS) (44, 49) and may be mediated by activation of c-Src-dependent serine kinase by shear stress (50). Tsao and coworkers (45) have shown that NO mediates the steady shear stress inhibition of oxLDL and LPS/TNF–α-induced superoxide production, NF–κB activation, VCAM-1 expression and endothelial-monocyte adhesion. Under appropriate conditions NO may reduce intracellular oxidative stress (45). Thus, elaboration of NO may be one mechanism by which endothelial cells modulate the level of intracellular ROS and regulate redox-sensitive gene expression in response to changes in endothelial shear stresses. Cumulatively, these data support the notion that modulation of endothelial cell redox state by shear stress may contribute to altered endothelial gene expression and contribute to the focal nature of atherosclerosis.

NADPH Oxidase

Stimulation of various mammalian cell types with cytokines, phorbol esters or growth factors results in an oxidative stress response due to the production of ROS. In both endothelial cells and vascular smooth muscle cells, NADPH oxidase is an important source of superoxide (16, 51). Cytokines and growth factors such as TNF–α, IL-1β, angiotensin II and interferon–γ activate membrane bound NADPH oxidase and stimulate the production of superoxide in endothelial cells (16, 51-53).

Diphenylene iodonium, an inhibitor of NADPH oxidase, has been shown to abrogate superoxide production in response to TNF–α in endothelial cells (54). The notion that ROS generated via NADPH oxidase may function as signaling molecules to modulate vascular gene expression is supported by the observation that NADPH oxidase inhibitors block cytokine-induced VCAM-1 and ICAM-1 gene expression in human aortic endothelial cells (54) and attenuate angiotensin II-mediated activation of VCAM-1 and MCP-1 in vascular smooth muscle cells (55). Consequently, the generation of ROS via NADPH oxidase in response to pro-inflammatory stimuli may regulate the expression of a variety of redox-sensitive genes in the vasculature.

Nitric Oxide

The free radical NO is produced by multiple cell types including endothelial cells, macrophages, smooth muscle cells, and fibroblasts and has been shown to be an important factor in the regulation of many biological responses. NO produced by the endothelium exhibits a number of anti-atherogenic properties including modulation of vasomotor tone and inhibition of platelet aggregation and smooth muscle cell proliferation (see Chapter 9) (56). Based on the cell type or concentration relative to superoxide, NO has been shown to both augment (57, 58) and inhibit (59, 60) oxygen-radical mediated tissue damage and lipid peroxidation. Thus, NO exhibits a dual redox function based on its interaction with other ROS. Several studies have demonstrated NO inhibits induction of vascular inflammatory gene expression including VCAM-1 (61, 62) and MCP-1 (63, 64). Furthermore, several studies have demonstrated that NO blocks the activity of cytokine-activated NF–κB in endothelial cells (61, 64, 65), thus providing a potential mechanism for NO suppression of vascular gene expression. NO may also modulate gene expression by reducing intracellular oxidative stress. NO has been shown to i) reduce superoxide generation in response to cytokines in endothelial cells (63), ii) inhibit oxidation of LDL and delay the formation of lipid peroxides (66) and iii) redirect the reactivity of partially reduced oxygen species (67). Thus, through direct modulation of intracellular oxidative stress NO can modulate signaling pathways (such as those involved in NF–κB activation) and regulate the expression of vascular inflammatory genes such as VCAM-1 and MCP-1.

Redox Modulation of Transcription Factor Activity

Transcription factors are the principal nuclear components that control gene expression. Regulation of transcription factor activity is mediated by post-translational modifications which, in turn, are controlled by a variety of signaling pathway. In this regard, vascular oxidative stress and ROS may be defined as second messenger molecules that regulate various intracellular signal transduction cascades and ultimately affect transcriptional activity. Indeed, in the vasculature ROS can affect multiple signal transduction pathways upstream of nuclear transcription factors, including modulation of Ca^{2+} signaling and protein kinase and phosphatase pathways (68-70). The role of protein kinases in mediating redox-sensitive signal transduction is summarized in Chapter 18.

The hypothesis that redox-sensitive signaling pathways regulate vascular inflammatory gene expression implies that ultimately, specific DNA binding proteins, or transcription factors, will be the target of such a signaling cascade. Transcription factors are central to any discussion of gene regulation, as they are the nuclear components that are modulated by upstream signaling events. By virtue of their ability to interact with very specific DNA sequences (which are unique to each transcription factor) in the regulatory regions of genes, transcription factors serve to modulate not only the magnitude of gene expression, but also the specificity of the signal. This specificity is determined in part by the presence or absence of a DNA binding site in the promoter region of the target gene.

The activity of many eukaryotic transcription factors has been reported to be modulated by redox changes and has been summarized in several excellent reviews (12, 68, 71, 72). Many of the reported studies demonstrate changes in the *in vitro* DNA binding activity of transcription factors in response to oxidants or reductants. Generally, highly conserved cysteine residues in the DNA binding regions of these proteins have been shown to be targets of redox modulation. These *in vitro* studies have generally shown that reducing environments increase, while oxidizing conditions inhibit, sequence-specific DNA binding. However, when intact cells have been used for study, it is generally observed that oxidizing agents activate and reducing conditions inhibit transcription factor activity. These observations present an intriguing paradox and suggest that *in vivo*, more complex regulatory networks mediated by ROS impart redox control of transcription factor activity.

Theoretically, redox-sensitive modulation of transcription factor activity can occur via: i) direct oxidative modification of the transcription factor itself by intracellular ROS or ii) postranslational modifications (ie. phosphorylation/dephosphorylation), by the effects of redox-regulated intracellular signaling cascades. Either mechanism can potentially affect various aspects of transcription factor function such as subcellular localization, DNA binding properties, and inherent transcriptional activity. Although redox regulation of many transcription factors has been documented, we will focus on the two best-characterized transcription factors subject to redox regulation in the vasculature, NF–κB and AP-1. In addition, we will discuss recent evidence implicating the potential role of the peroxisome proliferator-activated receptor (PPAR) family of transcriptional activators in oxidative stress.

Redox Regulation of AP-1

NF–κB and AP-1 are the most extensively studied transcriptional factors influenced by the cellular redox state (12, 72, 73). They have been implicated in transcriptional regulation of a wide range of genes involved in cellular inflammatory responses, tissue destruction and growth control. Homo- and heterodimers of members of the c-Jun and c-Fos proto-oncogene families constitute the transcription factor AP-1. At least three mammalian Jun proteins (c-Jun, Jun B and Jun D) and four Fos family members (c-Fos, Fra-1, Fra-2, and Fos B) have been identified (reviewed in 74). All of the Jun family proteins are capable of forming homo- and heterodimers. Fos proteins do not associate with each other but are capable of associating with any member of the Jun family to form stable heterodimers that have higher DNA binding activity than Jun-Jun homodimers (75). Both Jun:Jun and Fos:Jun forms of AP-1 bind to a specific DNA sequence (the TPA responsive element, TRE) in promoters of many inducible genes. The promoter for the c-Jun gene contains a TRE and is primarily activated by AP-1 in a positive autoregulatory fashion (74, 76). The promoter for c-Fos, however, does not contain a TRE and, therefore, is not subject to autoregulation by AP-1.

The activity of AP-1 is controlled by both transcriptional and postranslational mechanisms in response to a variety of extracellular stimuli including mitogens, phorbol esters and differentiation signals. In addition, AP-1 behaves as a redox-sensitive transcription factor in several cell types and is activated, to different extents, under pro-oxidant conditions generated by treatment with agents such as superoxide, H_2O_2, UV light, γ-irradiation and cytokines (77-81). In cell types of the vasculature, AP-1 is similarly activated by pro-oxidant stimuli. In endothelial cells, agents such as H_2O_2 (82), LDL (83), and oxLDL (84) activate AP-1 DNA binding activity. In smooth muscle cells, oxLDL (85), H_2O_2 (86) and the lipid peroxidation product 4-hydroxy-2-nonenal (87) have been shown to increase AP-1 expression or DNA binding activity. Furthermore, regulation of the vascular inflammatory genes MCP-1 and ICAM-1 by H_2O_2 is mediated by AP-1 binding elements in the promoters of these genes (88-89).

Little information is known about the exact mechanisms underlying ROS mediated AP-1 activation; however, phospholipase A_2, arachidonic acid, lipoxygenase, and protein kinase C have all been proposed for H_2O_2 induction of c-Fos (90) and c-Jun (91) expression in vascular smooth muscle cells. In addition, H_2O_2-induced AP-1 activation requires both tyrosine and serine/threonine phosphorylation (92) and it has been suggested that AP-1 activation under oxidative conditions may be, at least in part, mediated by phosphorylation of Jun proteins (93). Therefore, it appears that post-translational modifications following oxidative stress may modulate AP-1 activity.

Paradoxically, a number of antioxidants including dithiocarbamates, the antioxidant enzyme thioredoxin, and NAC have also been shown to stimulate the DNA binding and transcriptional activity of AP-1 (93). In monocytic cells, the upregulation of the β_2 integrin CD11c by PDTC was shown to involve a functionally important AP-1 site and correlated with increased levels of AP-1 DNA binding by PDTC (94). Similarly, PDTC-induced ICAM-1 expression correlated with increased AP-1 binding to the PDTC-responsive region of the ICAM-1 promoter in endothelial cells (95). On the other hand, antioxidants have also been shown to block AP-1 transcriptional activity in endothelial cells. The antioxidant enzyme thioredoxin peroxidase-1 blocked TNF-α-induced AP-1 activation in endothelial cells (96). Wung *et al.* (88) demonstrated that cyclic strain and H_2O_2-induced MCP-1 gene expression in endothelial cells was mediated by an AP-1 element in the MCP-1 promoter. NAC and catalase prevented cyclic strain- or H_2O_2-induced AP-1 binding and MCP-1 expression. Thus, conflicting evidence exists over the role of antioxidants in AP-1 activation. Unfortunately, little is known regarding the precise mechanisms involved in redox-mediated AP-1 activity, and it is possible that the mechanistic pathways may impact differently on individual target genes and in different cell types. In addition, since different antioxidants were used in these studies, it is possible that the loci of action of different forms of antioxidants may be specific to their chemical class. Likely, it is the ultimate balance of intracellular redox potential which will determine the effect on AP-1 activity in response to either an oxidative or an antioxidant challenge. Clearly, additional studies are needed to clarify the role of AP-1 in mediating redox-sensitive gene expression.

Redox Regulation of Nuclear Factor–κB

NF–κB is an inducible transcription factor complex composed of homo- or heterodimeric complexes of the Rel family of transcriptional activators. The predominant form of NF–κB exists as a heterodimer of the p50 and p65 subunits. In unstimulated cells, NF–κB is held in an "inactive" form by sequestration in the cytoplasm to the IκB family of inhibitor proteins. Agents that activate NF–κB induce specific phosphorylation of IκB via IκB kinase (IKK) activity, which direct IκB to a ubiquitination/proteosomal degradation pathway. Degradation of IκB thus unmasks the nuclear localization sequence of NF–κB and allows NF–κB to enter the nucleus and bind to specific DNA sequences in the regulatory regions of its target genes.

The NF–κB transcription factor family controls the expression of a multitude of genes involved in inflammation and proliferation. Recent studies suggest the involvement of NF–κB in a variety of acute and chronic inflammatory diseases such as sepsis, Crohn's disease, and rheumatoid arthritis (97). In addition, it is becoming increasingly apparent that NF–κB is involved in the pathogenesis of proliferative disorders of the vasculature including restenosis (98-100) and atherosclerosis (73). Studies have shown that activated NF–κB is present at increased levels in the fibrotic thickened intima-media and atheromatous areas of atherosclerotic lesions whereas little or no activated NF–κB is detected in non-diseased vessels (101). NF–κB was also shown to be activated by an atherogenic diet (102) and by other cellular products believed to be involved in atherogenesis including oxLDL (30, 103, 104) and AGE (105). In addition, several of the cytokines and growth factors found in the atherosclerotic lesion such as TNF–α and IL-1β activate NF–κB *in vitro* in relevant cell types such as macrophages, smooth muscle cells, endothelial cells and lymphocytes. Furthermore, many of the genes which are regulated by NF–κB encode for proteins such as TNF–α, IL-1, M-CSF, MCP-1, Tissue Factor, VCAM-1, ICAM-1, and E-selectin which function in regulating critical processes in atherogenesis. Cumulatively, these observations suggest a strong correlative role, if not a causal association, of NF–κB in the pathogenesis of atherosclerosis.

Given the widely held hypothesis implicating redox imbalances in the pathogenesis of vascular disorders such as atherosclerosis and restenosis, it is not surprising, that a substantial body of evidence indicates that activation of NF–κB in vascular cells may be controlled by the redox status of the cell (106). In fact, NF–κB was the first eukaryotic transcription factor shown to respond directly to oxidative stress. A common step in all the activation mechanisms which lead to IκB degradation and NF–κB nuclear translocation has been suggested to involve ROS (107-109). This conclusion was reached based upon the inhibition of NF–κB activation by several chemically distinct antioxidants including NAC, dithiocarbamates, vitamin E derivatives, glutathione peroxidase activators and various metal chelators. Many reports now exist demonstrating inhibition of NF–κB nuclear translocation by antioxidants, although the extent of this block appears to vary with the cell type and the nature of the signal (106, 109).

Additional support for the involvement of ROS as a common activator of NF–κB is provided by many studies demonstrating elevated levels of ROS by agents such as TNF–α, IL-1β, PMA, UV-light, gamma rays and lipid hydroperoxides. These agents are very potent NF–κB activating agents, and antioxidants have been shown to block both ROS production and resultant NF–κB activation (108). Further support for an essential role of ROS in NF–κB activation derives from experiments using exogenously added pro-oxidants. Initial work by Baeuerle and colleagues, among others, have shown that in some cells lines, H_2O_2 and peroxide containing molecules result in a rapid activation of NF–κB (107-109). Strong support for a role of H_2O_2 in NF–κB activation came from studies in a catalase-overexpressing cell line which exhibited suppressed activation of NF–κB in response to TNF–α (110). Addition of a catalase inhibitor restored the NF–κB response. Also, overexpression of cytosolic SOD which causes cytosolic H_2O_2 accumulation, potentiated the NF–κB response. Cumulatively, these observation have led to a general agreement that NF–κB activation is at least facilitated by some oxidative reactions.

The specific molecular targets involved in the translation of redox signals to NF-κB activation are unknown. It is unlikely that the NF–κB subunits themselves are directly activated by oxidation because only the reduced form of NF–κB binds to DNA *in vitro*, (111) and attempts to activate isolated NF–κB by oxidation *in vitro* were unsuccessful (107). Direct oxidative inactivation of IκB is also not likely to be involved in the redox-regulation of NF–κB since treatment of isolated NF–κB/IκB complexes with H_2O_2 *in vitro* failed to dissociate IκB or lead to NF–κB DNA binding (107, 112). Most evidence suggests that oxidative stresses induce, and antioxidants prevent, the cytoplasmic-nuclear translocation of NF–κB. Therefore, the most likely scenario is that the signaling cascade leading to the phosphorylation and subsequent degradation of IκB is regulated by redox processes. Indeed, it has recently been demonstrated that antioxidants inhibit IKK activity and prevent the phosphorylation and subsequent degradation of IκB (113-114).

Although the primary mechanism of activation of NF–κB by ROS appears to be release from IκB and its translocation to the nucleus, it is possible that ROS may modulate the activity of NF–κB by regulating post-translational modifications of the NF–κB subunits themselves or of other transcriptional cofactors which influence the transcriptional activity of NF–κB. Postranslational modifications of NF–κB subunits may influence i) DNA binding affinity and/or specificity, ii) multimerization specificity with other NF–κB subunits, or iii) transcriptional activity. Although phosphorylation has been shown to be important for some of these events (115-117), no evidence exists to demonstrate a role of ROS in these processes. Clearly, however, understanding the role of redox processes in controlling the multitude of signaling events regulating the activity of NF–κB will provide important mechanistic insights regarding redox modulation of transcriptional activity.

Peroxisome Proliferator-Activated Receptors

The peroxisome proliferator-activated receptors (PPARs) are composed of members of the nuclear hormone receptor superfamily of transcription factors, a large and diverse group of proteins that mediate ligand-dependent transcriptional activation and repression (118). PPARs are key players in lipid and glucose metabolism and are implicated in metabolic disorders predisposing to atherosclerosis, such as dyslipidemia and diabetes. Recent reports suggest that PPARs may play a role in inflammatory processes involved in the pathogenesis of atherosclerosis and restenosis by their ability to modulate monocytic gene expression (119-121). Furthermore, PPAR expression and functional activity has recently been observed in vascular cell types such as endothelial cells (122) and smooth muscle cells (123, 124).

PPARγ is one member of the PPAR family that has received considerable attention due to its role in regulating, among other things, energy balance and adipocyte differentiation. Identification of PPARγ as the receptor for the oral hypoglycemic thiazolidinedione drugs linked this receptor to glucose homeostasis (125, 126). Two recent reports suggest that PPARγ is involved in the development of monocytes along the macrophage lineage, in particular in the conversion of monocytes to foam cells. Tontonoz *et al.* demonstrated that oxLDL, but not the parent LDL particle, induced the expression of PPARγ in foam cells of atherosclerotic lesions (127). In addition, exposure of cells to PPARγ agonists increased the binding of oxLDL, but not LDL. It was further shown that increased oxLDL binding was the result of increased expression of the scavenger receptor CD36, but not two of the other oxLDL receptors, SRA-type I or type II. In a companion paper the nature of the endogenous ligand for PPARγ was examined and it was shown that oxLDL, but not native LDL, could serve as an endogenous ligand for PPARγ and could stimulate PPARγ-dependent transcription (119). This study identified the active components of the oxLDL particle as 9- and 13- hydroxyoctadecanoic acid by demonstrating that these compounds themselves could mimic oxLDL with respect to monocyte maturation, PPARγ expression, PPARγ-dependent transcription and induced CD36 expression. Together, these studies point towards a direct role of oxLDL and components in the activation of PPARγ-dependent gene expression and regulation of the oxLDL receptor, CD36. It remains to be determined if activation by oxidized fatty acids plays a significant role in PPARγ-mediated processes in other tissues. These observations suggest that activation of PPARγ by oxLDL in monocytes may contribute to foam cell conversion and thus potentiate early events the pathogenesis of atherosclerosis.

In contrast to the proposed role of PPARγ in potentially pro-atherogenic events, it has recently been proposed that activation of PPARα and PPARγ may mediate anti-inflammatory responses in the vessel wall. Two recent reports demonstrated that specific agonists of PPARγ suppress pro-inflammatory gene expression in monocytes (120, 121). In addition, Staels and coworkers (123) demonstrate that inflammatory responses in aortic smooth muscle cells (IL-1 induced production of IL-6, prostaglandin and COX-2) is blocked by specific activators of PPARα, but not PPARγ. Furthermore, Poynter and Daynes (128) demonstrated that activation of PPARα in aged mice restored the cellular redox balance to that of young animals. This was evidenced by a lowering of tissue lipid peroxidation, elimination of constitutively active NF–κB, and a loss in spontaneous inflammatory cytokine production following administration of PPARα activators. These effects were not observed in animals bearing a null mutation in PPARα. Also, administration of the antioxidant, vitamin E, to aged mice (that contain reduced levels of PPARα mRNA), resulted in an elevated expression of PPARα to levels seen in younger mice. This observation suggests that balancing the cellular redox state may provide a level of transcriptional regulation for PPARα.

These studies demonstrate that ligands for PPARs are effective in reducing levels of inflammatory cytokines and downstream markers of inflammation. It seems possible that suppression of these pro-inflammatory signals by PPAR-mediated inhibition of inflammatory gene expression may be one way to modulate or balance the oxLDL-mediated pro-inflammatory events associated with atherosclerosis. Thus, in a given cell, it is likely that the subtle balance between pro-inflammatory signals and suppression of these signals by transcriptional modulators (such as PPARs) will determine the inflammatory status of the cell. Future work is need clarify the role of oxLDL in PPAR-mediated signaling especially in vascular cell types. Cumulatively, these studies suggest that PPARs may mediate transcriptional responses to oxidative stress in the vasculature and may be involved in disease processes such as atherosclerosis and restenosis. It will be interesting to determine to what degree chemical antioxidants and therapeutic strategies aimed at modifying PPAR function play in modulating PPAR-mediated molecular and cellular events both *in vitro* and *in vivo*.

CONCLUSIONS

Alterations in the cellular redox status modify DNA binding and transactivation activities of a variety of transcriptional activators. This, in turn, leads to changes in expression of a variety of target genes with ultimate changes in cell function. Redox regulation of gene expression, therefore, is a robust regulatory system that allows cells to adapt to environmental changes. In considering the pathogenesis of atherosclerosis, a strong body of data supports the notion that ROS generated in response to environmental and physical risk factors modulate signal transduction processes ultimately leading to vascular inflammatory gene expression. Vascular inflammatory genes, such as VCAM-1, E-selectin and MCP-1, represent a subset of genes implicated in the pathogenesis of atherosclerosis whose regulation is characterized by a linkage between redox-sensitive signals and the nuclear regulatory apparatus. Mechanistically this might suggest that the proposed therapeutic benefits of antioxidants in atherosclerosis might be due to alterations in the molecular regulation of gene expression of endothelial, smooth muscle, and inflammatory cells. Therefore, as depicted in Figure 1, redox-sensitive regulation of vascular gene expression represents an intriguing paradigm for understanding not only the pathogenesis of atherosclerosis but also for the development of novel therapeutic treatment strategies. Hopefully, elucidation of precise redox-regulated signaling pathways as they relate to the expression of atherogenic genes will encourage the exploration of novel treatment modalities targeting these redox-sensitive pathways. This hypothesis establishes an important framework to begin to understand how modulation of redox-sensitive signaling process may be used to specifically alter the expression of genes involved in the pathogenesis of atherosclerosis and other diseases.

REFERENCES

1. Halliwell B, Gutteridge JMC. The importance of free radicals and catalytic metal ions in human disease. *Mol Asp Med.* 1985;8:89.
2. Medford RM. Antioxidants and endothelial expression of VCAM-1: A molecular paradigm for atherosclerosis. In: Gallo LL, ed. *Cardiovascular Disease.* New York, NY: Plenum Press; 1995;2:121.
3. Ross R. Atherosclerosis - an inflammatory disease. *New Engl J Med.* 1999;340:115.
4. Diaz MN, Frei B, Vita JA, Keaney JF. Antioxidants and atherosclerotic heart disease. *New Engl J Med.* 1997;337:408.
5. Ross R. Cell biology of atherosclerosis. *Ann Rev Physiol.*1995;57:791.
6. Gibbons GH, Dzau VJ. Molecular therapies for vascular diseases. *Science.* 1996;272:689.
7. Steinberg D, Parthasarathy S, Carew TE, Khoo JC, Witztum JL. Beyond cholesterol: modifications of low-density lipoprotein that increase its atherogenicity. *N Engl J Med.* 1989;320:915.
8. Alexander RW. Hypertension and the pathogenesis of atherosclerosis. Oxidative stress and the mediation of arterial inflammatory response: a new perspective. *Hypertension.* 1995;25:155.
9. Marui N, Offermann MK, Swerlick R, Kunsch C, Rosen CA, Ahmad M, Alexander RW, Medford RM. Vascular cell adhesion molecule-1 (VCAM-1) gene transcription and

expression are regulated through an antioxidant-sensitive mechanism in human vascular endothelial cells. *J Clin Invest.* 1993;92:1866.

10. Weber C, Erl W, Pietsch A, Strobel M, Ziegler-Heitbrock HW, Weber PC. Antioxidants inhibit monocyte adhesion by suppressing nuclear factor–κB mobilization and induction of vascular cell adhesion molecule-1 in endothelial cells stimulated to generate radicals. *Arterioscler Thromb.* 1994;14:1665.

11. Satriano JA, Shuldiner M, Hora K, Xing Y, Shan Z, Schlondorff D. Oxygen radicals as second messengers for expression of the monocyte chemoattractant protein, JE/MCP-1, and the monocyte colony-stimulating factor, CSF-1, in response to tumor necrosis factor-alpha and immunoglobulin G. Evidence for involvement of reduced nicotinamide adenine dinucleotide phosphate (NADPH)-dependent oxidase. *J Clin Invest.* 1993;92:1564.

12. Winyard PG, Blake DR. Antioxidants, redox-regulated transcription factors, and inflammation. *Adv in Pharm.* 1997;38:403.

13. Baynes JW. Role of oxidative stress in development of complications in diabetes. *Diabetes.* 1991;40:405.

14. Lander HM. An essential role for free radicals and derived species in signal transduction. *FASEB J.* 1997;11:118.

15. Chen XL, Medford RM. Oxidation-reduction sensitive regulation of inflammtory gene expression in the vasculature. In: Pearson JD, ed. *Vascular adhesionmolecules and inflammation.* Basel, Switzerland: Birkhauser Press; 1999 (in press).

16. Griendling KK, Minieri CA, Ollerenshw JD, Alexander RW. Angiotensin II stimulates NADH and NADPH oxidase activity in cultured vascular smooth muscle cells. *Circ Res.* 1994;74:1141.

17. Chen XL, Tummala PE, Olbrych MT, Alexander RW, Medford RM. Angiotensin II induces monocyte chemoattractant protein-1 gene expression in rat vascular smooth muscle cells. *Circ Res.* 1998;83:952.

18. Graier WF, Simecek S, Kukovetz WR, Kostner GM. High D-glucose-induced change in endothelial Ca^{2+} /EDRF signaling are due to generation of superoxide anions. *Diabetes.* 1996;45:1386.

19. Maziere C, Auclair M, Rose-Robert F, Leflon P, Maziere JC. Glucose-enriched medium enhances cell-mediated low dendity lipoprotein peroxidation. *FEBS lett.* 1995;363:277.

20. Pieper GM, Riaz ul Haq. Activation of nuclear factor–κB in cultured endothelial cells by increased glucose concentration: prevention by calphostin C. *J Cardiolvasc Pharm.* 1997;30:528.

21. Brownlee M, Cerami A, Vlassara H. Advanced glycosylation end products in tissue and the biochemical basis of diabetic complications. *N Engl J Med.* 1988;318:1315.

22. Schimidt AM, Hori O, Chen JX, Li JF, Crandall JZ, Cao R, Yan SD, Brett J, Stern D. Advanced glycation endproducts interacting with their endothelial receptor induce expression of vascular cell adhesion molecule (VCAM-1) in cultured human endothelial cells and in mice. A potential mechanism for the accelerated vasculopathy of diabetes. *J Clin Invest.* 1995;96:1395.

23. Yan SD, Schmidt AM, Anderson GM, Zhang J, Brett J, Zou YS, Pinksy D, Stern D. Enhanced cellular oxidative stress by the interaction of advanced glycation end products with their receptors/binding protein. *J Biol Chem.* 1994;269:9889.

24. Bierhaus AS, Chevion M, Chevion M, Hofmann P, Quehenberg T, Luther IT, Berentstein E, Tritschler H, Muller M, Wajl R, Ziegler R, Nowroth PP. Advanced glycation end product-induced activation of NF–κB is suppressed by α-lipoic acid in cultured endothelial cells. *Diabetes.* 1997;46:1481.

25. Lehr HA, Becker M, Marklund SL, Hubner C, Arfors KE, Kohlschutter A, Messmer K. Superoxide-dependent stimulation of leukocyte adhesion by oxidatively modified LDL *in vivo. Arterioscler Thromb.* 1992;12:824.

26. Witzum JL, Steinberg D. Role of oxidized low density lipoprotein in atherogenesis. *J Clin Invest.* 1991;88:1785.

27. Cominacini L, Ulisse G, Pasini AF, Davoli A, Campagnola M, Contessi GB, Pastorino A, Cascio VL. Antioxidants inhibit the expression of intercellular cell adhesion molecule-1 and vascular cell adhesion molecule-1 induced by oxidized LDL on human umbilical endothelial cells. *Free Rad Bio Med.* 1997;22:117.

28.   Khan BR, Parthasarathy SS, Alexander RW, Medford RM. Modified low density lipoprotein and its constituents augment cytokine-activated vascular cell adhesion molecule-1 gene expression in human endothelial cells. *J Clin Invest.* 1995;95:1262.

29.   Cominacini L, Garbin U, Fratta PA, Paulon T, Davoli A, Campagnola M, Marchi E, Pastorino AM, Gaviraghi G, Lo Cascio V. Lacidipine inhibits the activation of the transcription factor NF–κB and the expression of adhesion molecules induced by pro-oxidant signals on endothelial cells. *J Hypertens.* 1997;15:1633.

30.   Maziere C, Auclair M, Djavaheri-Mergny M, Packer L, Maziere JC. Oxidized low density lipoprotein induces activation of the transcription factor NF–κB in fibroblasts, endothelial and smooth muscle cells. *Biochem Mol Biol Int.* 1996;39:1201.

31.   Brand K, Eisele T, Kreusel U, Page M, Page S, Haas M, Gerling A, Kaltschmidt C, Neumann FJ, Mackman N, Baeurele PA, Walli AK, Neumeier D. Dysregulation of monocytic nuclear factor–κB by oxidized low-density lipoprotein. *Arterioscler Thromb Vasc Biol.* 1997;17:1901.

32.   Henriksson P, Hamberg M, Diczfalusy U. Formation of 15-HETE as a major hydroxyeicosatetraenoic acid in the atherosclerotic vessel wall. *Biochim Biophys Acta.* 1985;834:272.

33.   Yla-Herttuala S, Rosenfeld ME, Parthasarathy S, Sigal E, Sarkioja T, Witztum JL, Steinberg D. Gene expression in macrophage-rich human atherosclerotic lesions: 15-lipoxygenase and acetyl LDL receptor mRNA colocalize with oxidation-specific lipid-protein adducts. *J Clin Invest.* 1991;87:1146.

34.   Wolle J, Welch KA, Devall LJ, Cornicelli JA, Saxena U. Transient overexpression of human 15-lipoxygenase in aortic endothelial cells enhances tumor necrosis factor-induced vascular cell adhesion molecule-1 gene expression. *Biochem Biophy Res Com.* 1996;220:310.

35.   Lee S, Felts KA, Parry GC, Armacost LM, Cobb RR. Inhibition of 5-lipoxygenase blocks IL-1β-induced vascular adhesion molecule-1 gene expression in human endothelial cells. *J Immunol.* 1997;158:3401.

36.   Nerem RM. Hemodynamics and the vascular endothelium. *J Biomech Eng.* 1993;115:510.

37.   Chiu JJ, Wang KL, Chien S, Skalak R, Usami S. Effects of disturbed flow on endothelial cells. *J Biomech Eng.* 1998;120:2.

38.   Laurindo FRM, de Almedia Pedro M, Barbeiro HV, Pileggi F, Carvalho MHC, Augusto O, Lemos da Luz P. Vascular free radical release. *Ex vivo* and *in vivo* evidence for a flow-dependent endothelial mechanism. *Circ Res.* 1994;74:700.

39.   De Keulenaer GW, Chappell DC, Ishizaka N, Nerem RM, Alexander RW, Griendling KK. Oscillatory and steady laminar shear stress differentially affect human endothelial redox state. Role of a superoxide-production and NADH oxidase. *Circ Res.* 1998;82:1094.

40.   Hsieh HJ, Cheng CC, Wu ST, Chiu JJ, Wung BS, Wang DL. Increase of reactive oxygen species (ROS) in endothelial cells by shear flow and involvement of ROS in shear-induced c-Fos expression. *J Cell Physiol.* 1998;175:156.

41.   Chiu JJ, Wung BS, Shyy JYJ, Hsieh HJ, Wang DL. Reactive oxygen species are involved in shear stress-induced intercelluar adhesion molecule-1 expression in endothelial cells. *Arterioscler Thromb Vasc Biol.* 1997;17:3570.

42.   Wu AY, Yan C, Berk BC. Fluid shear stress generates oxidative stress in endothelial cells as assayed by aconitase. *Circulation.* 1998;98:I37. (Abst).

43.   Inoue N, Ramasamy S, Fukai T, Nerem RM, Harrison DG. Shear stress modulates expression of Cu/Zn superoxide dismutase in human aortic endothelial cells. *Circ Res.* 1996;79:32.

44.   Topper JN, Cai J, Falb D, Gimbrone MA. Identification of vascular endothelial genes differentially responsive to fluid mechanical stimuli: Cyclooxygenase-2, manganese superoxide dismutase, and endothelial cell nitric oxide synthase are selectively up-regulated by steady laminar shear stress. *Proc Natl Acad Sci USA.* 1996;93:10417.

45.   Tsao PS, Buitrago R, Chan JR, Cooke JP. Fluid flow inhibits endothelial adhesiveness, nitric oxide and transcriptional regulation of VCAM-1. *Circulation.* 1996;94:1682.

46.   Medford R, Erickson S, Chappell D, Offermann M, Nerem R, Alexander R. Laminar shear stress and redox sensitive regulation of human vascular endothelial cell VCAM-1 gene expression. *Circulation.* 1994;909(suppl I):I-83. (Abstr).

47.   Pohl U, Holtz J, Busse R, Bassenge E. Crucial role of endothelium in the vasodilator response to increase flow *in vivo. Hypertension.* 1986;8:37.
48.   Cooke JP, Rossitch E, Andon N, Loscalzo J, Dzau VJ. Flow activates an endothelial potassium channel to release an endogenous nitrovasodilator. *J Clin Invest.* 1991;88:1663.
49.   Uematsu M, Ohara Y, Navas JP, Nishida K, Murphy TJ, Alexander RW, Nerem RM, Harrison DG. Regulation of endothelial cell nitric oxide synthase mRNA expression by shear stress. *Am J Physiol.* 1995;269:C1371.
50.   Ueba H, Poppa V, Suero J, Okuda M, Berk BC. c-Src is required for flow-stimulated NO production in bovine aortic endothelial cells. *Circulation.* 1998;98:I313. (Abst.)
51.   Mohazzab KM, Kaminski PM, Wolin MS. NADH oxidoreductase is a major source of superoxide anion in bovine coronary artery endothelium. *Am J Physiol.* 1994;266:H2568.
52.   De Keulenaer GW, Alexander RW, Ushio-Fukai M, Ishizaka N, Griendling KK. Tumor necrosis factor alpha activates a p22 phox-based NADH oxidase in vascular smooth muscle. *Biochem J.* 1998;329:653.
53.   Matsubara T, Ziff M. Increased superoxide anion release from human endothelial cells in response to cytokines. *J. Immunol.* 1986;137:3295.
54.   Tummala PE, Chen X, Medford RM. Differential regulation of oxidation sensitive VCAM-1 gene expression and NF–κB activation by flavin binding proteins. *Circulation* 1996;94:I-45 (Abst.)
55.   Chen XL, Tummala PE, Laursen JB, Harrison DG, Alexander RW, Medford RM. Direct activation of aortic monocyte chemoattractant protein-1 gene expression *in vivo* and *ex vivo* by angiotensin II in experimental hypertension. *Circulation.* 1997;96:I-285. (Abst.)
56.   Moncada S, Palmer RM, Higgs EA. Nitric oxide: physiology, pathophysiology, and pharmacology. *Pharmacol Rev.* 1991;43:109.
57.   White CR, Brock TA, Chang LY, Crapo J, Briscoe P, Ku D, Bradley WA, Gianturco SH, Gore J, Freeman BA, Tarpey MM. Superoxide and peroxynitrite in atherosclerosis. *Proc Natl Acad Sci U S A.* 1994;91:1044.
58.   Beckman JS, Beckman TW, Chen J, Marshall PA, Freeman BA. Apparent hydroxyl radical production by peroxynitrite: implications for endothelial injury from nitric oxide and superoxide. *Proc Natl Acad Sci U S A.* 1990;87:1620.
59.   Rubanyi GM, Vanhoutte PM. Superoxide anions and hyperoxia inactivate endothelium-derived relaxing factor. *Am J Physiol.* 1986;250:H822.
60.   Gryglewski RJ, Palmer RMJ, Moncada S. Superoxide anion is involved in the breakdown of endothelium-derived vascular relaxing factor. *Nature (Lond)* 1986;320:454.
61.   Khan BV, Harrison DG, Olbrych MT, Alexander RW, Medford RM. Nitric oxide regulates vascular cell adhesion molecule 1 gene expression and redox-sensitive transcriptional events in human vascular endothelial cells. *Proc Natl Acad Sci USA.* 1996;93:9114.
62.   De Caterina R, Libby P, Peng HB, Thannickal VJ, Rajavashisth TB, Gimbrone MA, Shin WS, Liao JK. Nitric oxide decreases cytokine-induced endothelial activation: nitric oxide selectively reduces endothelial expression of adhesion molecules and pro-inflammatory cytokines. *J Clin Invest.* 1995;96:60.
63.   Tsao PS, Wang B, Buitrago R, Shyy JY, Cooke JP. Nitric oxide regulates monocyte chemotactic protein-1. *Circulation.* 1997;96:934.
64.   Zeiher AM, Fisslthaler B, Schray-Utz B, Busse R. Nitric oxide modulates the expression of monocyte chemoattractant protein 1 in cultured human endothelial cells. *Circ Res.* 1995;76:980.
65.   Peng HB, Libby P, Liao JK. Induction and stabilization of IκB–α by nitric oxide mediates inhibition of NF–κB. *J Biol Chem.* 1995;270:14214.
66.   Hogg N, Kalyanaramer B, Joseph J, Struck A, Parthasarathy S. Inhibition of low-density lipoprotein oxidation by nitric oxide. Potential role in atherogenesis. *FEBS Lett.* 1993; 334:170.
67.   Rubbo H, Darley UV, Freeman BA. Nitric oxide regulation of tissue free radical injury. *Chem Res Toxicol.* 1996;9:809.
68.   Suzuki YJ, Forman HJ, Sevanian A. Oxidants as stimulators of signal transduction. *Free Rad Biol Med.* 1997;22:269.
69.   Palmer HJ, Paulson KE. Reactive oxygen species and antioxidants in signal transduction and gene expression. *Nutrition Reviews.* 1997;55:353.

70.   Schulze-Osthoff K, Bauer MK, Vogt M, Wesselborg S.   Oxidative stress and signal transduction. *Internat J Vita Nutr Res.* 1997;67:336.

71.   Sen CK, Packer L.   Antioxidant and redox regulation of gene transcription. *FASEB J.* 1996;10:709.

72.   Sun Y, Oberley LW.   Redox regulation of transcriptional activators. *Free Rad Biol Med.* 1996;21:335.

73.   Brand K, Page S, Walli AK, Neumeier D, Baeuerle PA.   Role of nuclear factor–κB in atherogenesis. *Exp Phys.* 1997;82:297.

74.   Karin M.   Signal transduction and gene control. *Curr Opin Cell Biol.* 1991;3:467-473.

75.   Angel P, Karin M.   The role of Jun, Fos and the AP-1 complex in cell proliferation and transformation. *Biochim Biophys Acta.* 1991;1072:129.

76.   Chiu R, Boyle WJ, Meek J, Smeal T, Hunter T, Karin M.   The c-Fos protein interacts with c-Jun/AP-1 to stimulate transcription of AP-1 responsive genes. *Cell.* 1988;54:541.

77.   Crawford K, Zbinden I, Amstad P, Cerutti P.   Oxidant stress induces the proto-oncogenes c-Fos and c-myc in mouse epidermal cells. *Oncogene.* 1988;3:27.

78.   Shibanuma M, Kuroki T, Nose K.   Induction of DNA replication and expression of proto-oncogenes c-myc and c-Fos in quiescent Balb/3T3 cells by xanthine/xanthine oxidase. *Oncogene.* 1988;3:17.

79.   Devary Y, Gottilieb RA, Lau LF, Karin M.   Rapid and preferential activation of the c-Jun gene during the mammalian UV response. *Mol Cell Biol.* 1991;11:2804.

80.   Nose K, Shibanuma M, Kikuchi K, Kageyama H, Sakiyama S, Kuroki T.   Transcriptional activation of early-response genes by hydrogen peroxide in a mouse osteoblastic cell line. *Eur J Biochem.* 1991;201:99.

81.   Collart FR, Horio M, Huberman E.   Heterogeneity in c-Jun gene expression in normal and malignant cells exposed to either ionizing radiation or hydrogen peroxide. *Radiat Res.* 1995;142:188.

82.   Shono T, Ono M, Izumi H, Jimi SI, Matsushima K, Okamoto T, Kohno K, Kuwano M.   Involvement of the transcription factor NF–κB in tubular morphogenesis of human microvascular endothelial cells by oxidative stress. *Mol Cell Biol.* 1996;16:4231.

83.   Lin JH, Zhu Y, Liao HL, Kobari Y, Groszek L, Stemerman MB.   Induction of vascular cell adhesion molecule-1 by low-density lipoprotein. *Atherosclerosis.* 1996;127:185.

84.   Maziere C, Kjavaheri-Mergny M, Frye-Fressart V, Kelattre J, Maziere JC.   Copper and cell-oxidized low-density lipoprotein induces activator protein 1 in fibroblasts, endothelial and smooth muscle cells. *FEBS Lett.* 1997;409:351.

85.   Ares MP, Kallin B, Eriksson P, Nilsson J.   Oxidized LDL induces transcription factor activator protein-1 but inhibits activation of nuclear factor–κB in human vascular smooth muscle cells. *Arterioscler Thromb Vasc Biol.* 1995;15:1584.

86.   Rao GN, Berk BC.   Active oxygen species stimulate vascular smooth muscle cell growth and proto-oncogene expression. *Circ Res.* 1992;70:593.

87.   Ruef J, Rao GN, Li F, Bode C, Patterson C, Bhatnager A, Runge MS.   Induction of rat aortic smooth muscle cell growth by the lipid peroxidation product 4-hydroxy-2-nonenal. *Circulation.* 1998;97:1071.

88.   Wung BS, Cheng JJ, Hsieh HJ, Shyy YJ, Wang DL.   Cyclic strain-induced monocyte chemotactic protein-1 gene expression in endothelial cells involves reactive oxygen species activation of activator protein 1. *Circ Res.* 1997;81:1.

89.   Roebuck KA, Rahman A, Lakshminarayanan V, Janakidevi K, Malik AB. H_2O_2 and tumor necrosis factor-alpha activate intercellular adhesion molecule 1 (ICAM-1) gene transcription through distinct cis-regulatory elements within the ICAM-1 promoter. *J Biol Chem.* 1995;270:18966.

90.   Rao GN, Lassegue B, Griendling KK, Alexander RW, Berk BC.   Hydrogen peroxide-induced c-Fos expression is mediated by arachidonic acid release: Role of protein kinase C. *Nucleic Acids Res.* 1993;21:1259.

91.   Rao GN, Lassegue B, Griendling KK, Alexander RW.   Hydrogen peroxide stimulates transcription of c-Jun in vascular smooth muscle cells: Role of arachidonic acid. *Oncogene.* 1993;8:2759.

92. Barchowsky A, Munro SR, Morana SJ, Vincenti MP, Treadwell M. Oxidant-sensitive and phosphorylation-dependent activation of NF–κB and AP-1 in endothelial cells. *Am J Physiol.* 1995;269:L829.

93. Del Arco PG, Martinez-Martinez S, Calvo V, Armesilla AL, Redondo JM. Antioxidants and AP-1 activation: A brief overview. *Immunobiol.* 1997;198:273.

94. Aragones J, Lopez-Rodriquez C, Corbi A, del Arco PG, Lopez-Cabrera M, de Landazuri MO, Redondo JM. Dithiocarbamates trigger differentiation and induction of CD11c gene through AP-1 in the myeloid lineage. *J Biol Chem.* 1996;271:10924.

95. Munoz C, Castellanos MC, Alfranca A, Vara A, Esteban MA, Redondo JM, de Landazuri MO. Transcriptional up-regulation of intracellular adhesion molecule-1 in human endothelial cells by the antioxidant pyrrolidine dithiocarbamate involves the activation of activating protein-1. *J Immunol.* 1996;157:3587.

96. Shau H, Huang AC, Faris M, Nazarian R, de Vellis J, Chen W. Thioredoxin peroxidase (natural killer enhancing factor) regulation of activator protein-1 function in endothelial cells. *Biochem Biophys Res Commun.* 1998;249:683.

97. Baeuerle PA, Henkel T. Function and activation of NF–κB in the immune system. *Ann Rev Immunol.* 1996;12:141.

98. Autieri MV, Uye TL, Ferstein GZ, Ohlstein E. Antisense oligonucleotide to the p65 subunit of NF–κB inhibits vascular smooth muscle cell adherence and proliferation and prevents neointima formation in rat carotid arteries *Biochem Biophys Res Commun.* 1995;213:827.

99. Bellas RE, Lee JS, Sonenshein GE. Expression of a constitutive NF–κB-like activity is essential for proliferation of cultured bovine vascular smooth muscle cells. *J Clin Invest.* 1995; 96:2521.

100. Maruyama I, Shigeta K, Miyahara II, Nakajima T, Shin H, Ide S, Kitajima I. Thrombin activates NF–κB through thrombin receptor and results in proliferation of vascular smooth muscle cells: role of thrombin in atherosclerosis and restenosis. *Ann N Y Acad Sci.* 1997;811:429.

101. Brand K, Page S, Rogler G, Bartsch A, Brandl R, Knuechel R, Page M, Kaltschmidt C, Baeuerle PA, Neumeier D. Activated transcription factor NF–κB is present in the atherosclerotic lesion. *J Clin Invest.* 1996;97:1715.

102. Liao F, Andalibi A, deBeer FC, Fogelman AM, Susis AJ. Genetic control of inflammatory gene induction and NF–κB-like transcription factor activation in response to an atherogenic diet in mice. *J Clin Invest.* 1993;91:2572.

103. Parhami F, Fang ZT, Fogelman AM, Andalibi A, Territo MC, Berliner JA. Minimally modified low density lipoprotein-induced inflammatory responses in endothelial cells are mediated by cyclic adenosine monophosphate. *J Clin Invest.* 1993;92:471.

104. Rajavashisth TB, Yamada H, Mishra NK. Transcriptional activation of the macrophage-colony stimulating factor gene by minimally modified LDL. *Arterioscler Thromb Vasc Biol.* 1995;15:1591.

105. Yan SD, Schmidt AM, Andrson GM, Zhang J, Brett J, Zou YS, Pinsky D, Stern D. Enhanced cellular oxidant stress by the interaction of advanced glycation end products with their receptors/binding proteins. *J Biol Chem.* 1994;269:9889.

106. Suzuki YJ, Miauno M, Packer L. Signal transduction for NF–κB activation: Proposed location of antioxidant-inhibitable step. *J Immunol.* 1994;153:5008.

107. Schreck R, Rieber P, Baeuerle PA. Reactive oxygen intermediates as apparently widely used messengers in the activation of the NF–κB transcription factor and HIV-1. *EMBO J.* 1991;10:2247.

108. Schreck, R, Albermann K, Baeuerle PA. Nuclear factor κB: An oxidative stress-responsive transcription factor of eukaryotic cells (a review). *Free Radic Res Commun.* 1992;17:221.

109. Schreck R, Meier B, Mannel DN, Droge W, Baeuerle PA. Dithiocarbamates as potent inhibitors of nuclear factor κB activation in intact cells. *J Exp Med.* 1992;175:1181.

110. Schmidt KN, Traenckner EB, Meier B, Baeuerle PA. Induction of oxidative stress by okadaic acid is required for activation of transcription factor NF–κB. *J Biol Chem.* 1995;270:27136.

111. Hayashi T, Ueno Y, Okamoto T. Oxidoreductive regulation of nuclear factor kappa B. Involvement of a cellular reducing catalyst thioredoxin. *J Biol Chem.* 1993;268:11380.

112.   Grimm S, Baeuerle PA. The inducible transcription factor NF–κB: Structure-function relationship of its protein subunits. *Biochem J.* 1993;290:297.

113.   Spiecker M, Darlus H, Kaboth K, Hubner F, Liao JK. Differential regulation of endothelial cell adhesion molecule expression by nitric oxide donors and antioxidants. *J Leuk Biol.* 1998;63:732.

114.   Traenckner EB, Wilk S, Baeuerle PA. A proteasome inhibitor prevents activation of NF–κB and stabilizes a newly phosphorylated form of IκB–α that is still bound to NF–κB. *EMBO J.* 1994;15:5433.

115.   Schmitz ML, dos Santos Silva MA, Baeuerle PA. Transactivation domain 2 (TA2) of p65 NF–κB. Similarity to TA1 and phorbol ester-stimulated activity and phosphorylation in intact cells. *J Biol Chem.* 1995;270:15576.

116.   Zhong H, Su Yang H, Erdjument-Bromage H, Tempst P, Ghosh S. The transcriptional activity of NF–κB is regulated by the IκB-associated PKAc subunit through a cyclic AMP-independent mechanism. *Cell.* 1997;89:413.

117.   Bird TA, Schooley K, Dower SK, Hagen H, Virca GD. Activation of nuclear transcription factor NF–κB by interleukin-1 is accompanied by casein kinase II-mediated phosphorylation of the p65 subunit. *J Biol Chem.* 1997;272:32606.

118.   Mangelsdorf DJ, Thummel C, Beato M, Herrlich P, Schutz G, Umesono K, Blumberg B, Kastner P, Mark M, Chambon P, *et al.* The nuclear receptor superfamily: the second decade. *Cell.* 1995;83:835.

119.   Nagy L, Tontonoz P, Alvarez JGA, Chen H, Evans RM. Oxidized LDL regulates macrophage gene expression through ligand activation of PPARγ. *Cell.* 1998;93:229.

120.   Jiang C, Ting AT, Seed B. PPAR–γ agonists inhibit production of monocyte inflammatory cytokines. *Nature.* 1998;391:82.

121.   Ricote M, Li AC, Wilson TM, Kelly CJ, Glass CK. The peroxisome proliferator-activated receptor–γ is a negative regulator of macrophage activation. *Nature (Lond).* 1998;391:79.

122.   Marx N, Borucier T, Sukhova GK, Plutzky J. Human endothelial cells contain PPARs: evidence for PPARγ in atheroma and its regulation of PAI-1 expression. *Circlation.* 1998;98:I383. (Abst).

123.   Staels B, Koenig W, Habib A, Merval R, Lebret M, Torra IP, Delerive P, Fadel A, Chinetti G, Fruchart JC, Najib J, Maclouf J, Tedgui A. Activation of human aortic smooth muscle cells is inhibited by PPARα but not by PPARγ activators. *Nature.* 1998;393:790.

124.   Marx N, Schoenbeck U, Lazar MA, Libby P, Plutzky J. PPARγ in human vascular smooth muscle cells: inhibition of matrix metalloprotease expression, activity, and cell migration. *Circulation.* 1998; 98:I382. (Abst).

125.   Kliewer SA, Lenhard JM, Wilson TM, Patel I, Morris DC, Lehmann JM. A prostaglandin J2 metabolite binds peroxisome proliferator-activated receptor γ and promotes adipocyte differentiation. *Cell.* 1995;83:813.

126.   Forman BM, Tontonoz P, Chen J, Brun RP, Spiegelman BM, Evans RM. 15-deoxy-$\Delta^{12,14}$-prostaglandin J$_2$ is a ligand for the adipocyte determination factor PPARγ. *Cell.* 1995;83:803.

127.   Tontonoz P, Nagy L, Alvarez JGA, Thomazy VA, Evans RM. PPARγ promotes monocyte/macrophage activation and uptake of oxidized LDL. *Cell.* 1988;93:241.

128.   Poynter ME, Daynes RA. Peroxisome proliferator-acivated receptor α activation modulates cellular redox status, represes nuclear factor–κB signaling, and reduces inflammatory cytokine production in aging. *J Biol Chem.* 1998;273:32833.

9 ATHEROSCLEROSIS, OXIDATIVE STRESS, AND ENDOTHELIAL FUNCTION

John F. Keaney, Jr.

INTRODUCTION

Atherosclerosis and its associated vascular complications remain a major source of morbidity and mortality in western civilizations. In the United States alone, 5.8 million patients are discharged from the hospital annually with a diagnosis of cardiovascular disease (CVD) and in 1995 CVD claimed over 960,000 lives (1). This represents approximately 41% of all deaths in the United States and places cardiovascular disease as the number one cause of death in the United States, causing more deaths, in fact, than all types of cancer combined (1). In terms of economic costs, cardiovascular disease consumes approximately 20 billion dollars annually in direct health care costs and over 250 billion dollars annually if one includes lost productivity (1). Data from the World Health Organization indicate that continued global economic prosperity is likely to lead to an epidemic of CVD as developing countries acquire Western habits such as increased consumption of meat and tobacco (1). Thus, atherosclerosis is a major public health problem that consumes an enormous amount of resources.

Morphologically, atherosclerosis is a disease of large- and medium-sized arteries that is characterized by a progressive narrowing of the arterial lumen due to local thickening of the tunica intima, the inner most layer of the arterial wall. Early atherosclerotic lesions consist of fatty streaks, local intimal collections of lipid-laden macrophages known as foam cells (2). The persistence of fatty streaks leads to formation of fibrous plaques, lesions that are characterized by collections of foam cells covered by connective tissue. The subsequent migration and proliferation of smooth muscle cells from the media into the intima along with foam cell necrosis and a deposition of cellular debris and cholesterol crystals leads to the formation of advanced atherosclerotic lesions (2).

This process of atherogenesis and lesion progression may occur over several decades and remain clinically silent. In fact, the clinical manifestations of atherosclerosis such as stroke and myocardial infarction require the activation of atherosclerotic lesions characterized by plaque rupture, mural hemorrhage, platelet aggregation, vasoconstriction, and ultimately the formation of an occlusive thrombus (3). The precise mechanism(s) responsible for atherosclerotic lesion activation are not presently known with certainty, however, it is clear that lesion activation requires a fundamental lapse in the homeostatic mechanisms of the blood vessel (4,5).

VASCULAR HOMEOSTASIS

Normal vascular homeostasis insures adequate end organ perfusion through the precise control of blood flow, vascular tone, and the constitutive inhibition of thrombosis. The endothelium, situated at the interface between blood flow and the vascular wall, is an important component of vascular homeostasis. One major function of the endothelium is its role as a local site of integration for paracrine and autocrine signals. For example, the endothelium constitutively produces prostaglandin I_2 (PGI_2), a potent inhibitor of platelet activation (6). Endothelial cells also synthesize heparins and thrombomodulin, compounds that reduce thrombin activity on the endothelial surface (7,8) . The endothelium also exerts considerable control of fibrinolysis through the synthesis of tissue-type plasminogen activator and plasminogen activator inhibitor-1(PAI-1) (9). The normal balance of endothelial synthetic activity maintains a state that favors fibrinolysis.

Among the many synthetic products of the vascular endothelium, perhaps the most important with respect to vascular homeostasis is nitric oxide (NO). This free radical species is synthesized constitutively in the endothelium by the endothelial isoform of nitric oxide synthase (eNOS). The production of NO by the endothelium is critical for a number of important homeostatic functions. For example, endothelial elaboration of NO controls vascular tone (10), smooth muscle phenotype (11), as well as the adhesion and aggregation of both leukocytes (12) and platelets (13-15). The importance of endothelium-derived NO is readily apparent from observations that mice lacking eNOS exhibit spontaneous hypertension (16,17), defective vascular remodeling (18), and enhanced thrombotic responses (19). Moreover, patients with impaired NO bioactivity also exhibit spontaneous arterial thrombosis (20). Thus, available evidence indicates that NO is an important component of vascular homeostasis.

The biologic activity for NO is attributable to two main mechanisms. The first involves binding of NO to the heme component of soluble guanylyl cyclase resulting in enzymatic activation and an increase in the intracellular content of 3', 5'-cyclic guanosine monophosphate (cGMP) (21). This increase in intracellular cGMP has been implicated in both NO-mediated vasodilation (22,23) and inhibition of platelet activity (23,24). The second mechanism of NO bioactivity involves the formation of NO adducts. Specifically, under an aerobic conditions NO may form oxides of nitrogen that can react with thiol groups to form S-nitrosothiols (25,26). This chemistry has been implicated in NO-mediated activation of potassium channels (27), calcium channels (28,29), and the modulation of hemoglobin oxygen affinity (30).

Endothelial production of NO is now the subject of intense investigation. The endothelial isoform of NOS is distinguished from the neuronal (nNOS) and inducible (iNOS) isoforms by its predilection for the particulate fraction of cells (31). Unlike the other NOS isoforms, eNOS is specifically targeted to specialized invagination of the plasmalemma termed caveolae (32,33) via acetylation (31,33. The enzyme interacts with the "scaffolding" domain of caveolin-I (34) rendering it inactive (35). However, an increase in intracellular calcium releases eNOS from caveolin and permits interaction with calmodulin facilitating electron flow through the enzyme and the oxidation of L-arginine to form NO (35). Other protein-protein interactions also appear important for eNOS activity including association with heat-shock protein 90 (36).

The bioactivity of endothelium-derived NO is impaired in patients with frank atherosclerosis or known risk factors for atherosclerosis. For example, the vasodilatory responses to known stimuli for endothelium-derived NO production are abnormal in the coronary arteries of patients with atherosclerosis (37), diabetes (38) and hypertension (39). Such defects are not localized to the coronary circulation, as NO bioactivity is also impaired in the brachial artery (40,41) and resistance arterioles (39,42,43 in these patients. Abnormal NO-mediated arterial relaxation typically precedes overt clinical manifestations of vascular disease. Individuals with known atherosclerotic risk factors such as increased cholesterol (44,45), advanced age (44,45), cigarette smoking (46) all demonstrate impaired bioactivity of endothelium-derived NO. Patients with a family history of coronary atherosclerosis also demonstrate impaired NO bioactivity (47). Thus, both pre-clinical and clinical atherosclerotic vascular disease are characterized by impaired NO-dependent vascular homeostasis, and this defect is thought to play a large role in the clinical manifestations of atherosclerotic vascular disease (5,48).

OXIDATIVE STRESS AND IMPAIRED NO BIOACTIVITY

The precise mechanism producing impaired NO bioactivity in atherosclerosis is not known with certainty. However, a large body of evidence now indicates that excess vascular "oxidative stress" is one important mechanism responsible for reduced NO bioactivity. As a term, oxidative stress is not particularly precise but it has gained wide favor since its original introduction (see Chapter 1) to characterize an imbalance between oxidants and antioxidants in favor of the former. The fact that oxidative stress represents an imbalance between oxidants and antioxidants should not be under-emphasized. Increased oxidative stress may therefore result from either a relative abundance of oxidants or, alternatively a relative reduction in the availability of defense mechanisms to deal with oxidants (antioxidants). In the remainder of this chapter, we will consider sources of oxidative stress and antioxidant protection as they pertain to impaired NO bioactivity.

Superoxide and NO Bioactivity

Atherosclerosis is associated with both morphologic and functional alterations in the vasculature. It has been known for some time that atherosclerotic blood vessels demonstrate augmented responses to vasoconstrictor stimuli (49,50). Shortly after the seminal discovery of Endothelium-Derived Relaxing Factor (EDRF) by Furchgott (51), it also became clear that atherosclerosis and hypercholesterolemia were associated with altered endothelium-dependent arterial relaxation (52,53). Once it was known that EDRF is produced as NO (54), an intense effort was undertaken to determine the mechanisms responsible for impaired endothelial function in atherosclerosis. An important study in this regard, was the demonstration that atherosclerotic blood vessels remain capable of elaborating nitrogen oxides even in the face of atherosclerosis and hypercholesterolemia (55), suggesting that NO is somehow inactivated in these two pathologic states (Figure 1). One source of NO inactivation that has been identified is superoxide. Hypercholesterolemia and atherosclerosis are associated with an increase in the steady state flux of superoxide within the vascular wall (56,57).

An increase in the steady state flux of superoxide within the vascular wall has important implications for the bioactivity of NO. Superoxide and NO combine readily in a diffusion-limited reaction ($k = 1.9 \times 10^{10}$ M^{-1}•sec^{-1}) (58) to form peroxynitrite as depicted in reaction [1].

$$O_2^{•-} + NO \Rightarrow O\text{-}O\text{-}N{=}O^-$$ [1]

This reaction has physiologic relevance as it is known to occur *in vivo* (59,60) and serves to limit the bioactivity of NO. Although peroxynitrite has the capacity to activate the soluble form of guanylyl cyclase (61,62), it does so much less potently than authentic NO (62). Therefore, one could predict that any loss of authentic NO to peroxynitrite through the reaction of superoxide will effectively reduce any biologic activity of NO resulting from cGMP.

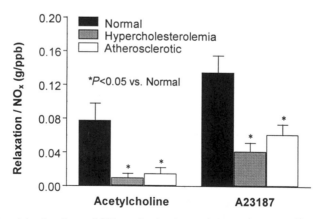

Figure 1. Arterial relaxation and NO production in rabbit aorta. Rabbits were treated with a 1% cholesterol diet for either 2-5 weeks (hypercholesterolemia) or 4 months (atherosclerotic). Arterial relaxation and chemiluminescence NO$_x$ (nitrite + nitrate) were determined in response to acetylcholine (1 µM) or calcium ionophore A23187 (10 µM). Reproduced from The Journal of Clinical Investigation (1990) 86:2109-2116 by copyright permission of the American Society for Clinical Investigation.

SOD and NO Bioactivity

As endothelial cells produce both NO and superoxide constitutively (63), small changes in the relative flux by this species should have important implications for the bioactivity of NO. Rubanyi and Vanhoutte have demonstrated that SOD improved the vascular relaxation response to endothelium-derived NO (Figure 2) (64). This observation applies to both acetylcholine-stimulated NO release as well as the basal endothelial production of NO (64,65). In addition, the exogenous addition of superoxide to bioassay systems results in impaired relaxation responses to endothelium-derived NO that is reversed by the inclusion of SOD (65,66).

If, indeed, the balance between NO and superoxide is rather fragile, one would predict that small changes in vascular SOD activity would have important implications for endothelium-dependent relaxation. Inactivation of Cu,Zn-SOD through copper chelation with diethyldithiocarbamate (DDC), an agent that chelates copper (67), results in impaired release of bioactive NO (68,69). In addition, DDC-treated arteries demonstrate impaired NO-mediated relaxation to the direct NO-dependent vasodilators nitroprusside (69) and nitroglycerin (68). These data make a compelling case that intact SOD activity is a prerequisite for normal NO bioactivity, although the capacity of DDC to form $Fe(DDC)_2$ and $Fe(DDC)_3$ complexes that scavenge NO (70) clouds the interpretation of such experiments. However, copper-deficient rats demonstrate impaired Cu,Zn-SOD activity (71,72) and impaired NO-

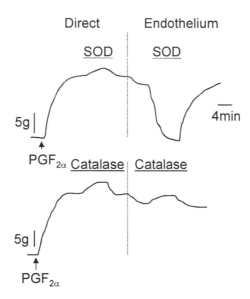

Figure 2. SOD enhances the relaxation from EDRF. The tracings demonstrate tension in a bioassay ring contracted with 4 µM prostaglandin $F_{2\alpha}$ (PG $F_{2\alpha}$) and superfused with the effluent from an arterial segment with endothelium. SOD (150 IU/mL) applied directly to the bioassay ring has no effect but evokes potent relaxation when applied to the segment with endothelium. Catalase has no effect. Reproduced with permission (64).

mediated arterial relaxation (72,73) that is associated with an increased vascular superoxide flux (72). Finally, adsorption of extracellular SOD type C onto rabbit arteries provides protection against impaired NO bioactivity due to superoxide (74). Thus, available evidence indicates that, on balance, vascular SOD activity is an important component of NO bioactivity.

In light of the above observations, one would predict that bolstering vascular SOD activity would improve NO-mediated arterial relaxation in atherosclerosis. In this context, the findings of Mugge and colleagues (75) merit consideration. These investigators treated atherosclerotic rabbits with parenteral polyethylene glycol-conjugated SOD for one week. Arteries harvested from treated animals demonstrated both an increase in vascular SOD activity and a striking improvement in NO-mediated arterial relaxation in response to acetylcholine and calcium ionophore, whereas non-atherosclerotic blood vessels did not (75). Similarly, acute treatment of arterial segments from atherosclerotic rabbits with liposome-encapsulated SOD also improved NO-mediated arterial relaxation (76). Taken together, these data suggest that an increased superoxide flux is responsible for some component of impaired NO-mediated arterial relaxation that is association with atherosclerosis and hypercholesterolemia.

Despite the consensus that ambient levels of vascular superoxide determine, in part, NO bioactivity, considerable controversy exists as to the source of superoxide. Normal rabbit arterial segments stained with nitroblue tetrazolium implicate the endothelial and adventitial layers of the vascular wall as sites of superoxide generation (77,78). Immunohistochemical data indicate that aortic adventitia principally contains an NADPH oxidoreductase activity (77) and known NADPH oxidase subunits such as p22^{phox}, gp91^{phox}, p47^{phox}, and p67^{phox} (78). In contrast, other studies in cultured endothelial cell homogenates indicate that an NADH oxidoreductase is the principal source of superoxide (79). Potential other sources of superoxide including PGH synthase (80), lipoxygenase (80), and xanthine oxidase(81) do not appear to contribute to vascular superoxide under non-pathologic conditions.

The source(s) of vascular superoxide in hypercholesterolemia and atherosclerosis are also not yet clear. In isolated segments of cholesterol-fed rabbit aorta, the flux of superoxide is significantly reduced with endothelial denudation or oxypurinol, an inhibitor of xanthine oxidase (56). These data suggest that hypercholesterolemia up-regulates endothelial xanthine oxidase activity (56), however, other investigators have demonstrated that hypercholesterolemia is associated with increased circulating xanthine oxidase that binds to the vascular endothelium (82). Studies in hypercholesterolemic patients demonstrate a partial improvement in NO-mediated arterial relaxation with oxypurinol (83), although the precise role of circulating xanthine oxidase has yet to be determined in human disease (see Chapter 12). When considering sources of superoxide, it is worth noting that all NOS isoforms are capable of reducing molecular oxygen to produce superoxide. Initially described for brain NOS under limiting concentrations of L-arginine (84), NOS-mediated superoxide production has since been reported for both eNOS (85) and iNOS (86). Such findings may have particular relevance for hypercholesterolemia-induced vascular superoxide generation as endothelial cells exposed to low-density lipoprotein exhibit enhanced superoxide anion generation from eNOS (87). Recent data demonstrating that tetrahydrobiopterin (88) or methyltetrahydrodrofolate (89), a cofactor for tetrahydrobiopterin synthesis, improve endothelium-derived NO bioactivity in hypercholesterolemic patients supports the notion that eNOS cofactor deficiency may contribute to endothelial dysfunction in atherosclerosis and hypercholesterolemia.

Combined evidence from biochemical, cell culture, and animal studies clearly indicates that the bioactivity of endothelium-derived NO is highly dependent upon the local availability of superoxide. However, it is also clear that the entire spectrum of endothelial dysfunction in hypercholesterolemia and atherosclerosis cannot be attributed solely to superoxide. For example, even in those studies that reported improved NO bioactivity with increased SOD activity (75,76) or with a reduced superoxide flux (56,82), the effect on NO bioactivity was incomplete. Consistent with these observations, chronic SOD inhibition appears to impair receptor-dependent stimuli for NO production to a greater extent than either non-receptor-dependent stimuli or authentic NO itself (72). Finally, the extent to which superoxide manipulation restores NO bioactivity in atherosclerosis is highly dependent upon the disease stage. Early pathologic stages tend to respond to SOD (75,76), whereas advanced atherosclerosis is largely SOD-insensitive (90). Taken together, these data indicate that increased vascular superoxide is not the sole abnormality responsible for the impairment of endothelium-derived NO bioactivity that accompanies atherosclerosis.

Lipid Peroxidation and NO Bioactivity

It is important to realize that superoxide is not the only source of oxidative stress in the setting of atherosclerosis. Peroxynitrite, the product of a facile interaction between superoxide and NO (reaction [1]) (91,92) is rapidly protonated at physiologic pH according to reaction [2] forming peroxynitrous acid, a potent oxidant (93).

$$H^+ + O\text{-}O\text{-}N{=}O^- \Rightarrow HO\text{-}O\text{-}N{=}O \qquad [2]$$

As an oxidant, peroxynitrite is quite promiscuous and can transfer oxygen atoms (93), oxidize sulfhydryls (94), initiate lipid peroxidation (95), and in the presence of CO_2, can oxidize and nitrate protein tyrosine residues (96,97). Thus, peroxynitrite formation represents one important means of propagating superoxide-mediated oxidative stress.

Peroxynitrite is not the only oxidizing species produced by superoxide. Superoxide is a much stronger reductant than oxidant (98) and has limited oxidizing activity at physiologic pH (99). However, in the presence of transition metal ions (Me^{n+}), superoxide may be converted to the hydroxyl radical (100), an extremely potent oxidant. This process involves the dismutation of superoxide to H_2O_2 (reaction [3]), followed by the reduction of H_2O_2 to the hydroxyl radical (˙OH) via the Haber-Weiss reaction (100), as shown in reactions [4] and [5] below.

$$2O_2^{\cdot-} + 2H^+ \Rightarrow H_2O_2 + O_2 \tag{3}$$
$$H_2O_2 + Me^{(n-1)+} \Rightarrow {}^{\cdot}OH + OH^- + Me^{n+} \tag{4}$$
$$O_2^{\cdot-} + Me^{n+} \Rightarrow O_2 + Me^{(n-1)+} \tag{5}$$

Since superoxide can also reduce transition metal ions (as shown in reaction [5]), only catalytic amounts of metals are required for the formation of ${}^{\cdot}OH$ from $O2^{\cdot-}$. Observations that ceruloplasmin contains redox-active copper (101) or catalytic quantities of iron can be isolated from atherosclerotic lesions suggest this reaction pathway is physiologically relevant (102). Admittedly, however, the availability of redox-active metals in vivo is a matter of some controversy (59,103).

Not all sources of oxidative stress in atherosclerosis are derived specifically from superoxide (see Chapter 2). Phagocytes secrete myeloperoxidase, a heme enzyme that, in the presence of hydrogen peroxide, produces a number of species capable of promoting lipid peroxidation including tyrosyl radical (104,105). Active myeloperoxidase is present in human atherosclerotic lesions (106) and LDL isolated from such lesions bear markers of myeloperoxidase activity (107), suggesting that myeloperoxidase is an important oxidant in atherosclerosis. Other potentially important sources of oxidative stress in atherosclerosis include lipoxygenase (108), homocyst(e)ine (109), and hypochlorous acid (110).

For a wide range of oxidants, membrane and lipoprotein lipids containing polyunsaturated fatty acids represent attractive oxidation targets due to the relatively low bond dissociation energy for *bis*-allylic methylene carbon-hydrogen bonds (75 – 80 kcal/mol) compared to the corresponding mono-allylic (~88 kcal/mol) and alkyl (101 kcal/mol) bonds (111). Oxidant-mediated hydrogen abstraction forms a carbon-centered radical that may initiate a chain reaction of lipid peroxidation via the formation of alkoxyl (LO${}^{\cdot}$) and lipid peroxyl radicals (LOO${}^{\cdot}$) and resulting accumulation of lipid hydroperoxides (LOOH) as shown in Figure 3 .

The process of lipid peroxidation is of some consequence for NO bioactivity. Like superoxide, lipid peroxyl radicals combine readily with peroxynitrite to form lipid peroxynitrite derivatives (113,114) effectively "quenching" bioactive NO. Lipid peroxidation within the vascular wall also leads to the formation of oxidized low-density lipoprotein (oxLDL) (115) that directly inactivates endothelium-derived NO (116) and reduces eNOS in endothelial cells (117). Indirect effects of lipid peroxidation are also important for NO bioactivity. The transfer of oxidized phospholipids from oxLDL to the endothelial cell plasma membrane stimulates protein kinase C (118) and impairs G-protein coupled signal transduction leading to abnormal NO-mediated arterial relaxation in response to receptor-dependent NO agonists (119). The precise molecular events that underlie such observations are not yet clear although recent observations eNOS function is dependent upon membrane targeting (120) and interaction with heat-shock protein 90 (36) prompt speculation that oxidized phospholipids may interrupt critical eNOS interactions.

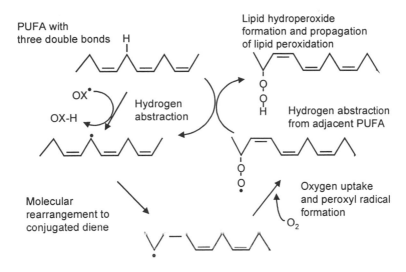

Figure 3. Representation of lipid peroxidation of polyunsaturated fatty acids (PUFAs). In this scheme a PUFA with three double bonds undergoes hydrogen abstraction by a one electron oxidant (OX') leading to conjugated diene formation with a carbon-centered radical. This radical spontaneously combines with O_2 to form a lipid peroxyl radical that abstracts a hydrogen atom from an adjacent PUFA thus propagating the chain reaction of lipid peroxidation. Adapted from (112).

The reaction between NO and lipid peroxyl radicals is thought to underlie observations that NO inhibits lipid peroxidation in cells (121) and lipoproteins (122). The role of peroxyl radicals in modulating NO bioactivity, however, has not been studied directly in any great detail. This lack of information may, in part, be related to the difficulty in producing a defined flux of lipid peroxyl radicals (LOO') in biologic systems. Most experiments have involved organic hydroperoxides (LOOH) that are assumed to produce lipid peroxidation through decomposition. For example, rabbit arteries exposed to the model organic hydroperoxides, cumene hydroperoxide or tert-butyl hydroperoxide, demonstrate an abrupt increase in tension and a reduction in smooth muscle cell cGMP production, suggesting an acute loss of endothelium-derived NO action (123). Platelet aggregation involves the formation of lipid hydroperoxides (124), and observations that inhibition of platelet aggregation by NO is potentiated by glutathione peroxidase suggests that reduction of lipid hydroperoxides enhances NO bioactivity (125).

Lipid-Soluble Antioxidants and NO Bioactivity

In light of the aforementioned evidence that lipid peroxidation impairs NO bioactivity, it follows that reducing vascular lipid peroxidation with lipid-soluble antioxidants should improve NO bioactivity. Lipid-soluble antioxidants are localized mainly to membranes and lipoproteins and include such compounds as α-tocopherol (vitamin E), beta-carotene, and ubiquinol-10. These three compounds represent the main lipid soluble antioxidants in humans and their main action is thought to be the inhibition of lipid peroxidation (126), although the activity of beta-carotene in this regard is controversial (127,128).

α-Tocopherol and β-Carotene

The activity of α-tocopherol and β-carotene with respect to NO bioactivity has been examined in animal models. Rabbits consuming a 1% cholesterol diet typically demonstrate impaired endothelium-derived NO bioactivity as assessed by arterial relaxation (52,129) that has been linked to an increase in vascular oxidative stress (56).   Cholesterol-fed rabbits treated with either β-carotene or α-tocopherol however, demonstrate near normal NO-mediated arterial relaxation responses to both acetylcholine and A23187 (130).   At least with α-tocopherol, this dietary treatment was associated with enhanced antioxidant protection as assessed by lipoprotein resistance to copper-mediated oxidation (130). There was no effect of either treatment on the lipoprotein profile or the extent of atherosclerosis (130). Similar studies in the coronary (131) and carotid (132) arteries of cholesterol-fed rabbits have also demonstrated that α-tocopherol preserves NO bioactivity. In rats, a species not normally susceptible to atherosclerosis, cholesterol-feeding has been associated with impaired endothelium-dependent arterial relaxation and this effect of cholesterol is abrogated by dietary vitamin E (133).   In a related study, hypercholesterolemic rats with a combined deficiency of α-tocopherol and selenium, a cofactor for glutathione peroxidase, produces impaired NO-bioactivity whereas cholesterol-feeding alone is ineffective (134).

The role of α-tocopherol in preserving NO bioactivity has not been limited solely to atherosclerosis and hypercholesterolemia. For example, streptozotocin-induced diabetic rats demonstrate impaired NO-mediated arterial relaxation in isolated aorta, however treatment with α-tocopherol significantly improves NO responses (135-137).   Similar observations have been reported in isolated perfused rat coronary arteries (138). To the extent that diabetes represents a state of heightened oxidative stress (139-141), these data provide additional evidence that antioxidant protection in vivo is important in maintaining normal NO bioactivity in the setting of chronic vascular disease.

Since LDL oxidation impairs NO bioactivity (119), and α-tocopherol inhibits LDL oxidation (142), it is reasonable to assume that α-tocopherol preserves NO bioactivity by eliminating LDL oxidation. Available evidence suggests that this observation may be overly simplistic. For example, cholesterol-fed rabbits treated with 2 different dietary regiments of α-tocopherol demonstrates strikingly different effects on NO bioactivity. At an α-tocopherol dose of 110 IU/d, NO-mediated arterial relaxation is preserved in cholesterol-fed rabbits and LDL is protected from copper-mediated oxidation ex-vivo (130,143). In contrast, a ten-fold increase in the daily dose of α-tocopherol produces worse NO bioactivity than cholesterol feeding alone despite excellent protection of LDL in ex-vivo copper-mediated oxidation assays (143). Thus, antioxidant protection of LDL alone is insufficient to preserve NO bioactivity in the cholesterol-fed rabbit model.

Although α-tocopherol is a very efficient scavenger of lipid peroxyl radicals, it is now clear that lipid peroxidation proceeds in the vascular wall despite the presence of α-tocopherol (144). In light of this knowledge, one must consider that α-tocopherol may favorably influence NO bioactivity principally through the protection of vascular cells against the deleterious effects of lipid peroxidation. Consistent with this notion, isolated arterial segments derived from α-tocopherol-deficient rabbits demonstrate impaired NO-mediated arterial relaxation upon exposure to oxLDL (145). In contrast, arterial segments derived from animals supplemented with α-tocopherol contain 100-fold more tocopherol and exhibit a marked resistance to the effects of oxLDL on NO bioactivity (145). Similar effects can be demonstrated using isolated endothelial cells in culture (147). Recent data has shed light on the mechanism of such observations. Exposure of arterial tissue to oxidized LDL results in protein kinase C stimulation (148,149) and incorporation of α-tocopherol into endothelial cells prevents this effect (Figure 4) (145). Since protein kinase C stimulation impairs NO bioactivity (118,149,150) and α-tocopherol prevents protein kinase C stimulation (145,151,152), these data suggest that α-tocopherol preserves NO bioactivity in atherosclerosis, in part, by preventing the stimulating of protein kinase C. It is worth noting that similar effects have been observed in smooth muscle cells (151) and platelets (152).

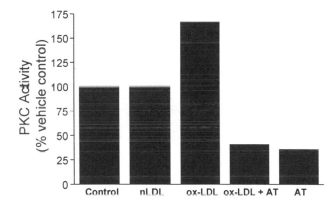

Figure 4. α-Tocopherol prevents protein kinase C stimulation due to oxidized LDL in endothelial cells. Human aortic endothelial cells were loaded with α-tocopherol (AT) or vehicle for 3d, washed, and incubated with oxidized LDL (oxLDL; 300 µg/ml), native LDL (nLDL; 300 µg/ml), or media (control) for 4 hours. After washing, protein kinase C activity was determined with an *in situ* assay (146). Reproduced from The Journal of Clinical Investigation (1996) 98:386-394 by copyright permission of the American Society for Clinical Investigation.

Probucol

The effect of lipid soluble antioxidants on NO bioactivity is not limited to α-tocopherol and β-carotene. Probucol is a cholesterol lowering compound that contains 2 phenolic hydroxy groups providing sufficient antioxidant activity.

Probucol is lipid soluble and transported primarily in lipoproteins (153) and in the setting of atherosclerosis it accumulates within the vascular wall (57,154). With respect to its antioxidant activity, probucol is a potent inhibitor of LDL oxidation in a variety of oxidizing system (153,155). Its notoriety is principally derived from its unequivocal activity to inhibit atherosclerosis in hypercholesterolemic rabbits (154,156,157) and cholesterol-fed primates (158). Curiously, probucol does not inhibit atherosclerosis in mouse models (159).

Probucol has been tested for its effect on endothelium-derived NO in cholesterol fed (57,160,161) and LDL receptor-deficient (162) rabbits. Uniform finding of these studies has been a lack of significant effect on plasma cholesterol levels. Moreover, probucol treatment, typically is 1% of the diet, did eliminate the increase in plasma (160,161) and aortic (57) lipid peroxides associated with cholesterol feeding as assessed by TBARS, or rather non-specific assay. More importantly, probucol treatment universally preserved NO bioactivity measured as endothelium-dependent arterial relaxation in response to either acetylcholine or A23187 (57, 160, 161). In the absence of cholesterol feeding, probucol does not appear to alter NO bioactivity (160), suggesting that its effect is limited to vascular disease states. Observations that probucol also improves NO bioactivity in alloxan-induced diabetes supports this contention (163).

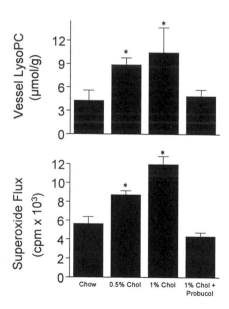

Figure 5. Probucol reduces vascular superoxide and lipid peroxidation in cholesterol-fed rabbits. Segments of thoracic aorta were harvested from animals fed diets consisting of standard chow (CTL), chow with 0.5% cholesterol (0.5% CHOL), chow with 1% cholesterol (1% CHOL), or chow with 1% cholesterol and 1% probucol. Vessel copper-zinc SOD activity was inhibited by incubating vessels with diethyldithiocarbamate for 30 minutes and prior to the assessment of superoxide using lucigenin chemiluminescence. Lysophosphatidylcholine (LysoPC) was determined by HPLC. * P<0.05 vs CTL by ANOVA. Reproduced from The Journal of Clinical Investigation (1995) 95:2520-2529 by copyright permission of the American Society for Clinical Investigation.

Although probucol potently inhibits LDL oxidation in ex-vivo assays (153,155), its mechanism of action in these animal models is independent of this effect. Arterial segments derived from cholesterol-fed rabbits typically demonstrate an increased vascular steady state superoxide flux (56). Probucol treatment, however, is associated with a reduction in this vascular flux of superoxide (57,161). This effect of probucol inhibits arterial wall lipid peroxidation (57,161) and accumulation of lysophosphatidylcholine (57) (Figure 5), two phenomena that have been linked to reduced NO bioactivity (72,164). Thus, probucol improves NO bioactivity in experimental animals principally through its effect on arterial tissues.

Human studies examining the effect of lipid soluble antioxidants on NO bioactivity are considerably less well developed than animal studies. Early studies examining the effect of antioxidants supplementation on NO bioactivity in resistance vessels have uniformly been negative (165-167). In contrast, the effect of lipid soluble antioxidant therapy on NO responses in conduit arteries has been in keeping with animal data. For example, postmenopausal women treated with α-tocopherol (168) and patients with remnant lipoprotein levels (169) have all demonstrated improved conduit artery NO responses with vitamin E treatment. The reader is directed to Chapter 12 for complete review of human studies examining the effect of antioxidants on vascular function.

Water-Soluble Antioxidants

It is important to note that the vascular wall contains both water- and lipid-soluble compartments. A main water soluble antioxidant in the arterial wall are glutathione (GSH) and ascorbic acid. Glutathione is typically present in plasma at concentrations below 1 μM (170), whereas ascorbic acid is normally considerably more abundant with concentrations ranging from 30 to 150 μM in plasma (112). In contrast, both compounds are abundant within the cell cytosol reaching concentrations that range from 1 to 5 mM (171,172). In addition, considerable evidence suggests that both intracellular compounds are required for normal function. All cells appear to demonstrate the active transport and/or synthase of GSH and vitamin C. Animals that are deprived or depleted of either compound become morbid and may die (173,174).

Glutathione

The potential role of intracellular GSH in the bioactivity and production of NO has been controversial. Early studies involving the manipulation of intracellular GSH in porcine (175) and bovine (176) endothelial cells produced concordant changes between GSH and the release of NO. Although consistent with the role for GSH in endothelial cell NO production, specific correlation between the intracellular thiol levels and the release of NO has been problematic. The release of NO from cultured bovine aortic endothelial cells by bradykinin is impaired by thiol alkylation with N-ethylmaleimide or oxidation of thiols with 2, 2'- dithiodipyridine. However, DTDP treatment was not clearly linked to a demonstrable reduction in endothelial cell GSH (176) suggesting that thiol levels per se may not be important for NO release. Proposed alternatives for the effect of DTDP included thiol oxidation state that may produce changes in calcium homeostasis (176). In a separate study with bovine cells, glutathione depletion using buthionine sulfoximine also failed to demonstrate any reduction in bioactive NO despite a > 90% reduction in GSH (69). Thus, these early studies in animals cells provided no consensus that intracellular GSH is important in endothelium-derived NO production.

Studies in human cells, however, have been more consistent with the role of intracellular GSH in NO production. The treatment of human umbilical vein endothelial cells with 1-chloro-2,4-dinitrobenzene (CDNB), a compound that covalently modifies GSH, was associated with a reduction in both intracellular GSH and endothelial NO elaboration (177). Conversely, increasing endothelial cell GSH with GSH ester increased cellular NO production and this correlated strongly with intracellular GSH (r = 0.92) (177).

Emerging data from human studies indicate that glutathione may have a role in modulating endothelium-derived NO. Patients with documented atherosclerosis and coronary artery disease are characterized by impaired NO-mediated arterial relaxation in the coronary circulation (37) and the brachial circulation (178). Treatment of such patients with L-2-oxo-4-thiazolidine carboxylate, an agent that selectively increases intracellular glutathione (179,180), is associated with improved NO bioactivity in the brachial artery (181). In patients with a vasospastic angina, intracoronary glutathione improves NO bioactivity in response to acetylcholine (182).

Although emerging evidence supports a role for glutathione and NO bioactivity, precise mechanisms responsible for this effect are not yet clear. Early studies with iNOS demonstrated that glutathione was necessary for optimal enzymatic activity (183). Subsequent studies have confirmed this effect for neuronal NOS (184,185). This effect of glutathione appears unique as other agents such as cysteine are considerably less effective (184,185). The precise events of this phenomenon are best understood for neuronal NOS, where thiol-mediated enhancement of enzymatic activity is associated with direct thiol binding to the heme moiety cooperatively with tetrahydrobiopterin (186). The precise mechanisms through which thiols operate are not clear although one possibility could include the prevention of NOS inactivation from peroxynitrite that is undoubtedly produced during simultaneously generation of NO and superoxide by the enzyme (85,187). Recent studies demonstrating a reduction in tissue GSH with hypercholesterolemia and enhanced oxidative damage would tend to support this contention (188).

The antioxidant properties of GSH may also be important for the efficiency of NO production and an indirect manner. For example, the NOS cofactor tetrahydrobiopterin, is subject to rapid autoxidation and GSH has been shown to be protective in this regard (189,190). In addition, L-arginine, the substrate for NO synthesis is transported into cells in a GSH-dependent manner (191). The maintenance of adequate NOS cofactor levels is particularly important as limiting concentrations of either L-arginine (84,85,192) or tetrahydrobiopterin (85,193) have been shown to limit enzymatic activity and facilitate the production of superoxide by NOS.

Ascorbic Acid

Ascorbic acid is among the most versatile antioxidants found in vivo. Its scavenges a wide range of biologically relevant oxidizing species including superoxide, aqueous peroxyl radicals, hydrogen peroxide, hydroxyl radical, and, perhaps hypochlorous acid (194-197), principally due to its potent antioxidant activity, the effect of ascorbic acid on NO bioactivity has been examined. In a large part, these studies have been done on humans and are contained in more detail in Chapter 12. For example, coronary artery disease patients treated with oral ascorbic acid demonstrate a significant improvement in NO bioactivity within the brachial artery (198). This effect is evident with plasma concentrations of ascorbic acid within the physiologic range. In contrast, other studies have typically used pharmacologic concentrations of ascorbic acid. For example, diabetic patients (199) and hypercholesterolemic patients (200) treated with high-dose intra-arterial ascorbic acid (about 10 mM) demonstrated enhanced NO- mediated vascular responses in forearm resistance vessels. Similar effects have also been observed with clinical conditions associated with atherosclerosis such as smoking (201), congestive heart failure (202), and hypertension (168,203).

The precise mechanisms responsible for the effect of ascorbic acid on NO bioactivity remains under investigation. At first glance, the fact that ascorbic acid scavenges superoxide prompts speculation that superoxide scavenging is responsible for improved NO bioactivity (168, 199-202). Direct studies in isolated arterial segments suggest that such speculation is unfounded. Isolated arteries exposed to superoxide readily demonstrate impaired NO-mediated arterial relaxation that readily improved with physiologic concentrations of SOD (about 1-3 μM) (64,66,204,205). However, ascorbic acid cannot substitute for SOD in these systems unless concentrations in excess of 10 mM are employed (Figure 6) (204). Although such concentrations may have been obtained in some human studies (199-201), these levels of ascorbic acid are not physiologically meaningful. In fact, such pharmacologic concentrations of ascorbic acid can be predicted based on available kinetic data considering that the interaction between superoxide and ascorbic acid occurs approximately 10^5 –fold less rapidly than the interaction of superoxide with NO (1.9×10^{10} $M^{-1} \cdot Sec^{-1}$) (58). Thus, simply superoxide scavenging appears to provide an incomplete explanation for the effect of ascorbic acid on NO bioactivity.

There are, however several actions of ascorbic acid that merit consideration. Ascorbic acid has been shown to increase the catalytic activity of neuronal NOS similar to glutathione (185). Treatment of either human (220) or porcine (A. Huang, J. Keaney, unpublished) endothelial cells with ascorbic acid potentiates endothelial cell NO synthesis. The mechanism for this observation is under investigation but may relate to enhanced hydroxylation of L-arginine. In addition, ascorbic acid may protect tetrahydrobiopterin from oxidation (190), although direct

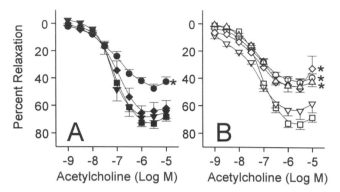

Figure 6. The effect of ascorbic acid and superoxide on NO bioactivity. (A) Contracted vessels (1 μM phenylephrine) were assayed for NO bioactivity as relaxation in response to acetylcholine in the presence of no additions (■), superoxide from pyrogallol (●), pyrogallol with 300 IU/ml SOD (♦), or 300 IU/ml SOD alone (▼). (B) NO bioactivity assayed as relaxation to acetylcholine in the presence of no additions (□),pyrogallol (○), or pyrogallol with 0.1 (△), 1.0 (◇), or 10 (▽) mM ascorbic acid. *$P<0.05$ vs no additions only by two-way ANOVA.

evidence to support this is not yet available. Finally, ascorbic acid has been shown to spare intracellular GSH (173,174,206), prompting speculation that ascorbic acid may influence NO bioactivity through mechanisms related to intracellular GSH.

OXIDATIVE STRESS AND OTHER ENDOTHELIAL FUNCTIONS

Despite the fact that NO is a major mediator of vascular homeostasis, it is important to realize that not all endothelial functions are derived from NO. As stated above, the endothelium synthesizes a number of lipid, protein, and glycosaminoglycan factors that contribute to the overall antithrombotic environment of the vascular surface. These functions of the endothelium have received considerably less attention for their sensitivity to oxidative stress than NO-mediated responses.

Nevertheless, there is data to indicate that oxidative stress alters other endothelial functions in a manner that would tend to support atherosclerosis and thrombosis. In this regard, oxLDL increases endothelin transcription and release from cultured endothelial cells (207). One implication for this effect of oxLDL would be to produce potent vasoconstriction (208) and smooth muscle cell proliferation (209), in keeping with the known bioactivity of endothelin. The oxidation of LDL phosphatidylcholine leads to LDL accumulation of lysophosphatidylcholine (210) that may transfer to endothelial cells both stimulating the release of PAI-1 and suppressing the release of tissue-type plasminogen activator, thereby favoring thrombosis over thrombolysis (211).

As the barrier between the plasma and vessel wall, the endothelium also serves the important function of regulating leukocyte traffic within the arterial wall. This function is mediated through the expression of cell surface adhesion molecules (see Chapter 8). Recent evidence has begun to link oxidative stress to the expression and activation of adhesion molecules. Thiol compounds with antioxidant activity such as N-acetylcysteine (NAC) or pyrrolidine dithiocarbamate (PDTC) inhibit endothelial cell expression of VCAM-1 by TNF-α (212). Conversely, endothelial cells exposed to oxLDL or oxidized fatty acids demonstrate enhanced expression of VCAM-1 in response to TNF-α (213). Expression of ICAM-1 and VCAM-1 by TNF-α is inhibited by a glutathione peroxidase mimic (214). This redox-sensitive regulation of adhesion molecule expression appears coupled to oxidative stress through the activity of transcription factors such as NF-κB (212). Even in the absence of cytokines, human arterial endothelial cells exposed to oxLDL alone express ICAM-1, VCAM-1 and E-selectin (215). Thus, oxidative stress appears to promote the adhesion of leukocytes to the endothelium through increased expression of endothelial adhesion molecules.

FUTURE DIRECTIONS

Without question, there are many other sources for oxidative stress in biologic systems, many of which will likely have important implications for endothelial function. At sites of inflammation including atherosclerosis, neutrophils secrete myeloperoxidase, a heme enzyme that produces a number of oxidizing species including hypochlorous acid (HOCL) and tyrosyl radical (104,105) (see Chapter 2). Emerging evidence also indicates that reactive nitrogen species such as nitrogen dioxide (NO_2) or nitryl chloride (CL-NO_2) may form as a consequence of peroxidase-catalyzed oxidation of nitrite (216) or the reaction of nitrite with HOCL (217). If one considers that tyrosyl radical has been shown to initiate lipid peroxidation in LDL (218) and that HOCL-modified LDL has been found in atherosclerotic lesions (219), it is reasonable to speculate that such oxidants may have important implications for endothelial function. Future studies with murine models may help tell us which oxidants are important not only for atherosclerosis, but for impaired vascular function as well.

REFERENCES

1.   American Heart Association. 1998 Heart and stroke statistical update. Internet. 1998. American Heart Association.
2.   Stary HC, Chandler AB, Glagov S, Guyton JR, Insull WJ, Rosenfeld ME, Schaffer SA, Schwartz CJ, Wagner WD, Wissler RW. A definition of initial, fatty streak, and intermediate lesions of atherosclerosis. A report from the Committee on Vascular Lesions of the Council on Arteriosclerosis, American Heart Association. *Circulation.* 1994;89:2462.
3.   Libby P. Molecular basis of the acute coronary syndromes. *Circulation.* 1995;91:2844.
4.   Keaney JF, Jr., Vita JA. Atherosclerosis, oxidative stress, and antioxidant protection in endothelium-derived relaxing factor action. *Prog Card Dis.* 1995;38:129.
5.   Levine GN, Keaney JF, Jr., Vita JA. Cholesterol reduction in cardiovascular disease. Clinical benefits and possible mechanisms. *N Engl J Med.* 1995;332:512.
6.   Radomski MW, Palmer RM, Moncada S. Comparative pharmacology of endothelium-derived relaxing factor, nitric oxide and prostacyclin in platelets. *Br J Pharmacol.* 1987;92:181.
7.   Ursini F, Maiorino M, Brigilius-Flohe R, Aumann KD, Roberi A, Schomburg D, Flohe L. Diversity of glutathione peroxidases. *Methods Enzymol.* 1995;252:38.
8.   Avissar N, Whitin JC, Annen PZ, Palmer IS, Cohen HJ. Antihuman plasma glutathione peroxidase antibodies: immunologic investigations to determine p;asma glutathione peroxidase protein and selenium content in plasma. *Blood.* 1989;73:318.

9.   Loskutoff DJ, Edgington DS. Synthesis of a fibrinolytic activator and inhibitor by endothelial cells. *Proc Natl Acad Sci USA.* 1977;74:3903.

10.   Quyyumi AA, Dakak N, Andrews NP, Husain S, Arora S, Gilligan DM, Panza JA, Cannon RO, III. Nitric oxide activity in the human coronary circulation. *J Clin Invest.* 1995;95:1747.

11.   Garg UC, Hassid A. Nitric oxide-generating vasodilators and 8-bromo-cGMP inhibit mitogenesis and proliferation of cultured rat vascular smooth muscle cells. *J Clin Invest.* 1989;83:1774.

12.   Kubes P, Kurose I, Granger DN. NO donors prevent integrin-induced leukocyte adhesion but not P-selectin-dependent rolling in postischemic venules. *Am.J.Physiol.* 1994;267:H931.

13.   Azuma H, Ishikawa M, Sekizaki S. Endothelium-dependent inhibition of platelet aggregation. *Br J Pharmacol.* 1986;88:411.

14.   Radomski MW, Palmer RM, Moncada S. Characterization of the L-arginine:nitric oxide pathway in human platelets. *Br J Pharmacol.* 1990;101:325.

15.   Freedman JE, Loscalzo J, Barnard MR, Alpert C, Keaney JF, Jr., Michelson AD. Nitric oxide released from activated platelets inhibits platelet recruitment. *J Clin Invest.* 1997;100:350.

16.   Huang PL, Huang Z, Mashimo H, Bloch KD, Moskowitz MA, Bevan JA, Fishman MC. Hypertension in mice lacking the gene for endothelial nitric oxide syntase. *Nature.* 1995;377:239.

17.   Shesely EG, Maeda N, Kim HS, Desai KM, Krege JH, Laubach VE, Sherman PA, Sessa WC, Smithies O. Elevated blood pressures in mice lacking endothelial nitric oxide synthase. *Proc Natl Acad Sci USA.* 1996;93:13176.

18.   Rudic RD, Shesely EG, Maeda N, Smithies O, Segal SS, Sessa WC. Direct evidence for the importance of endothelium-derived nitric oxide in vascular remodeling. *J Clin Invest.* 1998;101:731.

19.   Freedman, JE, Sauter, R, Ault KA, Huang PL, and Loscalzo J. Deficient platelet-derived nitric oxide and enhanced hemostasis in mice lacking the NOS3 gene. *Circulation* 1998;98:1-4.

20.   Freedman JE, Loscalzo J, Benoit SE, Valeri CR, Barnard MR, Michelson AD. Decreased platelet inhibition by nitric oxide in two brothers with a history of arterial thrombosis. *J Clin Invest.* 1996;97:979.

21.   Arnold WP, Mittal CK, Katsuki S, Murad F. Nitric oxide activates guanylate cyclase and increases guanosine 3',5'-cyclic monophosphate levels in various tissue preparations. *Proc Natl Acad Sci USA.* 1977;74:3203.

22.   Ignarro LJ, Burke TM, Wood KS, Wolin MS, Kadowitz PJ. Association between cyclic GMP accumulation and acetylcholine-elicited relaxation of bovine intrapulmonary artery. *J Pharmacol Exp Ther.* 1984;228:682.

23.   Moro MA, Russell RJ, Cellek S, Lizasoain I, Su Y, Darley-Usmar VM, Radomski MW, Moncada S. cGMP mediates the vascular and platelet actions of nitric oxide: Confirmation using an inhibitor of the soluble guanylyl cyclase. *Proc Natl Acad Sci USA.* 1995;93:1480.

24.   Radomski MW, Palmer RMJ, Moncada S. The role of nitric oxide and cGMP in platelet adhesion to the vascular endothelium. *Biochem Biophys Res Commun.* 1987;148:1482.

25.   Wink DA, Darbyshire JF, Nims RW, Saavedra JE, Ford PC. Reactions of the bioregulatory agent nitric oxide in oxygenated aqueous media: determination of the kinetics for oxidation and nitrosation by intermediates generated in the NO/O2 reaction. *Chem Res Toxicol.* 1993;6:23.

26.   Stamler JS, Singel DJ, Loscalzo J. Biochemistry of nitric oxide and its redox-activated forms. *Science.* 1992;258:1898.

27.   Bolotina VM, Najibi S, Palacino JJ, Pagano PJ, Cohen RA. Nitric oxide directly activates calcium-dependent potassium channels in vascular smooth muscle. *Nature.* 1994;368:850.

28.   Xu L, Eu JP, Meissner G, Stamler JS. Activation of the cardiac calcium release channel (ryonadine receptor by poly-S-nitrosylation. *Science.* 1998;279:234.

29.   Campbell DL, Stamler JS, Strauss HC: Redox modulation of L-type calcium channels in ferret ventricular myocytes. Dual mechanism regulation by nitric oxide and S-nitrosothiols. *J Gen Physiol.* 1996;108:277.

30.   Stamler JS, Jia L, Eu JP, McMahon TJ, Demchenko IT, Bonoventura J, Gernert K, Piantadosi CA. Blood flow regulation by S-nitrosohemoglobin in the physiological oxygen gradient. *Science.* 1997;276:2034.

31.   Busconi L, Michel T: Endothelial nitric oxide synthase. N-terminal myristoylation determines subcellular localization. *J Biol Chem.* 1993;268:8410.

32.   Shaul PW, Smart EJ, Robinson LJ, German Z, Yuhanna IS, Ying Y, Anderson R, Michel T. Acylation targets endothelial nitric-oxide synthase to plasmalemmal caveolae. *J Biol Chem.* 1996;271:6518.

33.   Garcia-Cardena G, Oh P, Liu J, Schnitzer JE, Sessa WC. Targeting of nitric oxide synthase to endothelial cell caveolae via palmitoylation: implications for nitric oxide signaling. *Proc Natl Acad Sci USA.* 1996;93:6448.

34.   Couet J, Li S, Okamoto T, Ikezu T, Lisanti MP. Identification of peptide and protein ligands for the caveolin-scaffoliding domain. implications for the interaction of caveolin with caveolae-associated proteins. *J Biol Chem.* 1997;272:6525.

35.   Michel JB, Feron O, Sase K, Prabhakar P, Michel T. Caveolin versus calmodulin. counterbalancing allosteric modulators of endothelial nitric oxide synthase. *J Biol Chem.* 1997;272:25907.

36.   Garcia-Cardena G, Fan R, Shah V, Sorrentino R, Cirino G, Papapetropoulos A, Sessa WC. Dynamic activation of endothelial nitric oxide synthase by Hsp90. *Nature.* 1998;392:821.

37.   Ludmer PL, Selwyn AP, Shook TL, Wayne RR, Mudge GH, Alexander RW, Ganz P. Paradoxical vasoconstriction induced by acetylcholine in atherosclerotic coronary arteries. *N Engl J Med.* 1986;315:1046.

38.   Nitenberg A, Valensi P, Sachs R, Dali M, Aptecar E, Attali JR. Impaiment of coronary vascular reserve and ACh-induced coronary vasodilation in diabetic patients with angiographically normal coronary arteries and normal left ventricular systolic function. *Diabetes.* 1993;42:1017.

39.   Panza JA, Casino PR, Kilcoyne CM, Quyyumi AA. Role of endothelium-derived nitric oxide in the abnormal endothelium-dependent vascular relaxation of patients with essential hypertension. *Circulation.* 1993,87.1468.

40.   Anderson TJ, Uehata A, Gerhard MD, Meredith IT, Knab S, Delagrange D, Lieberman EH, Gamz P, Creager MA, Yeung AC, Selwyn AP. Close relation of endothelial function in the human coronary and peripheral circulations. *J Am Coll Cardiol.* 1995;26:1235.

41.   Celermajer DS, Sorensen K, Ryalls M, Robinson J, Thomas O, Leonard JV, Deanfield JE. Impaired endothelial function occurs in the systemic arteries of children with homozygous homocystinuria but not in their heterozygous parents. *J Am Coll Cardiol.* 1993;22:854.

42.   Creager MA, Cooke JP, Mendelsohn ME, Gallagher SJ, Coleman SM, Loscalzo J, Dzau VJ. Impaired vasodilation of forearm resistance vessels in hypercholesterolemic humans. *J Clin Invest.* 1990;86:228.

43.   Johnstone MT, Gallagher MT, Scales KM, Cusco JA, Lee B, Creagher M. Endothelium-dependent vasodilation is impaired in patients with insulin-dependent diabetes mellitus. *Circulation.* 1992;86:I-618.

44.   Vita JA, Treasure CB, Nabel EG, McLenachan JM, Fish RD, Yeung AC, Vekshtein VI, Selwyn AP, Ganz P. Coronary vasomotor response to acetylcholine relates to risk factors for coronary artery disease. *Circulation.* 1990;81:491.

45.   Celermajer DS, Sorensen KE, Bull C, Ribinson J, Deanfield JE. Endothelium-dependent dilation in the systemic arteries of asymptomatic subjects relates to coronary risk factors and their interaction. *J Am Coll Cardiol.* 1994;24:1468.

46.   Kugiyama K, Yasue H, Ihgushi M, Motoyama T, Dawano H, Inobe Y, Hirachima O, Sugiyama S. Deficiency in nitric oxide bioactivity in epicardial coronary arteries of cigarette smokers. *J Am Coll Cardiol.* 1996;28:1161.

47.   Clarkson P, Celermajer DS, Powe AJ, Donald AE, Henry RMA, Deanfield JE. Endothelium-dependent dilatation is impaired in young healthy subjects with a family history of premature coronary disease. *Circulation.* 1997;96:3378.

48.   Diaz M, Frei B, Vita JA, Keaney JF, Jr. Antioxidants and atherosclerotic heart disease. *N Engl J Med.* 1997;337:408.

49.   Heistad DD, Armstrong ML, Marcus ML, Piegors KJ, Mark AL. Augmented responses to vasoconstrictor stimuli in hypercholesterolemic and atherosclerotic monkeys. *Circ Res.* 1984;54:711.

50.   Henry PD, Yokoyama M. Supersensitivity of atherosclerotic rabbit aorta to ergonovine mediated by a serotonergic mechanism. *J Clin Invest.* 1980;66:306.

51.   Furchgott RF, Zawadzki JV. The obligatory role of endothelial cells in the relaxation of arterial smooth muscle by acetylcholine. *Nature.* 1980;288:373.

52.   Jayakody RL, Senaratne MPJ, Thomson ABR, Kappagoda CT. Cholesterol feeding impairs endothelium-dependent relaxation of rabbit aorta. *Can J Physiol Pharmacol.* 1985;63:1206.

53. Freiman PC, Mitchell GG, Heistad DD, Armstrong ML, Harrison DG. Atherosclerosis impairs endothelium-dependent vascular relaxation to acetylcholine and thrombin in primates. *Circ Res.* 1986;58:783.

54. Ignarro LJ, Buga GM, Wood KS, Byrns RE, Chaudhuri G. Endothelium-derived relaxing factor produced and released from artery and vein is nitric oxide. *Proc Natl Acad Sci USA.* 1987;84:9265.

55. Minor RL, Jr., Myers PR, Guerra R, Jr., Bates JN, Harrison DG. Diet-induced atherosclerosis increases the release of nitrogen oxides from rabbit aorta. *J Clin Invest.* 1990;86:2109.

56. Ohara Y, Peterson TE, Harrison DG. Hypercholesterolemia increases endothelial superoxide anion production. *J Clin Invest.* 1993;91:2546.

57. Keaney JF, Jr., Xu A, Cunningham D, Jackson T, Frei B, Vita JA. Dietary probucol preserves endothelial function in cholesterol-fed rabbits by limiting vascular oxidative stress and superoxide generation. *J Clin Invest.* 1995;95:2520.

58. Kissner R, Nauser T, Bugnon P, Lye PG, Koppenol WH. Formation and properties of peroxynitrite as studied by laser flash photolysis, high-pressure stopped-flow technique, and pulse radiolysis. *Chem Res Toxicol.* 1997;10:1285.

59. Leeuwenburgh C, Hansen P, Shaish A, Holloszy JO, Heinecke JW. Markers of protein oxidation by hydroxyl radical and reactive nitrogen species in tissues of aging rats. *Am J Physiol.* 1998;274:R453.

60. Ischiropoulos H, Zhu L, Beckman JS. Peroxynitrite formation from macrophage-derived nitric oxide. *Arch Biochem Biophys.* 1992;298:446.

61. Mayer B, Schrammel A, Klatt P, Koesling D, Schmidt K. Peroxynitrite-induced accumulation of cyclic GMP in endothelial cells and stimulation of purified soluble guanylyl cyclase. Dependence on glutathione and possible role of S-nitrosation. *J Biol Chem.* 1995;270:17355.

62. Tarpey MM, Beckman JS, Ischiropoulos H, Gore JZ, Brock TA. Peroxynitrite stimulates vascular smooth muscle cell cyclic GMP synthesis. *FEBS Lett.* 1995;364:314.

63. Rosen GM, Freeman BA. Detection of superoxide generated by endothelial cells. *Proc Natl Acad Sci USA.* 1984;81:7269.

64. Rubanyi GM, Vanhoutte PM. Superoxide anions and hyperoxia inactivate endothelium-derived relaxing factor. *Am J Physiol.* 1986;250:H822.

65. Gryglewski RJ, Palmer RM, Moncada S. Superoxide anion is involved in the breakdown of endothelium-derived vascular relaxing factor. *Nature.* 1986;320:454.

66. Ignarro LJ, Byrns RE, Buga GM, Wood KS, Chaudhuri G. Pharmacological evidence that endothelium-derived relaxing factor is nitric oxide: use of pyrogallol and superoxide dismutase to study endothelium dependent and nitric oxide elicited vascular smooth muscle relaxation. *J Pharmacol Exp Ther.* 1988;244:181.

67. Heikkila RE, Cohen G. The inactivation of copper-zinc superoxide dismutase by diethyldithiocarbamate, in Anonymous Superoxide and Superoxide Dismutases. New York, Academic Press, 1977, p 367.

68. Omar HA, Cherry PD, Mortelliti MP, Burke-Wolin T, Wolin MS. Inhibition of coronary artery superoxide dismutase attenuates endothelium-dependent and -independent nitrovasodilator relaxation. *Circ Res.* 1991;69:601.

69. Mugge A, Elwell JK, Peterson TE, Harrison DG. Release of intact endothelium-derived relaxing factor depends on endothelial superoxide dismutase activity. *Am J Physiol.* 1991;260:C219.

70. Mulsch A, Mordvintcev P, Bassenge E, Jung F, Clement B, Busse R. In vivo spin trapping of glyceryl trinitrate-derived nitric oxide in rabbit blood vessels and organs. *Circulation.* 1995;92:1876.

71. Sarvazyan N, Askari A, Klevay LM, Huang WH. Role of intracellular SOD in oxidant-induced injury to normal and copper-deficient cardiac myocytes. *Am J Physiol.* 1995;268:H1115.

72. Lynch SM, Frei B, Morrow JD, Roberts LJ, II, Xu A, Jackson T, Reyna R, Klevay LM, Vita JA, Keaney JF, Jr. Vascular superoxide dismutase deficiency impairs endothelial vasodilator function through direct inactivation of nitric oxide and increased lipid peroxidation. *Arterioscler Thromb Vasc Biol.* 1997;17:2975.

73. Schuschke DA, Ree MWR, Saari JT, Miller FN. Copper deficiency alters vasodilation in the rat cremaster muscle microcirculation. *J Nutr.* 1992;122:1547.

74. Abrahamsson T, Brandt U, Marklund SL, Sjoqvist PO. Vascular bound recombinant extracellular superoxide dismutase type C protects against the detrimental effects of superoxide radicals on endothelium-dependent arterial relaxation. *Circ Res.* 1992;70:264.

75. Mugge A, Elwell JH, Peterson TE, Hofmeyer TG, Heistad DD, Harrison DG. Chronic treatment with polyethylene-glycolated superoxide dismutase partially restores endothelium-dependent vascular relaxations in cholesterol-fed rabbits. *Circ Res.* 1991;69:1293.

76. White CR, Brock TA, Chang LY, Crapo J, Briscoe P, Ku D, Bradley WA, Gianturco SH, Gore J, Freeman BA, Tarpey MM. Superoxide and peroxynitrite in atherosclerosis. *Proc Natl Acad Sci USA.* 1994;91:1044.

77. Pagano PJ, Ito Y, Tornheim K, Gallop P, Tauber AI, Cohen RA. An NADPH oxidase superoxide generating system in rabbit aorta. *Am J Physiol.* 1995;268:H2274.

78. Pagano PJ, Clark J, Cifuentes-Pagano ME, Clark SM, Callis GM, Quinn MT. Localization of a constitutively active, phagocyte-like NADPH oxidase in rabbit aortic adventitia: enhancement by angiotensin II. *Proc Natl Acad SciUSA.* 1997;94:14483.

79. Mojazzab H, Kaminski PM, Wolin MS: NADH oxidoreductase is a major source of superoxide anion in bovine coronary artery endothelium. *Am J Physiol.* 1994;266:H2568.

80. Kukreja RC, Kontos HA, Hess ML, Ellis EF. PGH synthase and lipoxygenase generate superoxide in the presence of NADH or NADPH. *Circ Res.* 1986;59:612.

81. Paler-Martinez A, Panus PC, Chumley PH, Ryan US, Hardy MM, Freeman DA. Endogenous xanthine oxidase does not significantly contribute to vascular endothelial production of reactive oxygen species. *Arch Biochem Biophys.* 1994;311:79.

82. White CR, Darley-Usmar V, Berrington WR, McAdams M, Gore JZ, Thompson JA, Parks DA, Tarpey MM, Freeman BA. Circulating plasma xanthine oxidase contributes to vascular dysfunction in hypercholesterolemic rabbits. *Proc Natl Acad Sci USA.* 1996;93:8745.

83. Cardillo C, Kilcoyne CM, Cannon RO, III, Quyyumi AA, Panza JA. Xanthine oxidase inhibition with oxypurinol improves endothelial fasodilator function in hypercholesterolemic but not in hypertensive patients. *Hypertension.* 1997;30:57.

84. Pou S, Pou WS, Bredt DS, Snyder SH, Rosen GM. Generation of superoxide by purified brain nitric oxide synthase. *J Biol Chem.* 1992;267:24173.

85. Vasquez-Vivar J, Kalyanaraman B, Martasek P, Hogg N, Masters BS, Karoui H, tordo P, Pritchard KA, Jr. Superoxide generation by endothelial nitric oxide synthase: the influence of cofactors. *Proc Natl Acad Sci USA.* 1998;95:9220.

86. Xia Y, Roman LJ, Masters BS, Zweier JL. Inducible nitric-oxide synthase generates superoxide from the reductase domain. *J Biol Chem.* 1998;273:22635.

87. Pritchard KA, Jr., Groszek L, Smalley DM, Sessa WC, Wu M, Villalon P, Wolin MS, Stemerman MB. Native low-density lipoprotein increases endothelial cell nitric oxide synthase generation of superoxide anion. *Circ Res.* 1995;77:510.

88. Stroes E, Kastelein J, Cosentino F, Erkelens W, Wever R, Koomans H, Luscher T, Rabelink T. Tetrahydrobiopterin restores endothelial function in hypercholesterolemia. *J Clin Invest.* 1996;99:41.

89. Verhaar MC, Wever RM, Kastelein JJ, van Dam T, Koomans HA, Rabelink TJ. 5-methyltetrahydrofolate, the active form of folic acid, restores endothelial function in familial hypercholesterolemia. *Circulation.* 1998;97:237.

90. Kagota S, Yamaguchi Y, Shinozuka K, Kunitomo M. Mechanisms of impairment of endothelium-dependent relaxation to acetylcholine in Watanabe heritable hyperlipidemic rabbit aortas. *Clin Exper Pharmacol Physiol.* 1998;25:104.

91. Beckman JS, Beckman TW, Chen J, Marshall PA, Freeman BA. Apparent hydroxyl radical production by peroxynitrite: implications for endothelial injury from nitric oxide and superoxide. *Proc Natl Acad Sci USA.* 1990;87:1620.

92. Saran M, Michel C, Bors W: Reaction of NO with O2-. Implications for the action of endothelium-derived relaxing factor (A2RF). *Free Radic Res Commun.* 1990;10:221.

93. Beckman JS, Crow JP. Pathological implications of nitric oxide, superoxide, and peroxynitrite formation. *Biochem Soc Trans.* 1993;21:330.

94. Moreno JJ, Pryor WA: Inactivation of a-1-proteinase inhibitor by peroxynitrite. *Chem Res Toxicol.* 1992;5:425.

95. Graham A, Hogg N, Kalyanaraman B, O'Leary V, Darley-Usmar V, Moncada S: Peroxynitrite modification of low-density lipoprotein leads to recognition by the macrophage scavenger receptor. *FEBS Lett.* 1993;330:181.

96. Landino LM, Crews BC, Timmons MD, Morrow JD, Marnett LJ. Peroxynitrite, the couling product of nitric oxide and superoxide, activates prostaglandin biosynthesis. *Proc Natl Acad Sci U.S.A.* 1996;93:15069.

97. Ischiropoulos H, Zhu L, Chen J, Tsai M, Martin JC, Smith CD, Beckman JS. Peroxynitrite-mediated tyrosine nitration catalyzed by superoxide dismutase. *Arch Biochem Biophys.* 1992;298:431.

98. Buettner GR. The pecking order of free radicals and antioxidants: lipid peroxidation, alpha-tocopherol, and ascorbate. *Arch Biochem Biophys.* 1993;300:535.

99. Lynch SM, Frei B: Mechanisms of copper-and iron-dependent oxidative modification of human low-density lipoprotein. *J Lipid Res.* 1993;34:1745.

100. Haber F, Weiss J: The catalytic decomposition of hydrogen peroxide by iron salts. *Proc Roy Soc London* 1934;147:332.

101. Ehrenwald E, Chisolm GM, Fox PL. Intact human ceruloplasmin oxidatively modifies low density lipoprotein. *J Clin Invest.* 1994;93:1493.

102. Smith C, Mitchinson MJ, Aruoma OI, Halliwell B. Stimulation of lipid peroxidation and hydroxyl radical generation by the contents of human atherosclerotic lesions. *Biochem J* 1992;286:901.

103. Semenkovich CF, Heinecke JW. The mystery of diabetes and atherosclerosis: time for a new plot. *Diabetes.* 1997;46:327.

104. Heinecke JW, Li W, Francis GA, Goldstein JA. Tyrosyl radical generated by myeloperoxidase catalyzes the oxidative cross-linking of proteins. *J Clin Invest.* 1993;91:2866.

105. Heinecke JW: Pathways for oxidation of low density lipoprotein by meloperoxidase: tyrosyl radical, reactive aldehydes, hypochlorous acid, and molecular chlorine. *Biofactors* 1997;6:145.

106. Daugherty A, Rateri DL, Dunn JL, Heinecke JW. Human atherosclerotic lesions contain myeloperoxidase, a phagocyte enzyme that catalyzes oxidation reactions. *Circulation.* 1993;88:I-32.

107. Hazen SL, Heinecke JW. 3-Chlorotyrosine, a specific marker of myeloperoxidase-catalyzed oxidation, is markedly elevated in low density lipoprotein isolated from human atherosclerotic intima. *J Clin Invest.* 1997;99:2075.

108. Folcik VA, Nivar-Aristy RA, Krajewski LP, Cathcart MK: Lipoxygenase contributes to the oxidation of lipids in human atherosclerotic plaques. *J Clin Invest.* 1995;96:504.

109. Loscalzo J. The oxidant stress of hyperhomocyst(e)inemia. *J Clin Invest.* 1996;98:5.

110. Malle E, Hazell L, Stocker R, Sattler W, Esterbauer H, Waeg G: Immunologic detection and measurement of hypochlorite-modified LDL with specific monoclonal antibodies. *Arterioscler Thromb Vasc Biol.* 1995;15:982.

111. Wagner BA, Buettner GR, Burns CP. Free radical-mediated lipid peroxidation in cells: oxidizability is a function of cell lipid bis-allylic hydrogen content. *Biochemistry.* 1994;33:4449.

112. Keaney JF, Jr., Frei B. Antioxidant protection of low-density lipoprotein and its role in the prevention of atherosclerotic vascular disease, in Frei B (ed): *Natural antioxidants in human health and disease.* San Diego, Academic Press, 1994, p 303.

113. Padmaja S, Huie RE: The reaction of nitric oxide with organic peroxyl radicals. *Biochem Biophys Res Commun.* 1993;195:539.

114. Rubbo H, Radi R, Trujillo M, Telleri R, Kalyanaraman B, Barnes S, Kirk M, Freeman BA: Nitric oxide regulation of superoxide and peroxynitrite-dependent lipid peroxidation. Formation of novel nitrogen-containing oxidized lipid derivatives. *J Biol Chem.* 1994;269:26066.

115. Ylä-Herttuala S, Palinski W, Rosenfeld ME, Parthasarathy S, Carew TE, Butler S, Witztum JL, Steinberg D: Evidence for the presence of oxidatively modified low density lipoprotein in atherosclerotic lesions of rabbit and man. *J Clin Invest.* 1989;84:1086.

116. Chin JH, Azhar S, Hoffman BB: Inactivation of endothelium-derived relaxing factor by oxidized lipoproteins. *J Clin Invest.* 1992;89:10.

117. Liao JK, Shin WS, Lee WY, Clark SL. Oxidized low-density lipoprotein decreases the expression of endothelial nitric oxide synthase. *J Biol Chem.* 1995;270:319.

118. Ohgushi M, Kugiyama K, Fukunaga K, Murohara T, Sugiyama S, Miyamoto E, Yasue H: Protein kinase C inhibitors prevent impairment of endothelium-dependent relaxation by oxidatively modified LDL. *Arterioscler Thromb.* 1993;13:1525.

119. Kugiyama K, Kerns SA, Morrisett JD, Roberts R, Henry PD: Impairment of endothelium-dependent arterial relaxation by lysolecithin in modified low-density lipoproteins. *Nature.* 1990;344:160.

120. Liu J, Garcia-Cardena G, Sessa WC. Palmitoylation of endothelial nitric oxide synthase is necessary for optimal stimulatted release of nitric oxide: implications for caveolae localization. *Biochemistry.* 1996;35:13277.

121. Wink DA, Hanbauer I, Krishna MC, DeGraff W, Gamson J, Mitchell JB. Nitric oxide protects against cellular damage and cytotoxicity from reactive oxygen species. *Proc Natl Acad Sci USA.* 1993;90:9813.

122. Hogg N, Kalyanaraman B, Joseph J, Struck A, Parthasarathy S. Inhibition of low-density lipoprotein oxidation by nitric oxide. Potential role in atherogenesis. *FEBS Lett.* 1993;334:170.

123. Zembowicz A, Hatchett RJ, Jakubowski AM, Gryglewski RJ. Involvement of nitric oxide in the endothelium-dependent relaxation induced by hydrogen peroxide in rabbit aorta. *Br J Pharmacol.* 1993;110:151.

124. Okuma M, Steiner M, Bladini MG. Studies on lipid peroxides in platelets. II. Effect of aggregating agents and platelet antibody. *J Lab Clin Med.* 1971;77:728.

125. Freedman JE, Frei B, Welch GN, Loscalzo J. Glutathione peroxidase potentiates the inhibition of platelet function by S-nitrosothiols. *J Clin Invest.* 1995,96.394.

126. Esterbauer H, Striegl G, Puhl H, Oberreither S, Rotheneder M, el-Saadani M, Jürgens J. The role of vitamin E and carotenoids in preventing oxidation of low density lipoprotein. *Ann NY Acad Sci.* 1989;570:254.

127. Jialal I, Norkus EP, Cristol L, Grundy SM. Beta-carotene inhibits the oxidative modification of low density lipoprotein. *Biochim Biophys Acta.* 1991;1086:134.

128. Gaziano IM, Hatta A, Flynn M, Johnson EJ, Krinsky NI, Ridker PM, Hennekens CH, Frei B. Supplementation with beta-carotene in vivo and in vitro does not inhibit low density lipoprotein (LDL) oxidation. *Atherosclerosis* 1995;112:187.

129. Verbeuren TJ, Jordaens FH, Zonnekeyn LL, VanHove CE, Coene MC, Herman AG. Effect of hypercholesterolemia on vascular reactivity in the rabbit *Circ Res.* 1986;58:553.

130. Keaney JF, Jr., Gaziano JM, Xu A, Frei B, Curran-Celentano J, Shwaery GT, Loscalzo J, Vita JA. Dietary antioxidants preserve endothelium-dependent vessel relaxation in cholesterol-fed rabbits. *Proc Natl Acad Sci USA.* 1993;90:11880.

131. Andersson TLG, Matz J, Ferns GAA, Änggård EE. Vitamin E reverses cholesterol-induced endothelial dysfunction in the rabbit coronary circulation. *Atherosclerosis* 1994;111:39.

132. Stewart-Lee AL, Forster LA, Nourooz-Zadeh J, Ferns GAA, Änggård EE. Vitamin E protects against impairment of endothelium-mediated relaxations in cholesterol-fed rabbits. *Arterioscler Thromb.* 1994;14:494.

133. Lutz M, Cortez J, Vinet R. Effects of dietary fats, alpha-tocopherol and beta-carotene supplementation on aortic ring segment responses in the rat. *Int J Vit Nutr Res* 1995;65:225.

134. Raij L, Jagy J, Coffee K, DeMaster EG. Hypercholesterolemia promotes endothelial dysfunction in vitamin E- and selenium-deficient rats. *Hypertension.* 1993;22:56.

135. Keegan A, Walbank H, Cotter MA, Cameron NE. Chronic vitamin E treatment prevents defective endothelium-dependent relaxation in diabetic rat aorta. *Diabetologia* 1995;38:1475.

136. Karasu C, Ozansoy G, Bozkurt O, Erdogan D, Omeroglu S. Changes in isoprenaline-induced endothelium-dependent and -independent relaxations of aorta in long-term STZ-diabetic rats: reversal effect of dietary vitamin E. *Gen Pharm* 1997;29:561.

137. Karasu C, Ozansoy G, Bozkurt O, Erdogan D, Omeroglu S. Antioxidant and triglyceride-lowering effects of vitamin E associated with the prevention of abnormalities in the reactivity and morphology of aorta from streptozotocin-diabetic rats. Antioxidants in Diabetes-Induced Complications (ADIC) Study Group. *Metabolism* 1997;46:872.

138. Rosen P, Ballhausen T, Stockklauser K. Impairment of endothelium dependent relaxation in the diabetic rat heart: mechanisms and implications. *Diabetes Res Clin Pract* 1996;31 Suppl:S143.

139. Gopaul NK, Änggård EE, Mallet AI, Betteridge DJ, Wolff SP, Nourooz-Zadeh J. Plasma 8-epi-PGF2alpha levels are elevated in individuals with non-insulin dependent diabetes mellitus. *FEBS Lett.* 1995;368:225.

140. Davi G, Ciabottoni G, Consoli A, Messetti A, Falco A, Santarone S, Pennese E, Vitacolonna E, Bucciarelli T, Costantini F, Capani F, Patrono C. In vivo formation of 8-iso-prostaglandin

F2alpha and platelet activation in diabetes mellitus. effects of improved metabolic control. *Circulation.* 1998;98:in press

141.   Keaney JF, Jr., Loscalzo J. Oxidative stress, diabetes, and platelet activation. *Circulation.* 1999;98:in press

142.   Dieber-Rotheneder M, Puhl H, Waeg H, Striegl G, Esterbauer H. Effect of oral supplementation with D-alpha-tocopherol on the vitamin E content of human low density lipoproteins and resistance to oxidation. *J Lipid Res.* 1991;32:1325.

143.   Keaney JF, Jr., Gaziano JM, Xu A, Frei B, Curran-Celentano J, Shwaery GT, Loscalzo J, Vita JA. Low-dose α-tocopherol improves and high-dose α-tocopherol worsens endothelial vasodilator function in cholesterol-fed rabbits. *J Clin Invest.* 1994;93:844.

144.   Suarna C, Dean RT, May J, Stocker R: Human atherosclerotic plaque contains both oxidized lipids and relatively large amounts of α-tocopherol and ascorbate. *Arterioscler Thromb Vasc Biol.* 1995;15:1616.

145.   Keaney JF, Jr., Guo Y, Cunningham D, Shwaery GT, Xu A, Vita JA. Vascular incorporation of α-tocopherol prevents endothelial dysfunction due to oxidized LDL by inhibiting protein kinase C stimulation. *J Clin Invest.* 1996;98:386.

146.   Williams B, Schrier RW. Characterization of glucose-induced in situ protein kinase C activity in cultured vascular smooth muscle cells. *Diabetes.* 1992;41:1464.

147.   Jay MT, Chirico S, Siow RC, Bruckdorfer KR, Jacobs M, Leake DS, Pearson JD, Mann GE. Modulation of vascular tone by low density lipoproteins: effects on L-arginine transport and nitric oxide synthesis. *Exp Physiol* 1997;82:349.

148.   Kugiyama K, Ohgushi M, Sugiyama S, Murohara T, Fukunaga K, Miyamoto E, Yasue H. Lysophosphatidylcholine inhibits surface receptor-mediated intracellular signals in endothelial cells by a pathway involving protein kinase C activation. *Circ Res.* 1992;71:1422.

149.   Sugiyama S, Kugiyama K, Ohgushi M, Fujimoto K, Yasue H. Lysophosphatidylcholine in oxidized low-density lipoprotein increases endothelial susceptibility to polymorphonuclear leukocyte-induced endothelial dysfunction in porcine coronary arteries: role of protein kinase C. *Circ Res.* 1994;74:565.

150.   Flavahan NA, Shimokawa H, Vanhoutte PM. Inhibition of endothelium-dependent relaxations by phorbol myristate acetate in canine coronary arteries: role of a pertussus toxin-sensitive G-protein. *J Pharmacol Exp Ther.* 1991;256:50.

151.   Boscoboinik D, Szewczyk A, Hensey C, Azzi A. Inhibition of cell proliferation by α-tocopherol. *J Biol Chem.* 1991;266:6188

152.   Freedman JE, Farhat JH, Loscalzo J, Keaney JF, Jr. α-Tocopherol inhibits aggregation of human platelets by a protein kinase C-dependent mechanism. *Circulation.* 1996;94:2434.

153.   Marshall FN: Pharmacology and toxicology of probucol. *Artery* 1982;10:7.

154.   Shaish A, Daugherty A, O'Sullivan F, Schonfeld G, Heinecke JW: Beta-carotene inhibits atherosclerosis in hypercholesterolemic rabbits. *J Clin Invest.* 1995;96:2075.

155.   Parthasarathy S, Young SG, Witztum JL, Pittman RC, Steinberg D: Probucol inhibits oxidative modification of low density lipoprotein. *J Clin Invest.* 1986;77:641.

156.   Carew TE, Schwenke DC, Steinberg D: Antiatherogenic effect of probucol unrelated to its hypocholesterolemic effect: evidence that antioxidants in vivo can selectively inhibit low density lipoprotein degradation in macrophage-rich fatty streaks and slow the progression of atherosclerosis in the Watanabe heritable hyperlipidemic rabbit. *Proc Natl Acad Sci USA.* 1987;84:7725.

157.   Kita T, Nagano Y, Yokode M, Ishii K, Kume N, Ooshima A, Yoshida H, Kawai C: Probucol prevents the progression of atherosclerosis in Watanabe heritable hyperlipidemic rabbit, an animal model for familial hypercholesterolemia. *Proc Natl Acad Sci USA.* 1987;84:5928.

158.   Sasahara M, Raines EW, Chait A, Carew TE, Steinberg D, Wahl PW, Ross R: Inhibition of hypercholesterolemia-induced atherosclerosis in the nonhuman primate by probucol. Is the extent of atherosclerosis related to resistance of LDL to oxidation? *J Clin Invest.* 1994;94:155.

159.   Zhang SH, Reddick RL, Avdievich E, Surles LK, Jones RG, Reynolds JB, Quarfordt SH, Maeda N. Paradoxical enhancement of atherosclerosis by probucol treatment in apolipoprotein E-deficient mice. *J Clin Invest.* 1997;99:2858.

160.   Simon BC, Haudenschild CC, Cohen RA. Preservation of endothelium-dependent relaxation in atherosclerotic rabbit aorta by probucol. *J Cardiovasc Pharmacol.* 1993;21:893.

161.   Inoue N, Ohara Y, Fukai T, Harrison DG, Nishida K: Probucol improves endothelial-dependent relaxation and decreases vascular superoxide production in cholesterol-fed rabbits. *Am J Med Sci.* 1998;315:242.

162.   Hoshida S, Yamashita N, Igarashi J, Aoki K, Kuzuya T, Hori M. Long-term probucol treatment reverses the severity of myocardial injury in watanabe heritable hyperlipidemic rabbits. *Arterioscler Thromb Vasc Biol* 1997;17:2801.

163.   Tesfamariam B, Cohen RA. Free radicals mediate endothelial cell dysfunction caused by elevated glucose. *Am J Physiol.* 1992;263:H321.

164.   Flavahan NA. Atherosclerosis or lipoprotein-induced endothelial dysfunction: potential mechanisms underlying reduction in A2RF/nitric oxide activity. *Circulation.* 1992;85:1927.

165.   McDowell IFW, Brennan GM, McEneny J, Young IS, Nicholls DP, McVeigh GE, Bruce I, Trimble ER, Johnston GD: The effect of probucol and vitamin E treatment on the oxidation of low-density lipoprotein and forearm vascular responses in humans. *Eur J Clin Invest.* 1994;24:759.

166.   Elliott TG, Barth JD, Mancini J. Effects of vitamin E on endothelial function in men after myocardial infarction. *Am J Cardiol.* 1995;76:1188.

167.   Gilligan DM, Sack MN, Guetta V, Casino PR, Quyyumi AA, Rader DJ, Panza JA, Cannon RO, III. Effect of antioxidant vitamins on low density lipoprotein oxidation and impaired endothelium-dependent vasodilation on patients with hypercholesterolemia. *J Am Coll Cardiol.* 1994;24:1611.

168.   Koh KK, Blum A, Schenke WH, Hathaway I., Mincemoyer R, Panza JA, Cannon RO, III. Vitamin E improves endothelium-dependent vasodilator responsiveness comparable to estrogen in postmenopausal women. *Circulation* 1998;98:III-3468.

169.   Motoyama T, Kugiyama K, Doi H, Kawano K, Moriyama Y, Sakamoto T, Takazoe K, Yoshimura M, Hirai N, Ota Y. Vitamin E treatment improves impairment of endothelium-dependent vasodilation in patients with high remnant lipoprotein levels. *Circulation* 1998;98:III-904.

170.   Wendel A, Cikryt P. The level and half-life of glutathione in human plasma. *FEBS Lett.* 1980,120.209.

171.   Bray TM, Taylor CG. Tissue glutathione, nutrition, and oxidative stress. *Can J Physiol Pharmacol.* 1993;71:746.

172.   Bergsten P, Yu R, Kehrl J, Levine M. Ascorbic acid transport and distribution in human B lymphocytes. *Arch Biochem Biophys.* 1994;317:208.

173.   Martensson J, Han J, Griffith EW, Meister A. Glutathione ester delays the onset of scurvy in ascorbate-deficient guinea pigs. *Proc Natl Acad Sci USA.* 1993;90:317.

174   Martensson J, Meister A. Glutathione deficiency decreases tissue ascorbate levels in newborn rats: ascorbate spares glutathione and protects. *Proc Natl Acad Sci USA.* 1991;88.4656.

175.   Murphy ME, Piper HM, Watanabe H, Sies H: Nitric oxide production by cultured aortic endothelial cells in response to thiol depletion and replenishment. *J Biol Chem.* 1991;266:19378.

176.   Hecker M, Seigle I, Macarthur H, Sessa WC, Vane JR. Role of intracellular thiols in release of EDRF from cultured endothelial cells. *Am J Physiol.* 1992;262:H888.

177.   Ghigo D, Alessio P, Foco A, Bussolino F, Costamagna D, Heller R, Garbarino G, Pescarmona GP, Bosia A. Nitric oxide synthesis is impaired in glutathione depleted human umbilical vein endothelial cells. *Am J Physiol.* 1993;265:C728.

178.   Celermajer DS, Sorensen KE, Gooch VM, Spiegelhalter DJ, Miller OI, Sullivan ID, Lloyd JK, Deanfield JE. Non-invasive detection of endothelial dysfunction in children and adults at risk of atherosclerosis. *Lancet.* 1992;340:1111.

179.   Williamson JM, Meister A. Stimulation of hepatic glutathione formation by administration of L-2-oxothiazolidine-4-carboxylate: a 5-oxo-L-prolinase substrate. *Proc Natl Acad Sci USA.* 1981;78:936.

180.   Boesgaard S, Aldershvile J, Poulsen HE, Loft S, Anderson ME, Meister A. Nitrate tolerance in vivo is not associated with depletion of arterial or venous thiol levels. *Circ Res.* 1994;74:115.

181.   Vita JA, Frei B, Holbrook M, Gokce N, Leaf C, Keaney JF, Jr. L-2-Oxothiazolidine-4-carboxylic acid revereses endothelial dysfunction in patients with coronary artery disease. *J Clin Invest.* 1998;101:1408.

182.   Kugiyama K, Ohgushi M, Motoyama T, Hirashima O, Soejima H, Misumi K, Yoshimura M, Ogawa H, Sugiyama S, Yasue H. Intracoronary infusion of reduced glutathione improves

endothelial vasomotor response to acetylcholine in human coronary circulation. *Circulation* 1998;97:2299.

183. Stuehr DJ, Kwon NS, Nathan CF. FAD and GSH participate in macrophage synthesis of nitric oxide. *Biochem Biophys Res Commun.* 1990;168:558.
184. Komori Y, Hyun J, Chiang K, Fukuto JM. The role of thiols in the apparent activation of rat brain nitric oxide synthase (NOS). *J Biochem.* 1995;117:923.
185. Hofmann H, Schmidt HHHW. Thiol dependence of nitric oxide synthase. *Biochemistry.* 1995;34:13443.
186. Gorren ACF, Schrammel A, Schmidt K, Mayer B. Thiols and neuronal nitric oxide synthase: complex formation, competitive inhibition, and enzyme stabilization. *Biochemistry.* 1997;36:4360.
187. Fitzgerald DJ, Roy L, Catella F, FitzGerald GA: Platelet activation in unstable coronary disease. *N Engl J Med.* 1986;315:983.
188. Ma XL, Lopez BL, Liu GL, Christopher TA, Gao F, Guo Y, Feuerstein GZ, Ruffolo J, Barone FC, Yue TL. Hypercholesterolemia impairs a detoxification mechanism againt peroxynitrite and renders the vascular tissue more susceptible to oxidative injury. *Circ Res.* 1997;80:894.
189. Howells DW, Hyland K. Direct analysis of tetrahydrobiopterin in ceribrospinal fluid by high-perfomrmance liquid chromatography with redox electrochemistry: prevention of autoxidation during storage and analysis. *Clin Chim Acta.* 1987;167:23.
190. Heales S, Hyland K. Determination of quinonoid dihydrobiopterin by high-performance liquid chromatrography and electrochemical detection. *J Chromatogr.* 1989;494:77.
191. Patel JM, Abeles AJ, Block ER. Nitric oxide exposure and sulfhydryl modulation alter L-arginine transport in cultured pulmonary artery endothelial cells. *Free Radic Biol Med.* 1996;20:629.
192. Xia Y, Dawson VL, Dawson TM, Snyder SH, Zweier JL. Nitric oxide synthase generates superoxide and nitric oxide in arginine-depleted cells leading to peroxynitrite-mediated cell injury. *Proc Natl Acad Sci USA.* 1996;93:6770.
193. Heinzel B, John M, Klatt P, hme E, Mayer B. Ca2+/calmodulin-dependent formation of hydrogen peroxide by brain nitric oxide synthase. *Biochem J.* 1992;281:627.
194. Nishikimi M. Oxidation of ascorbic acid with superoxide anion generated by the xanthine-xanthine oxidase system. *Biochem Biophys Res Commun.* 1975;63:463.
195. Bodannes RS, Chan PC. Ascorbic acid as a scavenger of singlet oxygen. *FEBS Lett.* 1979;105:195.
196. Halliwell B, Wasil M, Grootveld M. Biologically significant scavenging of the myeloperoxidase-derived oxidant hypochlorous acid by ascorbic acid. Implications for antioxidant protection in the inflamed rheumatoid joint. *FEBS Lett.* 1987;213:15.
197. Frei B, England L, Ames BN. Ascorbate is an outstanding antioxidant in human blood plasma. *Proc Natl Acad Sci USA.* 1989;86:6377.
198. Levine GN, Frei B, Koulouris SN, Gerhard MD, Keaney JF, Jr., Vita JA. Ascorbic acid reverses endothelial dysfunction in patients with coronary artery disease. *Circulation.* 1996;96:1107.
199. Ting HH, Timimi FK, Boles KS, Creager SJ, Ganz P, Creager MA. Vitamin C improves endothelium-dependent vasodilation in patients with non-insulin-dependent diabetes mellitus. *J Clin Invest.* 1996;97:22.
200. Ting HH, Timimi FK, Haley EA, Roddy MA, Ganz P, Creager MA. Vitamin C improves endothelium-dependent vasodilation in forearm resistance vessels of humans with hypercholerolemia. *Circulation.* 1997;95:2617.
201. Heitzer T, Just H, Munzel T. Antioxidant vitamin C improves endothelial dysfunction in chronic smokers. *Circulation.* 1996;94:6.
202. Hornig B, Arakawa N, Kohler C, Drexler H. Vitamin C improves endothelial function of conduit arteries in patients with chronic heart failure. *Circulation.* 1998;97:363.
203. Motoyama T, Kawano H, Hirai N. Vitamin E administration improves impairment of endothelium-dependent vasodilation in patients with coronary spastic angina. *Circulation* 1998;98:III-4464.
204. Jackson TS, Xu A, Vita JA, Keaney JF, Jr. Ascorbic acid prevents the interaction of nitric oxide and superoxide only at very high physiologic concentrations. *Circ Res.* 1998;83:916.
205. O'Keefe JH, Jr., Stone GW, McCallister BD, Jr., Maddex C, Ligon R, Kacich RL, Kahn J, Cavero PG, Hartzler GO, Mccallister BD. Lovistatin plus probucol for prevention of restenosis after percutaneous transluminal coronary angioplasty. *Am J Cardiol.* 1996;77:649.

206. Jain A, Martensson J, Mehta T, Krauss AN, Auld PA, Meister A. Ascorbic acid prevents oxidative stress in glutathione-deficient mice: effects on lung type 2 cell lamellar bodies, lung survactant, and skeletal muscle. *Proc Natl Acad Sci USA*. 1992;89:5093.

207. Boulanger CM, Tanner FC, Bea ML, Hahn AWA, Werner A, Luscher TF. Oxidized low density lipoproteins induce mRNA expression and release of endothelin from human and porcine endothelium. *Circ Res*. 1992;70:1191.

208. Yanagisawa M, Kurihara H, Kimura S, Tomobe Y, Kobayashi M, Mitsui Y, Yazaki Y, Goto K, Masaki T. A novel potent vasoconstrictor peptide produced by vascular endothelial cells. *Nature*. 1988;332:411.

209. Masaki T, Yanagisawa M, Goto K. Physiology and pharmacology of endothelins. *Med Res Rev*. 1992;12:391.

210. Steinbrecher UP, Parthasarathy S, Leake DS, Witztum JL, Steinberg D. Modification of low density lipoprotein by endothelial cells involves lipid peroxidation and degradation of low density lipoprotein phospholipids. *Proc Natl Acad Sci USA*. 1984;81:3883.

211. Kugiyama K, Sakamoto T, Misumi I, Sugiyama S, Ohgushi M, Ogawa H, Horiguchi M, Yasue H. Transferable lipids in oxidized low-density lipoprotein stimulate plasminogen activator inhibitor-1 and inhibit tissue-type plasminogen activator release from endothelial cells. *Circ Res*. 1993;73:335.

212. Marui N, Offermann MK, Swerlick R, Kunsch C, Rosen CA, Ahmad M, Alexander RW, Medford RM. Vascular cell adhesion molecule-1 (VCAM-1) gene transcription and expression are regulated through an antioxidant-sensitive mechanism in human vascular endothelial cells. *J Clin Invest*. 1993;92:1866.

213. Khan BV, Parthasarathy SS, Alexander RW, Medford RM. Modified low density lipoprotein and its constituents augment cytokine activated vascular dell adhesion molecule-1 gene expression in human vascular endothelial cells. *J Clin Invest*. 1995;95:1262.

214. D'Alessio P, Moutet M, Coudrier E, Darquenne S, Chaudiere J. ICAM-1 and VCAM-1 expression induced by TNF-alpha are inhibited by a glutathione peroxidase mimic. *Free Radic Biol Med*. 1998;24:979.

215. Amberger A, Maczek C, Jurgens G, Michaelis D, Schett G, Trieb K, Eberl T, Jindal S, Xu Q, Wick G. Co-expression of ICAM-1, VCAM-1 ELAM-1 and Hsp60 in human arterial and venous endothelial cells in response to cytokines and oxidized low-density lipoproteins. *Cell Stress & Chap*. 1997;2:94.

216. van der Vliet A, Eiserich JP, Halliwell B, Cross CE. Formation of reactive nitrogen species during peroxidase-catalyzed oxidation of nitrite. *J Biol Chem*. 1997;272:7617

217. Eiserich JP, Cross CE, Jones AD, Halliwell B, van der Vliet, A. Formation of nitrating and chlorinating species by reaction of nitrite with hypocholorous acid. *J Biol Chem*. 1996;271:19199.

218. Savenkova MI, Meuller DM, Heinecke JW. Tyrosyl radical generated by myeloperoxidase is a physiological catalyst for the initiation of lipid peroxidation in low density lipoprotein. *J Biol Chem*. 1994;269:20394.

219. Hazell LJ, Arnold L, Flowers D, Waeg G, Malle E, Stocker R. Presence of hypochlorite-modified proteins in human atherosclerotic lesions. *J Clin Invest*. 1996;97:1535

220. Heller R, Münscher-Paulig,F.; Gräbner,R; Till,U. Ascorbic acid potentiates nitric oxide synthesis in endothelial cells. *J Biol. Chem* 1999;274:8254..

10 OXIDANTS AND ANTIOXIDANTS IN PLATELET FUNCTION

Jane E. Freedman

INTRODUCTION

Epidemiological studies have shown that dietary antioxidant consumption is inversely associated with the development of coronary artery disease. The precise mechanisms that underlie these observations, however, are not clear. While the beneficial effects of antioxidants have been attributed to the prevention of oxidative modification of low-density lipoprotein (LDL) and the inhibition of atherogenesis, other factors may also be important. Platelet function is dependent upon the balance between oxidative stress and antioxidant protection and, importantly, platelets have been implicated in the development of atherosclerosis, as well as in the acute occlusion of coronary vessels (1, 2).

While dramatic changes in the platelet redox status occur during normal aggregation, the introduction of additional oxidative stress is prothrombotic. Modulation of platelet redox status, as well as the addition of exogenous antioxidants, inhibits platelet aggregation *in vitro* and *in vivo* and both the water- and lipid-soluble antioxidant status of platelets may be important in regulating platelet function. In this chapter, the local platelet balance between oxidative stress and antioxidant protection and its effect on platelet function and vascular homeostasis will be further discussed.

PLATELETS AND ATHEROTHROMBOTIC VASCULAR DISEASE

Thrombus formation within a coronary vessel is the precipitating event in myocardial infarction and unstable angina as shown in angiographic (3) and pathologic (4) studies. The angiographic severity of coronary stenoses does not adequately predict sites of subsequent acute coronary syndromes. For this reason, plaque rupture in relatively mildly stenosed vessels and subsequent thrombus formation is believed to underlie the majority of coronary syndromes (1,5).

In the normally intact endothelium, activation and recruitment of platelets is tightly regulated. Adhesion of platelets to the endothelium is prevented by several mechanisms including endothelial cell production of prostacyclin and nitric oxide

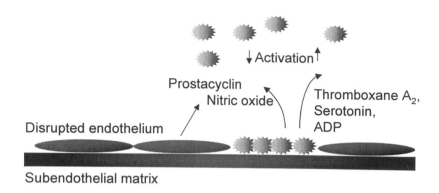

Figure 1. Atherosclerotic Plaque Disruption and Thrombus Formation

(NO) (6, 7). Both superficial intimal injury caused by endothelial denudation and deep intimal injury caused by plaque rupture expose collagen and von Willebrand factor to platelets (1). Platelets then adhere directly to collagen or indirectly via the binding of von Willebrand factor to the glycoprotein Ib/IX matrix. As shown in Figure 1, local platelet activation (by tissue factor-mediated thrombin generation or by collagen) stimulates further thrombus formation and additional platelet recruitment by supporting cell-surface thrombin formation and releasing potent platelet agonists such as ADP, serotonin, and thromboxane A_2 (8). Thrombus forms as platelets aggregate via the binding of bivalent fibrinogen to glycoprotein IIb/IIIa. In support of these mechanisms, increased platelet-derived thromboxane and prostaglandin metabolites have been detected in patients with acute coronary syndromes (9). The importance of platelet activation in acute coronary syndromes is further supported by the clear clinical benefit of treatment with aspirin for both primary and secondary prevention of acute coronary events (10, 11).

Recent epidemiological studies have shown that antioxidants play a role in the prevention of cardiovascular disease in humans. Plasma antioxidant levels inversely correlate with the development of angina pectoris (12), and dietary antioxidant consumption is inversely associated with the development of clinical coronary artery disease (13). The precise mechanism(s) accounting for this benefit of antioxidants in coronary disease activity remains unknown. Clearly, animal and cell culture data suggest that antioxidants preserve NO bioactivity in the face of oxidative stress. Since oxidative stress may alter platelet function, it is also conceivable that the benefits of antioxidants may be a consequence of their enhancing or promoting the antiplatelet effects of NO derived from both endothelial cells and platelets. In support of this hypothesis, patients with coronary artery disease have been found to have decreased plasma and platelet antioxidant activities that were associated with enhanced platelet aggregation responses (14).

REACTIVE OXYGEN SPECIES AND PLATELET-MEDIATED THROMBOSIS

Evidence suggests that oxidative stress is important to normal platelet function. Platelet aggregation is associated with a burst of oxygen consumption (15) and a marked rise in glutathione disulfide (16). While dramatic changes in platelet NO redox status occurs during normal aggregation, conditions that provoke oxidative stress without inducing a florid aggregation response have also been shown to be prothrombotic. Reactive oxygen species contribute causally to many pathophysiologic conditions, including atherosclerosis, and have been detected in both resting and activated platelets.

Reactive oxygen species derived from both platelets and other vascular sources have been shown to alter platelet responses (Table 1). Superoxide is produced by platelets (17,18), as are hydroperoxy derivatives of long-chain fatty acids such as 12-hydroperoxy-eicosotetranoic acid (12-HpETE). Superoxide, in particular, is known to augment platelet aggregation responses (19). Low (μM) concentrations of hydrogen peroxide, in the presence of plasma, inhibit platelet function (20) although concentrations under 50 μM also cause platelet injury as measured by platelet serotonin release (21). While high (mM) concentrations of hydrogen peroxide have been shown to stimulate platelet aggregation through tyrosine phosphorylation (22), the physiological relevance of levels greater than 1 mM is questionable (22a).

Table 1. Reactive Oxygen Species and Platelet Function

Reactive Oxygen Species	Effect on Platelet Function	Ref
Superoxide anion	Prothrombotic	(17, 18)
Hydrogen peroxide (μM)	Pro/anti-thrombotic	(20,21)
Hydrogen peroxide (mM)	Prothrombotic	(22)
Hydroxyl radical	Prothrombotic	(23)

In platelets, reactive oxygen species may cause activation through regulation of protein kinase C (PKC). Platelet aggregation and increased fibrinogen binding sites induced by exposure to ultraviolet B radiation appear to be mediated by activation of platelet PKC via reactive oxygen species (24). Therefore, antioxidant metabolism of both exogenous and platelet-derived reactive oxygen species may influence platelet PKC activity and, potentially, platelet function.

ANTIOXIDANTS AND PLATELET-MEDIATED THROMBOSIS

Antioxidants may indirectly inhibit platelets through scavenging of reactive oxygen species, many of which alter platelet function. Hydroperoxides produced by the platelet such as prostaglandin G_2, 12-HpETE, and phospholipid hydroperoxides are metabolized by the selenium-dependent enzyme, glutathione peroxidase. Glutathione peroxidase is tightly coupled to the hexose monophosphate shunt through reduced nicotinamide adenine dinucleotide phosphate (NADPH), which restores reduced glutathione concentrations and re-establishes the platelet thiol redox state via glutathione reductase. Glutathione depletion in platelets leads to attenuated glutathione peroxidase activity and increased lipid peroxidation (25).

Despite the different subcellular locations of water- and lipid-soluble antioxidants, these antioxidant pathways in platelets are closely linked. Glutathione depletion in platelets leads to attenuated glutathione peroxidase activity, decreased levels of α-tocopherol, and increased lipid peroxidation (25). Tocopherol oxidation in platelets can be blocked by preincubation of platelets with ascorbate (26). In α-tocopherol-depleted platelet lysates, the addition of either ascorbate or glutathione causes significant tocopherol regeneration (27).

There is ample *in vivo* evidence to suggest that antioxidant status is an important determinant of platelet function. In normal individuals, selenium supplementation leads to increased plasma glutathione peroxidase activity and a prolongation of the bleeding time (28). Platelets of selenium-deficient rats have increased aggregation in response to arachidonic acid (29). Decreased human platelet antioxidant content is associated with enhanced platelet activation responses in many clinically relevant settings, including smoking, diabetes mellitus, and aging (30-32). Normal aging is associated with both increased platelet aggregation (30) as well as decreased antioxidant content or enzyme activity, including glutathione peroxidase (31). Smoking-induced platelet hyperactivity is linked to increased formation of lipid hydroperoxides and normalization of platelet aggregation ensues with the addition of exogenous antioxidants (32). There is also clinical evidence to suggest that antioxidant status is important in normal platelet function in patients with cardiovascular disease as decreased plasma and platelet antioxidant activity is associated with increased platelet aggregability (14).

The Role of α-Tocopherol in Platelet Function and Thrombosis

A clinical study demonstrating that vitamin E supplementation is associated with increased hemorrhagic stroke has renewed interest in the platelet inhibitory properties of α-tocopherol (33). Inhibition of platelet aggregation by α-tocopherol was first demonstrated by Higashi and Kikuchi (34). Subsequently, Steiner and Anastasi demonstrated dose-dependent inhibition of platelet aggregation and 5-hydroxytryptamine release by α-tocopherol in response to ADP, epinephrine, and collagen (35). α-Tocopherol has been shown to inhibit the platelet release reaction (35) and may interfere with prostanoid metabolism (36). The role of α-tocopherol in modulating platelet function had not gained wide acceptance because earlier studies used supraphysiologic levels of α-tocopherol and studies in patients supplemented with α-tocopherol have not demonstrated decreased platelet aggregation (37).

In platelets, membrane-bound PKC plays a central role in the cell signaling process that subsequently leads to platelet secretion and aggregation. Membrane-bound diacylglycerol triggers the translocation of inactive PKC from the platelet cytosol to the platelet membrane (38). Protein kinase C activation also contributes to platelet adhesion in response to shear stress (39).

In other cell types, antioxidants such as α-tocopherol inhibit cellular proliferation and PKC activity by altering phorbol ester binding and by decreasing PKC translocation (40). We have found that α-tocopherol inhibits platelet function both *in vitro* and *in vivo* through a PKC-dependent mechanism (41). In this study, the platelet α-tocopherol levels achieved with *in vitro* loading (117.6 ± 15.3 pmol/10^8 platelets) were comparable to the levels measured after *in vivo* α-tocopherol supplementation (160.5 ± 70.5 pmol/10^8 platelets). This finding suggests that *in vitro* loading of platelets using supraphysiological levels of α-tocopherol is a reasonable means of increasing platelet α-tocopherol to comparable levels as observed *in vivo*. In this study, platelet incorporation of α-tocopherol via oral supplementation (400 to 1200 IU/day) correlated with marked inhibition of PMA-mediated platelet aggregation ($r=0.67$; $P<0.01$). Both *in vitro* loading and oral supplementation with α-tocopherol were associated with inhibition of platelet aggregation through a PKC-dependent mechanism as is shown by the inhibition in phosphorylation of a 47 kD PKC substrate (Figure 2).

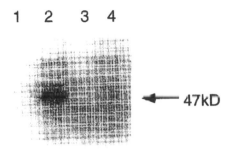

Figure 2. Oral α-tocopherol supplementation inhibits platelet PKC-dependent protein phosphorylation. Platelet-rch plasma from a normal subject was incubated with ^{32}[P]orthophosphate, gel-filtered, and stimulated with vehicle (lane 1) or 27 nmol/L PMA (lane 2) followed by SDS-PAGE autoradiography. Lanes 3 and 4 represent vehicle and PMA stimulation of similarly treated platelets from the same subject after 14 days or oral supplementation with α-tocopherol (1200 IU/d). In this individual, platelet α-tocopherol content increased from 49.2 to 124.5 pmol/10^8 platelets. Data are representative of two independent experiments on two subjects. (36)

OXIDANTS AND ANTIOXIDANTS IN NITRIC OXIDE-INDUCED PLATELET INHIBITION

Adhesion of platelets to the endothelium is prevented by several mechanisms including endothelial cell production of prostacyclin and NO (6,7). Nitric oxide inhibits platelet activation (42,43) and prevents thrombosis (44). Exogenous NO has been shown to inhibit the normal activation-dependent increase in the expression of platelet surface glycoproteins, including P-selectin and the integrin glycoprotein IIb/IIIa (45).

Constitutive nitric oxide synthase (cNOS) has also been identified in both human platelets and megakaryoblastic cells (46,47). As with exogenous NO, platelet aggregation is sensitive to endogenous NO production. Platelet aggregation is enhanced by inhibitors of cNOS and inhibited by the cNOS substrate, L-arginine (48). *In vivo*, systemic infusion of the cNOS inhibitor L-N^G-monomethyl arginine (L-NMMA) caused no change in vessel tone, but a reduction in bleeding time (49) and enhanced platelet reactivity to various agonists (50). Platelet NO production has been described with both resting (51) and aggregating platelets (52-54). Nitric oxide release from activated human platelets using indirect methods has been estimated at 11.2 pmol NO/min/10^8 cells, indicating that the magnitude of platelet NO release may be comparable to that of endothelial cells (51). While platelet-derived NO appears to inhibit the primary aggregation response only modestly, we have recently shown that NO release from activated human platelets markedly inhibits platelet recruitment and thus, may attenuate the progression of intra-arterial thrombosis (54). In addition, activated platelets from patients with acute coronary syndromes produce significantly less NO compared to patients with stable coronary artery disease (55). This observation suggests that impaired platelet-derived NO may contribute to the development of acute coronary syndromes by influencing platelet function or recruitment and, indirectly, thrombus formation.

Although investigation into the relation between platelet-derived NO production and cardiovascular disease has been limited, the role of endothelium-derived NO in this regard has been extensively characterized (see Chapter 9). Endothelium-derived NO bioactivity is impaired in animal models of atherosclerosis and in isolated atherosclerotic human coronary arteries (56). In addition, it is well established that cardiovascular disease and coronary risk factors including cholesterol level, male gender, family history, and age, are associated with impaired NO-mediated, endothelium-dependent, vasodilation in coronary arteries (57).

Superoxide and NO-Induced Platelet Inhibition

A prominent feature of both abnormal platelet and endothelial function in the setting of cardiovascular disease is oxidative stress. Excessive vascular superoxide production has been demonstrated in hypercholesterolemia as well as other disease states associated with endothelial dysfunction (58, see also Chapters 9, 12, and 13). Superoxide produced by the vasculature or platelets can evoke an oxidative stress characterized by lipid peroxidation, cellular activation, and vascular dysfunction. Superoxide (in the presence of transition metals) promotes lipid peroxidation leading to the generation of lipid alkoxyl and peroxyl radicals that propagate radical chain reactions (59). This process can be terminated by NO through the reaction of NO with lipid peroxyl radicals to form non-radical products (60) such as lipid peroxynitrites with a resultant loss in NO bioactivity (58,61). Similarly, superoxide and NO readily combine in a diffusion-limited reaction (k=1.9 x 10^{10} $M^{-1} \cdot s^{-1}$) that competes favorably on a kinetic basis with the dismutation reaction catalyzed by SOD (62).

Thus, NO is readily inactivated by oxidative stress. A logical extension of these observations is that NO bioactivity is dependent upon platelet antioxidant status. Platelets have a number of antioxidant defenses including SOD. Human platelets contain approximately 1 femtogram of SOD/platelet, or about one-fifth of that present in leukocytes. Approximately 77% of platelet SOD is believed to be Cu,Zn-SOD, while the remainder is Mn-SOD.

Experimental evidence suggests that SOD is important in normal platelet function and the prevention of thrombosis. Studying platelet-mediated cyclic flow variations in rabbit carotid arteries, Meng and colleagues showed that platelet-mediated thrombosis could be attenuated by intravenous infusion of SOD (63). Infusion of the nitric oxide synthase inhibitor L-NMMA, restored the cyclic thrombotic response. These findings were confirmed by changes in cyclic guanosine 3',5'-monophosphate (cGMP) levels in platelets isolated from these animals. Thus, this study suggests that dismutation of superoxide decreases platelet-dependent thrombus formation by potentiation of endogenous NO bioactivity.

Consistent with these observations, in a model of endothelium-injured canine coronary arteries, Ikeda and colleagues demonstrated that platelet-mediated cyclic flow variation was attenuated by intravenous infusion of SOD and catalase (64). Additionally, an infusion of xanthine and hypoxanthine or hydrogen peroxide significantly increased cyclical flow variation, suggesting that reactive oxygen species contribute to platelet activation and thrombosis.

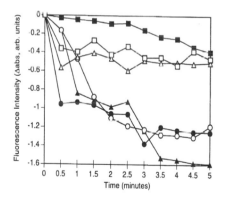

Figure 3. Increased hydrogen peroxide generation in plasma samples from two children with a history of arterial thrombosis. The generation of hydrogen peroxide in the presence of homocysteine was detected by extinction of scopoletin fluorescence during its oxidation by horseradish peroxidase over a 5-min period in the presence of plasma (4% vol/vol) from the patient 1 (closed circle), patient 2 (closed triangle), sister (closed square), mother (open circle), father (open triangle), or a pooled pediatric control (open square) (62).

Glutathione Peroxidase and NO-Mediated Inhibition of Platelet Function

Platelet aggregation leads to the formation of reactive oxygen species that modulate the thrombotic response, in part, by inactivating NO. Therefore, endogenous antioxidant enzymatic mechanisms that metabolize reactive species should attenuate the prothrombotic effects of these free radical species. In addition to SOD, one enzyme responsible for ROS metabolism is glutathione peroxidase. This enzyme is classically thought of as a selenocysteine-containing protein that reduces peroxides to their corresponding alcohols using glutathione as an obligate co-substrate. Since peroxides can decompose into lipid peroxyl radicals, elimination of lipid peroxides represents an important means of limiting peroxyl radicals that inactivate NO (60).

As with other antioxidants, there is evidence that glutathione peroxidase activity has important implications for platelet function. Glutathione peroxidase potentiates the inhibitor effect of NO on platelet aggregation by reducing lipid hydroperoxides (65). Evidence also indicates this function of glutathione peroxidase is important for normal blood homeostasis as defects in this system can lead to a clinical thrombotic disorder we found in two brothers with thrombotic strokes in childhood (66). In these children, aggregometry and flow cytometry studies indicated that their platelets were hyper-aggregatory due to an abnormality in their plasma. In the presence of their plasma, NO failed to inhibit aggregation or surface expression of P-selectin on normal platelets. The increase in hydrogen peroxide generation in the presence of their plasma (Figure 3), as well as the decrease in plasma cGMP and NO levels in these patients was probably secondary to metabolism or destruction of NO as glutathione peroxidase activity was decreased in their plasma and their NO-dependent coagulation abnormality normalized after addition of exogenous glutathione peroxidase (Figure 4).

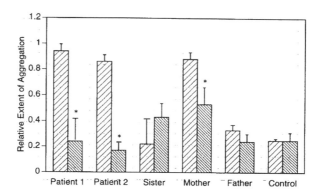

Figure 4. Glutathione peroxidase enhances platelet inhibition by S-nitroso-glutathione in two patients with thrombotic strokes. Gel-filtered platelets from a normal adult donor were incubated with plasma from a family member or from a pooled pediatric control. S-nitroso-glutathione (5 μM) was added for 1 min and aggregation induced with ADP. Relative extent of platelet aggregation was determined in the presence (second set of bars) or absence (first set of bars) of glutathione peroxidase (5 U/ml). Data are expressed as a percent of control aggregation for each subject with ADP alone. (For patient 1, patient 2, and mother, $P<0.05$ compared to S-nitrosoglutathione alone (62).

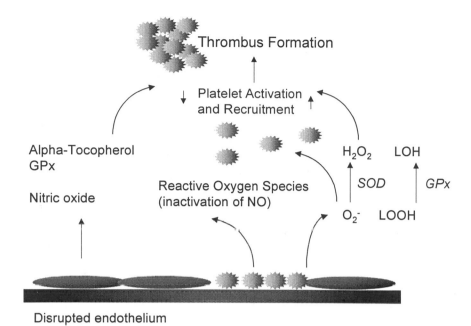

Figure. 5. Scheme for the interaction of reactive oxygen species and antioxidants in platelet-mediated atherothrombosis.

In summary, ischemic heart disease is caused by vessel injury and subsequent thrombus formation. Normally, platelet activation is limited by endothelial production of NO and prostacyclin but, in the atherosclerotic vessel, this process may be impaired as is suggested by the attenuated endothelium-dependent vascular reactivity seen in cardiovascular disease. Atherosclerotic coronary disease is associated with enhaced oxidative stress. The increase in oxidant stress and decrease in antioxidant levels found in cardiovascular disease are also associated with abnormal platelet function. Antioxidants, such as the lipid-soluble α-tocopherol, inhibit platelet aggregation, while reactive oxygen species increase platelet function both directly and through inactivation of the platelet inhibitor NO

Therefore, in the setting of cardiovascular disease, the interaction between reactive oxygen species, antioxidants, and NO contributes to increased platelet aggregability and thrombus formation (Figure 5). Through metabolism of both exogenous and endogenous reactive oxygen species produced by the resting and aggregating platelet, antioxidants may alter platelet function. Thus, the regulation of reactive oxygen species and antioxidant status plays an important role in platelet function, thrombosis, and the clinical expression of cardiovascular disease.

REFERENCES

1.   Davies MJ, Thomas AC. Thrombosis and acute coronary-artery lesions in sudden cardiac ischemic death. *N Engl J Med.* 1984;310:1137.

2.   David M. A macro and micro view of coronary vascular insult with ischemic heart disease. *Circulation.* 1990;82:1138.

3.   DeWood MA, Spores J, Notske R, Mouser LT, Burroughs R, Golden MS, Lang HT. Prevalence of total coronary occlusion during the early hours of transmural myocrdial infarction. *N Engl J Med.* 1980;303:897.

4.   Falk E. Unstable angina with fatal outcome: dynamic coronary thrombosis leading to infarction and/or sudden death. Autopsy evidence of recurrent mural thrombosis with peripheral embolization culminating in total vascular occlusion. *Circulation.* 1985;71:699.

5.   Falk E. Plaque rupture with severe pre-existing stenosis precipitating coronary thrombis. *Brit Heart J.* 1983;1983:127.

6.   de Graff JC, Banga JD, Moncada S, Palmer RMJ, de Groot PG, Sixma JJ. Nitric oxide functions as an inhibitor of platelet adhesion under flow conditions. *Circulation.* 1992;85:2284.

7.   Radomski MW, Palmer MJ, Moncada S. The role of nitric oxide and cGMP in platelet adhesion to vascular endothelium. *Biochem Biophysic Res Comm.* 1987;148:1482.

8.   Santol MT, Valles J, Marcus AJ, Safier M, Brodkman J, Islan N, Ullman HL, Eirosa AM, Aznar J. Enhancement of platelet reactivity and modulation of eicosanoid production by intact erythrocytes. *J Clin Invest.* 1991;87:571.

9.   Fitzgerald DJ, Roy L, Catella F, FitzGerald GA: Platelet activation in unstable coronary disease. *N Engl J Med.* 1986;315:983.

10.   The RISC Group. Risk of myocardial infarction and death during treatment with low dose aspirin and intravenous heparin in men with unstable coronary artery disease. *Lancet.* 1990;336:827.

11.   Antiplatelet Trialists Collaboration. Collaborative overview of randomized trials of antiplatelet therapy: I. Prevention of death, myocardial infarction, and sroke by prolonged antiplatelet therapy in various categories of patients. *Brit Med J.* 1994;308:81.

12.   Riemersma RA, Wood DA, Macintyre CCH, Elton RA, Gey KF, Oliver MF: Risk of angina pectoris and plasma concentrations of vitamins A, C, E, and carotene. *Lancet.* 1991;337:1.

13.   Rimm EB, Stampfer MJ, Ascherio A, Giovannucci E, Colditz GA, Willett WC: Vitamin E consumption and the risk of coronary heart disease in men. *N Eng J Med.* 1993;328:1444.

14.   Buczynski AB, Wachowicz B, Dedziora-Kornatowska K, Tkaczewski W, Kedziora J. Changes in antioxidant enzyme activities, aggregability, and malonyldialdehyde concentrations in blood platelet from patients with coronary heart disease. *Atherosclerosis.* 1993;100:223.

15.   Bressler N, Broekman M, Marcus A. Concurrent studies of oxygen consumption and aggregation in stimulated human platelets. *Blood.* 1979;53:167.

16.   Burch JW, Burch PT: Glutathione disulfide production during arachidonic acid oxygenation in human platelets. *Prostaglandins.* 1990;39:123.

17.   Marcus AJ, Silk ST, Safier LB, Ullman HL. Superoxide production and reducing activity in human platelets. *J Clin Invest.* 1977;59:149.

18.   Freedman JE, Keaney JF, Jr.: NO and superoxide detection in human platelets. In: Packer L, ed. Nitric Oxide, Part C: Biological and Antioxidants Activities. Vol 301. San Diego, CA: Academic Press, 1998.

19.   Handin RI, Karabin R, Boxer GJ: Enhancement of platelet function by superoxide anion. *J Clin Invest.* 1987;59:149.

20.   Stuart M, Holmsen H. Hydrogen peroxide, an inhibitor of platelet function: effect on adenine nucleotide metabolism, and the release reaction. *Am J Hematol.* 1977;2:53.

21.   Handin RI, Karabin R, Boxer GJ: Enhancement of platelet function by superoxide anion. *J Clin Invest.* 1977;59:959.

22.   Rodvien R, Lindon J, Levine P. Physiology and ultrastructure of the blood platelet following exposure to hydrogen peroxide. *Brit J Haematol.* 1976;33:19.

22a.   Irani K, Pham Y, Coleman LD, Roos C, Cooke GE, Miodovnik A, Karim N, Wildhide CC, Goldscmidt-Clermont PJ. Priming of platelet $\alpha_1\beta_3$ by oxidants is associated with tyrosine phosphorylation of β_3. *Arterioscler Thromb Vasc Biol* 1998;18:1698.

23.	Marcus A. Pathways of oxygen utilization by stimulated platelets and leukocytes. *Semin Hamatol*. 1979;16:188.

24.	Kooy M, Akkerman W, Van Asbeck S, Borghuis L, Van Prooijen H. UVB radiation exposed fibrinogen binding sites on platelets by activating protein kinase C via reactive oxygen speces. *Brit J Haematol*. 1992;83:253.

25.	Calzada C, Vericei E, Lagarde M. Decrease in platelet reduction glutathione increases lipoxygenase activity and decreasee vitamin E. *Lipids*. 1991;26:696.

26.	Vatassery G, Smith W, Quack H. Ascorbate acid, glutathione and synthetic antioxidants prevent the oxidation of vitamin E in platelets. *Lipids*. 1989;24:1043.

27.	Chan AC, Tran K, Raynor T, Ganz PR, Chow CK: Regeneration of vitamin E in human platelets. *J Biol Chem*. 1991;266:17290.

28.	Schiavon R, Freeman G, Guidi G, Perona G, Zatti M, Kakkar V. Selenium enhances prostacyclin production by cultured endothelial cells: possible explanation for increased bleeding times in volunteers taking selenium as a dietary supplement. *Thrombosis Res*. 1984;34:389.

29.	Schoene N, Morris V, Levander O. Altered arachidonic acid metabolism in platelets and artas from selenium-deficient rats. *Nutrtion Res*. 1986;6:75.

30.	Johnson M, Ramey E, Ramwell P. Sex and age differences in human platelet aggregation. *Nature*. 1975;253:355.

31.	Vericel E, Rey C, Calzada C, Haond P, Capuy P, Lagarde M. Age-related changes in arachidonic acid peroxidation and glutathione-peroxidase activity in human platelets. *Prostaglandins*. 1992;43:75.

32.	Blache D. Involvement of hydrogen and lipid peroxidase in acute tobacco smoking-induced platelet hyperactivity. *Am J Physiol*. 1995;268:H679.

33.	The Alpha-Tocopherol Beta-Carotene Cancer Prevention Study Group. The effect of vitamin E and beta carotene on the incidence of lung cander and other cancers in male smokers. *N Engl J Med*. 1994;330:1029.

34.	Higashi O, Kikuchi Y: Effects of vitamin E on the aggregation and the lipid peroxidation of platelets exposed to hydrogen peroxide. *Tohoku J Exp Med*. 1974,112.271.

35.	Steiner M, Anastasi J: Vitamin E: an inhibitor of the platelet release reaction. *J Clin Invest* 1976;57:732.

36.	Jandak J, Steiner M, Richardson P. Alpha-tocopherol, an effective inhibitor of platelet adhesion. *Blood*. 1982;73:141.

37.	Steiner M: Effect of α-tocopherol administration on platelet function in man. *Thromb Haemost*. 1983;49:73.

38.	Baldassare JJ, Henderson P, Burns D, Loomis C, Fischer GJ: Translocation of protein kinase C isoenzymes thrombin-stimulated human platelets - correlation with 1,2 diacylglycerol levels. *J Biol Chem*. 1992;267:15585.

39.	Kroll MH, Hellums JD, Guo Z, Durante W, Razdan D, Hrbolich JK, Schafer AI: Protein kinase C is activated in platelets subjected to pathological shear stress. *J Biol Chem*. 1993;268:3520.

40.	Mahoney CW, Azzi A: Vitamin E inhibits protein kinase C activity. *Biochem Biophys Res Commun*. 1988;154:694.

41.	Freedman JE, Farhat JH, Loscalzo J, Keaney JF, Jr.: α-Tocopherol inhibits aggregation of human platelets by a protein kinase C-dependent mechanism. *Circulation*. 1996;94:2434.

42.	Stamler J, Mendelsohn ME, Amarante P, Smick D, Andon N, Davies PF, Cooke JP, Loscalzo J. N-Acetylcysteine potentiates platelet inhibition by enodhtleium-derived relaxing factor. *Circ Res*. 1989;65:789.

43.	Cooke JP, Stamler J, Andon N, Davies PF, McKinley G, Loscalzo J: Flow stimulates endothelial cells to release nitrovasodilator that is potentiated by reduced thiol. *Am J Physiol*. 1990;259:H804.

44.	Shultz PJ, Raij L: Endogenously synthesized nitric oxide prevents endotoxin-induced glomerular thrombosis. *J Clin Invest*. 1992;90:1718.

45.	Michelson AD, Benoit SE, Furman MI, Breckwoldt WL, Rohter MJ, Barnard MR, Loscalzo J: Effects of endotheium-derived relaxing factor/nitric oxide on platelet surface glycoproteins. *Am J Physiol*. 1996;39:H1640.

46.	Mehta JL, Chen LY, Kone BC, Mehta P, Turner P: Identification of constitutive and inducible forms of nitric oxide synthase in human platelets. *J Lab Clin Med*. 1995;125:370.

47.   Sase K, Michel T: Expression of constitutive endothelial nitric oxide synthase in human blood platelets. *Life Sci.* 1995;57:2049.
48.   Chen LY, Mehta JL: Variable effects of L-arginine-nitric oxide pathway in human neutrophils and platelets may relate to different nitric oxide synthase isoforms. *J Pharmacol Exp Ther.* 1996;267:253.
49.   Simon DI, Stamler JS, Loh E, Loscalzo J, Francis SA, Creager MA: Effect of nitric oxide synthase inhibition on bleeding time in humans. *J Cardiovasc Pharmacol.* 1995;26:339.
50.   Bodzenta-Lukaszyke A, Gabryelewicz A, Lukaszyke A, Bielawiec M, Konturek JW, Domschke W. Nitric oxide synthase inhibition and platelet function. *Thromb Res.* 1994;75:667.
51.   Zhou Q, Hellermann GR, Solomonson LP: nitric oxide release from resting human platelets. *Thromb Res.* 1995;77:87.
52.   Malinski T, Radomski MW, Taha Z, Moncada S: Direct electrochemical measurement of nitric oxide released from human platelets. *Biochem Biophys Res Comm.* 1993;194:960.
53.   Radomski MW, Palmer RMJ, Moncada S. An L-arginine/nitric oxide pathway present in human platelets regulates aggregation. *Proc Natl Acad Sci USA.* 1990;87:5193.
54.   Freedman JE, Loscalzo J, Barnard MR, Alpert C, Keaney JF, Jr., Michelson AD: Nitric oxide released from activated platelets inhibits platelet recruitment. *J Clin Invest.* 1997;100:350.
55.   Freedman JE, Ting B, Hankin B, Loscalzo J, Keaney JF, Jr., Vita JA: Impaired platelet production of nitric oxide predicts the presence of acute coronary syndromes. *Circulation.* 1998;In press.
56.   Bossaller C, Habib GB, Yamamoto H, Williams C, Wells S, Henry PD. Impaired muscarinic endothelium-dependent relaxation and cyclic guanosine 5-monophosphate formation in atherosclerotic human coronary artery and rabbit aorta. *J Clin Invest.* 1986;170.
57.   Vita JA, Treasure CB, Nabel EG, McLenachan JM, Fish RD, Yeung AC, Vekshtein VI, Selwyn AP, Ganz P: Coronary vasomotor response to acetylcholine relates to risk factors for coronary artery disease. *Circulation.* 1990;81:491.
58.   Ohara Y, Peterson TE, Harrison DG: Hypercholesterolemia increases endothelial superoxide anion production. *J Clin Invest.* 1993;91:2546.
59.   Lynch SM, Frei B: Mechanisms of copper-and iron-dependent oxidative modification of human low-density lipoprotein. *J Lipid Res.* 1993;34:1745.
60.   Rubbo H, Radi R, Trujillo M, Telleri R, Kalyanaraman B, Barnes S, Kirk M, Freeman BA: Nitric oxide regulation of superoxide and peroxynitrite-dependent lipid peroxidation. Formation of novel nitrogen-containing oxidized lipid derivatives. *J Biol Chem.* 1994;269:26066.
61.   Gryglewski RJ, Palmer RM, Moncada S: Superoxide anion is involved in the breakdown of endothelium-derived vascular relaxing factor. *Nature.* 1986;320:454.
62.   Kissner R, Nauser T, Bugnon P, Lye PG, Koppenol WH: Formation and properties of peroxynitrite as studied by laser flash photolysis, high-pressure stopped-flow technique, and pulse radiolysis. *Chemical Res Toxicol.* 1997;10:1285.
63.   Meng YY, Trachtenburg J, Ryan US, Abendschein DR: Potentiation of endogenous nitric oxide with superoxide dismutase inhibits platelet-mediated thrombosis in injured and stenotic arteries. *J Am Coll Cardiol.* 1995;25:269.
64.   Ikeda H, Koga Y, Od T, Kuwano K, Nakayama H, Ueno T, Toshima H, Michael L, Entman M. Free oxygen radicals contribute to platelet aggregation and cyclic flow variations in stenosed and endothelium-injred canine coronary arteries. *J Am Coll Cardiol.* 1994;24:1749.
65.   Freedman JE, Frei B, Welch GN, Loscalzo J: Glutathione peroxidase potentiates the inhibition of platelet function by S-nitrosothiols. *J Clin Invest.* 1995;96:394.
66.   Freedman JE, Loscalzo J, Benoit SE, Valeri CR, Barnard MR, Michelson AD: Decreased platelet inhibition by nitric oxide in two brothers with a history of arterial thrombosis. *J Clin Invest.* 1996;97:979.

11 ANTIOXIDANTS AND ATHEROSCLEROSIS: ANIMAL STUDIES

John F. Keaney, Jr.

INTRODUCTION

Atherosclerosis and its clinical sequelae such as myocardial infarction and stroke represent a major source of morbidity and mortality in the developed world, claiming over 960,000 lives annually in the United States alone (1). A wealth of data now links serum cholesterol, in particular low-density lipoprotein (LDL) cholesterol (2) to the development of atherosclerosis. Despite this causative association between LDL cholesterol and atherosclerosis, isolated LDL particles typically fail to demonstrate atherogenic effects *in vitro* (3). For example, the loading of tissue macrophages with LDL cholesterol is tightly regulated (3). In contrast, the oxidation of LDL lipids is associated with a number of structural changes within LDL that support its unregulated uptake into macrophages leading to foam cell formation, the hallmark of an early atherosclerotic lesion (3,4). *In vitro* studies also indicate that oxidized LDL (oxLDL) possesses many other proatherogenic properties that are reviewed in detail in Chapter 4. Consistent with an important role for oxLDL in atherosclerosis, its formation has been identified *in vivo* (5,6). Despite this demonstration that oxLDL occurs *in vivo*, data directly attributing a causative role of oxLDL in atherosclerosis has been difficult to obtain. This chapter will review available evidence on antioxidants and atherosclerosis from the perspective that oxLDL is an important factor in the atherogenic process. The implications of the "oxidative modification hypothesis" of atherosclerosis with respect to vascular antioxidant status will be reviewed, and animal intervention trials investigating the effect of antioxidant manipulation on atherosclerosis will be discussed.

ANTIOXIDANT STATUS AND THE OXIDATIIVE MODIFICATION HYPOTHESIS

There is considerable evidence that lipid peroxidation occurs within the vascular wall during atherosclerosis. Glavind first identified the presence of lipid hydroperoxides within atherosclerotic lesions (7). Although this original study did not specify the type of lipid hydroperoxide, later investigation revealed both oxidized free (8,9) and a esterified (10-12) cholesterol oxidation products in atherosclerotic lesions. Subsequent studies have also shown that peroxidation of fatty acids as well (13-16). Since a number of antioxidants are known to limit LDL oxidation in *ex vivo* assays (see Chapters 3 and 5), one implication of these data is that antioxidant defenses of the vascular wall may be impaired.

Experimental evidence examining the extent of antioxidant defenses in the arterial wall during atherosclerosis is somewhat limited. Human studies, for example, tend to be limited to advanced stages of atherosclerosis. Since the oxidative modification hypothesis links oxidative events to early events in atherosclerosis, one might expect that examining late stages of the disease would provide limited insight. Available data is also limited by the lack of any systematic studies linking antioxidant status in the arterial wall to the stages of atherosclerotic lesions. Nevertheless, it is worthwhile reviewing the available data on vascular antioxidant defenses in the setting of atherosclerosis.

Conceptually, one can divide vascular antioxidant defenses into two distinct categories that are outlined in great detail in Chapter 3. One category, the enzymatic antioxidants include superoxide dismutase, catalase, and glutathione peroxidase. The second category includes the low molecular weight lipid- and water-soluble antioxidants. The major water-soluble antioxidants are ascorbic acid, glutathione, and in the extracellular space, urate. The major change-breaking lipid-soluble antioxidant compounds in the vascular wall are α-tocopherol (vitamin E) β-carotene, and Ubiquinol-10.

With respect to enzymatic antioxidants, Table 1 contains 14 published studies examining vascular antioxidant status and atherosclerosis. Human studies have primarily involved comparison of normal aorta or non-diseased arteries such as the internal mammary artery with areas of aorta or carotid artery that contain atherosclerotic lesions. In general, these human studies have demonstrated a trend towards a decrease in enzymatic antioxidant status in the late stages of atherosclerosis versus normal arterial sites (17-20). Given that such studies are limited to measurements performed at a single point in time, it is unclear whether the reported reduction in enzymatic antioxidants is in fact causative or a consequence of late atherosclerosis.

A number of animal models have also been used to examine the relationship enzymatic antioxidants status and atherosclerosis. In contrast to the results reported in humans, these studies are considerably more mixed. For example, studies in rabbits fed a high-fat diet have demonstrated a decrease in SOD activity (21), whereas studies in cholesterol-fed rabbits have demonstrated either no change (22) or an increase (23-25) in SOD activity. In contrast, studies using cholesterol-fed Japanese quail have typically demonstrated either no change (26) or a decrease (27) in SOD activity. The data is similarly mixed for glutathione-related enzymatic antioxidants. Out of eight animals studies, only two have demonstrated a decrease in glutathione peroxidase activity (27,28), whereas five have demonstrated a

Table 1. Enzymatic antioxidant status and atherosclerosis.

Study	Model	Activity in lesions compared with corresponding control					
		Glutathione peroxidase		GSH reductase	GSH transferase	SOD	Catalase
		Se (+)	Se (-)				
Human studies							
Lankin (17)	Normal aorta vs. lesions	↓	↓	↓	↓		
Dubick (18)	Normal aorta vs. lesions					↓[a]	
Mezzetti (19)	IMA vs. aortic lesion	↓	↓	↓	↑		
Lapenna (20)	IMA vs. carotid lesion	↓	↑	↓	↔		
Animal Studies							
Wang (28)	Cholesterol-fed quail	↓					
Del Duccio (23)	Cholesterol-fed rabbits	↑[h]		↓	↓	↑	↓
Mugge (22)	Cholesterol-fed rabbits					↔	
Mantha (24)	Cholesterol-fed rabbits	↑[b]				↑	↑
Godin (27)	Cholesterol-fed quail	↓[b]				↑	
Godin (26)	Cholesterol-fed quail[c]	↑[b]		↔		↔	
Mantha (25)	Cholesterol-fed rabbit	↑				↑	↑
Cheng (29)	Cholesterol-fed quail	↔[b]		↓	↔		
Toborek (21)	High-fat fed rabbits[d]	↑[b]		↑		↓	
Fukai (30)	Atherosclerotic mice[e]					↑[f]	

[a]Only Cu,Zn-SOD activity was decreased (Check on this). [b]Selnium-dependence not reported in the present study. [c]Data is reported only for males, as females did not demonstrate atherosclerotic lesions. [d]Data are reported only for corn oil vs. low-fat control, other sources of fat (corn oil + cholesterol, chicken fat, beef tallow, or lard) did not produceany changes in activity. [e]Both apo E null and cholesterol-fed LDL receptor null mice were employed. The change in SOD activity was restricted to extracellular type C SOD.

corresponding increase (21, 23-26) with another showing no change (29). As shown in Table 1, the studies are somewhat heterogeneous using three different animal models and the precise mechanisms for determination of glutathione-peroxidase activity differed. In contrast to the situation with glutathione peroxidase, studies of glutathione reductase and glutathione-S-transferase have generally demonstrated a decrease in activity in atherosclerosis (23,29) with one study showing an increase in glutathione reductase (21). Thus, there is no consensus concerning any changes in enzymatic antioxidant of the vascular wall during atherosclerosis.

The situation with low molecular weight antioxidants is somewhat more straightforward. Suarna and colleagues (31) have published an in-depth

Table 2. Antioxidant levels of normal and atherosclerotic vessels.

| Study | Model | Ratio plaque/corresponding control | | | |
		Vitamin E	Ubiquinol	Ascorbic acid	Urate
Suarna (31)					
	Surgical specimens	1.5	1	9.8	29
Killion (32)	Surgical specimens	0.9 – 4.0	ND	ND	ND
Carpenter (33)	Necropsy specimens	0.19	ND	ND	ND

All values for vitamin E and ubiquinol represent ratios derived from lipid-standardized values. The corresponding values for ascorbic acid and urate are protein-corrected. ND, not determined.

examination of the antioxidant content of atherosclerotic plaques and normal vessel segments in humans. As shown in Table 2, there was no deficiencies of any main lipid-soluble antioxidants in atherosclerotic plaques. In fact, if anything there was an excess of antioxidants that was particularly notable for ascorbic acid and urate. Although not shown in the table, all atherosclerotic lesions also contained detectable quantities of oxidized lipids indicating that lipid peroxidation was an on-going process. A similar study was published by Killian and colleagues focusing exclusively on vitamin E again, demonstrating no deficiency in diseased vessels (32). These two studies stand in stark contrast to the findings of Carpenter and colleagues (33), who described a reduction in lesion α-tocopherol (corrected for total cholesterol content). This latter study employed necropsy specimens raising the possibility that α-tocopherol may have undergone some oxidation prior to sample processing. Nevertheless, in humans the preponderance of evidence does not indicate a deficiency of low-molecular weight antioxidants in the presence of even advanced atherosclerosis. Animal studies have not provided much additional insight since tissue antioxidant levels have been difficult to interpret as atherosclerosis is typically produced by high-fat feeding leading to considerable variation in lipoprotein levels and lipid-soluble vitamin absorption.

In summary, available data provides no clear indication that any particular component of vascular antioxidant defenses are lacking in the setting of atherosclerosis. Admittedly, the tools available to address this question are limited, and gross antioxidant determinations in homogenized arterial samples may not adequately reflect events at a subcellular level. Notwithstanding these constraints, let us turn our attention to interventional studies in which antioxidants have been tested as agents to inhibit the development and/or progression of atherosclerosis.

ANTIOXIDANTS AND ATHEROSCLEROSIS: INTERVENTION STUDIES

One important corollary to the oxidative modification hypothesis is the notion that agents which limit the oxidation of LDL should also inhibit the development of atherosclerosis. This corollary has been tested in a number of animal models using a variety of structurally distinct antioxidant compounds. Although a considerable fraction of such intervention studies actually predate the discovery of oxLDL, important insight into the activity of antioxidant compounds can still be garnered from such studies and they will be included here.

Vitamin E

Early studies demonstrating that experimental animals lacking vitamin E exhibit abnormal capillaries and increased tissue cholesterol levels (34,35) prompted Dam to study the effect of vitamin E on atherosclerosis in cholesterol-fed rabbits. Vitamin E in the diet limited the mortality associated with high-fat feeding, but did not alter the extent of aortic cholesterol deposition. Subsequently, Stamler and colleagues (36) reported similar findings in cholesterol-fed chicks that were confirmed by others (37). One problem with these studies was the dual effect of vitamin E on both cholesterol and lesion accumulation.

More recent studies in which the effect of vitamin E on both blood cholesterol and aortic atherosclerosis were determined are summarized in Table 3. These studies make a compelling argument that accounting for the effect of vitamin E on cholesterol is particularly important. Four studies in rabbits fed a high-fat diet (38-41) and one study in modified Watanabe Heritable Hyperlipidemic (WHHL) rabbits (42) demonstrated a reduction in atherosclerosis by vitamin E accompanied by a significant reduction in blood cholesterol. In contrast, only one study demonstrating cholesterol reduction with vitamin E has failed to show any reduction in atherosclerosis (43). Thus, cholesterol reduction with vitamin E has generally produced a reduction in atherosclerosis.

As one can see from Table 3, in the absence of any effect on blood cholesterol, there is no clear consensus that vitamin E inhibits atherosclerosis in experimental animals. Of the 16 studies in which vitamin E had no effect on blood cholesterol, 10 demonstrated either no effect or an increase in atherosclerosis. These negative studies include models of high-fat diets in species such as quail (44) and rabbits (43, 45-49) and a genetic model of atherosclerosis (WHHL rabbits) (50-53). The remaining 6 studies that did demonstrate inhibition of atherosclerosis with vitamin E also involved a number of species such as chickens (54), rabbits (55, 56), monkeys (57), hamsters (58), and mice (59) consuming a cholesterol/high-fat diet.

The lack of any consistent vitamin E effect on animal models of atherosclerosis is difficult to explain. As stated above, there is no particular animal model that has consistently been associated with either a positive or negative effect of vitamin E on atherosclerosis. One important consideration in studies of vitamin E involves tissue levels. Some studies involve the initiation of vitamin E treatment with a high-fat diet concurrently. Clearly, under such conditions the maximum tissue concentration of vitamin E is not achieved until well into the study. A similar argument could be applied to the WHHL rabbit, a model of ongoing atherosclerosis. The precise events involved in initiation versus propagation of atherosclerosis may be distinct, and thus, distinctly sensitive to vitamin E if at all. In addition, the vitamin E status of animals at the initiation of many animals studies is not well controlled for. Some

Oxidative Stress and Vascular Disease

Table 3. Selected animal studies of vitamin E and atherosclerosis

Study	Model	Vitamin E dose	% Change compared to no supplement	
			Serum/plasma cholesterol	Lesion area
Brattsand (38)	Cholesterol-fed rabbits	125 mg/d	-19	-80 [a]
Wilson (39)	Butter-fed rabbits	10,000mg/kg diet	-75	-67 [b]
Morrissey (44)	0.5% Chol.-fed quail	22 mg/kg diet [d]	+27	-56 [b]
	1% Chol.-fed quail	22 mg/kg diet [d]	+42	+60 [b]
Westrope (40)	Coconut oil-fed rabbits	10,000 mg/kg diet	-57	-75
Godfried (60)	Cholesterol-fed rabbits	2,000 mg/kg diet	0	-16 [b]
	Cholesterol-fed rabbits [c]	10,000 mg/kg diet	-18	+66
Smith (54)	Cholesterol-fed chickens	1,000 IU/kg diet	0	-37
Wojcicki (45)	Cholesterol-fed rabbits	10 mg/kg/d*	0	0
Bocan (55)	Cholesterol-fed rabbits	500 mg/kg diet [d]	0	-46
Verlangieri (57)	Cholesterol-fed monkeys	79 mg/d	0	-30 [e]
Williams (42)	Modified WHHL rabbits [f]	5,000 mg/kg diet	-38	-32
Prasad (41)	Cholesterol-fed rabbits	40 mg/kg/d	-23	-73
Willingham (50)	WHHL rabbits	2,000 mg/kg diet	-19	0
Morel (46)	Cholesterol-fed rabbits	10,000 mg/kg diet [d]	0	0
Kleinveld (51)	WHHL rabbits	250 mg/kg diet	0	0
Keaney (47)	Cholesterol-fed rabbits	1,000 mg/kg diet	0	+26 [g]
		10,000 mg/kg diet	0	+160 [g]
Parker (58)	Chol.-fed hamsters [h]	1,000 mg/kg diet	0	0
	Chol.-fed hamsters [h]	1,000 mg/kg diet	0	0
	Chol.-fed hamsters [i]	1,000 mg/kg diet*	+15	-81
Freubis (61)	WHHL rabbits	1,000 mg/kg diet*	0	0
Shaish (48)	Cholesterol-fed rabbits	100 mg/kg diet	0	0
Kleinveld (52)	Oleate-fed WHHL rabbits	250 mg/kg diet	0	0
	Linoleate-fed WHHL rabbits	250 mg/kg diet	0	0
Chen (56)	Cholesterol-fed rabbits	40 mg/kg/d	0	-44
Tijburg (49)	Cholesterol-fed rabbits	300 mg/kg diet	0	0
Fruebis (53)	WHHL rabbits	1,000 mg/kg diet [k]	0	0
Schwenke (43)	Cholesterol-fed rabbits	1,375 mg/kg diet	-17	0
Crawford (59)	Cholesterol-fed LDLR-deficient mice [j]	1,000 mg/kg diet [l,d]	0	-60
Pratico (109)	ApoE (-/-) mice	2,000 mg/kg diet	0	-66

All values for changes in cholesterol and lesion area are at study termination unless otherwise indicated. [a]Diet also contained 25 mg vitamin A palmitate daily. [b]Atherosclerosis measured as incidence of aortic lesions. [c]New Zealand White. [d]Diet also contained supplemental vitamin C. [e]Atherosclerosis determined as percent carotid stenosis by ultrasound. [f]Watanabe heritable hyperlipidemic rabbits that lack functional LDL receptors. [g]Atherosclerosis measured as intimal thickness. [h]Chow-based diet providing 88 mg/kg diet before supplementations. [i]Synthetic diet deficient in vitamins C,E, and K as well as carotenoids, equivalent results were also observed for 0.8% cholesterol supplementation of this diet. [j]LDL receptor-deficient mice. [k]Diet also contained 500 mg/kg probucol analog and 250 mg/kg probucol. [l]Diet also contained 5,000 mg/kg diet β-carotene. *Indicates that tocopherol-stripped chow was used in the control group.

studies choose as a control diet vitamin E stripped ingredients whereas others opt for laboratory chow that already contains substantial quantities of vitamin E (40 –80 mg/kg diet). Despite such considerations, however, no consistent effect of vitamin E on atherosclerosis can be implied from available literature.

Probucol

Probucol is a cholesterol lowering agent that shares considerable structural homology with the food preservative and antioxidant butylated hydroxytoluene (62). Early studies investigating the cholesterol lowering properties of this drug found that it inhibited the development of atherosclerosis in rabbits (63, 64) and monkeys (65) principally as a consequence of its lipid-lowering effect. It was at this time that the oxidative modification hypothesis of atherosclerosis was under development and Parthasarathy found that probucol, at physiologic concentrations, inhibited the oxidative modification of LDL (66). Based on this finding, two studies were performed in WHHL rabbits demonstrating inhibition of atherosclerosis in association with the antioxidant protection of LDL (67,68) (Table 4). Kita and colleagues (67) demonstrated both inhibition of copper-mediated LDL oxidation and atherosclerosis in WHHL rabbits, however, interpretation of this study was complicated by a 17% reduction in cholesterol due to probucol. This issue was nicely addressed by Carew and colleagues (68) who compared the effect of probucol with that of lovastatin, a cholesterol-lowering agent without antioxidant properties. Despite a similar cholesterol-lowering effect as lovastatin, probucol demonstrated an additional 48% reduction in atherosclerosis compared to lovastatin. The authors interpreted this finding as evidence that probucol reduces atherosclerosis through the antioxidant protection of LDL. In support of this argument, probucol treatment also resulted in a reduction in the fractional degradation of LDL within the aortic wall (68)

There is other experimental evidence to support the notion that probucol inhibits atherosclerosis, at least in part, through its antioxidant activity. Mao and colleagues treated WHHL rabbits with both probucol and a structural analog of probucol (MDL 29,311) that does not lower plasma cholesterol (69). Both compounds provided significant antioxidant protection of LDL against copper-mediated oxidation in *ex vivo* assays. Probucol, as expected, significantly lowered serum cholesterol by 23% and this was associated with a 69% reduction in atherosclerosis. However, MDL 29,311 also inhibited atherosclerosis but without lowering cholesterol significantly bolstering the idea that enhanced LDL antioxidant protection reduces atherosclerosis. As shown in Table 4, a number of other studies with probucol in both cholesterol-fed animals and WHHL rabbits have demonstrated a reduction in atherosclerosis with variable effect on serum cholesterol. It should be noted, however that even in studies where no significant effect on cholesterol was reported, there was a trend towards cholesterol reduction and those studies may have lacked statistical power to demonstrate the hypocholesterolemic effect of probucol. The observations of Sasahara and coworkers further strengthened the relation between LDL antioxidant protection by probucol and reduced atherosclerosis. These investigators treated cholesterol-fed monkeys with probucol (16 mg/kg/day) and observed a 43% reduction in atherosclerosis that was directly

Table 4. Animal studies of probucol and atherosclerosis

Study	Model	Probucol dose	Serum/plasma cholesterol	Lesion area
			% Change compared to no supplement	
Wissler (65)	Cholesterol-fed monkeys	60 mg/kg/d	-26	-12
Tawara (64)	Cholesterol-fed rabbits	5,000mg/kg diet	-41	-54
Kita (67)	Young WHHL rabbits[a]	10,000 mg/kg diet	-17	-87
Carew (68)	Young WHHL rabbits	10,000 mg/kg diet	-12	-65
	Young WHHL rabbits[b]	10,000 mg/kg diet	0	-48
Stein (75)	Cholesterol-fed rabbits[c]	10,000 mg/kg diet	0	0
Daugherty (76)	Cholesterol-fed rabbits	10,000 mg/kg diet	0	-9
Finckh (77)	Young WHHL rabbits	10,000 mg/kg diet	-28	-63
Daugherty (78)	Mature WHHL rabbits	10,000 mg/kg diet	-17	0
Mao (69)	Modified WHHL rabbits	10,000 mg/kg diet	-23	-69
Nagano (79)	Young WHHL rabbits	10,000 mg/kg diet	0	-74
	Mature WHHL rabbits	10,000 mg/kg diet	0	-54
Bocan (55)	Cholesterol/coconut & peanut oil-fed rabbits	500 mg/kg diet	-47	0
Yamaguchi (80)	Cholesterol-fed mice	10,000 mg/kg diet	-25	-19
Bocan (81)	Cholesterol-fed quail	500 mg/kg diet	0	-62
Sasahara (70)	Cholesterol-fed monkeys	60 mg/kg/d	0	-43
Fruebis (82)	Young WHHL rabbits	10,000 mg/kg diet	-26	-46
Kleinveld (51)	Mature WHHL rabbits	250 mg/kg diet	-20	0
Morel (46)	Cholesterol-fed rabbits	10,000 mg/kg diet	-40[d]	-67
Parker (58)	Cholesterol -fed hamsters[e]	2,000 mg/kg diet	0	-41
Braesen (83)	WHHL rabbits	10,000 mg/kg diet		
Shaish (48)	Cholesterol-fed rabbits	10,000 mg/kg diet	0	-31
Del Rio (84)	Cholesterol-fed rabbit	10,000 mg/kg diet	0	-91
Kogushi (85)	WHHL rabbits	10,000 mg/kg diet	0	-70
Zhang (71)	Apo E (-/-) mice fed chow	5,000 mg/kg diet	-40	+241
	Apo E (+/-) mice fed high-fat diet	5,000 mg/kg diet	-21	+208
Hoshida (86)	Young WHHL rabbits	10,000 mg/kg diet	0	-47
Fruebis (53)	Young WHHL rabbits	910 mg/kg diet[f]	+9	-52
Wu (87)	Cholesterol-fed rabbits	10,000 mg/kg diet	-47	-74
Oshima (88)	Mature WHHL rabbits	10,000 mg/kg diet	-14	-39
Schwenke (43)	Cholesterol-fed rabbits	3,800 mg/kg diet	-40	-81
Bird (72)	Cholesterol-fed LDL-receptor (-/-) mice	5,000 mg/kg diet[g]	-48	+268
		250 mg/kg diet	-26	+64
Cynshi (73)	Young WHHL rabbits	10,000 mg/kg diet	0	-30
	Chol.-fed C57BL/6J mice	10,000 mg/kg diet	-50	+158
	LDLR (-/-) mice	10,000 mg/kg diet	NR	+23[g]

[a]Young is < 3 months of age. [b]Control group in this series included lovastatin-treated animals to match cholesterol-reduction with that of probucol. [c]Dietary cholesterol was manipulated to match cholesterol in the control and probucol groups. [d]VLDL measurement only. [e]Synthetic diet deficient in vitamins C,E, and K as well as carotenoids, results reported for 0.8% cholesterol supplementation of this diet. [f]Amount was varied to match antioxidant protection of LDL with a combined antioxidant group (see Table 3). [g]Results are reported for male mice only. NR = not reported

correlated with LDL resistance to copper-mediated oxidation (70). Thus, there is considerable evidence linking the antiatherosclerotic effect of probucol to its antioxidant activity in a number of models.

The success of probucol in reducing atherosclerosis in rabbits, monkeys, and hamsters stands in stark contrast to the experience with mice. In three separate studies (see Table 4) probucol has been found to accelerate atherosclerosis in mice (71-73). Zhang and colleagues (71) studied the effect of dietary probucol (0.5% by weight) on atherosclerosis in apolipoprotein E-knockout (apoE -/-) mice. Animals treated with probucol demonstrated a significant reduction in total cholesterol on the order of 21% to 40%. Despite this reduction in cholesterol, probucol-treated animals demonstrated a 2 - 2.4 fold increase in atherosclerosis. This effect of probucol to promote atherosclerosis has been confirmed in a second mouse model deficient in the LDL receptor (LDLR-/-) model (72). Bird and colleagues found that either 0.5 % or 0.025% probucol by weight in the diet promoted atherosclerosis in LDLR-/- mice regardless of the sex of the animals, the cholesterol levels, or the duration of high-fat feeding. This increase in atherosclerosis ranged from 1.3-fold to 2.9-fold in female mice and from 3.6-fold to 3.7-fold in males (72). Qualitatively similar results were also reported by Cynshi and coworkers (73). This pro-atherogenic action of probucol is all the more remarkable considering that all three studies also demonstrated effective protection of lipoproteins against *ex vivo* copper-mediated oxidation (71-73). Thus, in contrast to the experience in rabbits, antioxidant protection of lipoproteins was not associated with an inhibition of atherosclerosis and, in fact promoted atherosclerosis. Possible mechanisms for such observations might include alternative metabolism of probucol in mice versus other experimental models, or some fundamental difference between the pathogenesis of atherosclerosis in murine models versus other models.

N, N'-Diphenyl Phenylenediamine (DPPD)

DPPD is a synthetic aniline compound that inhibits the oxidation of LDL *in vitro*. This compound has been tested for its effect to inhibit atherosclerosis in two animal models. Sparrow and colleagues (74) treated cholesterol-fed rabbits with 1% by weight DPPD. Animals were treated in this manner for 71 days at which point both atherosclerosis and the extent to which DPPD protected LDL against oxidation were also determined. DPPD treatment was associated with a reduction in atherosclerotic lesion area from 42% to 12% and a concomitant reduction in tissue cholesterol content. There was no effect of DPPD on total cholesterol, although isolated LDL from DPPD-treated rabbits demonstrated marked protection against oxidation in response to copper (74).

These data were interpreted to indicate a link between antioxidant protection of lipoproteins and a reduction in atherosclerosis. A similar study has been performed in apoE -/- mice in which Tangirala and colleagues treated the mice with a high-fat diet containing either vehicle or 0.5% DPPD by weight (108). Similar to the study of Sparrow and colleagues, these investigators found no effect of DPPD on plasma lipoprotein levels but did observe a marked antioxidant effect of DPPD on isolated LDL. After six months of consuming a high-fat diet, control animals demonstrated approximately 22% of the aorta covered by atherosclerotic lesions while DPPD treated animals exhibited only 14% coverage. Thus, in this study of murine atherosclerosis, DPPD treatment both protected LDL against oxidation and reduced the extent of atherosclerosis.

Other Lipid-Soluble Antioxidants

The experience with other lipid-soluble antioxidant in atherosclerosis is less extensive then that outlined above for vitamin E, probucol, or DPPD. Carotenoids such as β-carotene are the second most abundant lipid-soluble antioxidant in human plasma and lipoproteins (89). However, the activity of these agents against LDL oxidation is minimal at best (90-92). A limited number of studies have examined the effects of carotenoids on atherosclerosis. The intramuscular injections of the carotenoid crocetin has been shown to decrease the severity of atherosclerotic lesions in cholesterol-fed rabbits in association with reduced cholesterol and triglyceride levels (93). More recently, Shaish and colleagues (48) examined the effects of β-carotene on atherosclerosis in cholesterol-fed rabbits. These investigators found that the all-*trans* form of β-carotene reduced atherosclerosis lesion coverage in the aortic arch from approximately 69% to 43%. In contrast, the 9-*cis* form of β-carotene had no effect and there was no effect of either compound on antioxidant protection of LDL. The precise mechanisms responsible for this observation are not clear, although those authors speculated that some stereospecific interaction with retinoic acid receptors in the arterial wall may be responsible.

Two synthetic antioxidants butylated hydroxy toluene (BHT) and butylated hydroxyanisole (BHA) are commonly used as food preservatives. Both of these compounds have been tested for their activity against atherosclerosis in animal models. Wilson and colleagues (39) found that combined supplementation of BHT and BHA (0.1% of the diet by weight each) prevented atherosclerosis in butter-fed rabbits. Similarly, Bjorkhem (94) found that BHT reduced atherosclerosis in cholesterol-fed rabbits when provided as 1% of the diet by weight. A similar protective effect against lesion formation was found with BHT in rabbits following balloon injury of the aorta (95), although the adequacy of this balloon-injured model for atherosclerosis remains a matter of question.

Recently, Cynshi and colleagues reported the antioxidant activity of a synthetic compound (BO-653) based upon vitamin E and probucol (73). These investigators designed an antioxidant compound with the radical trapping activity of vitamin E and the lipophilicity of probucol. In WHHL rabbits and two separate strains of cholesterol fed mice, this compound demonstrated significant activity to inhibit atherosclerosis. Interestingly, the same study used probucol as a comparison and probucol inhibited atherosclerosis in the WHHL rabbits but enhanced atherosclerosis in the mouse models of atherosclerosis (Table 4). Undoubtedly, considerable effort will be directed at synthetic antioxidants in the future looking for a compound that has broad activity as both an antioxidant and an anti-atherogen.

Vitamin C

Vitamin C is the main water-soluble antioxidant in human plasma and interstitial fluid. *In vitro*, vitamin C protects LDL from oxidation (96,97) and has the capacity to regenerate vitamin E from its oxidized form. In animal studies of vitamin C in the vasculature, the guinea pig has traditionally been the animal of choose because it is unable to synthesize ascorbic acid, similar to humans. Willis (98) was among the first to examine the effect of vitamin C on atherosclerosis, using the scorbutic guinea pig as a model. Willis found that sub-intimal lipid lesions developed in guinea pigs as early as 15 days after institution of a vitamin C-free diet. Subsequent addition of vitamin C to the diet reversed the situation. Similarly, feeding animals 500 mg cholesterol daily increased lesion formation during acute vitamin C deficiency. A similar finding was subsequently reported by Fujinami and coworkers who performed a 2 x 2 factorial study of vitamin C and 5% coconut oil by weight in guinea pigs on a scorbutic diet (99). Animals consuming coconut oil without vitamin C developed early atherosclerotic lesions, whereas animals on vitamin C did not.. Neither of the aforementioned studies was unable to maintain animals on a scorbutic diet and perform chronic cholesterol feeding as typical complications of scurvy would develop such as loss of appetite, growth retardation, hemorrhage, and anemia. Thus, early data indicated that vitamin C deficiency induced histologic features of early atherosclerosis, although chronic studies of cholesterol feeding were not feasible.

The complications of scurvy usually resulted in the death of guinea pigs after about 28 days of vitamin C deficiency. Ultimately, this problem was overcome by Ginter who developed a model of marginal vitamin C deficiency based on the depletion of vitamin C tissue stores and then marginal vitamin C supplementation (0.5 mg/day) that just prevents the development of scurvy (100). Animals treated in this manner can survive for long periods of time with no appreciable co-morbid conditions, allowing the study of more chronic disease states, such as atherosclerosis. Ginter and colleagues found that guinea pigs on the marginally scorbutic diet for 80 days along with 0.3% cholesterol by weight leads to in increased accumulation of cholesterol in the aorta without frank atherosclerotic lesions (101). More prolonged exposure to the same cholesterol-containing diet in marginally scorbutic guinea pigs does result in the development of atherosclerotic lesions that is inhibited by excess vitamin C (50 mg/day).

Similar findings have been reported in animal models other than guinea pigs. Verlangieri and colleagues (102) examined the effect of vitamin C on atherosclerosis in Dutch-belted rabbits fed 0.5% cholesterol by weight over 6 weeks. Using intimal area as an index of atherosclerosis, they found that vitamin C 100 mg/kg inhibited the development of atherosclerosis by 84% without any effect on plasma lipid parameters. A similar result was also reported with vitamin C (150 mg/d) in albino rabbits treated on a 0.3% cholesterol diet, although atherosclerosis was only inhibited by ~23% (103).

Although vitamin C has been shown to limit TBARS in scorbutic rats (104), a specific link to atherosclerosis has not been demonstrated. One must be cognizant of the many activities of vitamin C within the vascular wall. For example, vitamin C is required for the hydroxylation of lysyl and prolyl residues in collagen (105). Predictably, the levels of cross-linked collagen are reduced in animals rendered deficient in vitamin C. The precise extent to which this contributes to the development of atherosclerosis is not known. Similarly, glycosaminoglycans are metabolized differently in the presence of vitamin C deficiency and the precise implication of glycosaminoglycan metabolism on atherosclerosis is not known (106). Finally, vitamin C status also has important implications for cholesterol metabolism. Specifically, cholesterol oxidation is reduced in vitamin C deficiency resulting in increased hepatic cholesterol accumulation as a direct consequence of impaired bile acid production (107). Thus, vitamin C influences a number of biochemical processes that may have a direct on atherosclerosis, although the precise extent to which any of these processes contribute to the effect of vitamin C on atherosclerosis is still unknown.

SUMMARY AND CONCLUSIONS

As one can infer from the data reviewed in this chapter, there is considerable evidence to suggest that antioxidant status and/or antioxidant therapy has some effect for the development of atherosclerosis in experimental animals. This data is strongest for lipid-soluble antioxidants such as probucol, DPPD, and BO653. Likewise there is also data to support the idea that vitamin C status is an important determinant of the severity of atherosclerosis in experimental guinea pigs, and some rabbit studies. Until recently, the oxidative modification hypothesis of atherosclerosis provided the only convenient model to explain the observation that antioxidant treatment reduces atherosclerosis. According to this hypothesis (see Chapter 4), oxidation of LDL in the arterial wall is the critical step allowing for foam cell formation and the initiation of atherosclerosis. It is now apparent that both the initiation and progression of atherosclerosis involves a number of redox-sensitive events that go beyond the oxidative modification of LDL. Endothelial expression of leukocyte adhesion molecules, endothelial dysfunction, and platelet activation all involve redox-sensitive signals that are independent of LDL oxidation. This realization may help to explain the inconsistent results of some antioxidants (vitamin E and probucol) on atherogenesis despite equivalent LDL antioxidant protection. Considerably more investigation will be needed to precisely determine which component(s) of vascular oxidative stress are critical for the development of atherosclerosis and the clinical expression of atherosclerotic vascular disease.

REFERENCES

1.   American Heart Association. 1998 Heart and stroke statistical update. Internet. 1998. American Heart Association.
2.   Wilson PW, Garrison RJ, Castelli WP, Feinleib M, McNamara PM, Kannel WB. Prevalence of coronary heart disease in the Framingham Offspring Study: role of lipoprotein cholesterols. *Am J Cardiol.* 1980;46:649.

3. Goldstein JL, Ho YK, Basu SK, Brown MS. Binding site on macrophages that mediates uptake and degradation of acetylated low density lipoprotein, producing massive cholesterol deposition. *Proc Natl Acad Sci USA.* 1979;76:333.
4. Henriksen T, Mahoney EM, Steinberg D. Enhanced macrophage degradation of low density lipoprotein previously incubated with cultured endothelial cells: recognition by receptor for acetylated low density lipoproteins. *Proc Natl Acad Sci USA.* 1981;78:6499.
5. Palinski W, Rosenfeld ME, Ylä-Herttuala S, Gurtner GC, Socher SS, Butler SW, Parthasarathy S, Carew TE, Steinberg D, Witztum JL. Low density lipoprotein undergoes oxidative modification *in vivo*. *Proc Natl Acad Sci USA.* 1989;86:1372.
6. Ylä-Herttuala S, Palinski W, Rosenfeld ME, Parthasarathy S, Carew TE, Butler S, Witztum JL, Steinberg D. Evidence for the presence of oxidatively modified low density lipoprotein in atherosclerotic lesions of rabbit and man. *J Clin Invest.* 1989;84:1086.
7. Glavind J., Hartmann S, Clemmesen J, Jessen KE, Dam H. Studies on the role of lioperoxides in human pathology, II: the presence of peroxidized lipids in the atherosclerotic aorta. *Acta Path Microbiol Immunol Scand.* 1952;30:1.
8. Brooks CJ, Harland WA, Steel G. Squalene, 26-hydroxycholesterol and 7-ketocholesterol in human atheromatous plaques. *Biochim Biophys Acta* 1966;125:620.
9. Gilbert JD, Harland WA, Steel G, Brooks CJ. The isolation and identification of 5 alpha-cholestan-3 beta-ol from the human atheromatous aorta. *Biochim Biophys Acta* 1969;187:453.
10. Harland WA, Gilbert JD, Steel G, Brooks CJ. Lipids of human atheroma. The occurrence of a new group of polar sterol esters in various stages of human atherosclerosis. *Atherosclerosis* 1971;13:239.
11. Brooks CJ, Steel G, Gilbert JD, Harland WA. Lipids of human atheroma. Characterisation of a new group of polar sterol esters from human atherosclerotic plaques. *Atherosclerosis* 1971;13:223.
12. Gilbert JD, Brooks CJ, Harland WA. Lipids of human atheroma. VII. Isolation of diesters of cholest-5-ene-3 ,26-diol from extracts of advanced atherosclerotic lesions of human aorta. *Biochim Biophys Acta.* 1972;270:149.
13. Harland WA, Gilbert JD, Brooks CJ. Lipids of human atheroma. 8. Oxidised derivatives of cholesteryl linoleate. *Biochim Biophys Acta.* 1973;316:378.
14. Carpenter KLH, Taylor SE, Ballantine JA, Fussell B, Halliwell B, Mitchinson MJ. Lipids and oxidised lipids in human atheroma and normal aorta. *Biochim Biophys Acta.* 1993;1167:121.
15. Chisolm GM, Ma G, Irwin KC, Martin LL, Gunderson KG, Linberg LF, Morel DW, DiCorleto PE. 7 beta-hydroperoxycholest-5-en-3 beta-ol, a component of human atherosclerotic lesions, is the primary cytotoxin of oxidized human low density lipoprotein. *Proc Natl Acad Sci USA.* 1994;91:11452.
16 Kuhn H, Belkner J, Wiesner R, Schewe T, Lankin VZ, Tikhaze AK. Structure elucidation of oxygenated lipids in human atherosclerotic lesions. *EICOSANOIDS* 1992;5:17.
17. Lankin VZ, Vikhert AM, Kosykh VA, Tikhaze AK, Galakhov IE, Orekhov AN, Repin VN. Enzymatic detoxication of superoxide anion-radicals and lipoperoxides in intima and media of atherosclerotic aorta. *Biomed Biochim Acta.* 1984;43:797.
18. Dubick MA, Hunter GC, Casey SM, Keen CL. Aortic ascorbic acid, trace elements, and superoxide dismutase activity in human aneurysmal and occlusive disease. *Proc Soc Exp Biol Med.* 1987;184:138.
19. Mezzetti A, Lapenna D, Calafiore AM, Proietti-Franceschilli G, Porreca E, De Cesare D, Neri M, Di Ilio C, Cuccurullo F. Glutathione-related enzyme activities and lipoperoxide levels in human internal mammary artery and ascending aorta. Relations with serum lipids. *Arterioscler Thromb.* 1992;12:92.
20. Ceriello A, Giacomello R, Stel G, Motz E, Taboga C, Tonutti L, Pirisi M, Falleti E, Bartoli E. Hyperglycemia-induced thrombin formation in diabetes. *Diabetes.* 1995;44:924.
21. Toborek M, Feldman DL, Hennig B. Aortic antioxidant defense and lipid peroxidation in rabbits fed diets supplemented with different animal and plant fats. *J Am Coll Nutr.* 1997;16:32.
22. Mugge A, Elwell JH, Peterson TE, Hofmeyer TG, Heistad DD, Harrison DG. Chronic treatment with polyethylene-glycolated superoxide dismutase partially restores endothelium-dependent vascular relaxations in cholesterol-fed rabbits. *Circ Res.* 1991;69:1293.

23.   Del Boccio G, Lapenna D, Porreca E, Pennelli A, Savini F, Feliciani P, Ricci G, Cuccurullo F. Aortic antioxidant defence mechanisms: time-related changes in cholesterol-fed rabbits. *Atherosclerosis* 1990;81:127.

24.   Mantha SV, Prasad M, Kalra J, Prasad K. Antioxidant enzymes in hypercholesterolemia and effects of vitamin E in rabbits. *Atherosclerosis* 1993;101:135.

25.   Mantha SV, Kalra J, Prasad K. Effects of probucol on hypercholesterolemia-induced changes in antioxidant enzymes. *Life Sci* 1996;58:503.

26.   Godin DV, Garnett ME, Cheng KM, Nichols CR. Sex-related alterations in antioxidant status and susceptibility to atherosclerosis in Japanese quail. *Can J Cardiol.* 1995;11:945.

27.   Godin DV, Cheng KM, Garnett ME, Nichols CR. Antioxidant status of Japanese quail: comparison of atherosclerosis-susceptible and -resistant strains. *Can J Cardiol.* 1994;10:221.

28.   Wang J, Lu YC, Guo ZZ, Zhen EZ, Shi F. Lipid peroxides, glutathione peroxidase, prostacyclin and cell cycle stages in normal and atherosclerotic Japanese quail arteries. *Atherosclerosis* 1989;75:219.

29.   Cheng KM, Aggrey SE, Nichols CR, Garnett ME, Godin DV. Antioxidant enzymes and atherosclerosis in Japanese quail: heritability and genetic correlation estimates. *Can J Cardiol.* 1997;13:669.

30.   Fukai T, Galis ZS, Meng XP, Parthasarathy S, Harrison DG. Vascular expression of extracellular superoxide dismutase in atherosclerosis. *J Clin Invest.* 1998;101:2101.

31.   Suarna C, Dean RT, May J, Stocker R. Human atherosclerotic plaque contains both oxidized lipids and relatively large amounts of α-tocopherol and ascorbate. *Arterioscler Thromb Vasc Biol.* 1995;15:1616.

32.   Killion SL, Hunter GC, Eskelson CD, Dubick MA, Putnam CW, Hall KA, Luedke CA, Misiorowski RL, Schilling JD, McIntyre KE. Vitamin E levels in human atherosclerotic plaque: the influence of risk factors. *Atherosclerosis* 1996;126:289.

33.   Carpenter KL, Cheeseman KH, van d, V, Taylor SE, Walker MK, Mitchinson MJ. Depletion of alpha-tocopherol in human atherosclerotic lesions. *Free Radic Res* 1995;23:549.

34.   Heinrich MR, Mattil HA. Lipids of muscle and brain in rats deprived of tocopherol. *Proc Soc Exp Biol Med.* 1943;52:344.

35.   Morgulis S, Wilder VM, Spencer HC, Eppstein SH. Studies on the lipid content of normal and dystrophic rabbits. *J Biol Chem.* 1938;124:755.

36.   Stamler J, Pick R, Katz LN. Failure of vitamin E, vitamin B$_{12}$, and pancreatic extracts to influence plasma lipids and atherogenesis in cholesterol-fed chicks. *Circulation* 1954;8:455.

37.   Beeler DA, Rogler JC, Quackenbush FW. Effects of certain dietary lipids on plasma cholesterol and atherosclerosis in the chick. *J Nutr.* 1962;78:184.

38.   Brattsand R. Actions of vitamins A and E and some nicotinic acid derivatives on plasma lipids and on lipid infiltration of aorta in cholesterol-fed rabbits. *Atherosclerosis* 1975;22:47.

39.   Wilson RB, Middleton CC, Sun GY. Vitamin E, antioxidants and lipid peroxidation in experimental atherosclerosis on rabbits. *J Nutr.* 1978;108:1858.

40.   Westrope KL, Miller RL, Wilson RB. Vitamin E in a rabbit model of endogenous hypercholesterolemia and atherosclerosis. *Nutr Reports Intl.* 1982;25:83.

41.   Prasad K, Kalra J. Oxygen free radicals and hypercholesterolemic atherosclerosis: effect of vitamin E. *Am Heart J.* 1993;125:958.

42.   Williams RJ, Motteram JM, Sharp CH, Gallagher PJ. Dietary vitamin E and the attenuation of early lesion development in modified Watanabe rabbits. *Atherosclerosis* 1992;94:153.

43.   Schwenke DC, Behr SR. Vitamin E combined with selenium inhibits atherosclerosis in hypercholesterolemic rabbits independently of effects on plasma cholesterol concentrations. *Circ Res.* 1998;83:366.

44.   Morrissey RB, Donaldson WE. Cholesterolemia in Japanese quail: response to a mixture of vitamins C and E and choline chloride. *Artery* 1979;5:182.

45.   Wojcicki J, Rozewicka B, Barcew-Wisziewska B, Samochowiec L, Juzwaik S, Kadlubowska D, Tustanowski T, Juzyszyn Z. Effect of selenium and vitamin E on the development of experimental atherosclerosis in rabbits. *Atherosclerosis* 1991;87:9.

46.   Morel DW, de la Llera-Moya M, Friday KE: Treatment of cholesterol-fed rabbits with dietary vitamins E and C inhibits lipoprotein oxidation but not development of atherosclerosis. *J Nutr.* 1994;124:2123.

47.   Keaney JF, Jr., Gaziano JM, Xu A, Frei B, Curran-Celentano J, Shwaery GT, Loscalzo J, Vita JA. Low-dose α-tocopherol improves and high-dose α-tocopherol worsens endothelial vasodilator function in cholesterol-fed rabbits. *J Clin Invest.* 1994;93:844.

48. Shaish A, Daugherty A, O'Sullivan F, Schonfeld G, Heinecke JW. Beta-carotene inhibits atherosclerosis in hypercholesterolemic rabbits. *J Clin Invest.* 1995;96:2075.
49. Tijburg LB, Wiseman SA, Meijer GW, Weststrate JA. Effects of green tea, black tea and dietary lipophilic antioxidants on LDL oxidizability and atherosclerosis in hypercholesterolaemic rabbits. *Atherosclerosis* 1997;135:37.
50. Willingham AK, Bolanos C, Bohannan E, Cenedella RJ. The effects of high levels of vitamin E on the progression of atherosclerosis in the Watanabe heritable hyperlipidemic rabbit. *J Nutr Biochem.* 1993;4:651.
51. Kleinveld HA, Demacker PNM, Stalenhoef AFH. Comparative study on the effect of low-dose vitamin E and probucol on the susceptibility of LDL to oxidation and the progression of atherosclerosis in Watanabe heritable hyperlipidemic rabbits. *Arterioscler Thromb.* 1994;14:1386.
52. Kleinveld HA, Hak-Lemmers HL, Hectors MP, de Fouw NJ, Demacker PN, Stalenhoef AF. Vitamin E and fatty acid intervention does not attenuate the progression of atherosclerosis in watanabe heritable hyperlipidemic rabbits. *Arterioscler Thromb Vasc Biol.* 1995;15:545.
53. Fruebis J, Bird DA, Pattison J, Palinski W. Extent of antioxidant protection of plasma LDL is not a predictor of the antiatherogenic effect of antioxidants. *J Lipid Res* 1997;38:2455.
54. Smith TL, Kummerow FA. Effect of dietary vitamin E on plasma lipids and atherogenesis in restricted ovulator chickens. *Atherosclerosis* 1989;75:105.
55. Bocan TM, Mueller SB, Brown EQ, Uhlendorf PD, Mazur MJ, Newton RS. Antiatherosclerotic effects of antioxidants are lesion-specific when evaluated in hypercholesterolemic New Zealand white rabbits. *Exp Mol Pathol.* 1992;57:70.
56. Chen L, Haught WH, Yang B, Saldeen TG, Parathasarathy S, Mehta JL. Preservation of endogenous antioxidant activity and inhibition of lipid peroxidation as common mechanisms of antiatherosclerotic effects of vitamin E, lovastatin and amlodipine. *J Am Coll Cardiol.* 1997;30:569.
57. Verlangieri AJ, Bush MJ. Effects of d-alpha-tocopherol supplementation on experimentally induced primate atherosclerosis. *J Am Coll Nutr.* 1992;11:131.
58. Parker RA, Sabrah T, Cap M, Gill BT. Relation of vascular oxidative stress, α-tocopherol, and hypercholesterolemia to early atherosclerosis in hamsters. *Arterioscler Thromb Vasc Biol.* 1995;15:349.
59. Crawford RS, Kirk EA, Rosenfeld ME, LeBoeuf RC, Chait A. Dietary antioxidants inhibit development of fatty streak lesions in the LDL receptor-deficient mouse. *Arterioscler Thromb Biol.* 1998;18:1506.
60. Godfried SL, Combs GF, Saroka JM, Dillingham LA. Potentiation of atherosclerotic lesions in rabbits by a high dietary level of vitamin E. *Br J Nutr.* 1989;61:607.
61. Fruebis J, Carew TE, Palinski W. Effect of vitamin E on atherogenesis in LDL receptor-deficient rabbits. *Atherosclerosis* 1995,117.217.
62. Marshall FN. Pharmacology and toxicology of probucol. *Artery* 1982;10:7.
63. Kritchevsky D, Kirn HK, Tepper SA. Influence of 4,4-(isopropylidenedithio)bis(2,6-di-t-butylphenol)(DH-581) on experimental atherosclerosis in rabbits. *Proc Soc Exp Biol Med.* 1971;136:1216.
64. Tawara K, Ishihara M, Ogawa H, Tomikawa M. Effect of probucol, pantethine and their combinations on serum lipoprotein metabolism and on the incidence of atheromatous lesions in the rabbit. *Jpn J Pharmacol.* 1986;41:211.
65. Wissler RW, Vesselinovitch D. Combined effects of cholestyramine and probucol on regression of atherosclerosis in rhesus monkey aortas. *Appl Pathol.* 1983;1:89.
66. Parthasarathy S, Young SG, Witztum JL, Pittman RC, Steinberg D. Probucol inhibits oxidative modification of low density lipoprotein. *J Clin Invest.* 1986;77:641.
67. Kita T, Nagano Y, Yokode M, Ishii K, Kume N, Ooshima A, Yoshida H, Kawai C. Probucol prevents the progression of atherosclerosis in Watanabe heritable hyperlipidemic rabbit, an animal model for familial hypercholesterolemia. *Proc Natl Acad Sci USA.* 1987;84:5928.
68. Carew TE, Schwenke DC, Steinberg D. Antiatherogenic effect of probucol unrelated to its hypocholesterolemic effect: evidence that antioxidants *in vivo* can selectively inhibit low density lipoprotein degradation in macrophage-rich fatty streaks and slow the progression of atherosclerosis in the Watanabe heritable hyperlipidemic rabbit. *Proc Natl Acad Sci USA.* 1987;84:7725.

69.   Mao SJT, Yates MT, Parker RA, Chi EM, Jackson RL. Attenuation of atherosclerosis in a modified strain of hypercholesterolemic Watanabe rabbits with the use of a probucol analogue (MDL 29,311) that does not lower serum cholesterol. *Arterioscler Thromb.* 1991;11:1266.

70.   Sasahara M, Raines EW, Chait A, Carew TE, Steinberg D, Wahl PW, Ross R. Inhibition of hypercholesterolemia-induced atherosclerosis in the nonhuman primate by probucol: I. Is the extent of atherosclerosis related to resistance of LDL to oxidation? *J Clin Invest.* 1994;94:155.

71.   Zhang SH, Reddick RL, Avdievich E, Surles LK, Jones RG, Reynolds JB, Quarfordt SH, Maeda N. Paradoxical enhancement of atherosclerosis by probucol treatment in apolipoprotein E-deficient mice. *J Clin Invest.* 1997;99:2858.

72.   Bird DA, Tangirala RK, Fruebis J, Steinberg D, Witztum JL, Palinski W. Effect of probucol on LDL oxidation and atherosclerosis in LDL receptor-deficient mice. *J Lipid Res* 1998;39:1079.

73.   Cynshi O, Kawabe Y, Suzuki T, Takashima Y, Kaise H, Nakamura M, Ohba Y, Kato Y, Tamura K, Hayasaka A, Higashida A, Sakaguchi H, Takeya M, Takahashi K, Inoue K, Noguchi N, Niki E, Kodama T. Antiatherogenic effects of the antioxidant BO-653 in three different animal models. *Proc Natl Acad Sci USA.* 1998;95:10123.

74.   Sparrow CP, Doebber TW, Olszewski J, Wu MS, Ventre J, Stevens KA, Chao Y. Low density liopoprotein is protected from oxidation and the pregression of atherosclerosis is slowed in cholesterol-fed rabbits by the antioxidant N,N'diphenyl-phenylenediamine. *J Clin Invest.* 1992;89:1885.

75.   Stein Y, Stein O, Delplanque B, Fesmire JD, Lee DM, Alaupovic P. Lack of effect of probucol on atheroma formation in cholesterol-fed rabbits kept at comparable plasma cholesterol levels. *Atherosclerosis* 1989;75:145.

76.   Daugherty A, Zweifel BS, Schonfeld G. Probucol attenuates the development of aortic atherosclerosis in cholesterol-fed rabbits. *Br J Pharmacol.* 1989;98:612.

77.   Finckh B, Niendorf A, Rath M, Beisiegel U. Antiatherosclerotic effect of probucol in WHHL rabbits: are there plasma parameters to evaluate this effect? *Eur J Clin Pharmacol.* 1991;40:Suppl-80.

78.   Daugherty A, Zweifel BS, Schonfeld G. The effects of probucol on the progression of atherosclerosis in mature Watanabe heritable hyperlipidaemic rabbits. *Br J Pharmacol* 1991;103:1013.

79.   Nagano Y, Nakamura T, Matsuzawa Y, Cho M, Ueda Y, Kita T. Probucol and atherosclerosis in the Watanabe heritable hyperlipidemic rabbit--long-term antiatherogenic effect and effects on established plaques. *Atherosclerosis* 1992;92:131.

80.   Yamaguchi Y, Kitagawa S, Imaizumi N, Kunitomo M, Fujiwara M. Enhancement of aortic cholesterol deposition by dietary linoleic acid in cholesterol-fed mice: an animal model for primary screening of antiatherosclerotic agents. *J Pharmacol Toxicol Methods* 1993;30:169.

81.   Bocan TM, Mazur MJ, Mueller SB, Charlton G, Kieft KA, Krause BR. Atherosclerotic lesion development in hypercholesterolemic Japanese quail following probucol treatment: a biochemical and morphologic evaluation. *Pharmacol Res* 1994;29:65.

82.   Fruebis J, Steinberg D, Dresel HA, Carew TA. A comparison of the antiatherogenic effects of probucol and of a structural analogue of probucol in low density lipoprotein receptor-deficient rabbits. *J Clin Invest.* 1994;94:392.

83.   Braesen JH, Beisiegel U, Niendorf A. Probucol inhibits not only the progression of atherosclerotic disease, but causes a different composition of atherosclerotic lesions in WHHL-rabbits. *Virchows Arch.* 1995;426:179.

84.   Del Rio M, Chulia T, Ruiz E, Tejerina T. Action of probucol in arteries from normal and hypercholesterolaemic rabbits. *Br J Pharmacol* 1996;118:1639.

85.   Kogushi M, Tanaka H, Ohtsuka I, Yamada T, Kobayashi H, Saeki T, Takada M, Hiyoshi H, Yanagimachi M, Kimura T, Yoshitake S, Saito I. Anti-atherosclerotic effect of E5324, an inhibitor of acyl-CoA:cholesterol acyltransferase, in Watanabe heritable hyperlipidemic rabbits. *Atherosclerosis* 1996;124:203.

86.   Hoshida S, Yamashita N, Igarashi J, Aoki K, Kuzuya T, Hori M. Long-term probucol treatment reverses the severity of myocardial injury in watanabe heritable hyperlipidemic rabbits. *Arterioscler Thromb Vasc Biol.* 1997;17:2801.

87.   Wu YJ, Hong CY, Lin SJ, Wu P, Shiao MS. Increase of vitamin E content in LDL and reduction of atherosclerosis in cholesterol-fed rabbits by a water-soluble antioxidant-rich fraction of Salvia miltiorrhiza. *Arterioscler Thromb Biol.* 1998;18:481.

88. Oshima R, Ikeda T, Watanabe K, Itakura H, Sugiyama N. Probucol treatment attenuates the aortic atherosclerosis in Watanabe heritable hyperlipidemic rabbits. *Atherosclerosis* 1998;137:13.
89. Keaney JF, Jr., Frei B. Antioxidant protection of low-density lipoprotein and its role in the prevention of atherosclerotic vascular disease, in Frei B (ed): *Natural antioxidants in human health and disease*. San Diego, Academic Press, 1994, pp 303-352.
90. Jialal I, Norkus EP, Cristol L, Grundy SM. Beta-carotene inhibits the oxidative modification of low density lipoprotein. *Biochim Biophys Acta*. 1991;1086:134.
91. Gaziano JM, Hatta A, Flynn M, Johnson EJ, Krinsky NI, Ridker PM, Hennekens CH, Frei B. Supplementation with beta-carotene *in vivo* and *in vitro* does not inhibit low density lipoprotein (LDL) oxidation. *Atherosclerosis* 1995;112:187.
92. Hatta A, Frei B. Oxidative modification and antioxidant protection of human low density lipoprotein at high and low oxygen partial pressures. *J Lipid Res*. 1995;36:2383.
93. Gainer JL, Jones JR. The use of crocetin in experimental atherosclerosis. *Experientia* 1975;31:548.
94. Byorkhem I, Henriksson-Freyschuss A, Breuer O, Diczfalusy U, Berglund L, Henriksson P. The antioxidant butylated hydroxytoluene protects against atherosclerosis. *Arterioscler Thromb*. 1991;11:15.
95. Freyschuss A, Sitko-Rahm A, Swidenborg J, Henriksson P, Bj, Berglund L, Nilsson J. Antioxidant treatment inhibits the development of intimal thickening after balloon injury of the aorta in hypercholesterolemic rabbits. *J Clin Invest*. 1993;91:1282.
96. Jialal I, Vega GL, Grundy SM. Physiologic levels of ascorbate inhibit oxidative modification of low density lipoprotein. *Atherosclerosis* 1990;82:185.
97. Retsky KL, Freeman MW, Frei B. Ascorbic acid oxidation product(s) protect human low density lipoprotein against atherogenic modification. Anti- rather than prooxidant activity of vitamin C in the presence of transition metal ions. *J Biol Chem*. 1993;268:1304.
98. Willis GC. An experimental study of the intimal ground substance in atherosclerosis. *Can Med Assoc J*. 1953;69:17.
99. Fujinami T, Okado K, Senda K, Sugimura M, Kishikawa M. Experimental atherosclerosis with ascorbic acid deficiency. *Jap Circ J*. 1971;35:1559.
100. Ginter E, Ondreicka R, Bobek P, Simko V. The influence of chronic vitamin C deficiency on fatty acid composition of blood serum, liver triglycerides, and cholesterol esters in guinea pigs. *J Nutr*. 1969;99:261.
101. Ginter E, Babala J, Cerven J. The effect of chronic hypovitaminosis C on the metabolism of cholesterol and atherogenesis in guinea pigs. *J Atheroscler Res*. 1969;10:341.
102. Verlangieri AJ, Jollis TM, Mumma RO. Effects of ascorbic acid and its 2-sulfate on rabbit aortic intimal thickening. *Blood Vessels*. 1977;14:157.
103. Beetens JR, Coene MC, Veheyen A, Zonnekeyn L, Herman AG. Vitamin C increases the prostacyclin production and decreases the vascular lesions in experimental atherosclerosis in rabbits. *Prostaglandins* 1986;32:335.
104. Kimura H, Yamada Y, Morita Y, Ikeda J, Matsuo T. Dietary ascorbic acid depresses plasma and low density lipoprotein lipid peroxidation in genetically scorbutic rabbits. *J Nutr*. 1992;122:1904.
105. Wilson JD. Disorders of vitamins: deficiency, escess, and errors of metabolism, in Petersdorf RG, Adams RD, Braunwald E, Isselbacher KJ, Martin JB, Wilson JD (eds): *Harrison's principals of internal medicine*. New York, McGraw Hill, 1983, pp 461-472.
106. Bannerjee S, Ghosh PK. Hexosamine and hydroxyproline contents of tissues in scurvy. *Proc Soc Exp Biol Med*. 1961;107:275.
107. Ginter E, Nemec R, Cerven J, Mikus L. Quantification of lowered cholesterol oxidation in guinea pigs with latent vitamin C deficiency. *Lipids* 1973;8:135.
108. Tangirala RK, Casanada F, Miller E, Witztum JL, Steinberg D, Palinski W. Effect of the antioxidant N,N'-diphenyl 1,4-phenylenediamine (DPPD) on atherosclerosis in apo E-deficient mice. *Atheroscler. Thromb. Vasc. Biol*. 1995;15:1625-2630.
109. Pratico D,

12 HUMAN STUDIES OF ANTIOXIDANTS AND VASCULAR FUNCTION

Elizabeth S. Biegelsen and Joseph A. Vita

INTRODUCTION

Antioxidants are commonly consumed by patients for the prevention and treatment of cardiovascular disease (CVD) based upon recent clinical studies that suggest an association between increased intake of certain antioxidant vitamins and reduced risk for CVD. It is important to realize, however, that the putative mechanisms of any benefit remain uncertain. Investigations in animal models indicate that increased oxidative stress contributes to the atherogenic process and to the development of vascular dysfunction. In such models, antioxidant treatment has often been shown to limit the extent of atherosclerosis and maintain normal vascular function. If applicable to humans, these effects could explain the clinical benefits of antioxidants.

Recently, investigators have examined the effects of antioxidant therapy on atherosclerosis and endothelial function in human subjects. This chapter will first outline the clinical importance of atherosclerosis progression and endothelial dysfunction, and will then review in detail the available studies on the effects of natural and synthetic antioxidants on these parameters. The effects of low-molecular weight lipid-soluble and water-soluble antioxidants, as well as enzymatic antioxidants, will be considered in turn. These studies provide important insight into how antioxidants affect the development and clinical expression of CVD in humans and may guide their future therapeutic use.

ANTIOXIDANTS, ATHEROSCLEROSIS PROGRESSION AND CLINICAL EXPRESSION OF CVD

According to the well-accepted oxidative modification hypothesis of atherosclerosis reviewed in Chapter 4, oxidative modification of low-density lipoprotein (LDL) is a key step in the atherogenic process, ultimately leading to foam cell formation (1). Oxidized LDL (oxLDL) also promotes intimal inflammation and vascular dysfunction, which contribute to the development of an atherosclerotic plaque (1). As discussed in Chapter 13, some epidemiological studies suggest that increased intake of antioxidant vitamins is associated with decreased risk for CVD. Since antioxidants are capable of inhibiting LDL oxidation, many investigators have assumed that antioxidants cause this reduction in clinical events by inhibiting the formation and progression of atherosclerotic lesions. However, this assumption may be overly simplistic. For example, inhibition of LDL oxidation does not necessarily correlate with a reduction in atherogenesis in animal models (2). In addition, it has been difficult to demonstrate any effect of antioxidant intake on lesion severity or progression in humans (3), despite profound effects on clinical events (4).

Another problem with this paradigm is the assumption that clinical expression of atherosclerosis relates to the severity or progression of lesions. In fact, it is now recognized that atherosclerosis is a dynamic disease. Most clinical events do not result from gradual progression of lesions, and lesion severity does not predict risk for acute clinical events (5-7). Instead, acute myocardial infarction, unstable angina, and stroke usually occur following rupture of a relatively mild atherosclerotic plaque in the coronary or cerebral circulation with subsequent thrombosis and vasospasm, leading to an acute reduction or obstruction of blood flow (7). The physical and biological factors that lead to plaque rupture and influence the severity of the subsequent thrombotic and vasoconstrictor response remain uncertain, but these factors clearly reflect a loss of normal homeostatic mechanisms in the vasculature (5). These observations have prompted a number of investigators to examine the effects of antioxidants on vascular function as an alternative explanation for the apparent beneficial effects of antioxidants. The next section provides a brief review of the functions of the vascular endothelium under normal and atherosclerotic conditions, with particular attention to the impact of oxidative stress on vascular function. This section will be followed by a detailed discussion of antioxidants in cardiovascular disease.

Vascular Dysfunction In CVD

Normal Endothelial Function

Under normal conditions, the endothelium exerts vasodilator, antithrombotic, anti-inflammatory, and growth-inhibiting effects on the vessel wall through the release of a number of paracrine factors, including nitric oxide (NO). Endothelium-derived NO (EDNO) is synthesized from L-arginine by a constitutive endothelial isoform of NO synthase (eNOS) (8). Nitric oxide relaxes vascular smooth muscle primarily by stimulating guanylyl cyclase activity and increasing intracellular cyclic-3',5'-guanosine monophosphate (cGMP) concentration (9). Several endogenous factors such as shear stress (10), thrombin and serotonin (11), catecholamines, and muscarinic receptor agonists, such as methacholine and acetylcholine (12) stimulate the synthesis and release of NO. In general, the vasodilator effects of EDNO serve to limit arterial shear stress and oppose the direct vasoconstrictor effects of these factors on the underlying smooth muscle. In addition to NO, endothelial cells synthesize a number of other vasodilator and vasoconstrictor substances that contribute to the maintenance of normal vasomotor tone including prostacyclin (PGI_2) (13), endothelium-derived hyperpolarizing factor (14), adenosine (15), and endothelin (16).

The normal endothelium modulates other homeostatic functions in the vasculature. For example, nitric oxide and PGI_2 inhibit platelet function (17). Endothelial cells also inhibit thrombosis via synthesis of heparan sulfate proteoglycans, which exhibit anticoagulant activity (18), and through the action of thrombomodulin, which reduces thrombin activity at the endothelial surface (19). Fibrinolysis is subject to modulation by the endothelium through the secretion of tissue-type plasminogen activator (t-PA) and plasminogen activator inhibitor-1 (PAI-1) (20), which maintain a pro-thrombolytic state. The growth of vascular smooth muscle cells is regulated by endothelium-derived growth inhibitors including NO, PGI_2, and heparan sulfate (21-24). Finally, the normal endothelium serves as a barrier to inflammatory cells, in part through the action of EDNO (25).

Endothelial Dysfunction in Atherosclerosis

In the setting of atherosclerosis, the normal regulatory functions of the vascular endothelium are impaired (5, 23). Impairment of the endothelium-dependent vasodilator response in atherosclerosis and related disease states has been well-documented in humans. Ludmer and colleagues demonstrated that an intracoronary infusion of acetylcholine produced coronary artery dilation in healthy young subjects with angiographically normal coronary arteries (26). In contrast, acetylcholine produced "paradoxical" constriction in subjects with angiographic evidence of coronary atherosclerosis, while the vasodilator response to nitroglycerin was maintained (26). These findings are now understood largely to reflect a loss of acetylcholine-mediated release of EDNO and the ensuing unopposed vasoconstrictor effects of acetylcholine on vascular smooth muscle. Similar observations were subsequently made in isolated vascular tissue from hypercholesterolemic animals and from human subjects with coronary artery disease (27). Loss of the normal vasodilator response of epicardial coronary arteries to muscarinic agonists may precede the development of coronary atherosclerosis in patients with coronary risk factors, particularly hypercholesterolemia (28). This observation supports animal studies indicating that loss of EDNO action contributes to the development of atherosclerosis (25).

Since this chapter will focus in large part on the effects of antioxidants on EDNO action in human subjects, a further word about the methodology for study of endothelial vasomotor function is appropriate. While clinically relevant, the coronary circulation is not readily available for study in subjects who do not require cardiac catheterization. For this reason, investigators have developed invasive and non-invasive methods for examination of EDNO bioactivity in the peripheral circulation. In normal patients, infusion of acetylcholine or methacholine into the brachial artery causes EDNO-mediated vasodilation of forearm resistance vessels and an increase in forearm blood flow, as assessed by venous occlusion plethysmography. This response is impaired in patients with atherosclerotic risk factors such as diabetes mellitus (29), hypercholesterolemia (30), hypertension (31), and patients with clinically evident atherosclerosis (32).

Nitric oxide bioactivity can also be assayed as endothelium-dependent, flow-mediated vasodilation of the conduit brachial artery using non-invasive vascular ultrasound. With this method, vessel diameter is measured at baseline and during reactive hyperemia induced by transient cuff occlusion of limb blood flow (33). The increase in flow leads to increased shear stress at the endothelial surface and, as a consequence, stimulation of EDNO release. Depending on the extent of hyperemia and arterial size, the brachial artery dilates 6 - 15% on average in normal subjects (33). The response is largely blocked by an intra-arterial infusion of the NO synthase inhibitor N^G-monomethyl-L-arginine (L-NMMA), confirming that flow-mediated dilation of the brachial artery depends on NO synthesis (34,35). Brachial artery flow-mediated dilation is impaired in subjects with coronary risk factors and in patients with documented coronary artery disease (36). Recent reports have shown close correlation between noninvasive measurements of brachial artery flow-mediated dilation and coronary vasodilation in response to acetylcholine (37).

Although less well studied in human subjects, there is experimental evidence that the fibrinolytic and anti-inflammatory properties of the endothelium are also impaired in the setting of atherosclerosis and hypercholesterolemia. Atherosclerosis is associated with a reduction in the activity of t-PA, largely due to an increase in PAI-1 activity (38). Expression of intracellular adhesion molecule-1 (ICAM-1) is increased in the endothelium of atherosclerotic plaques in humans (39), and increased circulating levels of ICAM-1 (40) and C-reactive protein (41) are associated with increased CVD risk. Thus, endothelial dysfunction in hypercholesterolemia and atherosclerosis appears to be a generalized abnormality that includes impaired NO bioactivity, thrombosis, and inflammation (5).

There is growing evidence that endothelial dysfunction may contribute to the clinical expression of coronary artery disease. In patients with stable angina, loss of EDNO bioactivity may lead to pathological constrictor responses that potentiate ischemia in the setting of exercise (42) or mental stress (43). EDNO action is more severely impaired in patients with unstable angina than in patients with chronic stable angina (44) and in an infarct-related stenosis of the coronary artery compared to a non-infarct-related stenosis (45). Experimental studies suggest that accumulation of inflammatory cells in atherosclerotic plaques may promote rupture via expression of matrix metalloproteinases that degrade collagen (6). Thus, endothelial dysfunction may contribute to the risk for plaque rupture and to the severity of the resulting thrombosis and vasospasm that obstruct the arterial lumen (5).

Oxidative Stress and Endothelial Dysfunction

As detailed in Chapter 9, there is firm evidence that oxidative stress, defined as an excess of endogenous oxidants when compared to antioxidants, contributes to endothelial dysfunction in atherosclerosis. In this regard, studies have focused particularly on the importance of increased production of superoxide anion and on the accumulation of oxLDL in the vasculature. Regarding superoxide anion, it is known that superoxide and NO react rapidly to form peroxynitrite, thus reducing the biological activity of NO (46). Vascular production of superoxide anion is increased in experimental hypercholesterolemia, and specific superoxide scavengers restore EDNO action in these models (47-49).

There also is good evidence that oxLDL may impair the biological activity of EDNO as well as other functions of the endothelium. Ox-LDL is cytotoxic to endothelial cells (50) and may inactivate NO directly (51). oxLDL impairs the release of EDNO from endothelial cells by interrupting G-protein-dependent signal transduction (52) and decreasing expression of eNOS in cultured human endothelial cells (53). Regarding other functions of the endothelium, oxLDL stimulates production of endothelin (54) and tissue factor (55). In addition, products of LDL oxidation such as lysophosphatidylcholine may stimulate expression of ICAM-1 (56) and PAI-1 (57) and increase vascular production of superoxide anion (58). Thus, oxLDL impairs the vasodilator, antithrombotic, and antiinflammatory functions of the endothelium. Consistent with this notion, Heitzer and colleagues demonstrated a significant inverse correlation between EDNO bioactivity in forearm resistance vessels and plasma antibodies against oxLDL in patients with coronary artery disease and a history of cigarette smoking (59). Overall, the available evidence suggests a causal link between increased oxidative stress and endothelial dysfunction in atherosclerosis.

ANTIOXIDANT THERAPY IN PATIENTS WITH CVD

In light of the extensive evidence that increased oxidative stress contributes to both lesion formation and endothelial dysfunction in atherosclerosis, it seems reasonable to consider that antioxidant supplementation might have clinical benefit against CVD. Naturally occurring antioxidants may be divided into low-molecular-weight compounds, both lipid-soluble and water-soluble, enzymatic antioxidants, and non-enzymatic protein antioxidants; these are reviewed extensively in Chapter 3. This chapter will review the human studies of antioxidants and vascular function, beginning with low-molecular-weight, lipid-soluble compounds, such as α-tocopherol, phenolic estrogens, and flavonoids, as well as probucol, a synthetic lipid-soluble antioxidant. Next the chapter will discuss the data for water-soluble antioxidants, such as ascorbic acid and glutathione. Finally, studies employing enzymatic antioxidants, specifically superoxide dismutase and glutathione peroxidase, will be reviewed. For each antioxidant, we will briefly review the evidence for clinical benefit, summarize the basic data suggesting effects on vascular function, and discuss in detail the clinical studies of vascular function conducted in humans.

α-Tocopherol

α-Tocopherol (the primary component of vitamin E) is the predominant antioxidant in lipoproteins and cell membranes. It is a potent scavenger of reactive oxygen species that initiate or propagate lipid peroxidation (60). Following supplementation in human subjects, α-tocopherol accumulates in LDL and increases its resistance to oxidation (61). In addition, α-tocopherol may have direct effects on cellular function such as the release of EDNO, resistance to the adverse effects of oxidized LDL, reduced platelet aggregation, and reduced monocyte adhesion (2).

Clinical Events

As reviewed in Chapter 13, epidemiological studies support a link between an increase in the intake of α-tocopherol and a reduction in cardiovascular disease (62). However, randomized clinical trials conducted in patients with known coronary disease have demonstrated mixed results. In the Cambridge Heart Antioxidant Study (CHAOS), 2002 patients with angiographically proven coronary artery disease were randomized to receive 400-800 IU/day of α-tocopherol or placebo and followed for a median of 510 days. α-Tocopherol treatment reduced the combined endpoint of cardiovascular death and non-fatal myocardial infarction by 47 percent (4). There was an impressive 77% reduction in the risk of non-fatal myocardial infarction in the α-tocopherol group that was apparent after only 200 days of treatment. In contrast, the α-Tocopherol, β-Carotene Cancer Prevention Study (ATBC) showed no reduction in cardiovascular disease with α-tocopherol treatment in male smokers with a prior myocardial infarction (63). However, the dose of α-tocopherol in that trial (50 mg) was much lower than in the CHAOS trial, and lower than the protective dose range suggested by prior cohort studies (100 – 250 IU) (64,65). Thus, treatment with an adequate dose of α-tocopherol appears to reduce CVD risk.

Investigators have also examined the effects of α-tocopherol on symptoms of peripheral vascular disease and have obtained similar results. For example, 50 mg/day of α-tocopherol was found to have no effect on the severity of claudication in subjects enrolled in the ATBC study (66). In contrast, two older trials did show a reduction in symptoms of intermittent claudication following long term α-tocopherol treatment (300 – 1600 mg/d for 10 – 40 months) in patients with established peripheral vascular disease (67,68).

In addition to the reduction in clinical events, some trials have also shown an association between increased intake of α-tocopherol and decreased extent of atherosclerosis. For example, in the Atherosclerosis Risk in Communities Study (ARIC), increased intake of α-tocopherol was associated with reduced carotid artery intimal thickness in older women, but not in other subgroups (69). A subgroup analysis of patients in the Cholesterol Lowering Atherosclerosis Study (CLAS) showed that daily supplementation of more than 100 IU of α-tocopherol was associated with a reduction in coronary artery lesion progression, particularly when combined with lipid lowering therapy (70). Although statistically significant, the changes in lesion severity in that study were very small, and it is difficult to attribute the large reduction in CVD events to those effects.

Effects on Vascular Function: Basic Evidence

The mechanisms of the beneficial effect of α-tocopherol on CVD remain unclear. Since oxidative modification of LDL is a key event in the atherogenic process and since α-tocopherol inhibits LDL oxidation, investigators have hypothesized that α-tocopherol may slow progression or cause regression of atheroslcerotic lesions. Although the results are somewhat mixed, a number of studies in animal models support this contention (71). However, data from human studies such as CHAOS suggest that antioxidants may influence CAD risk by mechanisms other than preventing formation or progression of atheroslcerotic lesions (4). As has been proposed for cholesterol-lowering agents (5,72), it is possible that antioxidants not only affect the severity of stenosis, but also the biology of the lesion itself, including endothelial vasomotor function and other properties of the vascular endothelium.

As reviewed in Chapter 9, it is well established that α-tocopherol has a beneficial effect on endothelial vasomotor function in animal models of atherosclerosis. For example, several investigators have demonstrated that α-tocopherol preserves normal acetylcholine-induced arterial relaxation in hypercholesterolemic rabbits (73-75). α-Tocopherol also preserves endothelium-dependent dilation in experimental models of diabetes mellitus (76). These effects likely relate both to antioxidant protection of LDL and to direct tissue effects of α-tocopherol (2).

In addition to its effects on endothelial vasomotor function, α-tocopherol has been shown to inhibit leukocyte adhesion to the endothelial surface. In human endothelial cell culture, loading the cells with α-tocopherol inhibited cytokine-induced monocyte binding (77). Similarly, monocytes from healthy subjects treated with 8 weeks of supplemental α-tocopherol (1200 IU/day) were less adherent to resting and activated endothelial cells than at baseline or after a 6 week washout phase (78).

Effects on Vascular Function: Human Data

Despite the strong evidence for a beneficial effect of α-tocopherol on EDNO action in cell culture and in experimental animals, studies of this issue in human subjects have provided varied results (see Table for a list of available studies of antioxidant treatment and endothelial vasomotor function in human subjects). Gilligan and colleagues examined the effect of 4 weeks of supplemental α-tocopherol (800 IU/d), given in conjunction with β-carotene (30 mg/d) and ascorbic acid (1000 mg/d), on LDL oxidation and endothelial function in hypercholesterolemic patients (79). They

Table. Clinical studies of antioxidants and endothelial vasomotor function.

Study	Vascular Bed	Condition	N	Effect
α-Tocopherol				
Gilligan (79)	Forearm	HC	19	Negative
Elliot (32)	Forearm	MI	12	Negative
Chowienczyk (80)	Forearm	HC/CAD	20	Negative
McDowell (81)	Forearm	HC	24	Negative
Green (84)	Forearm	HC	7	Positive
Neunteufl (82)	Brachial	HC	7	Positive
Motoyama (83)	Brachial	VA	30	Positive
β-Carotene				
Gilligan (79)	Forearm	HC	19	Negative
Estrogen				
Lieberman (100)	Brachial	PM	13	Positive
Reis (102)	Coronary	PM	22	Positive
Probucol				
Anderson (124)	Coronary	CAD	49	Positive
McDowell (81)	Forearm	HC	24	Negative
Ascorbic Acid				
Levine (135)	Brachial	CAD	46	Positive
Ito (137)	Brachial	CAD	10	Positive
Plotnick (139)	Brachial	PPH	20	Positive
Ting (140)	Forearm	DM	10	Positive
Ting (142)	Forearm	HC	11	Positive
Taddei (143)	Forearm	HTN	14	Positive
Hornig (138)	Forearm	CHF	15	Positive
Heitzer (145)	Forearm	TOB	10	Positive
Solzbach (146)	Coronary	HTN	22	Positive
Kugiyama (147)	Coronary	VAS	32	Positive
Glutathione				
Vita (166)	Brachial	CAD	48	Positive
Kugiyama (167)	Coronary	VAS	26	Positive
N-acetylcysteine				Negative
Creager (169)	Forearm	Normals	29	Negative
Superoxide Dismutase				
Garcia (175)	Forearm	HTN	20	Negative
Garcia (176)	Forearm	HC	20	Negative
Meredith (178)	Coronary	CAD	8	Positive

Abbreviations: CAD, coronary artery disease; CHF, congestive heart failure; DM, diabetes mellitus; HC, hypercholesterolemia; HTN, hypertension; PPH, post-prandial hypertriglyceridemia; TOB, tobacco use; VAS, vasospastic angina.

observed a reduction in the susceptibility of LDL to oxidation, which correlated strongly with plasma α-tocopherol levels. However, there was no improvement in endothelium-dependent vasodilation as measured by forearm blood flow responses to acetylcholine. Likewise, 3 months of supplemental α-tocopherol (800 IU/d) failed to improve forearm blood flow responses to acetylcholine, which were abnormal at baseline in patients with recent myocardial infarction (32). Chowienczyk and colleagues also observed no improvement in the forearm blood flow responses to acetylcholine following 8 weeks of α-tocopherol (400 IU/d) in patients with mild hypercholesterolemia and coronary artery disease (80). Similarly, McDowell and colleagues found no effect on forearm microvascular responses in hypercholesterolemic patients on simvastatin therapy who were randomized to 8 weeks of α-tocopherol (400 IU), probucol, or placebo (81).

In contrast to these carefully performed negative studies, several studies and preliminary reports suggest that α-tocopherol treatment improves EDNO bioactivity function in human subjects. In a cross-over study of seven patients with hypercholesterolemia, Neunteufl and colleagues reported that the combination of α-tocopherol (300 IU/d) and simvastatin therapy for eight weeks was associated with a more marked improvement in brachial artery flow-mediated dilation when compared to simvastatin alone (82). In patients with vasospastic angina, Motoyama and colleagues reported that α-tocopherol (300 mg/d) improved brachial artery flow-mediated dilation. That improvement was associated with an increase in plasma levels of α-tocopherol and a reduction in plasma thiobarbituric acid reactive substances (TBARS), suggesting a reduction in lipid peroxidation (83). In a recent study, Green and colleagues reported improved forearm blood flow responses to acetylcholine following four weeks of α-tocopherol (1000 IU/d) in hypercholesterolemic subjects (84). Heitzer and colleagues reported a beneficial effect of four months of α-tocopherol treatment on endothelium-dependent vasodilation of forearm microvessels in subjects with a history of both hypercholesterolemia and cigarette smoking, but not in patients with either hypercholesterolemia or smoking alone (85). In that preliminary study, the improvement in endothelial function was associated with a reduction in plasma antibodies against oxidized LDL.

It is notable that nearly all of the studies which measure the effect of α-tocopherol on forearm blood flow responses fail to show improvement, while the studies of the effect of α-tocopherol on brachial artery flow-mediated dilation demonstrate beneficial effects. This raises the possibility that α-tocopherol may affect conduit vessels to a greater extent than resistance vessels. Other reasons for the discrepant results of the above studies could relate to differences in the studied patient population, concurrent therapy, duration of treatment, or α-tocopherol dose. There is a clear need for a larger scale, well-controlled study of this question.

In summary, despite the evidence of beneficial effects of α-tocopherol on atherogenesis and vascular cell function in experimental models, it remains uncertain whether α-tocopherol exerts similar benefits in human subjects. The idea that α-tocopherol acts to improve endothelial function has also been difficult to confirm in human subjects, although the available studies have been limited to relatively short-term therapy (1-4 months) and have largely been restricted to examination of forearm microvessels. On the other hand, there is accumulating evidence that α-tocopherol improves brachial artery flow-mediated dilation, another measure of endothelial vasomotor function. Further study is needed to elucidate the specific mechanisms of the beneficial effects of α-tocopherol against CVD.

Estrogen

Clinical Events

Premenopausal women have a lower incidence of coronary artery disease than men of similar age (86). Further, epidemiological studies suggest that estrogen replacement therapy is associated with a reduced risk of cardiac disease among post-menopausal women (87) and with increased survival of women with proven coronary atherosclerosis (88). In the Cardiovascular Health Study, a population-based study of CVD in the elderly, estrogen replacement therapy was associated with less carotid artery intimal thickness and lower risk for significant carotid stenosis (89).

Despite these highly suggestive findings, a recent randomized, placebo-controlled study of hormone replacement therapy casts doubt on the overall benefit of estrogen for secondary prevention of CVD. The Heart and Estrogen/Progestin Replacement Study (HERS) randomized 2763 post-menopausal women with coronary heart disease to treatment with either placebo or estrogen plus progestin for four years; this study failed to demonstrate a reduction in CVD risk (90). It remains unknown whether estrogen without progesterone or longer-term hormone replacement therapy is beneficial. It is also unclear whether estrogen replacement therapy will have benefit for primary prevention of CVD.

Antioxidant Effects of Estrogen

Despite the recent negative findings of HERS, there continues to be great interest in the mechanisms for reduced cardiovascular disease in pre-menopausal women. It is well known that estrogen therapy reduces LDL cholesterol and increases HDL cholesterol (91). However, the available epidemiological studies suggest that only 25 to 50% of the reduction in CVD risk is due to these alterations in the lipid profile (92). One alternative mechanism for the beneficial effects of estrogen may relate to its antioxidant properties. Supraphysiological concentrations of phenolic estrogens are known to directly inhibit oxidative modification of LDL by copper ions, monocytes, and endothelial cells (93). 17β-estradiol, the most common endogenous form of estrogen, is also the most potent antioxidant (93). More recently, Shwaery and colleagues demonstrated that physiologic concentrations of 17β-estradiol in a plasma milieu provide antioxidant protection *in vitro*, possibly via the formation of fatty acid esters of 17β-estradiol (94). Sack and colleagues demonstrated that acute and chronic treatment of post-menopausal women with physiological concentrations of 17β-estradiol provides antioxidant protection of LDL (95).

Estradiol may also have cellular effects on vascular cells that relate to oxidative stress. For example, in cultured endothelial cells, estradiol inhibits production of superoxide anion and increases the biologic activity of EDNO (96). In addition, 17β-estradiol provides protection against oxLDL-mediated cytotoxicity (97) and inhibits cytokine-induced expression of endothelial cell leukocyte adhesion molecules including E-selectin, VCAM-1, and ICAM-1 (98).

Effect on Vascular Function: Basic Evidence

The antioxidant effects of estrogens may lead to favorable effects on vascular endothelial function. With regard to endothelial vasomotor function, 17β-estradiol preserved EDNO bioactivity in ovariectomized, hypercholesterolemic swine (99). This effect correlated with an increase in the resistance of LDL to *ex vivo* oxidation (99) supporting the hypothesis that 17β-estradiol preserves endothelial function in hypercholesterolemia by virtue of its antioxdidant activity.

Effect on Vascular Function: Human Data

Several studies have investigated the effect of estrogen on endothelial function in humans. In post-menopausal women, estrogen therapy improved flow-mediated, endothelium-dependent vasodilation of the brachial artery (100), and the effect was not attenuated by concomitant treatment with progesterone (101). In the coronary circulation of women with baseline endothelial dysfunction, short-term estrogen administration inhibited acetylcholine-mediated vasoconstriction (102). It should be emphasized that a definite link between the antioxidant properties of estrogen and improvement in endothelial vasomotor function has not been established in humans. It is likely that the beneficial effects of estrogen are multi-factorial.

Flavonoids

Flavonoids are a class of polyphenolic compounds found in certain foods including tea, apples, onions (103), and red wine (104). These compounds have the ability to scavenge reactive oxygen species, such as superoxide anion and lipid peroxyl radicals (105).

Clinical Events

Several studies have suggested that increased flavonoid intake is associated with decreased risk of CVD (62). A Finnish cohort study demonstrated that very low flavonoid consumption (<2.1-2.4 mg/d) was associated with increased total and CVD mortality (106). Similarly, the Zutphen Elderly Study demonstrated a dose-related relationship between flavonoid intake and CVD mortality after five (103) and ten (107) years of follow-up in a group of 805 Dutch men over age 65 years. In contrast, Rimm and colleagues found no significant association between flavonoid intake and CVD in a much larger population of male health professionals age 40 – 75 years in the United States (34,789) (108). The reason for these discrepant results is unclear, but could relate to the somewhat lower daily flavonoid intake in the Health Professionals Follow-up Study (20 mg/d) compared to the Zutphen Elderly study (26 mg/d) or other differences in the two populations.

Effect on Vascular Function

The potential mechanism of benefit of flavonoid intake against CVD remains unknown. Flavonoids have been shown to inhibit LDL oxidation (109), although in a careful study involving human subjects, tea consumption did not affect the susceptibility of isolated LDL to oxidation *ex vivo* (110). Several animal studies support a reduction in atherosclerosis extent with flavonoid treatment (111,112). To date, there are no studies in humans that have examined the effect of flavonoid consumption on atherosclerosis severity or vascular function.

Probucol

Probucol is a dimer of butylated hydroxytoluene (BHT) and was originally formulated as a lipid-lowering agent. It is a potent inhibitor of LDL oxidation by virtue of its ability to effectively donate hydrogen atoms (113). Probucol has been shown to limit atherogenesis in certain animal models (114-116), and provided some of the earliest evidence to support the oxidative modification hypothesis of atherosclerosis (1). These results prompted a number of clinical trials designed to examine the effects of probucol on the vasculature in CVD.

Clinical Events

The Probucol Quantitative Regression Swedish Trial (PQRST) is a large well-controlled study performed to examine the effects of probucol on the progression or regression of femoral atherosclerosis in human subjects. This study randomized 274 patients with femoral atherosclerosis to probucol (1 g/day) or placebo for three years (3). All subjects also received dietary recommendations and cholestyramine treatment if the total serum cholesterol was >250 mg/dl. The effect of treatment on femoral arterial lesion severity was examined using quantitative angiography. Overall, there was no beneficial effect of probucol. In fact, the control group, which received lipid-lowering therapy, demonstrated significant regression of atherosclerosis, while the probucol group did not. This apparent adverse effect of active treatment has been attributed in part to the HDL-lowering effect of probucol (117). Probucol has also been shown to reduce the rate of restenosis following coronary angioplasty in humans (118). This will be discussed in detail in Chapter 19.

Effect on Vascular Function: Basic Evidence

Probucol was has been shown to limit atherogenesis in the Watanabe Hereditable Hyperlipidemic rabbit (114,115), and in cholesterol-fed monkeys (119), where extent of lesion formation correlated inversely with the resistance of isolated LDL to oxidation. In addition to inhibiting atherogenesis in these animal models, probucol may also act to prevent the development of endothelial dysfunction. For example, probucol treatment preserves EDNO action in hypercholesterolemic (120) and diabetic rabbits (121). In hypercholesterolemic rabbits, improved endothelial function with probucol treatment is associated with a reduction in vascular production of superoxide anion and a reduction in vascular tissue levels of lysophosphatidylcholine and TBARS, reflecting a reduction in lipid peroxidation. In addition, probucol treatment resulted in increased resistance of isolated LDL to *ex vivo* oxidation (122). In human subjects, probucol treatment is associated with incorporation of the compound into LDL and increased resistance of LDL to *in vitro* oxidation (123).

In addition to its beneficial effects on EDNO-dependent vasomotion, probucol also influences leukocyte adhesion to the endothelial surface. Pretreatment of isolated human endothelial cells with probucol inhibits monocyte adhesion following cytokine activation (77). Thus, probucol may improve endothelial function through improvements in the vasomotor and anti-inflammatory functions of the vascular endothelium. Probucol may exert these effects via several mechanisms including antioxidant protection of LDL as well as direct effects on the vasculature.

Effect on Vascular Function: Human Data

The beneficial effect of probucol treatment on vascular endothelial function has also been demonstrated in human subjects (Table). Anderson and colleagues studied 49 patients with elevated cholesterol levels and randomized them either to a cholesterol-lowering diet, lovastatin and cholestyramine, or lovastatin and probucol (500 mg bid). The vasomotor response to intracoronary acetylcholine infusion was assessed at baseline and after one year of therapy. The group of patients treated with lovastatin and probucol showed more improvement in coronary artery endothelium-dependent vasomotion than the groups treated with lipid-lowering agents alone or diet alone (Figure 1) (124). The improvement in coronary endothelial function was shown to correlate with a reduction in the susceptibility of LDL to *ex vivo* oxidation (125), a finding consistent with an antioxidant mechanism for the beneficial effect of probucol. Another study examined the effect of probucol and simvastatin on endothelial function in forearm resistance vessels and observed no beneficial effect despite significant protection of LDL against *ex vivo* oxidation (81). Thus, the response to probucol treatment may depend on several factors including the duration of therapy and the specific vascular bed.

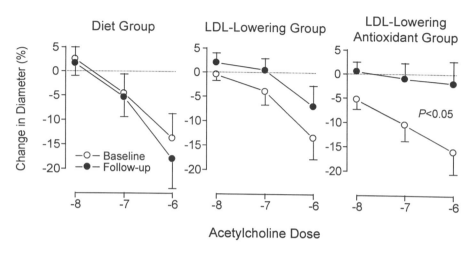

Figure 1: The effect of lovastatin and probucol on coronary artery endothelial function. Patients with coronary artery disease were randomized to treatment with diet, lovastatin plus cholestyramine, or lovastatin plus probucol for one year. As demonstrated, intracoronary acetylcholine produced dose-dependent coronary vasoconstriction at baseline, and the response was unchanged by diet treatment (left panel). One year of lovastatin plus cholestyramine produced a trend for less constriction to acetylcholine that did not achieve statistical significance (middle panel). However, the combination of lovastatin plus probucol significantly decreased the constrictor response to acetylcholine, a finding consistent with an improvement in the bioactivity of EDNO (right panel). Reproduced by permission from Anderson and colleagues (124).

In summary, despite the fact that probucol failed to induce regression of femoral atherosclerosis, it has a number of effects that are relevant to vascular function in human atherosclerosis including improved EDNO bioactivity, reduced adhesion of inflammatory cells, and decreased proliferation of smooth muscle cells. In fact, of all the lipid-soluble antioxidants, the data for a beneficial effect is strongest for probucol. Unfortunately, probucol also reduces HDL cholesterol, and thus it is unlikely that this agent will prove beneficial for the long-term treatment of patients with CVD.

Ascorbic Acid

Ascorbic acid is an important water-soluble antioxidant in intra- and extracellular fluids. Its biological activity derives from its strong reducing potential. Ascorbic acid is a scavenger of reactive oxygen species including superoxide anion and a potent inhibitor of lipid peroxidation (60). Although still somewhat controversial, there is accumulating evidence that ascorbic acid status relates to human CVD.

Clinical Events

Several case-control studies have shown that lower plasma and tissue ascorbic acid levels are associated with increased risk of cardiovascular disease. In Scottish men, low plasma concentrations of ascorbic acid were related to an increased risk of angina, although this effect was no longer significant after adjustment for cigarette smoking (126). In an angiographic study, Ramirez and Flowers found that leukocyte ascorbic acid levels were lower in patients with coronary artery disease (127). Recently, Vita and colleagues demonstrated an independent association between low plasma ascorbic acid levels and a recent unstable coronary syndrome in patients with coronary artery disease referred for catheterization (128).

Two prospective cohort studies have also suggested that ascorbic acid status relates to CVD. In Finnish men, a very low plasma ascorbic acid concentration (<11.4 µM)) correlated with an increased risk of acute myocardial infarction (129). The National Health And Nutrition Examination Survey (NHANES) follow-up study demonstrated a correlation between increased ascorbic acid intake (>50 mg/day) and decreased cardiovascular mortality (130). However, neither the Nurses' Health Study (64) nor the Health Professionals' Follow-up Study (65) showed an increase in major coronary events with lower intakes of ascorbic acid. In those more recent studies, the lowest quartile of ascorbic acid intake was relatively high. Since tissue stores become saturated with an ascorbic acid intake of only 100 mg/d, it is possible that the negative findings may be explained by a failure to separately consider the group of subjects with a sufficiently low ascorbic acid intake as was done in NHANES (131). To date, no randomized clinical trial has addressed the question of whether ascorbic acid treatment is beneficial for the prevention of CVD.

Several clinical trials have examined the relationship between ascorbic acid intake and atherosclerosis severity. The ARIC study demonstrated an inverse association between ascorbic acid intake and carotid artery wall thickness in men and women aged 55-64, but not in subjects aged 45-54 (69). In contrast, the Cholesterol Lowering and Atherosclerosis Study, a randomized trial evaluating the effect of cholesterol-lowering therapy on angiographic progression of disease, found that increased ascorbic acid intake in diet or supplements bore no relationship to the change in severity of coronary atherosclerosis over a two year period (70).

Effect on Vascular Function: Basic Evidence

Since ascorbic acid is a potent inhibitor of LDL oxidation in plasma (132), investigators have speculated that ascorbic acid treatment inhibits atherogenesis. Although there is evidence that scorbutic animals demonstrate increased lesion formation that can be reversed by ascorbic acid, there is little evidence that supplementation of non-deficient animals has any effect (71). In addition to its ability to inhibit LDL oxidation, other actions of ascorbic acid contribute to its effect on vascular function. Ascorbic acid is a scavenger of several reactive oxygen species, including superoxide anion (60).   At high physiologic concentrations, ascorbic acid prevents the superoxide-induced impairment of EDNO-mediated arterial relaxation (133).   Ascorbic acid also plays an important role in the maintenance of intracellular redox status, and may thereby improve EDNO action (134).

Effect on Vascular Function: Human Data

In contrast to the lack of evidence for an effect on lesion severity, there now is extensive and strong evidence that ascorbic acid improves vascular function in human atherosclerosis and associated disease states (Table).   In a randomized, placebo-controlled study of 46 patients with proven coronary artery disease, Levine and colleagues demonstrated an acute improvement in EDNO-dependent, flow-mediated dilation of the brachial artery two hours after a single two gram oral dose of ascorbic acid (135).   Ascorbic acid had no effect on nitroglycerin-mediated dilation, suggesting that the observed improvement related to an improvement in the bioactivity or production of EDNO.   In that study, ascorbic acid produced a 2.5 fold increase in plasma ascorbic acid concentration (46 ± 8 to 114 ± 11 μM), which was within the normal physiological range of 30 to 150 μM (60).   The acute beneficial effect of ascorbic acid on brachial artery flow-mediated dilation was confirmed in a second randomized, placebo-controlled study of patients with coronary disease (Figure 2) (136).   In that recent study, improvement in brachial artery flow-mediated dilation was sustained after 30 days of oral ascorbic acid treatment (500 mg/d).   Ito

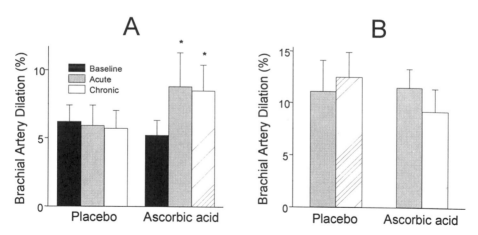

Figure 2: The effect of acute and chronic ascorbic acid treatment on brachial artery flow-mediated dilation (A) and nitroglycerin-mediated dilation (B) in patients with coronary artery disease and baseline flow-mediated dilation of less than 10%.   Brachial artery ultrasound was performed at baseline (black bars), two hours after a two gram oral dose of ascorbic acid (gray bars), and following one month of oral supplementation of 500 mg/d of ascorbic acid (hatched bars).   Ascorbic acid had a significant effect on flow-mediated dilation acutely, and this effect persisted following chronic therapy (P=0.002 by repeated measures ANOVA).   Ascorbic acid had no effect on nitroglycerin-mediated dilation (B), suggesting that the observed effect of ascorbic acid relates to an improvement in the bioavailability of EDNO. Reproduced with permission (136).

and colleagues also described acute improvement in brachial artery flow-mediated dilation one hour after a one gram intravenous dose of ascorbic acid in patients with CAD and stable angina (137). One prior study by Gilligan and colleagues failed to demonstrate a beneficial effect of ascorbic acid treatment. That study observed no improvement in forearm microvascular endothelial function following four weeks of ascorbic acid treatment (1 g/d) in combination with α-tocopherol and β-carotene in subjects with hypercholesterolemia (79). The reasons for these discrepant results are unclear, but could relate to the effects of concomitant treatment with other vitamins or to differences between conduit arteries and the microvasculature.

Physiological concentrations of ascorbic acid may also improve endothelial function in disease states other than atherosclerosis. Hornig and colleagues demonstrated improved flow-mediated dilation of the radial artery of patients with congestive heart failure (CHF) after 4 weeks of oral ascorbic acid therapy (2 g/day) (138). However, the etiology of CHF was not specified in that study, and it is possible that CAD was the underlying cause. In a study involving patients with idiopathic dilated cardiomyopathy, where the lack of CAD was confirmed by angiography, acute administration of ascorbic acid had no effect on brachial artery flow-mediated dilation (137).

An acute impairment of endothelial vasodilator function has been reported to occur following a high-fat meal (139). In that setting, oral administration of ascorbic acid (1 gram), together with 800 IU of α-tocopherol preserved brachial artery flow-mediated dilation (139). Since it is likely that a single dose of α-tocopherol had only a minor effect on plasma concentration, the observed effect may be attributed largely to ascorbic acid.

In addition to the studies involving physiological concentrations of ascorbic acid, several studies have examined the effects of an acute high-dose intra-arterial infusion of ascorbic acid on endothelial vasomotor function. In patients with non-insulin-dependent diabetes mellitus, Ting and colleagues observed an acute improvement in the forearm blood flow response to methacholine during intra-arterial ascorbic acid infusion at a rate of 24 mg/min, a dose calculated to produce local concentrations of 1 to 10 mM (140) (Figure 3). Similar findings were observed in the forearm microcirculation of patients with insulin-dependent diabetes mellitus (141), hypercholesterolemia (142), hypertension (143,144), congestive heart failure (138), and cigarette smoking (145). In the coronary circulation of patients with hypertension, acute intravenous infusion of three grams of ascorbic acid produced an improvement in flow-mediated dilation and in the vasomotor response to acetylcholine (146). Plasma levels of ascorbic acid were not measured in that study, but were probably in the 1 to 10 mM range. Finally, high-dose intra-arterial ascorbic acid infusion also blunted the vasoconstrictor response to intracoronary acetylcholine infusion in patients with vasospastic angina (147).

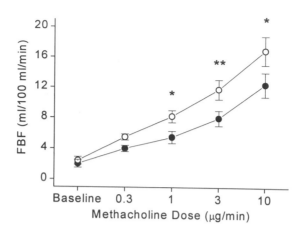

Figure 3: The effect of intra-arterial ascorbic acid on endothelial vasodilator function in forearm microvessels of patients with non-insulin-dependent diabetes mellitus. Forearm blood flow (FBF) responses at baseline and during intra-arterial infusion of methacholine were measured using venous occlusion plethysmography. Dose-response curves are shown for intra-arterial infusions of methacholine alone (filled circles) and methacholine plus ascorbic acid (open circles). Ascorbic acid was infused at a rate of 24 mg/min to achieve an estimated local concentration of 1 to 10 mM. The forearm blood flow response to methacholine was significantly augmented during simultaneous infusion of methacholine and ascorbic acid (P = 0.002 by ANOVA). Adapted by permission from Ting and colleagues (140).

Ascorbic acid has a number of actions that might explain its beneficial effects on endothelial vasomotor function. Ascorbic acid is known to scavenge superoxide anion (60), which in turn is known to react rapidly with EDNO and eliminate its biological activity (46). Since hypercholesterolemia (48,122), diabetes mellitus (121), and hypertension (148) are all associated with excess generation of superoxide anion, many investigators have assumed that ascorbic acid improves EDNO action in these disease states by scavenging superoxide and preventing inactivation of EDNO. However, on a kinetic basis, one would predict that only supra-physiological concentrations of ascorbic acid would be effective in this regard. The bimolecular rate constant for the reaction between ascorbic acid and NO (3.3×10^5 $M^{-1}s^{-1}$) (149) is approximately 10^5 less than the rate constant for the reaction between superoxide and NO (1.9×10^{10} $M^{-1}s^{-1}$) (150). Based on an estimated local NO concentration of 0.1 to 1 µM adjacent to the endothelial surface (151), an ascorbic acid concentration of 10 to 100 mM would be required to prevent EDNO inactivation. Jackson and colleagues recently confirmed this prediction using an *in vitro* model of superoxide-mediated endothelial dysfunction (133). Thus, superoxide scavenging could account for the effects of an acute intra-arterial infusion that produces local concentrations of approximately 10 mM (140-144). This mechanism is unlikely to be important in the studies involving lower, more physiologically relevant concentrations of ascorbic acid (135-139).

Ascorbic acid is also a potent inhibitor of LDL oxidation in plasma (132) and extracellular fluids (152). Since oxLDL interferes with EDNO action by a number of mechanisms, it is possible that ascorbic acid acts by preventing the formation of oxidized LDL. In the acute studies that involved ascorbic acid treatment over a period of 30 minutes to two hours (135-137), it is unlikely that a there was a significant reduction in lipid peroxidation. It is possible that this mechanism was important for the improvement in endothelial vasomotor function after 30 days of oral ascorbic acid treatment (136), however the improvement in brachial artery flow-mediated dilation was not associated with a change in plasma F_2-isoprostanes, a systemic marker of lipid peroxidation (136). Although this systemic marker may not reflect the extent of lipid peroxidation within the vessel wall, this finding argues against an effect of ascorbic acid on the formation of oxLDL under these conditions.

In addition to scavenging reactive oxygen species and inhibiting LDL oxidation, ascorbic acid may also improve the bioactivity of EDNO by influencing intracellular redox state. In this regard, ascorbic acid has been shown to enhance the activity of isolated neuronal nitric oxide synthase, possibly by recycling or preventing the oxidation of the essential cofactor tetrahydrobiopterin (153). Recent data suggests that ascorbic acid has a similar effect on nitric oxide production by endothelial NO synthase (179) consistent with observations that direct tetrahydrobiopterin administration improves endothelium-dependent forearm vasodilation in patients with hypercholesterolemia (154). Ascorbic acid may also augment release of NO from S-nitrosoglutathione or other nitrosothiols, thus increasing NO bioavailability (155). Finally, ascorbic acid may act by sparing intracellular glutathione (134), which can augment EDNO bioactivity by several mechanisms as will be discussed below.

In summary, the evidence for a beneficial effect of antioxidant therapy on vascular function in humans is strongest for ascorbic acid. Brief intra-arterial infusion of high concentrations of ascorbic acid improves endothelium-dependent vasodilation in patients with risk factors for coronary disease. The pharmacokinetics of these studies is consistent with the ability of ascorbic acid to scavenge superoxide anion. This observation provides insight into the causes of vascular dysfunction in disease states such as hypercholesterolemia, diabetes mellitus, and hypertension. Perhaps more clinically relevant are the studies that demonstrated improved endothelial vasomotor function following oral ascorbic acid supplementation; these studies achieved physiological concentrations of ascorbic acid. The above studies of the effect of ascorbic acid on vascular function may explain the observation that adequate ascorbic acid intake is associated with a decrease in CVD risk. Moreover, these studies provide a potential rationale for recommending ascorbic acid supplementation in patients with coronary artery disease, particularly acute coronary syndromes, where ascorbic acid levels are decreased. The specific role of ascorbic acid supplements for CVD is currently being examined in several large prospective studies.

Glutathione

Glutathione (L-γ-glutamyl-L-cysteinyl-glycine) is a tripeptide thiol that is present in high concentration inside cells (1 to 10 mM). Together with ascorbic acid, glutathione is the major intracellular water-soluble antioxidant and plays a central role in the regulation of cellular redox state (134). The availability of reduced glutathione is important for maintaining the reduced state of critical protein thiols. In addition, glutathione plays a major role in the catabolism of lipid hydroperoxides and hydrogen peroxide through the action of glutathione peroxidase (156). Glutathione and ascorbic acid interact in the regulation of intracellular redox state, and each antioxidant is capable of sparing the other as a reducing agent in a number of important cellular functions (134).

Effect on Vascular Function: Basic Evidence

There is accumulating experimental evidence that glutathione status is important for the bioactivity of EDNO. Early studies using bovine or porcine cells suggested that depletion of glutathione does not affect EDNO production (47, 157). However in studies involving manipulation of glutathione concentration in cultured human endothelial cells, Ghigo and colleagues found an extremely strong correlation between EDNO production and cellular glutathione concentration (158). Although the precise mechanism for this effect in human endothelial cells remains unclear, there is evidence that glutathione may increase or maintain the activity of neuronal and inducible NO synthase (159-160). In addition, increased availability of glutathione may lead to stabilization of EDNO through the formation of S-nitrosothiols (161). Finally, endothelial transport of the NO synthase substrate L-arginine is sensitive to adequate glutathione levels (162). The finding that glutathione status is important for EDNO activity is likely to be relevant to atherosclerosis: Ma and colleagues observed a reduction in total glutathione concentration in vascular tissue of hypercholesterolemic rabbits (163). Furthermore, exposure to oxidized LDL decreases glutathione concentration in cultured endothelial cells (164).

Effect on Vascular Function: Human Data

Several studies have examined the importance of glutathione status for the bioactivity of EDNO in human subjects. Using L-2-oxo-4-thiazolidine carboxylate (OTC), a cysteine prodrug that enhances intracellular glutathione levels (165), Vita and colleagues examined the effect of glutathione on EDNO bioactivity in patients with coronary artery disease. A single oral dose of OTC improved brachial artery flow-mediated dilation (166), strongly supporting the hypothesis that intracellular glutathione availability is relevant to the bioactivity of EDNO in human vascular disease. Several investigators have examined the effects of short-term intra-arterial glutathione infusion on vascular function, an intervention that primarily increases extra-cellular glutathione. In the coronary circulation of patients with vasospastic angina, intracoronary glutathione infusion improved endothelium-dependent vasodilation, as assessed by the vasomotor response to acetylcholine (167). There also is preliminary evidence that intra-arterial glutathione infusion improves acetylcholine-mediated vasodilation in the femoral circulation of patients with atherosclerosis (168). It remains uncertain whether these observations are attributable to extracellular metabolism of glutathione to its component amino acids and cellular uptake of cysteine. However, a recent study demonstrated that intra-arterial infusion of N-acetylcysteine, which increases extracellular cysteine concentration, had no effect on endothelial vasomotor function in normal subjects (169). The effect of N-acetylcysteine in atherosclerosis or related disease states remains unknown.

Glutathione status could contribute to other aspects of vascular dysfunction to or the atherogenic process. For example, it is known that intracellular thiol status influences expression of adhesion molecules (170). However, no published studies have addressed these issues in humans or in experimental animals. Direct glutathione treatment is unlikely to have significant clinical utility given the requirement for parental administration.

Enzymatic Antioxidants

Enzymatic and protein antioxidants play a central role in the protection of cells against the adverse effects of oxidative stress. Although not extensively studied in human subjects, there is evidence that genetic variation in the availability or activity of enzymatic antioxidants may be relevant to cardiovascular disease. Marklund and colleagues observed that a specific mutation in the heparin-binding domain of extracellular superoxide dismutase results in a bimodal distribution of the plasma concentrations of this antioxidant enzyme; plasma levels also varied with other known coronary risk factors (171). In a report of two cases of patients with arterial thrombosis, Freedman and colleagues provided evidence that decreased availability of plasma glutathione peroxidase was associated with a decrease in NO bioactivity (172).

There is animal evidence that administration of Cu-Zn superoxide dismutase improves EDNO action in hypercholesterolemia (49) and hypertension (173), particularly when administered in liposomes or other some other form that facilitates access to the vascular wall. Several studies have examined the effects of superoxide dismutase administration in human subjects. In a preliminary report involving humans with coronary artery disease, Meredith and colleagues demonstrated an improvement in endothelium-dependent dilation during intracoronary administration of recombinant human Cu-Zn superoxide dismutase (174). However, Garcia and colleagues found that intra-arterial superoxide dismutase infusion had no effect on forearm endothelial vasomotor function in patients with hypertension (175) or hypercholesterolemia (176). Finally, an intravenous infusion of recombinant superoxide dismutase failed to reduce ischemia-reperfusion injury as assessed by a reduction in infarct size in patients undergoing PTCA for acute myocardial infarction (177). All of these studies involving infusion of enzymatic superoxide dismutase are limited because it is unclear whether the compound had access to the intimal space during the period of treatment. An alternative approach that would result in intracellular delivery or increased cellular expression of superoxide dismutase would potentially have a greater effect on vascular function.

SUMMARY

Epidemiological studies suggest that increased intake of antioxidants such as α-tocopherol and ascorbic acid may reduce the risk for CVD. A single randomized trial further supports the potential benefits of α-tocopherol in the secondary prevention of coronary artery disease. Since formation of oxLDL is a key step in the atherogenic process and antioxidants may limit LDL oxidation, some investigators have assumed that antioxidants act by preventing the formation and progression of atherosclerotic lesions. However, the evidence supporting a beneficial effect of antioxidants on the progression or regression of atherosclerotic lesions is extremely limited. We now understand that the clinical expression of atherosclerosis often relates to plaque activation and rupture, rather than to gradual progression of lesion severity. In this chapter, we reviewed the accumulating evidence that antioxidants may restore normal homeostatic mechanisms of the vasculature and thereby reduce the risk of plaque rupture and its consequences. In particular, we have focused on the beneficial effects of antioxidants on the regulatory functions of the vascular endothelium.

The epidemiological evidence of benefit is strongest for α-tocopherol, and there is convincing experimental evidence that this lipid-soluble antioxidant has a beneficial effect on vascular function. However, the available human studies of the vascular effects of α-tocopherol have been conflicting. These studies are limited because they are relatively short in duration of treatment and because they focus primarily on forearm microvessels. Of the other lipid-soluble antioxidants, probucol has been shown to have the greatest impact on vascular function in humans; however, it is unlikely to have clinical utility because it also lowers HDL cholesterol. Among the water-soluble antioxidants, there is extensive human evidence that ascorbic acid improves vascular function in human subjects, but the mechanisms of benefit remain unclear. The improvement in vascular endothelial function with oral ascorbic acid treatment supports the idea that in addition to inhibiting the formation of oxLDL, antioxidants also act through direct cellular effects. The possible role for altered expression of enzymatic antioxidants remains largely unexplored to date.

Human studies of antioxidant action provide important insights into the causes of vascular dysfunction in atherosclerosis. In general, the findings support the extensive experimental work implicating increased oxidative stress as an important causative mechanism in atherosclerosis. The human studies reviewed in this chapter provide a rationale for the ongoing trials of antioxidants for the management of CVD. In addition, these studies may lead to innovative approaches for improving the care of patients with cardiovascular disease.

REFERENCES

1. Quinn MT, Parthasarathy S, Fong LG, Steinberg D. Oxidatively modified low density lipoproteins: a potential role in recruitment and retention of monocyte/macrophages during atherogenesis. *Proc Natl Acad Sci USA*. 1987;84:2995.

2. Diaz MN, Frei B, Vita JA, Keaney JF Jr. Antioxidants and atherosclerotic heart disease. *N Engl J Med*. 1997;337:408.

3. Walldius G, Erikson U, Olsson AG, Bergstrand L, Hadell K, Johansson J, Kaijser L, Lassvik C, Molgaard J, Nilsson S. The effect of probucol on femoral atherosclerosis: the Probucol Quantitative Regression Swedish Trial (PQRST). *Am J Cardiol*. 1994;74:875.

4. Stephens NG, Parsons A, Schofield PM, Kelly F, Cheeseman K, Mitchinson MJ. Randomised controlled trial of vitamin E in patients with coronary disease: Cambridge Heart Antioxidant Study (CHAOS). *Lancet*. 1996;347:781.

5. Levine GN, Keaney JF Jr, Vita JA. Cholesterol reduction in cardiovascular disease: Clinical benefits and possible mechanisms. *N Engl J Med*. 1995;332:512.

6. Libby P. Molecular basis of the acute coronary syndromes. *Circulation*. 1995;91:2844.

7. Fuster V, Badimon L, Badimon JJ, Chesebro JH. The pathogenesis of coronary artery disease and the acute coronary syndromes (Part 1). *N Engl J Med*. 1992;326:242.

8. Palmer RM, Ashton DS, Moncada S. Vascular endothelial cells synthesize nitric oxide from L-arginine. *Nature*. 1988;333:664.

9. Ignarro LJ, Buga GM, Wood KS, Byrns RE, Chaudhuri G. Endothelium-derived relaxing factor produced and released from artery and vein is nitric oxide. *Proc Natl Acad Sci USA*. 1987;84:9265.

10. Young MA, Vatner SF. Regulation of large coronary arteries. *Circ Res*. 1986;59:579.

11. Shimokawa H, Aarhus L, Vanhoutte PM. Porcine coronary arteries with regenerated endothelium have a reduced endothelium-dependent responsiveness to aggregating platelets and serotonin. *Circ Res*. 1987;61:256.

12. Furchgott R. Role of endothelium in responses of vascular smooth muscle. *Circ Res*. 1983;53:557.

13. Oates JA, Fitzgerald GA, Branch RA, Jackson EK, Knapp HR, Roberts LJ 2d. Clinical implications of prostaglandin and thromboxane A2 formation. *N Engl J Med*. 1988;319:689.

14. Chen G, Suzuki H, Weston AH. Acetylcholine releases endothelium-derived hyperpolarizing factor and EDRF from rat blood vessels. *Br J Pharmacol*. 1988;95:1165.

15. Pearson JD, Gordon JL. Vascular endothelial and smooth muscle cells in culture selectively release adenine nucleotides. *Nature*. 1979;281:384.

16. Yanagisawa M, Kurihara H, Kimura S, Tomobe Y, Kobayashi M, Mitsui Y, Yazaki Y, Goto K, Masaki T. A novel potent vasoconstrictor peptide produced by vascular endothelial cells. *Nature*. 1988;332:411.

17. Radomski MW, Palmer RM, Moncada S. Comparative pharmacology of endothelium-derived relaxing factor, nitric oxide and prostacyclin in platelets. *Br J Pharmacol*. 1987,92.181.

18. Marcum JA, Rosenberg RD. Heparin-like molecules with anticoagulant activity are synthesized by cultured endothelial cells. *Biochem Biophys Res Commun*. 1985;126:365.

19. Esmon NL, Owen WG, Esmon CT. Isolation of a membrane bound cofactor for thrombin-catalyzed activation of protein C. *J Biol Chem*. 1982;257:859.

20. Loskutoff D, Edgington T. Synthesis of a fibrinolytic activator and inhibitor by endothelial cells. *Proc Natl Acad Sci USA*. 1977;74:3903.

21. Berk BC, Alexander RW. Commentary: Vasoactive effects of growth factors. *Biochem Pharmacol*. 1989;38:219.

22. Gibbons GH, Dzau VJ. The emerging concept of vascular remodeling. *N Engl J Med*. 1994;330:1431.

23. Gokce N, Keaney JF Jr, Vita JA. Endotheliopathies: Clinical manifestations of endothelial dysfunction, in Loscalzo J, Shafer AI (eds): *Thrombosis and Hemorrhage*, Second ed., Williams and Wilkins, 1998, pp. 901-924.

24. Garg UC, Hassid A. Nitric oxide-generating vasodilators and 8-bromo-cyclic guanosine monophosphate inhibit mitogenesis and proliferation of cultured rat vascular smooth muscle cells. *J Clin Invest*. 1989;83:1774.

25.   Cooke JP, Singer AH, Tsao P, Zera P, Rowan RA, Dillingham ME. Antiatherogenic effects of L-arginine in hypercholesterolemic rabbits. *J Clin Invest.* 1992;90:1168.

26.   Ludmer PL, Selwyn AP, Shook TL, Wayne RR, Mudge GH, Alexander RW, Ganz P. Paradoxical vasoconstriction induced by acetylcholine in atherosclerotic coronary arteries. *N Engl J Med.*1986;315:1046.

27.   Bossaller C, Habib GB, Yamamoto H, Williams C, Wells S, Henry PD. Impaired muscarinic endothelium-dependent relaxation and cyclic guanosine 5'-monophosphate formation in atherosclerotic human coronary artery and rabbit aorta. *J Clin Invest.* 1987;79:170.

28.   Vita JA, Treasure CB, Nabel EG, McLenachan JM, Fish RD, Yeung AC, Vekshtein VI, Selwyn AP, Ganz P. Coronary vasomotor response to acetylcholine relates to risk factors for coronary artery disease. *Circulation.* 1990;81:491.

29.   Johnstone MT, Creager SJ, Scales KM, Cusco JA, Lee BK, Creager MA. Impaired endothelium-dependent vasodilation in patients with insulin-dependent diabetes mellitus. *Circulation.* 1993;88:2510.

30.   Creager MA, Cooke JP, Mendelsohn ME, Gallagher SJ, Coleman SM, Loscalzo J, Dzau VJ. Impaired vasodilation of forearm resistance vessels in hypercholesterolemic humans. *J Clin Invest.* 1990;86:228.

31.   Panza JA, Quyyumi AA, Brush JE, Epstein SE. Abnormal endothelium-dependent vascular relaxation in patients with essential hypertension. *N Engl J Med.* 1990;323:22.

32.   Elliot TG, Barth JD, Mancini GBJ. Effects of Vitamin E on Endothelial Function in Men After Myocardial Infarction. *Am J Cardiol.* 1995;76:1188.

33.   Vita JA, Keaney JF Jr. Ultrasound assessment of endothelial vasomotor function, in Lanzer P, Lipton M (eds): *Diagnostics of vascular diseases: Principals and technology*, Second ed. Berlin, Springer, 1996, pp. 249-259.

34.   Lieberman EH, Gerhard MD, Uehata A, Selwyn AP, Ganz P, Yeung AC, Creager MA. Flow-induced vasodilation of the human brachial artery is impaired in patients <40 years of age with coronary artery disease. *Am J Cardiol.* 1996;78:1210.

35.   Joannides R, Haefeli WE, Linder L, Richard V, Bakkali EH, Thuillez C, Luscher TF. Nitric oxide is responsible for flow-dependent dilatation of human peripheral conduit arteries *in vivo*. *Circulation.* 1995;91:1314.

36.   Lieberman EH, Uehata A, Polak J, Ganz P, Selwyn AP, Creager MA, Yeung AC. Flow-mediated vasodilation is impaired in the brachial artery of patients with coronary disease or diabetes mellitus (abst.). *Clin Res.* 1993;41:217A.

37.   Anderson TJ, Uehata A, Gerhard MD, Meredith IT, Knab S, Delagrange D, Leiberman E, Ganz P, Creager MA, Yeung AC, Selwyn AP. Close relation of endothelial function in the human coronary and peripheral circulations. *J Am Coll Cardiol.* 1995;26:1235.

38.   Ridker PM, Vaughan DE, Stampfer MJ, Manson JE, Hennekens CH. Endogenous tissue-type plasminogen activator and risk of myocardial infarction. *Lancet.* 1993;341:1165.

39.   Collins T. Endothelial Nuclear Factor-□B and the Initiation of the Atherosclerotic Lesion. *Lab Invest.* 1993;68:499.

40.   Ridker PM, Hennekens CH, Roitman-Johnson B, Allen J. Plasma concentration of soluble intercellular adhesion molecule 1 and risks of future myocardial infarction in apparently healthy men. *Lancet.* 1998;351:88.

41.   Ridker PM, Cushman M, Stampfer MJ, Tracy RP, Hennekens CH. Inflammation, aspirin, and the risk of cardiovascular disease in apparently healthy men. *N Engl J Med.* 1997;336, No. 14:973.

42.   Gordon JB, Ganz P, Nabel EG, Fish RD, Zebede J, Mudge GH, Alexander RW, Selwyn AP. Atherosclerosis influences the vasomotor response of epicardial coronary arteries to exercise. *J Clin Invest.* 1989;83:1946.

43.   Yeung AC, Vekshtein VI, Krantz DS, Vita JA, Ryan TJ Jr, Ganz P, Selwyn AP. The effect of atherosclerosis on the vasomotor response of coronary arteries to mental stress. *N Engl J Med.* 1991;325:1551.

44.   Bogaty P, Hackett D, Davies G, Maseri A. Vasoreactivity of the culprit lesion in unstable angina. *Circulation.* 1994;90:5.

45.   Okumura K, Yasue H, Matsuyama K, Ogawa H, Morikami Y, Obata K, Sakaino N. Effect of acetylcholine on the highly stenotic coronary artery: difference between the constrictor response of the infarct-related coronary artery and that of the noninfarct-related artery. *J Am Coll Cardiol.*

1992;19:752.

46.   Gryglewski RJ, Palmer RM, Moncada S. Superoxide anion is involved in the breakdown of endothelium-derived vascular relaxing factor. *Nature.* 1986;320:454.

47.   Mugge A, Elwell JK, Peterson TE, Harrison DG. Release of intact endothelium-derived relaxing factor depends on endothelial superoxide dismutase activity. *Am J Physiol.* [Cell Physiol. 29] 1991;260:C219.

48.   Ohara Y, Peterson TE, Harrison DG. Hypercholesterolemia increases endothelial superoxide anion production. *J Clin Invest.* 1993;91:2546.

49.   Mugge A, Elwell JH, Peterson TE, Hofmeyer TG, Heistad DD, Harrison DG. Chronic treatment with polyethylene-glycolated superoxide dismutase partially restores endothelium-dependent vascular relaxations in cholesterol-fed rabbits. *Circ Res.* 1991;69:1293.

50.   Morel DW, Hessler GM, Chisolm GM. Low density lipoprotein cytotoxicity induced by free radical peroxidation of lipid. *J Lipid Res.* 1983;24:1070.

51.   Chin JH, Azhar S, Hoffman BB. Inactivation of endothelium-derived relaxing factor by oxidized lipoproteins. *J Clin Invest.* 1992;89:10.

52.   Kugiyama K, Kerns SA, Morrisett JD, Roberts R, Henry PD. Impairment of endothelium-dependent arterial relaxation by lysolecithin in modified low-density lipoproteins. *Nature.* 1990;344:160.

53.   Liao JK, Shin WS, Lee WY, Clark SL. Oxidized low-density lipoprotein decreases the expression of endothelial nitric oxide synthase. *J Biol Chem.* 1995;270:319.

54.   Boulanger CM, Tanner FC, Bea ML, Hahn AW, Werner A, Luscher TF. Oxidized low density lipoproteins induce mRNA expression and release of endothelin from human and porcine endothelium. *Circ Res.* 1992;70:1191.

55.   Weis JR, Pitas RE, Wilson BD, Rodgers GM. Oxidized low-density lipoprotein increases cultured human endothelial cell tissue factor activity and reduces protein C activation. *FASEB J.* 1991;5:2459.

56.   Kume N, Cybulsky MI, Gimbrone MA Jr. Lysophosphatidylcholine, a component of atherogenic lipoproteins, induces mononuclear leukocyte adhesion molecules in cultured human and rabbit arterial endothelial cells. *J Clin Invest.* 1992;90:1138.

57   Kugiyama K, Sakamoto T, Misumi I, Sugiyama S, Ohgushi M, Ogawa H, Horiguchi M, Yasue H. Transferable lipids in oxidized low-density lipoprotein stimulate plasminogen activator inhibitor-1 and inhibit tissue-type plasminogen activator release from endothelial cells. *Circ Res.* 1993;73:335.

58.   Ohara Y, Peterson TE, Zheng B, Kuo JF, Harrison DG. Lysophosphatidylcholine increases vascular superoxide anion production via protein kinase C activation. *Arterioscler Thromb.* 1994;14:1007.

59.   Heitzer T, Yla-Herttuala S, Luoma J, Kurz S, Munzel T, Just H, Olschewski M, Drexler H. Cigarette smoking potentiates endothelial dysfunction of forearm resistance vessels in patients with hypercholesterolemia. Role of oxidized LDL. *Circulation.* 1996;93:1346.

60.   Briviba K, Sies H. Nonenzymatic antioxidant defense systems, in Frei B (ed): *Natural antioxidants in human health and disease.* San Diego, Academic Press, 1994, pp. 107-128.

61.   Reaven PD, Khouw A, Beltz WF, Parthasarathy S, Witztum JL. Effect of dietary antioxidant combinations in humans. protection of LDL by vitamin E but not beta carotene. *Arterioscler Thromb.* 1993;13:590.

62.   Gaziano JM, Manson JE, Hennekens CH. Natural antioxidants and cardiovascular disease: Observational epidemiologic studies and randomized trials, in Frei B (ed): *Natural antioxidants in human health and disease.* San Diego, CA, Academic Press, Inc., 1994, pp. 387-409.

63.   Rapola JM, Virtamo J, Ripatti S, Huttunen JK, Albanes D, Taylor PR, Heionen OP. Randomised trial of a-tocopherol and B-carotene supplements on incidence of major coronary events in men with previous myocardial infarction. *Lancet.* 1997;349:1715.

64.   Stampfer MJ, Hennekens CH, Manson JE, Colditz GA, Rosner B, Willett WC. Vitamin E consumption and the risk of coronary disease in women. *N Engl J Med.* 1993;328:1444.

65.   Rimm EB, Stampfer MJ, Ascherio A, Giovannucci E, Colditz GA, Willett WC. Vitamin E consumption and the risk of coronary heart disease in men. *N Engl J Med.* 1993;328:1450.

66.   Tornwall ME, Virtamo J, Haukka JK, Aro A, Albanes D, Edwards BK, Huttunen JK. Effect of a-tocopherol (vitamin E) and b-carotene supplementation on the incidence of intermittent claudication in male smokers. *Arterioscler Thromb Vasc Biol.* 1997;17:3475.

67. Williams HTG, Fenna D, MacBeth RA. Alpha Tocopherol in the treatment of intermittent claudication. *Surg Gyn Obstetrics.* 1971;48:662.

68. Haeger K. Long-time treatment of intermittent claudication with vitamin E. *Am J Clin Nutr.* 1974;27:1179.

69. Kritchevsky SB, Shimakawa T, Tell GS, Dennis B, Carpenter M, Eckfeldt JH, Peacher-Ryan H, Heiss G. Dietary antioxidants and carotid artery wall thickness: The ARIC study. *Circulation.* 1995;92:2142.

70. Hodis HN, Mack WJ, LaBree L, Cashin-Hemphill L, Sevanian A, Johnson R, Azen SP. Serial coronary angiographic evidence that antioxidant vitamin intake reduces progression of coronary artery atherosclerosis. *JAMA* 1995;273:1849.

71. Lynch SM, Frei B. Antioxidants as antiatherogens: Animal studies, in Frei B (ed): *Natural antioxidants in human health and disease.* San Diego, CA, Academic Press, 1994, pp. 353-386.

72. Loscalzo J. Regression of coronary atherosclerosis. *N Engl J Med.* 1990;323:1337.

73. Keaney JF Jr, Gaziano JM, Xu A, Frei B, Curran-Celentano J, Shwaery GT, Loscalzo J, Vita JA. Dietary antioxidants preserve endothelium-dependent vessel relaxation in cholesterol-fed rabbits. *Proc Natl Acad Sci USA.* 1993;90:11880.

74. Andersson TLG, Matz J, Ferns GAA, Anggard EE. Vitamin E reverses cholesterol-induced endothelial dysfunction in the rabbit coronary circulation. *Atherosclerosis.* 1994;111:39.

75. Steward-Lee AL, Forster LA, Nourooz-Zadeh J, Ferns GAA, Anggard EE. Vitamin E protects against impairment of endothelium-mediated relaxations in cholesterol-fed rabbits. *Arterioscler Thromb.* 1994;14:494.

76. Keegan A, Walbank H, Cotter MA, Cameron NE. Chronic vitamin E treatment prevents defective endothelium-dependent relaxation in diabetic rat aorta. *Diabetologia.* 1995;38:1475.

77. Faruqi R, De La Motte C, Dicorleto PE. a-tocopherol inhibits agonist-induced monocytic cell adhesion to cultured human endothelial cells. *J Clin Invest.* 1994;94:592.

78. Devaraj S, Li D, Jialal I. The Effects of Alpha Tocopherol Supplementation on Monocyte Function. *J Clin Invest.* 1996;98:756.

79. Gilligan DM, Sack MN, Guetta V, Casino PR, Quyyumi AA, Rader DJ, Panza JA, Cannon RO. Effect of antioxidant vitamins on low density lipoprotein oxidation and impaired endothelium-dependent vasodilation in patients with hypercholesterolemia. *J Am Coll Cardiol.* 1994;24:1611.

80. Chowienczyk PJ, Kneale BJ, Brett SE, Paganga G, Jenkins BS, Ritter JM. Lack of effect of vitamin E on L-arginine responsive endothelial dysfunction in patients with mild hypercholesterolemia and coronary artery disease. *Clin Sci.* 1998;94:129.

81. McDowell IF, Brennan GM, McEneny J, Young IS, Nicholls DP, McVeigh GE, Bruce I, Trimble ER, Johnston GD. The effect of probucol and vitamin E treatment on the oxidation of low-density lipoprotein and forearm vascular responses in humans. *Eur J Clin Invest.* 1994;24:759.

82. Neunteufl T, Kostner K, Katzenschlager R, Zehetgruber M, Maurer G. Additional benefit of vitamin E supplementation to simvastatin therapy on vasoreactivity of the brachial artery of hypercholesterolemic men. *J Am Coll Cardiol.* 1998;32:711.

83. Motoyama T, Kawano H, Kugiyama K, Hirashima O, Ohgushi M, Tsunoda R, Moriyama Y, Miyao Y, Yoshimura M, Ogawa H, Yasue H. Vitamin E administration improves impairment of endothelium-dependent vasodilation in patients with coronary spastic angina. *J Am Coll Cardiol.* 1998;32:1672.

84. Green D, O'Driscoll G, Rankin JM, Maiorana AJ, Taylor RR. Beneficial effect of vitamin E administration on nitric oxide function in subjects with hypercholesterolaemia. *Clin Sci.* 1998;95:361.

85. Heitzer T, Yla-Herttuala S, Wild E, Munzel T, Drexler H. Effect of vitamin E on endothelial function and plasma autoantibodies in patients with increased oxidative stress. *Circulation.* 1997;96:I-417.

86. Barrett-Connor E, Bush TL. Estrogen and coronary heart disease in women. *JAMA.* 1991;265:1861.

87. Stampfer MJ, Colditz GA, Willett WC, Manson JE, Rosner B, Speizer FE, Hennekens CH. Postmenopausal estrogen therapy and cardiovascular disease. Ten-year follow-up from the nurses' health study. *N Engl J Med.* 1991;325:756.

88. Sullivan JM, Vander Zwaag R, Hughes JP, Madduck V, Kroetz FW, Ramanathan KB, Mirvis DM. Estrogen replacement and coronary artery disease. Effect on survival in post-menopausal women. *Arch Intern Med.* 1990;150:2557.

89.   Jonas HA, Kronmal RA, Psaty BM, Manolio TA, Meilahn EN, Tell GS, Tracy RP, Robbins JA, Anton-Culver H. Current estrogen-progestin and estrogen replacement therapy in elderly women: association with carotid atherosclerosis. CHS Collaborative Research Group. Cardiovascular Health Study. *Ann Epidemiol.* 1996;6:314.

90.   Hulley S, Grady D, Bush T, Furberg C, Herrington D, Riggs B, Vittinghoff E. Randomized trial of estrogen plus progestin for secondary prevention of coronary heart disease in women. *JAMA.* 1998;280:605.

91.   Walsh BW, Schiff I, Rosner B, Greenberg L, Ravnikar V, Sacks FM. Effects of postmenopausal estrogen replacement on the concentrations and metabolism of plasma lipoproteins. *N Engl J Med.* 1991;325:1196.

92.   Bush TL, Barrett-Connor E, Cowan LD, Criqui MH, Wallace RB, Suchindran CM, Tyroler HA, Rifkind BM. Cardiovascular mortality and noncontraceptive use of estrogen in women: results from the Lipid Research Clinics Program Follow-up Study. *Circulation.* 1987;75:1102.

93.   Mazière C, Auclair M, Ronoveaux MF, Salmon S, Santus R, Mazière JC. Estrogens inhibit copper and cell-mediated modification of low density lipoprotein. *Arteriosclerosis.* 1991;89:175.

94.   Shwaery GT, Vita JA, Keaney JF Jr. Antioxidant protection of LDL by physiological concentrations of 17-beta estradiol. *Circulation.* 1997;95:1378.

95.   Sack MN, Rader DJ, Cannon RO 3rd. Oestrogen and inhibition of oxidation of low-density lipoproteins in postmenopausal women. *Lancet.* 1994;343:269.

96.   Arnal JF, Clamens S, Pechet C, Negre-Salvayre A, Allera C, Girolami JP, Salvayre R, Bayard F. Ethinylestradiol does not enhance the expression of nitric oxide synthase in bovine endothelial cells but increases the release of bioactive nitric oxide by inhibiting superoxide anion production. *Proc Natl Acad Sci USA.* 1996;93:4108.

97.   Nègre Salvayre A, Pieraggi MT, Mabile L, Salvayre R. Protective effect of 17-beta-estradiol against the cytotoxicity of minimally oxidized LDL to cultured bovine aortic endothelial cells. *Atherosclerosis.* 1992;99:207.

98.   Caulin-Glaser T, Watson CA, Pardi R, Bender JR. Effects of 17beta-estradiol on cytokine-induced endothelial cell adhesion molecule expression. *J Clin Invest.* 1996;98:36.

99.   Keaney JF Jr, Shwaery GT, Xu A, Nicolosi RJ, Loscalzo J, Foxall TL, Vita JA. 17beta-estradiol preserves endothelial vasodilator function and limits LDL oxidation in hypercholesterolemic swine. *Circulation.* 1994;89:2251.

100.   Lieberman EH, Gerhard MD, Uehata A, Walsh BW, Selwyn AP, Ganz P, Yeung AC, Creager MA. Estrogen improves endothelium-dependent, flow mediated vasodilation in post menopausal women. *Ann Intern Med.* 1994;121:936.

101.   Gerhard M, Walsh MW, Tawakol A, Haley EA, Creager SJ. Estradiol therapy combined with progesterone and endothelium-dependent vasodilation in postmenopausal women. *Circulation.* 1998;98:1158.

102.   Reis SE, Gloth ST, Blumenthal RS, Resar JR, Zacur HA, Gerstenblith G, Brinker JA. Ethinyl estradiol acutely attenuates abnormal coronary vasomotor responses to acetylcholine in postmenopausal women. *Circulation.* 1994;89:52.

103.   Hertog MGL, Feskens EJM, Hollman PCH, Martijn B, Kromhout D. Dietary antioxidant flavonoids and risk of coronary heart disease: the Zutphen Elderly Study. *Lancet.* 1993;342:1007.

104.   Frankel EN, Kanner J, German JB, Parks E, Kinsella JE. Inhibition of oxidation of human low-density lipoprotein by phenolic substances in red wine. *Lancet.* 1993;341:454.

105.   Korkina LG, Afanas'ev IB. Antioxidant and chelating properties of flavonoids, in Sies H (ed). *Antioxidants in disease mechanisms and therapy.* San Diego, CA, Academic Press, 1997, pp. 151-163.

106.   Knekt P, Jarvinen R, Reunanen A, Maatela J. Flavonoid intake and coronary mortality in Finland: a cohort study. *Br Med J.* 1996;312:478.

107.   Hertog MGL, Feskens EJM, Kromhout D. Antioxidant flavanols and coronary heart disease risk. *Lancet.* 1997;349:699.

108.   Rimm EB, Katan MB, Ascherio A, Stampfer MJ, Willett WC. Relation between intake of flavonoids and risk for coronary heart disease in male health professionals. *Ann Intern Med.* 1996;125:384.

109.   Ishikawa T, Suzukawa M, Ito T, Yoshida H, Ayaori M. Effect of tea flavonoid supplementation on the susceptibility of low-density lipoprotein to oxidative modification. *Am J Clin Nutr.*

1997;66:261.

110. van het Hof KH, de Boer HS, Wiseman SA, Lien N, Westrate JA, Tiburg LBM. Consumption of green or black tea does not increase the resistance of LDL to oxidation in humans. *Am J Clin Nutr.* 1997;66:1125.

111. Hayek T, Furman B, Vaya JR, Rosenblat M, Belinky P, Coleman R, Elis A, Aviram M. Reduced progression of atherosclerosis in apoplipoprotein E-deficient mice following consumption of red wine or its polyphenols quercetin or catechin, is associated with reduced susceptibility of LDL to oxidation and aggregation. *Arterioscler Thromb Vasc Biol.* 1997;17:2744.

112. Xu R, Yokoyama WH, Irving D, Rein D, Walzem RL, German JB. Effect of dietary catechin and vitamin E on aortic fatty streak accumulation in hypercholesterolemic hamsters. *Atherosclerosis.* 1998;137:29.

113. Keaney JF Jr, Frei B. Antioxidant protection of low-density lipoprotein and its role in the prevention of atherosclerotic vascular disease, in Frei B (ed): *Natural antioxidants in human health and disease.* San Diego, Academic Press, 1994, pp. 303-352.

114. Carew TE, Schwenke DC, Steinberg D. Antiatherogenic effect of probucol unrelated to its hypocholesterolemic effect: evidence that antioxidants *in vivo* can selectively inhibit low density lipoprotein degradation in macrophage-rich fatty streaks and slow the progression of atherosclerosis in the Watanabe heritable hyperlipidemic rabbit. *Proc Natl Acad Sci USA.* 1987;84:7725.

115. Kita T, Nagano Y, Yokode M, Ishii K, Kume N, Ooshima A, Yoshida H, Kawai C. Probucol prevents the progression of atherosclerosis in Watanabe heritable hyperlipidemic rabbit, an animal model for familial hypercholesterolemia. *Proc Natl Acad Sci USA.* 1987;84:5928.

116. Shankar R, Sallis JD, Stanton J, Thomson R: Influence of probucol on early experimental atherogenesis in hypercholesterolemic rats. *Atherosclerosis.* 1989;78:91.

117. Johansson J, Olsson AG, Bergstrand L, Elinder LS, Nilsson S, Erikson U, Molgaard J, Holme I, Walldius G. Lowering of HDL2b by probucol partly explains the failure of the drug to affect femoral atherosclerosis in subjects with hypercholesterolemia. A Probucol Quantitative Regression Swedish Trial (PQRST) Report. *Arterioscler Thromb Vasc Biol* 1995;15:1049.

118. Tardif JC, Cote G, Lesperance J, Bourassa M, Lambert J, Doucet S, Bilodeau L, Nattel S, de Guise P. Probucol and multivitamins in the prevention of restenosis after coronary angioplasty. *N Engl J Med.* 1997;337:365.

119. Sasahara M, Raines E, Chait A, Carew TE, Steinberg D, Wahl PW, Ross R. Inhibition of hypercholesterolemia-induced atherosclerosis in the non-human primate by probucol: I. Is the extent of atherosclerosis related to resistance of LDL to oxidation? *J Clin Invest.* 1994;94:155.

120. Simon BC, Haudenschild CC, Cohen RA. Preservation of endothelium-dependent relaxation in atherosclerotic rabbit aorta by probucol. *J Cardiovasc Pharmacol.* 1993;21:893.

121. Tesfamariam B, Cohen RA. Free radicals mediate endothelial cell dysfunction caused by elevated glucose. *Am J Physiol.* 1992;263:H321.

122. Keaney JF Jr, Xu A, Cunningham DC, Jackson T, Frei B, Vita JA. Dietary probucol preserves endothelial function in cholesterol-fed rabbits by limiting vascular oxidative stress and superoxide production. *J Clin Invest.* 1995;95:2520.

123. Reaven PD, Parthasarathy S, Beltz WF, Witztum JL. Effect of probucol dosage on plasma lipid and lipoprotein levels and on protection of low density lipoprotein against *in vitro* oxidation in humans. *Arterioscler Thromb.* 1992;12:318.

124. Anderson TJ, Meredith IT, Yeung AC, Frei B, Selwyn A, Ganz P. The effect of cholesterol lowering and antioxidant therapy on endothelium-dependent coronary vasomotion. *N Engl J Med.* 1995;332:488.

125. Anderson TJ, Meredith IT, Charbonneau F, Yeung AC, Frei B, Selwyn AP, Ganz P. Endothelium-dependent coronary vasomotion relates to susceptibility of LDL to oxidation in humans. *Circulation.* 1996;93:1647.

126. Riemersma RA, Wood DA, Macintyre CCH, Elton RA, Gey KF, Oliver MF. Risk of angina pectoris and plasma concentrations of vitamins A, C, E, and carotene. *Lancet.* 1991;337:1.

127. Ramirez J, Flowers NC. Leukocyte ascorbic acid and its relationship to coronary artery disease in man. *Am J Clin Nutr.* 1980;33:2079.

128. Vita JA, Keaney JF Jr, Raby KE, Morrow JD, Freedman JE, Lynch S, Koulouris SN, Hankin BR, Frei B. Low plasma ascorbic acid independently predicts the presence of an unstable coronary syndrome. *J Am Coll Cardiol.* 1998;31:980.

129. Nyyssöncn K, Parviainen MT, Salonen R, Tuomilehto J, Salonen JT. Vitamin C deficiency and risk of myocardial infarction: prospective population study of men from eastern Finland. *Br Med J.* 1997;314:634.

130. Enstrom JE, Kanim LE, Klein MA. Vitamin C intake and mortality among a sample of the United States population. *Epidemiology.* 1992;3:194.

131. Levine M, Conry-Cantilena C, Wang Y, Welch RW, Washko PW, Dhariwal KR, Park JB, Lazarev A, Graumlich JF, King J, Cantilena LR. Vitamin C pharmacokinetics in healthy volunteers: Evidence for a recommended dietary allowance. *Proc Natl Acad Sci USA.* 1996;93:3704.

132. Frei B, England L, Ames BN. Ascorbate is an outstanding antioxidant in human blood plasma. *Proc Natl Acad Sci USA.* 1989;86:6377.

133. Jackson TS, Xu A, Vita JA, Keaney JF Jr. Ascorbate prevents the interaction of superoxide and nitric oxide only at high physiologic concentrations. *Circ Res.* 1998;83:916.

134. Meister A. Glutathione-ascorbic acid antioxidant system in animals. *J Biol Chem.* 1994;269:9397.

135. Levine GN, Frei B, Koulouris SN, Gerhard MD, Keaney JF Jr, Vita JA. Ascorbic acid reverses endothelial vasomotor dysfunction in patients with coronary artery disease. *Circulation.* 1996;96:1107.

136. Gokce N, Keaney JF Jr., Frei B, Holbrook M, Olesiak M, Zachariah BJ, Leeuwenburgh C, Heinecke JW, Vita JA. Long-term ascorbic acid administration reverses endothelial vasomotor dysfunction in patients with coronary artery disease. *Circulation.* 1999;99:3234.

137. Ito K, Akita H, Kanazawa K, Yamada S, Terashima M. Comparison of effects of ascorbic acid on endothelium-dependent vasodilation in patients with chronic congestive heart failure secondary to idiopathic dilated cardiomyopathy versus patients with effort angina pectoris secondary to coronary artery disease. *Am J Cardiol.* 1998;82:762.

138. Hornig B, Arakawa N, Kohler C, Drexler H. Vitamin C improves endothelial function of conduit arteries in patients with chronic heart failure. *Circulation.* 1998;97:363.

139. Plotnick GD, Corretti MC, Vogel RA. Effect of antioxidant vitamins on the transient impairment of endothelium-dependent brachial artery vasoactivity following a single high-fat meal. *JAMA.* 1997;278:1682.

140. Ting HH, Timimi FK, Boles KS, Creager SJ, Ganz P, Creager MA. Vitamin C improves endothelium-dependent vasodilation in patients with non-insulin-dependent diabetes mellitus. *J Clin Invest.* 1996;97:22.

141. Timimi FK, Ting HH, Haley EA, Roddy MA, Ganz P, Creager MA. Vitamin C improves endothelium-dependent vasodilation in patients with insulin-dependent diabetes mellitus. *J Am Coll Cardiol.* 1998;31:552.

142. Ting HH, Timimi FK, Haley EA, Roddy MA, Ganz P, Creager MA. Vitamin C improves endothelium-dependent vasodilation in forearm resistance vessels of humans with hypercholesterolemia. *Circulation.* 1997;95:2617.

143. Taddei S, Virdis A, Ghiadoni L, Magagna A, Salvetti A. Vitamin C improves endothelium-dependent vasodilation by restoring nitric oxide activity in essential hypertension. *Circulation.* 1997;97:2222.

144. Sherman DL, Keaney JF Jr, Hankin B, Mannion T, Jewett T, Coffman JD, Vita JA. Ascorbic acid improves endothelial function in essential hypertension. *Circulation.* 1998;98:I-376 (abstract).

145. Heitzer T, Just H, Munzel T. Antioxidant vitamin C improves endothelial dysfunction in chronic smokers. *Circulation.* 1996;94:6.

146. Solzbach U, Hornig B, Jeserich M, Just H. Vitamin C improves endothelial dysfunction of epicardial coronary arteries in hypertensive patients. *Circulation.* 1997;96:1513.

147. Kugiyama K, Motoyama T, Hirashima O, Ohgushi M, Soejima H, Misumi K, Kawano H, Miyao Y, Yoshimura M, Ogawa H, Matsumura T, Sugiyama S, Yasue H. Vitamin C attenuates abnormal vasomotor reactivity in spasm coronary arteries in patients with coronary spastic angina. *J Am Coll Cardiol.* 1998;32:103.

148. Rajagopalan S, Kurz S, Munzel T, Tarpey M, Freeman BA, Griendling KK, Harrison DG. Angiotensin II-mediated hypertension in the rat increases vascular superoxide production via membrane NADH/NADPH oxidase activation. *J Clin Invest.* 1996;97:1916.

149. Gotoh N, Niki E. Rates of interactions of superoxide with vitamin E, vitamin C, and related

compounds as measured by chemiluminescence. *Biochim Biophys Acta*.1992;1115:201.

150.   Huie RE, Padmaja S. The reaction of NO with superoxide. *Free Radic Res Commun.* 1993;18:195.

151.   Malinski T, Taha Z, Grunfeld S, Patton S, Kapturczak M, Tomboulian P. Diffusion of nitric oxide in the aorta wall monitored in situ by porphyrinic microsensors. *Biochem Biophys Res Commun.* 1993;193:1076.

152.   Dabbagh AJ, Frei B. Human suction blister interstitial fluid prevents metal ion-dependent oxidation of low density lipoprotein by macrophages and in cell-free systems. *J Clin Invest.* 1995;96:1958.

153.   Howells DW, Hyland K. Direct analysis of tetrahydrobiopterin in cerebrospinal fluid by high-performance liquid chromatography with redox electrochemistry: Prevention of autooxidation during storage and analysis. *Clin Chim Acta.* 1987;167:23.

154.   Stroes E, Kastelein J, Cosentino F, Erkelens W, Wever R, Koomans H, Luscher T, Rabelink T. Tetrahydrobiopterin restores endothelial function in hypercholesterolemia. *J Clin Invest.* 1997;99:41.

155.   Kashiba-Iwatsuki M, Yamaguchi M, Inoue M. Role of ascorbic acid in the metabolism of S-nitroso-glutathione. *FEBS Lett.* 1996;389:149.

156.   Anderson ME. Glutathione and glutathione delivery compounds, in Sies H (ed): *Antioxidants in disease mechanisms and therapy*, Advances in Pharmacology ed. San Diego, CA, Academic Press, 1997, vol 38, pp. 65-78.

157.   Murphy ME, Piper H-M, Watanabe H, Sies H. Nitric oxide production by cultured aortic endothelial cells in response to thiol depletion and replenishment. *J Biol Chem.* 1991;266:19378.

158.   Ghigo D, Alessio P, Foco A, Bussolino F, Costamagna C, Heller R, Garbarino G, Pescarmona GP, Bosia A. Nitric oxide synthesis is impaired in glutathione-depleted human umbilical vein endothelial cells. *Am J Physiol.* 1993;265:C728.

159.   Komori Y, Hyun J, Chiang K, Fukuto JM. The role of thiols in the apparent activation of rat brain nitric oxide synthase (NOS). *J Biochem.* 1995;117:923.

160.   Stuehr DJ, Kwon NS, Nathan CF. FAD and GSH participate in macrophage synthesis of nitric oxide. *Biochem Biophys Res Commun.* 1990;168:558.

161.   Stamler JS, Singel DJ, Loscalzo J. Biochemistry of nitric oxide and its redox-activated forms. *Science.* 1992;258:1898.

162.   Patel JM, Abeles AJ, Block ER. Nitric oxide exposure and sulfhydryl modulation alter L-arginine transport in cultured pulmonary artery endothelial cells. *Free Rad Biol Med.* 1996;20:629.

163.   Ma XL, Lopez BL, Liu GL, Christopher TA, Gao F, Guo Y, Feuerstein GZ, Ruffolo RR Jr, Barone FC, Yue TL. Hypercholesterolemia impairs a detoxification mechanism against peroxynitrite and renders the vascular tissue more susceptible to oxidative injury. *Circ Res.* 1997;80:894.

164.   Kuzuya M, Naito M, Funaki C, Hayashi T, Asai K, Kuauya F. Protective role of intracellular glutathione against oxidized low density lipoprotein in cultured endothelial cells. *Biochem Biophys Res Commun.* 1989;163:1466.

165.   Porta P, Aebi S, Summer K, Lauterburg BH. L-2-oxothiazolidine-4-carboxylic acid, a cysteine prodrug: Pharmacokinetics and effects on thiols in plasma and lymphocytes in humans. *J Pharmacol Exp Ther.* 1991;257:331.

166.   Vita JA, Frei B, Holbrook M, Gokce N, Leaf C, Keaney JF Jr. L-2-oxothiazolidine-4-carboxylic acid reverses endothelial dysfunction in patients with coronary artery disease. *J Clin Invest.* 1998;101:1408.

167.   Kugiyama K, Ohgushi M, Motoyama T, Hirashima O, Soejima H, Misumi K, Yoshimura M, Ogawa H, Sugiyama S, Yasue H. Intracoronary infusion of reduced glutathione improves endothelial vasomotor response to acetylcholine in human coronary circulation. *Circulation.* 1998;97:2299.

168.   Prasad A, Padder F, Andrews NP, Husain M, Mincemoyer R, Panza JA, Quyyumi AA. Glutathione and N-acetylcysteine improve endothelial dysfunction in humans. *Circulation.* 1998;96:I-251 (abstract).

169.   Creager MA, Roddy MA, Boles K, Stamler JS. N-acetylcysteine does not influence the activity of endothelium-derived relaxing factor *in vivo. Hypertension.* 1997;29:668.

170.   Marui N, Offermann MK, Swerlick R, Kunsch C, Rosen C, Ahmad M, Alexander RW, Medford RM. Vascular Cell Adhesion Molecule-1 (VCAM-1) Gene Transcription and Expression Are

Regulated through an Antioxidant-sensitive Mechanism in Human Vascular Endothelial Cells. *J Clin Invest.* 1993;92:1866.

171. Marklund SL, Nilsson P, Israelsson K, Schampi I, Peltonen M, Asplund K. Two variants of extracellular-superoxide dismutase: relation to cardiovascular risk in an unselected middle-aged population. *J Intern Med.* 1997;242:5.

172. Freedman JE, Loscalzo J, Benoit SE, Valeri CR, Barnard MR, Michelson AD. Decreased platelet inhibition by nitric oxide in two brothers with a history of arterial thrombosis. *J Clin Invest.* 1996;97:979.

173. Nakazono K, Watanabe N, Matsuno K, Sasaki J, Sato T, Inoue M. Does superoxide underlie the pathogenesis of hypertension? *Proc Natl Acad Sci USA.* 1991;88:10045.

174. Meredith IT, Anderson TJ, Yeung AC, Lieberman EH, Dyce MC, Gonenne A, Uehata A, Selwyn AP, Ganz P. Superoxide dismutase restores endothelial vasodilator function in human coronary arteries *in vivo. Circulation.* 1993;88:I-467.

175. Garcia C, Kilcoyne CM, Cardillo C, Cannon RO III, Quyyumi AA, Panza JA. Effect of copper-zinc superoxide dismutase on endothelium-dependent vasodilation in patients with essential hypertension. *Hypertension.* 1995;26:863.

176. Garcia CE, Kilcoyne CM, Cardillo C, Cannon RO 3rd, Quyyumi AA, Panza JA. Evidence that endothelial dysfunction in patients with hypercholesterolemia is not due to increased extracellular nitric oxide breakdown by superoxide anions. *Am J Cardiol.* 1995;76:1157.

177. Flaherty JT, Pitt B, Gruber JW, Heuser RR, Rothbaum DA, Burwell LR, George BS, Kereiakes DJ, Deitchman D, Gustafson N, Drinker JA, Becker LC, Mancini J, Topol E, Werns SW. Recombinant human superoxide dismutase (h-SOD) fails to improve recovery of ventricular function in patients undergoing coronary angioplasty for acute myocardial infarction. *Circulation.* 1994;89:1982.

178. Ross R. The pathogenesis of atherosclerosis: a perspective for the 1990s. *Nature.* 1993;362:801.

179. Heller R, Münscher-Paulig,F.; Gräbner,R; Till,U. Ascorbic acid potentiates nitric oxide synthesis in endothelial cells. *J Biol. Chem* 1999;274.8254

13 ANTIOXIDANTS AND CARDIOVASCULAR DISEASE

J. Michael Gaziano

INTRODUCTION

Oxidative stress is thought to have an important role in the pathogenesis of cardiovascular disease. The preceding chapters of this book have reviewed the scientific basis of this hypothesis, involving oxidation of low-density lipoprotein (LDL) and subsequent effects on endothelial structure and function, recruitment of monocyte/macrophages, and development of foam cells in an atheroma. Because antioxidant compounds are found in certain foods, the possibility that diets high in these compounds can help prevent cardiovascular disease has long been considered. Over one hundred observational and epidemiological studies, from the 1950s to the present, have examined the role of dietary antioxidants in cardiovascular disease. Many of these studies suggest that diets high in vitamin C, β-carotene, and α-tocopherol may reduce moderately the incidence of atherosclerosis, stroke, and ischemic heart disease.

However, several important factors complicate the study of diet in cardiovascular disease. First, risks and benefits of various aspects of diet accrue over years or even decades, and eating habits change over time. Quantitative assessment of diet is generally based on self reports, and until recently, accurate means of assessing micronutrient data were unavailable. Finally, dietary habits tend to be imbedded in cultural practices and associated with many lifestyle factors, making it difficult to separate the specific effects of diet on cardiovascular disease versus the effects of related lifestyle factors.

Two types of epidemiologic studies have examined the relation between diet and cardiovascular disease: observational studies and randomized controlled studies. Observational studies are excellent for formulating and testing hypotheses and are relatively efficient. With a case-control or cohort design, they can even control for known potential confounding variables. However, they cannot control for unknown confounding variables, and their ability to a establish a small to moderate effect associated with a specific variable is questionable because the degree of uncontrolled confounding variables may be as large or larger than the postulated effect. In such cases, large-scale, randomized controlled trials are necessary to obtain reliable data. Assuming a large enough population size, randomization evenly distributes confounding variables among treatment groups, and enables investigators to much more accurately assess a small to moderate potential benefit of a proposed intervention.

DIETARY ANTIOXIDANTS

In vitro and *in vivo* studies have identified three abundant dietary antioxidants: vitamin C (ascorbic acid), vitamin E, and β-carotene. Vitamin C is a water-soluble antioxidant found in many fresh fruits and vegetables that can scavenge or quench peroxyl and superoxide radicals involved in oxidative damage (1,2). Vitamin C may also regenerate oxidized vitamin E (3), a lipid-soluble compound found in vegetable oils, cereal grains, egg yolk, liver, milk fat, nuts, and green vegetables. Alpha-tocopherol, the most potent antioxidant component of vitamin E, accumulates in lipid membranes and circulating lipids, where it terminates lipid peroxidation (4). Dietary supplementation with vitamin E reduces production of pentane, a byproduct of oxidation of omega-6 fatty acids measured in the breath (5). B-carotene is the most abundant of the carotenoids, which are found in high concentrations in fresh fruits and vegetables such as carrots, squash, melons, spinach, and broccoli. B-carotene is a lipid-soluble antioxidant that can neutralize singlet oxygen (6), prevent lipid oxidation *in vitro* (7) and under certain conditions, is also a chain-breaking antioxidant like vitamin E. B-carotene is concentrated in circulating lipids and in atherosclerotic plaque (8). These three dietary antioxidants have been the most widely studied in epidemiological studies and trials.

Descriptive Studies

Several descriptive or ecological studies -- the simplest of observational-type studies -- have suggested that consumption of fresh fruits and vegetables is inversely correlated with risks of cardiovascular disease (Table 1). Two studies in the United Kingdom found an inverse association between the per capita consumption of fresh fruits and vegetables and risk of cardiovascular disease (CVD) (9,10). In the United States, the dramatic decline in CVD mortality (approximately 2% per year over the last 25 years) has been attributed, in part, to the increased availability and consumption of fresh fruits and vegetables (11). In addition, American per capita consumption of vitamin C intake has been inversely associated with CVD mortality rates (12).

In a study of 16 European countries, Gey *et al.* found an inverse association between mortality rates due to ischemic heart disease and lipid-standardized α-tocopherol levels ($r^2 = 0.44$, P = 0.02), but not vitamin C and β-carotene levels (13,14,15). Similarly, in a study of four European populations, Riemersma found a nonsignificant inverse association between vitamin E intake and cardiovascular mortality (16). Although the results of these studies are suggestive, descriptive studies do not take into account important potential confounding variables, such as other dietary or lifestyle characteristics, genetics, or differing availability of health care resources.

Table 1. Descriptive Studies of Dietary Antioxidants

Variable	Population	Major finding	Reference
Per capita fruit and vegetable consumption	United Kingdom	Higher consumption of fruit and vegetables associated with lower rates of CVD.	(9)
Per capita fruit and vegetable consumption	United Kingdom	Higher consumption of fruit and vegetables associated with lower rates of ischemic heart disease.	(10)
Per capita vitamin C consumption	United States	Higher consumption of vitamin C associated with lower CVD mortality.	(12)
Lipid-standardized α-tocopherol, vitamin C and β-carotene levels	16 European countries	Higher levels of α-tocopherol associated with lower ischemic heart disease	(13,14,15)
Vitamin E intake	4 European countries	Increased vitamin E intake associated with lower cardiovascular mortality	(16)

Case-Control Studies

Case-control studies have the advantage of being able to control for potential confounding variables. Two case-control or cross sectional studies reported a significant inverse association between plasma antioxidant levels and CVD (Table 2). Riemersma (17,18) found that angina patients had significantly lower plasma levels of vitamin C, lipid-standardized vitamin E, and carotene than healthy controls. After multivariate adjustment, the relative risk of angina between the lowest and highest quintiles of lipid-standardized vitamin E level was 2.98 (95% CI = 1.07-6.70). Vitamin C and β-carotene followed a similar trend, but these relationships were significantly attenuated by adjusting for cigarette smoking (relative risk = 1.63 [0.76-3.49] for vitamin C and 1.41 [0.63-3.13] for β-carotene). Vitamin A had no apparent relationship with angina. In the second study, Ramirez found significantly lower leukocyte ascorbic acid levels among those with angiographically documented coronary disease than in controls (P < 0.001) (19).

In the EURAMIC Study, a 1993 case-control study, adipose tissue levels of α-tocopherol and β-carotene were obtained in 683 cases of myocardial infarction and in 727 hospital-based controls (20). Mean levels of β-carotene were 0.35 μg/g in cases and 0.42 μg/g in controls, while α-tocopherol levels were 193 and 192 μg/g for cases and controls, respectively. The multivariate odds ratio in the lowest quintile β-carotene level compared to the highest was 1.78 (95% CI = 1.17-2.71) after controlling for a number of potential confounders, with a significant trend across quintiles (P for trend

= 0.001). The associations were strongest among current and former smokers. In contrast, low α-tocopherol levels were not associated with apparent increased risk; the odds ratio of myocardial infarction in the lowest compared to the highest category was 0.83 (95% CI = 0.57-1.21), and there was no significant trend across quintiles of α-tocopherol tissue levels (P for trend = 0.27).

Table 2. Case Control and Prospective Cohort Studies of Antioxidants in Cardiovascular Disease

Variable	Population	Major finding	Ref
Plasma antioxidant levels	Angina patients and healthy controls	Significantly lower levels of vitamin C, lipid-standardized vitamin E, and β–carotene in angina patients compared to controls.	(17,18)
Leukocyte ascorbic acid levels	Angiographic coronary disease and controls	Significantly lower leukocyte ascorbic acid levels in patients with coronary disease than in controls	(19)
Adipose tissue levels α-tocopherol and β-carotene (EURAMIC study)	683 cases of MI and 727 controls	Lower levels of β-carotene but not α-tocopherol associated with increased risk of MI, particularly current and former smokers.	(20)
Coronary risk factors (Nurses' Health Study)	121,000 female nurses in the US	Coronary disease reduced by 22% among the highest quintile of β-carotene intake, 34% in the highest quintile of vitamin E intake, and 20% for in the highest quintile of vitamin C intake. The highest quintile for combined intake of all three antioxidants had a 46% reduction in risk.	(22)
Consumption of dietary antioxidants (Health Professional Follow-up Study)	39,000 men	Coronary disease reduced by 25% in the highest quintile of β-carotene intake, 2% in the highest quintile of vitamin E intake, and increased by 29% among those in the highest intake of vitamin C.	(29)
Vitamin C intake (First National Health and Nutrition Examination Survey)	11,349 men and women aged 25-74	Those with the highest vitamin C intake had the lowest standardized cardiovascular mortality rate (relative risk 0.66).	(30)

Prospective Cohort Studies

Case-control studies are often more efficient and less costly than cohort studies, but are subject to selection and recall bias. In contrast, with prospective cohort studies , these biases are eliminated by collecting information before disease develops. Most, but not all, of the prospective cohort studies examining the role of dietary intake of antioxidants and cardiovascular disease suggest an inverse association (Table 2)

The Nurses' Health Study, involving 121,000 U.S. female nurses aged 30-55, is the largest prospective cohort study to examine the relationship of antioxidants with cardiovascular disease (21,22,23). Beginning in 1976, participants were followed for eight years with biennial questionnaires about a wide variety of coronary risk factors. In 1980 and 1984, questions were asked about consumption of certain foods during the previous year, with nine options ranging from "never" to "six or more times per day." The validity and reproducibility of the data obtained were documented and this information as well as the questionnaires themselves have been published (24,25). Intake scores were computed by multiplying how frequently each food was consumed by the nutrient content, as determined by U.S. Department of Agriculture and other published sources (26,27,28).

During eight years of follow-up (671,185 person-years), there were 552 cases of coronary disease, including 150 deaths and 437 non-fatal myocardial infarctions. Women in the highest quintile of β-carotene consumption had a 22% risk reduction (relative risk = 0.78, 95%CI = 0.59-1.03; P for trend across quintiles = 0.02) when compared to those in the lowest quintile. For vitamin E, the relative risk was 0.66 (95%CI – 0.50-0.87) in the highest quintile of intake (P for trend = 0.001), an effect attributable almost entirely to supplements, rather than diet. The relative risk for vitamin C was 0.80 (95%CI=0.58-1.10). Across quintiles, there was no significant trend after controlling for vitamin E and multi-vitamin intake, which were highly correlated with vitamin C consumption (P for trend = 0.15). When the intake of β-carotene, vitamin E, and vitamin C were combined into a total antioxidant score, the relative risk for coronary disease was 0.54 (95%CI=0.40-0.73) among those in the highest quintile compared to the lowest (P for trend = 0.001).

A more recent prospective cohort study, The Health Professionals' Follow-up Study, employed the same methodology as the Nurses' Health Study. Here, consumption of dietary antioxidants was examined over a four-year period beginning in 1986 with 39,000 men who had no history of vascular disease or other condition necessitating dietary changes (29). There were 667 major coronary events (360 revascularizations, 209 non-fatal myocardial infarctions, and 106 fatal myocardial infarctions) in four years. When men in the highest quintile of β-carotene intake were compared with those in the lowest quintile, the relative risk was 0.75 (95%CI = 0.57-0.99; P for trend = 0.04). Men in the highest quintile of vitamin E consumption had a relative risk of 0.68 (95%CI = 0.51-0.90; P for trend = 0.01) when compared with those in the lowest. The effect was largely confined to those who consumed more than 100 IU of vitamin E supplements daily for two or more years. The relative risk for vitamin C was 1.29 (P for trend = 0.10).

In the First National Health and Nutrition Examination Survey (NHANES-1), 11,349 men and women aged 25-74 were followed for a median of 10 years. Among those with the highest vitamin C intake, the standardized cardiovascular mortality rate was 34% lower (relative risk = 0.66, 95%CI = 0.53-0.82) than expected (30). Vitamin C supplements explained most of the association. In this study, vitamin C supplementation was not correlated with either vitamin E or multivitamins, a correlation that eliminated a crude association in the both the Nurses' Health Study and Health Professionals' Follow-up Study.

In the Massachusetts Elderly Cohort Study, lifestyle factors were related to health and functional status in the elderly. Dietary information was obtained through annual mailings and personal interviews in 1976 and 1980, with an average follow-up of 4.75 years (31). Of the 1,299 participants, 151 died of cardiovascular causes, including 47 fatal myocardial infarctions (MI). The relative risks of cardiovascular death from lowest to highest quartile of β-carotene were 1.00 (referent), 0.75, 0.65, and 0.57, respectively (P for trend = 0.016), after controlling for confounders such as age, gender, smoking, alcohol consumption, cholesterol intake, and functional status. The corresponding relative risks for fatal MI were 1.00 (referent), 0.77, 0.59, 0.32 (P for trend=0.02).

In the Swedish Cohort Study, 1462 Swedish women were followed prospectively for 12 years. After controlling for age, no correlation was found between vitamin C intake estimated from a 24 hour recall dietary history and cardiovascular mortality (32). The relatively small number of deaths on this cohort may have limited the power to detect small to moderate benefits.

Several studies measured plasma antioxidant levels at baseline for the entire cohort. In the Basel Prospective Study, baseline antioxidants were measured in 2974 middle-aged men who were followed for several years. The risk of death from coronary heart disease was increased among those in the lowest quartile of carotene (relative risk = 1.53; 95%CI = 1.07-2.20) and vitamin C (relative risk = 1.25; 95%CI = 0.77-2.01) level compared with those in the highest (33,34). In addition, low plasma concentrations of carotene accompanied by low plasma concentrations of vitamin C were associated with an elevated risk of ischemic heart disease mortality (relative risk = 1.96, 95% CI = 1.10-3.50). Risk of death from stroke was increased among those with both low β-carotene and low vitamin C levels (relative risk = 4.17; 95% CI = 1.68-10.33). There was no apparent relationship of lipid-standardized vitamin E levels with death from coronary heart disease or stroke.

In the Lipid Research Clinic Coronary Primary Prevention Trial, baseline carotenoid level after 14 years of follow-up was inversely correlated with risk of MI after adjustment for age, smoking, HDL, and LDL (35). In the Kupio Ischemic Heart Disease Study, plasma β-carotene and vitamin E levels were inversely related to progression of carotid artery wall thickness (36).

An alternative to measuring plasma antioxidant levels for an entire cohort is to collect and freeze baseline blood samples at the beginning of the trial. Subjects who later develop cardiovascular disease are matched with healthy controls, and their baseline blood samples are compared. In one such nested case-control study, Street *et al.* found a significant inverse association between baseline β-carotene levels and subsequent myocardial infarction (37). Two other nested case-control studies found no association between vitamin A and vitamin E levels and vascular mortality (38,39). However, the blood samples in these two studies were stored at -20° C, a temperature at which stability of antioxidants is questionable, and vitamin A level may not accurately reflect β-carotene status.

Table 3. Large-Scale Randomized Trials of Antioxidants

Trial	Treatment	Population	Mean Duration	Major finding
Chinese Cancer Prevention Study (41)	β-carotene, Vitamin E and Selenium	29,584 poorly nourished men and women	5 years	Reduction in total mortality largely due to reduction in total cancer.
Finnish Alpha-Tocopherol/B-Carotene Lung Cancer Prevention Study (ATBC) (42)	β-carotene and Vitamin E in a factorial design	29,133 male current and former smokers	6 years	β-carotene: No benefit on cancer or cardiovascular disease; Vitamin E: No benefit on cancer or cardiovascular disease or cancer.
Carotene/Retinol Cancer Prevention Trial (CARET) (45)	β-carotene and retinol	18,314 male smokers and asbestos workers	4 years	No benefit on cancer or cardiovascular disease
Physicians' Health Study (Physician's Health Study) (44)	β-carotene	22,071 healthy male physicians	12 years	No benefit on total epithelial cancers or cardiovascular disease
Cambridge Heart Antioxidant Study (CHAOS) (54)	Vitamin E	2,002 with coronary artery disease	14 years	Significant decrease in risk of MI; apparent increase in cardiovascular death

Randomized Trials

Overall, observational data suggest that consumption of dietary antioxidants may reduce risk of cardiovascular disease by 20 to 30%. Although this degree of potential benefit is highly significant, given that one in three Americans will eventually die of cardiovascular disease, it is also small enough to be explained by uncontrolled confounding variables. Observational studies cannot control for such variables because data on individuals are not obtained. Increased dietary intake of antioxidant vitamins could be a marker for other (even unknown) dietary or lifestyle practices. Alternatively, the benefits of antioxidant-rich food could be derived from other components of these foods. Thus, it is important to evaluate the antioxidant hypothesis further with randomized controlled trials, which, if they are of sufficient size and duration, can distribute evenly the effects of known and unknown variables. In a 1991 conference on antioxidants in the prevention of human atherosclerosis, the National Heart Lung and Blood Institute recommend randomized trials of vitamin C, vitamin E, and β-carotene in the primary and secondary prevention of cardiovascular disease (40). Three types of randomized trials have been conducted: primary prevention of CVD in the general population, targeted prevention among those with risk factors for CVD, and secondary prevention among people with existing CVD. To date, results of five recent large-scale trials have been published (Table 3) and further data is forthcoming from ongoing trials. These data supplement results of several smaller-scale secondary prevention trials, some dating back over four decades.

Primary Prevention Trials

The first large-scale randomized primary prevention trial of vitamin supplements in the prevention of cancer was conducted among a poorly-nourished population in Linxian, China (41). Overall, 29,584 men and women were randomized to one of eight treatment arms consisting of various combinations of nine vitamins and minerals. Overall mortality was significantly reduced among those assigned a cocktail of β-carotene (15 mg daily), α-tocopherol (30 mg daily) and selenium (50 μg daily), largely due to a reduction in stomach cancer mortality. Although cardiovascular mortality was also assessed, heart disease rates were relatively low. Less than 9% of the total deaths were due to ischemic heart disease. Cerebrovascular disease accounted for 26% of the total deaths, and there was a nonsignificant reduction in the risk of cerebrovascular disease mortality (relative risk = 0.90; 95% CI = 0.76-1.07). However, in this population, most strokes are likely to be hemorrhagic, which are not usually due to atherosclerotic disease.

The Alpha-Tocopherol Beta-Carotene (ATBC) Cancer Prevention Trial was the first large-scale randomized trial of antioxidant vitamins in a well-nourished population. This two by two factorial trial tested the effect of synthetic α-tocopherol (50 mg daily) and synthetic β-carotene (20 mg daily) in the prevention of lung cancer among 29,133 Finnish male smokers (42). After adjustment for testing multiple hypotheses, there were no increases or decreases in risk that could not be explained plausibly by chance. Nevertheless, some findings were unexpected. There was no reduction in the rate of lung cancer, risk of ischemic heart disease (relative risk = 0.95; 95% CI 0.85-1.05), or ischemic stroke mortality (relative risk = 0.84 95% CI 0.59-1.19) among those assigned to vitamin E. In a subsequent report, the risk of developing angina was lower among those receiving vitamin E (relative risk = 0.91; 95% CI 0.83-0.99) (43). However, the dose of vitamin E was not much higher than the US Recommended Daily Allowance (RDA). Some observational research suggests that higher dose supplementation may be required to reduce the risk of heart disease. The apparent benefits among those who took vitamin E supplements in the Nurses' Health Study (22) and the Health Professionals Follow-up Study(29) were largely confined to those who used an average daily dose of 100 IU or more.

There was an apparent increase in the risk of hemorrhagic stroke in the α-tocopherol treatment group compared to those assigned to placebo (relative risk = 1.50; 95% CI 1.03-2.20), a finding at variance with the lower stroke rates among those assigned antioxidant vitamins in the Linxian, China trial (41). Hemorrhagic stroke was not a prespecified endpoint, and while this finding could be attributed to an antiplatelet effect of vitamin E, it also could be the result of chance.

Unexpectedly, the incidence of lung cancer was increased among those assigned to receive β-carotene. Supplementation had no apparent protective effect with respect to deaths from ischemic heart disease and stroke; in fact there were slightly more ischemic heart disease deaths (relative risk = 1.12; 95% CI 1.00-1.25) among those assigned β-carotene. There was no reduction in risk of angina among the β-carotene group (relative risk = 1.06; 95%CI 0.97-1.16) (5).

The Physician's Health Study is a randomized, double-blind, placebo-controlled trial of β-carotene (50 mg on alternate days) among 22,071 US male physicians, aged 40 to 84, of whom 11% were current and 39% past smokers at baseline in 1982 (44). By December 31, 1995, the scheduled end of the trial, fewer than 1% were lost to morbidity and mortality follow-up and compliance was 78% among those assigned to active pills. After over 12 years of treatment and follow-up, among 11,036 participants randomized to β-carotene and 11,035 to placebo, there were virtually no early or late differences for cardiovascular disease deaths (relative risk = 1.09; 95% CI 0.93-1.27); myocardial infarction (relative risk = 0.96; 95% CI 0.84-1.09); stroke (relative risk = 0.96; 95% CI 0.83-1.11); or a composite of the previous three end points (relative risk = 1.00; 95% CI 0.91-1.09) between treatment groups. There was also no significant benefit or harm for total malignant neoplasms (relative risk = 0.98; 95% CI 0.91-1.06), cancer mortality (relative risk = 1.02; 95% CI 0.89-1.18) or lung cancer. Among current or past smokers, there were likewise no significant early or late effects of β-carotene on any of these end points. This large-scale randomized trial among apparently healthy well-nourished men provides substantial evidence that 12 years of β-carotene supplementation confers neither benefit nor harm with respect to CVD disease mortality or malignant neoplasms.

The B-Carotene and Retinol Efficacy Trial (CARET) involved 18,314 men and women at high risk of lung cancer due to cigarette smoking and/or occupational exposure to asbestos. A combined daily treatment of β-carotene (30 mg) and retinol (25,000 IU) was evaluated (45). Data were collected at annual clinic visits. The study was stopped prematurely when no benefit was detected over the projected funding period and there was a trend toward increased lung cancer in the treatment group. After four years of treatment and follow-up there was an excess of total deaths (relative risk = 1.17; 95% CI 1.03-1.33), a trend toward excess cardiovascular deaths (relative risk = 1.26; 95% CI 0.99-1.61) as well as excess cases of lung cancer among those assigned β-carotene and vitamin A. Data on specific other cardiovascular outcomes including nonfatal events are not yet available.

In the Skin Cancer Prevention Study, a multi-center, double-blind, placebo-controlled trial, investigators randomized 1805 men and women with history of skin cancer to 50 mg of β-carotene daily or placebo (46). More than 80% of participants reported taking more than 50% of their study pills after a median follow-up of 8.2 years by questionnaire and visits to dermatologists. Death certificates of all participants who died during the follow-up period were examined to ascertain the cause of death. There was no significant risk reduction in terms of total (relative risk = 1.05; 95% CI 0.83-1.32) or cardiovascular death (relative risk = 1.15; 95% CI 0.81-1.63).

Secondary Prevention Trials

Beginning in the 1950s, several small-scale trials have tested the effects of antioxidants among individuals with various forms of atherosclerotic disease including claudication and angina as well as following angioplasty. Benefits of supplemental vitamin E were observed in three studies of patients with claudication (47,48,49). However, the utility of these data is limited by the small sample sizes, high dropout rates, and lack of blinding. Two more recent trials found that vitamin E had an equivocal effect in the treatment of angina pectoris. In a nine week placebo-controlled trial among stable angina patients who consumed 3200 IU of vitamin E daily, angina pain score improved nonsignificantly (50). A double-blind crossover trial of 52 angina pectoris patients (51) receiving 1600 IU of vitamin E daily for six months found no apparent benefit of vitamin E treatment as measured by exercise tolerance, symptoms of angina pectoris, or left ventricular function. These studies provide no clear evidence that short term treatment with vitamin E benefits angina patients; however, both the small sample size and short duration of treatment may have limited their statistical power to detect small to moderate benefits.

One recent small-scale trial tested the effect of vitamin E supplementation on restenosis among 100 subjects after percutaneous transluminal coronary angioplasty (52). Restenosis is likely the result of an accelerated atherosclerotic process. Subjects were treated with 400 IU of vitamin E daily after angioplasty. There was an apparent, though not statistically significant, 30% reduction in the risk of restenosis as measured by later catheterization or exercise test.

A subgroup of the Physicians' Health Study was analyzed consisting of over 300 doctors who had chronic stable angina or a prior coronary revascularization procedure but no history of myocardial infarction or stroke (53). Among subjects who received β-carotene, there was a 51% reduction (relative risk = 0.49, 95%CI = 0.29-0.88) in risk of major coronary events, and a 54% reduction (relative risk = 0.46, 95%CI = 0.24-0.85) in risk of major vascular events after an average of five years of treatment. These findings were considerably attenuated with longer follow-up and in a similar subgroup of the ATBC trial, among those with angina at baseline, there was no reduction in risk of cardiovascular mortality or events for β-carotene or vitamin E (43).

In the Cambridge Heart Antioxidant Study (CHAOS), a randomized, double-blind, placebo-controlled trial, 2002 patients with angiographically proven coronary artery disease were assigned to supplemental vitamin E (n=1035; 546 patients treated with 800 IU and the remainder with 400 IU daily after a protocol change) or placebo (n=967) (54). Median follow-up was 510 days. Compared to those receiving placebo, those assigned to vitamin E had a significantly lower risk of subsequent nonfatal MI (relative risk = 0.53; 95% CI 0.11-0.47) and a combined endpoint of nonfatal MI and cardiovascular death (relative risk = 0.53; 95%CI 0.34-0.83). However, there was a nonsignificant excess of cardiovascular deaths (relative risk = 1.18; 95% CI 0.62-2.27). Due to the relatively small study sample size there were imbalances in various baseline characteristics between the two treatment groups including trends toward fewer women, lower cholesterol levels, and lower systolic blood pressure levels in the placebo group.

Ongoing Large-Scale Trials

More reliable data should soon be forthcoming that will further define the role of antioxidants in the prevention and treatment of atherosclerotic disease. Currently, several large-scale randomized trials are examining the role of dietary antioxidants in both primary and secondary prevention of cardiovascular disease and cancer. Three large-scale trials are testing antioxidant supplements among those without known atherosclerotic disease. The Women's Health Study (WHS) is testing vitamin E and low dose aspirin in the primary prevention of cardiovascular disease and cancer in 40,000 healthy, U.S. health professionals. The Heart Protection Study is testing a cocktail of vitamin E, β-carotene, and vitamin C in a factorial design with a cholesterol-lowering medicine among 20,000 higher-risk individuals with coronary risk factors but no known cardiovascular disease. The Physicians' Health Study will continue treatment with β carotene for an additional five years with willing participants and vitamin E, vitamin C, and a multivitamin will be added in a factorial design.

Three large-scale secondary prevention trials are currently underway. The Women's Antioxidant Cardiovascular Study (WACS) is a secondary prevention trial of vitamin C, vitamin E, and β-carotene in a factorial design which is has randomized approximately 8,000 female health professionals with reported cardiovascular disease or with several coronary risk factors. The Heart Outcomes Prevention Evaluation (HOPE) Study is testing vitamin E among 9,000 men and women with prior myocardial infarction or stroke or known peripheral vascular disease. The Gruppo Italiano per lo Studio della Sopravvivenza nell'Infarcto Miocardico (GISSI) is conducting an unblinded trial of vitamin E among those with a recent myocardial infarction. In addition, several small-scale angiographic trials are testing antioxidant supplements alone or in various combinations among individuals with coronary artery disease.

CONCLUSIONS

Antioxidants represent a promising but as yet unproven means to reduce risks of cardiovascular disease. Recent trials raise the possibility that some of the benefits suggested from observational epidemiology are overestimated (55). It remains possible that well-nourished populations may not derive as much benefit from supplementation as under-nourished populations. β-carotene supplementation appears to confer no overall benefit in the primary prevention of cardiovascular disease among well-nourished individuals. However, whether risk can be reduced among those with disease or lower baseline levels of β-carotene remains unclear. For vitamin E, both of the two primary prevention trials had methodological limitations. Recent trial data suggest that vitamin E may reduces reinfarction among those with coronary disease; however, this requires confirmation in the current ongoing large-scale randomized trials. These ongoing trials will provide valuable information upon which to make clinical decisions for individuals and to base policy for the health of the general public.

We must not forget, however, that even if all the postulated benefits of antioxidant vitamins in reducing cardiovascular disease are realized, these benefits are likely to be modest. Other factors, such as the proscription of harmful lifestyle practices have far greater benefits (56). Decreasing blood cholesterol by 10% reduces risk of coronary heart disease by 20-30%. Treating mild to moderate hypertension with drugs reduces diastolic blood pressure, on average, by 5 to 6 mmHg, yielding a 42% reduction in risk of stroke and a 16% reduction in coronary heart disease. Finally, smoking cessation reduces the risk of coronary heart disease by 50% within a few months. Three years after quitting, a former smoker's risk returns to that of a nonsmoker. Although it remains unclear whether antioxidant supplementation reduces the risks of cardiovascular disease, consumption of fruits and vegetables high in these micronutrients is an important part of a healthy diet.

References

1.   Niki E, Saito T, Kamiya Y The role of vitamin C as an antioxidant. *Chem Lett* 1983; 631-2.
2.   Som S, Raha C, Chatterje IB. Ascorbic acid: a scavenger of superoxide radical. *Acta Amino Enzymol* 1983; 5:243-50.
3.   Packer JE, Slater TF, Wilson RL. Direct observation of a free radical interaction between vitamin E and Vitamin C. *Nature* 1979; 278:737-8.
4.   Ingold KU, Webb AC, Witter D, Burton GW, Metcalf TA, Muller DPR. Vitamin E remains the major lipid-soluble, chain-breaking antioxidant in human plasma even in individuals suffering severe vitamin E deficiency. *Arch Biochem Biophys* 1987; 259:224-5.
5.   Lemoyne M, Van Gossum A, Kurian RT, Ostro M, Axler J, Jeejeebhoy KN. Breath pentane analysis as an index of lipid peroxidation: a functional test of vitamin E status. *Am J Clin Nutr* 1987; 46:267-72.
6.   Foote CS, Denny RW, Weaver L. Chang, Y Peters J. Quenching of singlet oxygen. *Ann N Y Acad Sci* 1970; 171:139-48.
7.   Burton GW, Ingold KU. β-carotene: An unusual type of lipid antioxidant. *Science* 1984; 224:569-73.
8.   Prince MR, LaMuraglia GM, MacNichol EF. Increased preferential absorption in human atherosclerotic plaque with oral β-carotene: implications for laser endarterectomy. *Circulation* 1988;78:338-44.
9.   Acheson RM, Williams DRR. Does consumption of fruit and vegetables protect against stroke? *Lancet* 1983;1:1191-93.
10.   Armstrong BK, Mann JL, Adelstein AM, Eskin F. Commodity consumption and ischemic heart disease mortality, with special reference to dietary practices *J Chronic Dis.* 1975; 36:673-7.
11.   Verlangieri AJ, Kapeghian JC, El-Dean S, Bush M. Fruit and vegetable consumption and cardiovascular disease mortality. *Med. Hypoth.* 1985; 16:7-15.
12.   Ginter, E. Decline of coronary mortality in the United States and vitamin C. *Am J Clin Nutr* 1979; 32:511-2.
13.   Gey KF, Brubacher GB, Stahelin. Plasma levels of antioxidant vitamins in relation to ischemic heart disease and cancer. *Am J Clin Nutr* 1987; 45:1368-77.
14.   Gey KF, Puska P. Plasma vitamins E and A inversely correlated to mortality from ischemic heart disease in cross-cultural epidemiology. *Ann N Y Acad Sci* 1989; 570:254-82.
15.   Gey KF, Stahelin HB, Puska P, Evans A. Relationship of plasma vitamin C to mortality from ischemic heart disease. *Ann N Y Acad Sci* 1987; 498:110-23.
16.   Riemersma RA, Oliver M, Elton MA, Alfthan G, Vartiainen E, Salo M, Rubba P, Mancici M, Georgi H, Vuilleumier J, Gey KF. Plasma antioxidants and coronary heart disease: vitamins C and E and selenium. *Eur J Clin Nutr* 1990; 44:143-50.
17.   Riemersma RA, Wood DA, Macintyre CHH, Elton RA, Gey KF, Oliver MF. Risk of angina pectoris and plasma concentrations of vitamins A,C,E, and carotene. *Lancet* 1991; 337:1-5.
18.   Riemersma RA, Wood DA, Macintyre CCH, Elton RA, Gey KF, Oliver MF. Low plasma Vitamin E and C increased risk of angina in Scottish men. *Ann N Y Acad Sci* 1989; 570:291-5.

19.   Ramirez J, Flowers NC. Leukocyte ascorbic acid and its relationship to coronary heart disease in man. *Am J Clin Nutr* 1980; 33:2079-87.

20.   Kardinaal AFM, Kok FJ, Ringstad J, Gomez-Aracena J, Mazaev VP, Kohlmeier L, Martin BC, Aro A, Kark JD, Delgado-Rodriguez M, Riemermsa RA, Huttunen JK, Martin-Moreno JM. Antioxidants in adipose tissue and risk of myocardial infarction: the EURAMIC study. *Lancet* 1993;342:1379-1384.

21.   Manson JE, Stampfer MJ, Willet WC, Colditz GA, Rosner B, Speizer FE, Hennekens CH. A prospective study of antioxidant vitamins and incidence of coronary heart disease in women. *Circulation* 1991; 84(4), suppl II.

22.   Stampfer MJ, Hennekens CH, Manson JE, Colditz GA, Rosner B, Willett WC. A prospective study of vitamin E consumption and risk of coronary disease in Women. *N Engl J Med* 1993;328:1444-1449.

23.   Manson JE, Stampfer MJ, Willett WC, Colditz GA, Rosner B, Speizer FE, Hennekens CH. A prospective study of vitamin C and incidence of coronary heart disease in women. *Circulation* 1992; 85:865.

24.   Willett WC, Sampson L, Stampfer MJ, *et al.* Reproducibility and validity of a semiquantitative food frequency questionnaire. *Am J Epidemiol* 1985; 122:51-65.

25.   Salvini S, hunter DJ, Sampson L, *et al.* Food-based validation of a dietary questionnaire: the effects of week-to-week variation in food consumption. *Int J Epidemiol* 1989; 18:858-67.

26.   Adams CF. Nutritive values of American foods. Washington, DC: United States Department of Agriculture, 1975. (No 456.)

27.   Consumer and Food Economics Institute. Composition of foods: fruits and fruit juices, raw, processed, prepared. Handbook 8-9. Washington, DC: US Department of Agriculture, 1982.

28   Willett WC, Stampfer MJ. Total energy intake: implications for epidemiologic analyses. *Am J Epidemiol* 1986; 124:17 27.

29.   Rimm EB, Stampfer MJ, Ascherio A, Giovannucci E, Colditz GA, Willett WC. Dietary intake and risk of coronary heart disease among men. *N Engl J Med* 1993;328:1450-1456.

30.   Enstrom JE, Kanim LE, Klein MA. Vitamin C intake and mortality among a sample of the United States population. *Epidemiology* 1992; 3:194-202.

31.   Gaziano JM, Manson JE, Branch LG, LaMott F, Colditz GA, Buring JE, Hennekens CH. Dietary β-carotene and decreased cardiovascular mortality in an elderly cohort. *J Am Coll Card* 1992;19:377.

32.   Lapidus L, Anderson H, Bengtson C, Bosceus I. Dietary habits in relation to incidence of cardiovascular disease and death in women; a 12 year follow-up of participants in the study of women in Gothenberg, Sweden. *Am J Clin Nutr* 1986; 44:444-8.

33.   Gey KF, Stahelin HB. Eicholzer M. Poor plasma status of carotene and vitamin C is associated with higher mortality from ischemic heart disease and stroke: Prospective Basel Study. *Clin Investig* 1993; 71:3-6.

34.   Eichholzer M, Stahelin HB, Gey KF. Inverse correlation between essential antioxidants in plasma and subsequent risk to develop cancer, ischemic heart disease and stroke, respectively: 12-year follow-up of the Prospective Basel Study. In: *Free radicals and aging*. Emerit I and Chance B, eds. Basel/Switzerland: Birkhauser Verlag 1992, 398-410.

35.   Morris DL, Kritchevsky SB, Davis CE. Serum carotenoids and coronary heart disease in the Lipid Research Clinics Coronary Primary Prevention Trial. *Circulation* 1993; 87(2):2 (abstr).

36.   Salonen JT, Nyyssonen K, Parviainen, Kantola M, Korpela H, Salonen R. Low plasma β-carotene, vitamin E and selenium levels associated with accelerated carotid atherogenesis in hypercholesterolemic eastern Finnish men. *Circulation* 1993; 87(2):1.

37.   Street DA, Comstock GW, Salkeld RM, Schuep W, Klag M. A population based case-control study of serum antioxidants and myocardial infarction. *Am J Clin Nutr* 1991;134:719-20.

38.   Kok FJ, de Bruijn AM, Vermeeren R, Hofman A, VanLaar A, deBruin M, Hermus RTJ, Valkenberg HA. Serum selenium, vitamin antioxidants and cardiovascular mortality: a 9 year follow-up study in the Netherlands. *Am J Clin Nutr* 1987;45:462-8.

39.   Salonen JT, Salonen R, Penttila I, Herranen J, Jauhiainen M, Kantola M, Lappetelainen R, Maenpaa P, Alfthan G, Puska P. Serum fatty acids, apolipoproteins, selenium and vitamin antioxidants and risk of death from coronary artery disease. *Am J Clin Nutr* 1985; 56:226-31.

40.   Steinberg D & Workshop Participants. 1992 Antioxidants in the prevention of human atherosclerosis: Summary of the proceedings of a national heart, Lung and Blood Institute Workshop: September 5-6, 1991, Bethesda, Maryland. *Circulation* 85 (6): 2337-2344.

41.   Blot WJ, Li JY, Taylor PR, Guo W, Dawsey S, Wang GQ, Yang CS, Zheng SF, Gail M, Li GY, Yu Y, Liu BQ, Tangrea J, Sun YH, Liu F, Fraumeni JF Jr, Zhang YH, Li B. Nutrition intervention trials in Linxian, China: Supplementation with specific vitamin/mineral combinations, cancer incidence, and disease-specific mortality in the general population. *J Natl Cancer Inst* 1993;85:1483-1492.

42.   The Alpha-Tocopherol, B-Carotene Cancer Prevention Study Group. The effect of vitamin E and β-carotene on the incidence of lung cancer and other cancers in male smokers. *N Engl J Med*, 1994;330;1029-35.

43.   Rapola JM, Virtamo J, Haukka JK, Heinonen, Albanes, Taylor PR, Huttunen JK. Effect of vitamin E and β-carotene on the incidence of angina pectoris: A randomized, double-blind, controlled trial. *JAMA* 1996:275:693-698.

44.   Hennekens CH, Buring JE, Manson JE, Stampfer M, Rosner B, Cook NR, Belanger C, LaMotte F, Gaziano JM, Ridker PM, Willett W, Peto R. Lack of effect of long term supplementation with β-carotene on the incidence of malignant neoplasms and cardiovascular disease. *N Engl J Med* 1996;334:1145-1149.

45.   Omenn GS, Goodman GE, Thornquist MD, Blames J, Cullen MR, Glass A, Keogh JP, Meyskens FL, Valanis B, Williams JH, Barnhart S, Hammer S. Effects of a combination of β-carotene and vitamin A on lung cancer and cardiovascular disease. *N Engl J Med* 1996;334:1150-1155.

46.   Greenberg ER, Baron JA, Karagas MR, Stukel TA, Nierenberg DW, Stevens MM, Mandel JS, Haile RW. Mortality associated with low plasma concentration of β-carotene and the effect of oral supplementation. *JAMA* 1996;275:660-703.

47.   Livingston PD, Jones C. Treatment of intermittent claudication with vitamin E. *Lancet* 1958; 2:602-4.

48.   Williams HTG, Fenna D, MacBeth RA. Alpha-tocopherol in the treatment of intermittent claudication. *Surg Gyn Obst* 1971; 132:662-6.

49.   Haeger K. Long-time treatment of intermittent claudication with Vitamin E. *Am J Clin Nutr* 1974; 27:1179-81.

50.   Anderson TW, Reid W. A double-blind trial of vitamin E in the treatment of angina pectoris. *Am Heart J* 10974; 93:444-449.

51.   Gillian RE, Mandell B, Warbasse JR. Quantitative evaluation of vitamin E in the treatment of angina pectoris. *Am Heart J* 1977; 93(4):444-9.

52.   DeMaio SJ, King, SB III, Lembo NJ, Roubin GS, Hearn JA, Bhagavan HN, Sgoutas DS. Vitamin E supplementation, plasma lipids and incidence of restenosis after percutaneous transluminal coronary angioplasty (PTCA). *J Am Coll Nutr* 1992;11:131-138.

53.   Gaziano JM, Manson JE, Ridker PM, Buring JE, Hennekens CH. B-carotene therapy for chronic stable angina. *Circulation* 1990; 82(4, Supplement III):III-202.

54.   Stephens NG, Parsons A, Schofield PM, Kelly F, Cheeseman, Mitchinson MJ, Brown MJ. Randomized controlled trial of vitamin E in patients with coronary disease: Cambridge Heart Antioxidant Study (CHAOS). *Lancet* 1996;347:781-786.

55.   Hennekens CH, Buring JE, Peto R, Antioxidant vitamins-benefits not yet proven. *N Engl J Med* 1994; 330-1080-1081.

56.   Manson JE, Tosteson H, Ridker PM, Satterfield S, Hebert P, O'Connor GT, Buring JE, Hennekens CH. The primary prevention of myocardial infarction. *N Engl J Med* 1992; 326:1406-1416.

14 GLYCATION AND GLYCOXIDATION IN DIABETIC VASCULAR DISEASE

Suzanne R. Thorpe, Timothy J. Lyons and John W. Baynes

INTRODUCTION

Elevated blood sugar is the hallmark of diabetes. Paradoxically, increased blood glucose occurs both when there is a complete absence of insulin in the body (type I, insulin dependent diabetes mellitus (IDDM)) and when there is an excess of circulating insulin (type II, non-insulin dependent diabetes mellitus (NIDDM)). Type I diabetes is generally associated with a young or juvenile onset, while Type II diabetes typically occurs with older age and obesity. However, individuals affected by either type of diabetes are at risk for developing a similar set of chronic complications. Microvascular disease in diabetes includes retinopathy, nephropathy and neuropathy. Macrovascular disease is associated with the 2-4 fold increased risk for atherosclerosis and ischemic heart disease observed in diabetic individuals. An unexpected finding in diabetes is that the tissues and cells in which complications occur, such as retinal and other vascular endothelial cells, renal mesangial cells and neural cells do not require insulin for glucose uptake. Because of the common occurrence of elevated circulating glucose, overlap in the complications associated with both type of diabetes, and development of complications in tissues freely permeable to glucose, much research has focused on mechanisms by which glucose itself may contribute to vascular disease in diabetes.

Like most chronic diseases, diabetes is widely believed to involve increased oxidative stress (1-4). Functionally oxidative stress is a condition characterized by an increase in the steady state concentration of reactive oxygen species. Increased oxidative stress and oxidative damage to tissues are general features of chronic disease, but a key issue is whether the increased stress and damage is the cause or the consequence of disease pathology. Recent insights into mechanisms of non-oxidative, carbohydrate-dependent modifications of proteins suggest that it may not be necessary to invoke increased oxidative stress as a significant factor in the etiology of diabetic vascular disease.

There are numerous chemical and metabolic hypotheses to explain the biochemical and molecular changes resulting from chronic hyperglycemia. Research in the authors' laboratories has focused primarily on chemical, non-enzymatic mechanisms contributing to diabetic vascular disease. We have studied chemical routes from reducing sugars to advanced glycation end-products (AGEs), with emphasis on glycoxidation products such as N^ϵ(carboxymethyl)lysine (CML) and pentosidine. However, as will become apparent, distinctions between chemical and metabolic sources of dysfunction in diabetes are likely to be somewhat arbitrary. There may be several pathways by which products of glucose metabolism lead to chemical modifications of proteins, and simultaneously pathways by which chemically modified proteins influence cellular metabolism. Below we provide background on the chemistry of both oxidative and non-oxidative modification of protein by reducing sugars. We will summarize evidence for increased carbohydrate-dependent and oxidative damage to protein in diabetes, emphasizing our studies on changes in skin collagen with age and in diabetes. Alternative mechanisms, independent of oxidation chemistry, will be considered for the increase in carbohydrate modifications that may contribute to pathology in diabetes. We will also describe how chemical, non-enzymatic reactions and metabolism may intersect to contribute synergistically to the pathogenesis of diabetic complications. Finally, because diabetes is a disorder of both carbohydrate and lipid metabolism, we will also consider the role of lipid peroxidation in chemical modification of proteins and development of diabetic complications.

CHEMISTRY OF GLYCATION AND GLYCOXIDATION REACTIONS

Glycation Involving Glucose

In its broadest definition, glycation refers to the chemical, non-enzymatic adduction of reducing sugars to protein. Glycation is one of the first steps in the browning or Maillard reaction, originally described by food chemists. The most common glycation reaction in the body is modification of the ε-amino group of lysine residues in protein by glucose, shown in Figure 1. The reaction begins with the reversible and rapid formation of a Schiff base, followed by a slower Amadori rearrangement, yielding a metastable, covalent adduct. In the case of glucose, the Amadori product is called fructose-lysine because the carbonyl functionality has moved from the C1-aldose position of glucose to the C2-ketose position, structurally related to fructose. Glycation involves dehydration and rearrangement reactions, neither of which involves oxidation chemistry.

Because tissue protein is bathed in 5 mM glucose (normal blood glucose concentration), fructose-lysine is formed continuously on protein throughout the body. The actual concentration of fructose-lysine on protein is determined both by the ambient glucose concentration and the rate of protein turnover. Overall rates of protein turnover are not significantly affected in diabetes so that the higher ambient glucose results in generally higher levels of fructose-lysine in protein isolated from diabetic compared to non-diabetic individuals. The observation that fructose-lysine

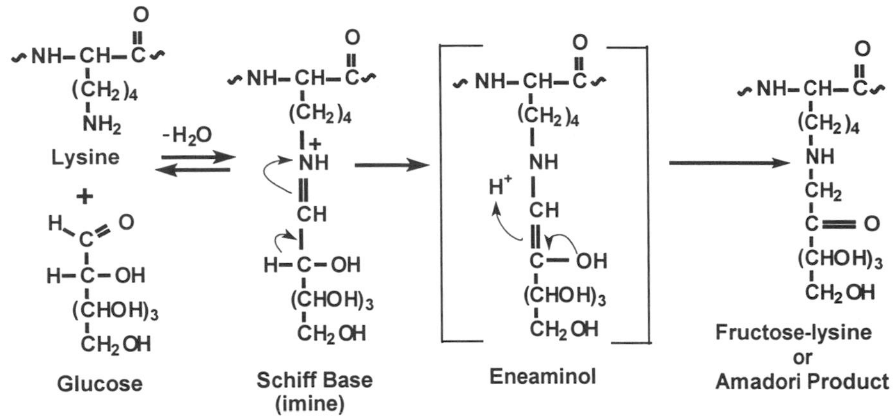

Figure 1. Glycation of lysine residues by glucose. The formation of a Schiff base (imine) between glucose and lysine involves a dehydration reaction. The chemically labile imine undergoes an Amadori rearrangement, via an eneaminol intermediate, to the more stable ketoamine adduct, fructose-lysine. None of the steps leading to the Amadori product requires the participation of oxygen or metal ion.

is a measure of glycemia has become a valuable tool for clinical management of diabetic patients. Thus, measurement of the concentration of glycated hemoglobin (HbA1c) provides an index of integrated glycemia during the previous 4-6 weeks. Increased glycation of long-lived, extracellular protein such as glomerular basement membrane (5), skin collagen (6) or lens crystallins (7) is welldocumented in diabetes, and also correlates with long-term glycemic control. Based on our analyses in liver cytosolic proteins from diabetic and non-diabetic rats, there is also an increase in hepatic intracellular protein glycation comparable to the increase in blood glucose (unpublished), consistent with the insulin-independent uptake of glucose in liver. The relatively rapid rate of intracellular protein turnover may limit long term deleterious effects of glycation on intracellular protein function, even during diabetic hyperglycemia

Glycation By Carbohydrates Other Than Glucose

3-Deoxyglucosone

Fructose-lysine undergoes both forward and reverse reactions. The reversal of the Amadori rearrangement through the Schiff base leads to the formation of the C2-epimers, glucose and mannose, and liberation of lysine (8). A biologically relevant, non-oxidative, forward rearrangement reaction of fructose-lysine also regenerates lysine and results in formation of 1- and 3-deoxyglucosones. 1-Deoxyglucosone have not been detected *in vivo*, however, 3-deoxyglycosone is increased 2-3 fold in plasma of diabetic and non-diabetic uremic subjects (9-12). The metabolic reduction product of 3-deoxyglycosones, 3-deoxyfructose, has also been measured in increased concentrations in plasma and urine of diabetic individuals (13).

Another source of 3-deoxyglucosone is the spontaneous β-elimination of phosphate from intracellular fructose-3-phosphate. Fructose-3-phosphate is formed by an enzymatic reaction catalyzed by fructose 3-phosphokinase (14). The greater flux of glucose through the polyol pathway during diabetic hyperglycemia will lead to an increase in intracellular fructose and fructose-3-phosphate, which has been noted in lens (14) and red cells in diabetes (15). The formation of 3-deoxyglucosone by both the Maillard reaction (from fructose-lysine) and metabolic pathways (from fructose-3-phosphate) illustrates the interplay between non-enzymatic and enzymatic chemistry in formation of reactive dicarbonyl sugars. The relative importance of these alternative pathways for increased formation of 3-deoxyglucosone in diabetes is unknown.

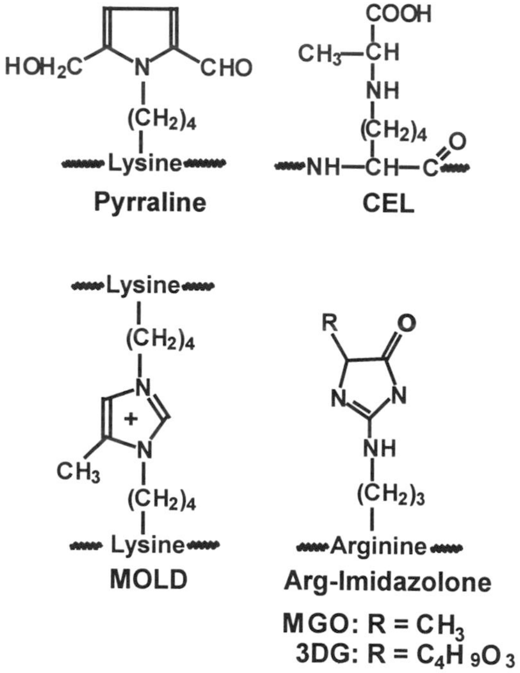

Figure 2. Structures of some glycated amino acids and a cross-link which may be formed under non-oxidative conditions. The precursor for pyrraline and 3-deoxyglucosone-Arg-imidazolone is 3-deoxyglucosone (3DG), and for N^{ε}(carboxyethyl)lysine (CEL), methylglyoxal lysine dimer (MOLD) and Arg-imidazolone is methylglyoxal (MGO). Neither precursors nor adducts require oxidation reactions for their formation.

Dicarbonyl sugars are more reactive than glucose with protein and 3-deoxyglucosone is a potent protein browning and cross-linking agent (16). Chemically characterized glycation products of 3-deoxyglucosone reaction with arginine and lysine include 3-deoxyglucosone-Arg-imidazolone (17) and pyrraline (18), respectively (Figure 2). These two compounds are dehydration and rearrangement products, formed under non-oxidative conditions. 3-deoxyglucosone-Arg-imidazolone, however, can be easily oxidized to 3-deoxyglucosone-Arg-dehydroimadizolone. 3-deoxyglucosone-Arg derivatives have been detected in tissues by immunohistochemistry, however, the antibody used could not distinguish between the two forms of the imidazolone adducts (17). Thus, it remains uncertain to what extent the increased concentration of 3-deoxyglucosone-Arg-imidazolone detected in diabetic erythrocytes, glomerular lesions, and in diabetic and non-diabetic atherosclerotic lesions in aorta, reflects the oxidized or non-oxidized derivative. Plasma proteins also contain pyrraline, and protein-bound pyrraline is increased in diabetes (18). Immunohistochemical techniques showed that pyrraline is found in interstitial connective tissue in both normal and diabetic kidneys (19). Recently free pyrraline has been measured in urine of both non-diabetic and diabetic individuals, and its concentration was correlated with glycemic control in diabetic subjects (20).

To the best of our knowledge, 3-deoxyglucosone is formed solely by non-oxidative mechanisms. It is not an oxidation but a dehydration product of glucose. The increase in 3-deoxyglucosone and its adducts to protein in diabetes indicates that not all dicarbonyl intermediates and products of the Maillard reaction are derived from oxidative chemistry.

Methylglyoxal

The dicarbonyl compound, methylglyoxal, does not fit the classic definition of a carbohydrate, a compound with the molecular formula $(CH_2O)_n$. However, chemically, methylglyoxal is closely related to carbohydrates and biochemically it is formed *in vivo* largely as a by-product of carbohydrate metabolism. methylglyoxal, like 3-deoxyglucosone, can be formed by non-oxidative β-elimination of phosphate from triose phosphate intermediates in anaerobic glycolysis. It is estimated that as much as 1% of triose phosphates produced during glycolysis are converted spontaneously to methylglyoxal (21). During diabetic hyperglycemia the greater flux of glucose through anaerobic glycolysis and the sorbitol pathway will also lead to an increase in formation of methylglyoxal (22). Methylglyoxal is also formed metabolically from catabolism of threonine and acetone. Increased concentrations of methylglyoxal and its detoxification product D-lactate have been reported in blood from diabetic subjects (23,24). Another potentially important source of methylglyoxal in diabetic subjects is catabolism of aminoacetone by semicarbizide sensitive amine oxidase yielding methylglyoxal, ammonia and H_2O_2 (25). This enzyme is elevated in plasma of IDDM and NIDDM subjects, and its activity is correlated with HbA1c concentrations (26). Of interest, enzymatic activity was highest in patients showing evidence of retinopathy and/ or nephropathy.   The authors concluded, however, that elevated semicarbizide sensitive amine oxidase may reflect progression of disease, rather than being predictive for any particular complication. Relevant to macrovascular disease the enzyme is also increased in patients with congestive heart failure and was increased with severity of disease (27). It may also be pertinent that semicarbizide sensitive amine oxidase increases toxicity to endothelial cells of other amines such as methylamine or allylamine by conversion to formaldehyde and acrolein, respectively (28).

In vitro studies have also shown that, unlike 3-deoxyglucosone, methylglyoxal may be formed by oxidative reactions. Thus, the production of methylglyoxal from the Schiff base (Figure 1) (29) and from oxidation of polyunsaturated fatty has been reported (30). The extent to which oxidation reactions contribute to methylglyoxal production *in vivo* is uncertain, since both oxidative (*e.g.* semicarbizide sensitive amine oxidase) and non-oxidative (*e.g.* triose phosphate degradation) routes to its formation are possible and are likely to occur simultaneously. However, as argued below, whatever the primary mechanism of methylglyoxal formation *in vivo*, impairment in the detoxification of this and other dicarbonyl compounds may be the critical factor in the pathogenesis of diabetic vascular disease.

Like glucose, methylglyoxal modifies lysine residues via formation of a Schiff base. The product formed is N^ϵ(carboxyethyl)lysine, via a Canizzaro rearrangement. N^ϵ(carboxyethyl)lysine increases in both lens protein and skin collagen with age (31). However, methylglyoxal reacts preferentially with arginine residues in protein, leading to formation of Arg-imidazolone and a fluorescent pyrimidine (Figure 2, 32,33). Based on immunochemical techniques the concentration of methylglyoxal-Arg adducts in serum proteins of diabetic subjects is increased and correlates with glycated hemoglobin (34). Both N^ϵ(carboxyethyl)lysine and Arg adducts of methylglyoxal are also formed in protein under oxidative conditions in vitro, from a variety of sugars including glucose, ascorbate, ascorbate oxidation products and pentoses (31,34). Even in these cases, it is possible that methylglyoxal formation is the result of non-oxidative reactions, *e.g.* reverse aldol reactions or dehydration of glyceraldehyde.

Proteins incubated with methylglyoxal exhibit an increase in fluorescence, brown color and cross-linking. One of these cross-links has been chemically characterized as an imidazolium salt, <u>m</u>ethylgly<u>o</u>xal lysine <u>d</u>imer (MOLD) (Figure 2, 35,36), which has been found in elevated amounts in plasma proteins in diabetic (35) and in non-diabetic uremic subjects (37) and in skin collagen of diabetic subjects (unpublished). MOLD also increases about 3-fold with age in lens protein (36), and represents the quantitatively most abundant non-enzymatic cross-link yet described in collagen. Yim *et al.*. (38), showed that methylglyoxal modification of alanine under mild conditions *in vitro,* and in the absence of metal ions and oxygen, led to formation of Maillard type fluorescence, generation of a radical cation cross-link and an methylglyoxal radical anion. In the presence of oxygen superoxide anion was also formed. If methylglyoxal cross-linking of protein occurs *in vivo* via a similar mechanism, it could explain how increased methylglyoxal modification of protein would be particularly damaging since it could occur in the absence of metal ion and also be a chronic source of reactive oxygen species. Thus, methylglyoxal formed under non-oxidative conditions may contribute to an increase in oxidative stress.

Other Carbohydrates

Fructose, dehyroascorbate, pentoses and phosphorylated sugars are also potent glycating agents, and are more reactive toward protein amino groups than glucose. There are, therefore, many possible precursors of protein modification by reducing sugars *in vivo,* many of which are increased in diabetes. Increases in a variety of forms of glycated protein during diabetic hyperglycemia provide additional substrates for oxidation, since carbohydrate-protein adducts, including the Amadori product, are more readily oxidized than the precursor sugar. One benefit, then, of efforts to maintain good blood glucose control may be in limiting the concentration of substrates for oxidation reactions. At the same time, as noted above for methylglyoxal and 3-deoxyglucosone, oxidation chemistry is not required for formation of modified and cross-linked protein. Therefore, some forms of protein damage need not be limited by the level of oxidative stress in tissues, but as discussed below, will depend largely on the concentration of reactive carbonyl compounds.

Glycoxidation Reactions

A critical factor in determining the concentration of fructose-lysine *in vitro* is whether glycation occurs under aerobic or anaerobic conditions. Zyzak *et al.* (8) showed that the half-life of fructose-lysine on collagen or model compounds was nearly 4-fold longer when incubations were conducted under anaerobic compared to aerobic conditions. *In vitro*, oxidative conditions promote, and anti-oxidative conditions prevent or markedly inhibit, the development of protein damage measured as increased browning, fluorescence or cross-linking (39). In the biomedical literature, forward reactions from the Amadori product or other glycation adducts have been referred to as advanced glycosylation reactions and the compounds formed are referred to as advanced glycosylation end-products (AGEs) (40,41).

The first structurally characterized AGEs were CML and pentosidine (Figure 3). Using combined gas chromatograph/ mass spectrometry or HPLC analyses, these compounds have been identified in acid hydrolysates of protein incubated *in vitro* under oxidative conditions, with a variety of sugars, including glucose, fructose, 3-deoxyglucosone, ascorbate and pentoses (16,42,43). CML and pentosidine increase 5-7 fold with chronological age in skin collagen (6), and their concentrations are further elevated in collagen from diabetic subjects (6, 44). CML is the most abundant AGE measured in protein from *in vivo* sources to date, and is also a major epitope detected by anti-AGE antibodies (45). Since oxygen was required for their

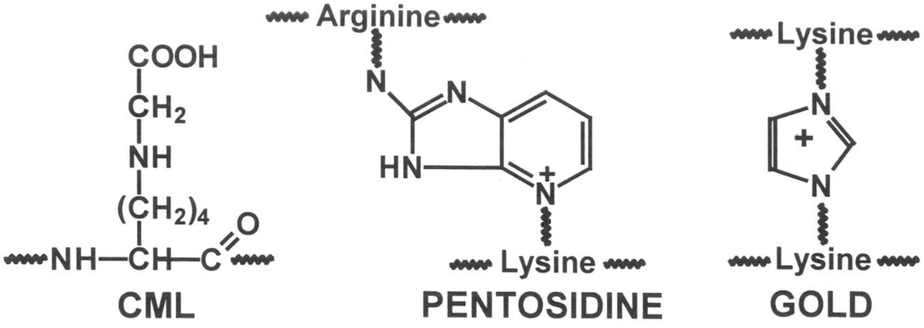

Figure 3. Structures of glycoxidation products. Oxidative reactions are required at some stage in the formation of glycoxidation products from glucose, either during generation of the precursor or conversion to the final adduct on protein. CML = N^{ε}(carboxyethyl)lysine; GOLD = glyoxal lysine dimer.

formation, Baynes coined the term "glycoxidation products" to describe the involvement of both glycation and oxidation reactions in their formation (46), and oxidation was invoked as a fixative of chemical modification. In a sense, glycoxidation products are a form of biological rust which cannot be repaired, but must be removed by protein turnover. For some proteins with slow turnover, such as collagen, the accumulated 'rust' may eventually affect functional properties.

CML was first identified as an oxidation product of the Amadori compound, fructose-lysine (42). A second route to formation of CML involves the dicarbonyl compound glyoxal, formed on autoxidation of glucose (see below, 47). Autoxidation reactions involve the direct oxidation of substrate by oxygen and typically require the participation of metal ions. Glyoxal reacts with lysine and forms CML via a Canizzaro rearrangement (47). Glyoxal can also be formed from glycoaldehyde (48). Glycoaldehyde has been reported as an oxidation product of Schiff bases (29,48) and can be formed oxidatively from the amino acid serine by action of the phagocyte enzyme myeloperoxidase (49). We have also shown that CML can be formed on protein during peroxidation of polyunsaturated fatty acids, in the absence of carbohydrate (50). In fact elevated levels of CML have been detected in atherosclerotic lesions of euglycemic individuals suggesting that in this instance the CML was derived from lipid rather than carbohydrate oxidation (51). The finding that CML can be produced during lipid peroxidation reactions emphasizes the potential role of dyslipidemia in diabetes as a source of 'AGE' formation. CML is thus both a glycoxidation and lipoxidation product, *i.e.* a modification of protein that is formed from during carbohydrate or lipid oxidation.

Recently we also characterized a glyoxal derived cross-link glyoxal lysine dimer (glyoxal lysine dimer, Figure 3,) and have now shown that this cross-link increases in lens protein with age, and is higher in skin collagen from old compared to young individuals (36). Whatever the precursor, CML and glyoxal lysine dimer are both formed as the result of oxidation reactions. Similarly, pentosidine contains 5 of the original 6 carbons of glucose, and is not formed under anaerobic conditions, so that an oxidative reaction must be involved in its formation. Even though pentoses, including ribose and arabinose, are much more ready sources of pentosidine formation of the cross-link from these sugars must also involve an oxidation reaction.

Autoxidation Versus Glycoxidation

Wolff proposed (52) that metal-dependent autoxidation of glucose would yield reactive dicarbonyl compounds, which in turn would react to form ketimine structures on protein. In experiments to determine products of glucose autoxidation during incubation of glucose in phosphate buffer, only two carbonyl compounds were detected, the two-carbon dicarbonyl glyoxal, and the five-carbon sugar arabinose (47). Since glyoxal is a more efficient precursor of CML and arabinose is a more efficient source of pentosidine than glucose, autoxidation of glucose rather than the Amadori compound, may make a major contribution to the formation of glycoxidation products on protein. Using $^{13}C_6$-glucose, Wells-Knecht *et al.* (53) showed that *in vitro* under conditions of high phosphate and glucose, autoxidation of the sugar, rather than oxidative cleavage of the Amadori adduct was the major source of CML. Under conditions of low phosphate and glucose concentrations approximating those of diabetic hyperglycemia, oxidation of the Amadori product became a greater source of CML. Elgawish *et al.* (54) studied CML production in glycated collagen implanted in the peritoneal cavity of diabetic rats and concluded that oxidative cleavage of the Amadori compound was the major route to CML formation *in vivo*. To the best of our knowledge autoxidation reactions, whether of glucose or the Amadori product, require the presence of both oxygen and metal ions. The availability of decompartmentalized metal ions in tissues may be rate limiting for the formation of autoxidation and glycoxidation products.

GLYCATION/ GLYCOXIDATION AND DIABETIC VASCULOPATHY

Glycation and Glycoxidation of Collagen

Our research initially focused on glucose as a reactive, α-hydroxyaldehyde capable of chemically modifying protein throughout the body. The working hypothesis was that increased glucose-dependent modification of protein occurring during diabetic hyperglycemia ultimately led to changes in protein structure and function, particularly affecting long-lived proteins. Thus, the loss of elasticity, increased thermal stability and resistance to enzymatic digestion, and development of fluorescence observed in structural proteins with age (55), and acceleration of the changes in diabetes (6), were attributed in part to glucose-dependent chemical modifications. Further, early studies also showed that glycated protein, even when removed from the presence of free glucose, continued to brown and cross-link (56), suggesting a mechanism whereby hyperglycemia, even if corrected, might continue to contribute to protein damage.

Decreased elasticity of arteries and arterioles is characteristic of diabetes (57) and may partly result from increased glucose-mediated protein cross-linking. Arterial stiffness and hypertension have been associated with skin collagen fluorescence and glycoxidation products in type I diabetic patients (58-61). Arterial stiffness and hypertension combined may alter endothelial shear stresses, predisposing vascular tissue to injury and atherogenesis, as well as to damage in the retinal and renal microcirculations. Further, collagen glycoxidation products may quench the activity of nitric oxide (62) causing abnormalities in vasomotor control. A generalized collagen abnormality in diabetes may, therefore, provide a common underlying mechanism contributing to micro- and macrovascular disease and explain in part, the identification of microalbuminuria as a risk factor for macrovascular disease. In addition, in diabetes, extravasated plasma proteins may also become bound to reactive glycoxidation products on vascular connective tissue. This process could contribute to sequestration of atherogenic lipoproteins such as low-density lipoproteins (LDL). (63). LDL trapped in vessel walls may undergo further glycoxidation and oxidation, increasing its atherogenicity and stimulating, via lipoxidation, further cross-linking of collagen (64). In this scenario interwoven chemical mechanisms contribute to vicious cycles of vascular damage in diabetes.

While the measurement of glycation and glycation products provides circumstantial evidence for a role of chemical, non-enzymatic modifications of protein in the pathogenesis of complications, ultimately the relationships are correlative in nature, rather than proof of a cause-effect relationship. Even if a cause-effect relationship existed, it is unclear which AGE or AGE precursors (glucose, Schiff base, Amadori product, etc.) should be identified as the source of pathology. Fructose-lysine, thought to be the harmless precursor of damaging glycoxidation products, could be a chronic source of reactive oxygen. Some studies found no association between levels of fructose-lysine in collagen and limited joint mobility, retinopathy, nephropathy, or arterial stiffness (65,66), suggesting that fructose-lysine in collagen does not contribute directly to the development complications. However, it may contribute indirectly, through its role as a precursor of AGEs. In support of this hypothesis we found that levels of fructose-lysine in skin collagen were independently associated with the presence of retinopathy and early nephropathy (microalbuminuria) (61). This finding is consistent with the work of Cohen *et al..* (67-69) described below concerning glycated albumin and diabetic nephropathy.
The follow discussion evaluates the evidence for chemical and metabolic sources of collagen damage in diabetes.

Oxidative Stress in Diabetes

Differences in systemic oxidative stress in diabetic subjects might modulate their risk for development of complications and, in part, explain the differential susceptibility to complications among individuals with comparable duration and severity of diabetes. Reactive oxygen species such as superoxide or hydroxyl radical are too short-lived to be readily measured, so that a number of indirect measures of oxidative chemistry have been used to assess oxidative stress in diabetes. These measures suggest that oxidative stress is increased in diabetes and contributes to the development of both microvascular complications and to premature atherosclerosis. For example, measurements have shown reduced antioxidant levels in plasma from diabetic compared to non-diabetic subjects, including α-tocopherol, reduced glutathione and superoxide dismutase and increased lipid peroxidation products (reviewed in 3,70). Further, plasma from poorly-controlled diabetic patients also showed reduced ability to trap peroxyl radicals (71). While other studies have not found changes in some of these parameters, all of them are indicators of short term oxidative stress. In contrast, in the studies summarized below, we found that elevated levels of glycoxidation and lipoxidation products in tissue samples from diabetic patients are proportionate to, or sometimes lower, than might be predicted from estimated increases in substrate concentrations. Thus, hyperglycemia alone may be sufficient to explain increased glycoxidation products without invoking increased oxidative stress.

In evaluating whether changes in markers of oxidative reactions support an increase in oxidative stress in diabetes, several issues must be considered. First, the presence of tissue ischemia resulting from vascular disease may increase oxidative damage, especially during episodes of reperfusion. Therefore, the presence of diabetic vascular complications, rather than the diabetic state itself, may increase oxidative stress. In agreement with this concept, Stringer (72) concluded that the increase in lipid peroxidation products in plasma of diabetic subjects was secondary to the presence of cardiovascular disease. Secondly, the products measured are derived from oxidation of a substrate, *e.g.* glucose or lipids. Thus, interpretation of results must take into account any alteration in substrate concentrations. In diabetes, levels of glucose and glycated residues in proteins are always increased, and dyslipidemia is frequent. The increase in glycoxidative or lipoxidative modification of protein could result from an increase in oxidizable substrate rather than an increase in oxidative stress. Finally, as described above many carbohydrate dependent modifications and damage to protein result from non-oxidative chemistry which itself may be affected by diabetes.

We have measured products of free radical-mediated oxidative damage to protein focusing on long-lived, slowly turning over proteins, including skin collagen and lens protein which serve to integrate the accumulation of oxidation products. Based on measurements in these long lived proteins, as well as red blood cell membrane protein and lipid, plasma LDL and urine, our data point to an alternative conclusion, *i.e.* that oxidative stress, at least in the extracellular environment, is *not* increased by the presence of diabetes (6,73). The experiments supporting this conclusion are described below.

Substrate Stress and Collagen Modification

Analogous to oxidative stress, substrate stress would result from an increase in carbohydrate or lipid precursors of AGEs, independent of an increase in levels of reactive oxygen species. To explore whether the increase in glycoxidation products in collagen could be explained solely on the basis of the increase in glycemia alone, we compared observed and predicted levels of CML, pentosidine and fluorescence in skin collagen of a group of type I diabetic subjects (6, Figure 4). The predicted level of AGEs and fluorescence was based on the age, duration of diabetes and long term glycemia of the subjects. The estimated values were calculated as a sum of adduct formed during 'normal' age-dependent accumulation, prior to the onset of diabetes, and an added contribution, depending on the degree of hyperglycemia and duration of diabetes. The degree of hyperglycemia was estimated from either the relative increase in glycated hemoglobin or collagen fructose-lysine values of patients compared to age-matched controls. If the observed values reflected the simple sum of glycoxidation products accumulating at rates proportional to glycemia, a ratio of 1 for observed/ predicted was expected. If oxidative stress were increased or decreased, the ratio would be higher or lower, respectively. Figure 4 shows that the mean ratio was significantly less than 1, whether glycemia was estimated from glycation of hemoglobin or collagen.

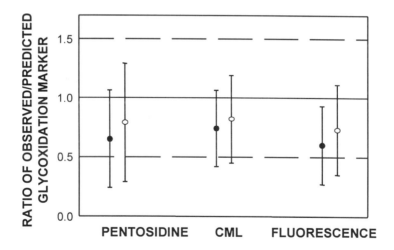

Figure 4. Ratio of observed to predicted levels of glycoxidation markers in skin collagen based on increase in glycemia alone. Predicted values were calculated based on patient age, duration of diabetes and average glycemia estimated from glycation of hemoglobin (•) or collagen (fructose-lysine) (o). Data are mean ± S.D., n = 39. Solid line = theoretical value if observed and predicted values were identical, *i.e.* without changes in oxidative stress; dashed lines at 0.5 and 1.5 represent theoretical value if oxidative stress were decreased or increased by 50%, respectively. Adapted from Dyer *et al.* (6).

The result of this analysis suggests that overall oxidative stress was not increased in these patients as a group. At the same time, the large standard deviations in all the measures suggest that there are wide variations among individual patients, and that a subset of patients may have experienced increased oxidative stress, placing them at added risk for development of complications. While many assumptions went into this analysis, a number of measurements in other tissues and fluids support the conclusion that levels of modified amino acids largely reflect increased formation of precursors, without the need to invoke increased oxidative stress. Thus, quantification of CML in LDL (unpublished) or in urine (74-76) from subjects with and without complications, also showed no increase in CML concentrations or modest decreases, in patients compared to non-diabetic individuals. Similarly, we measured both carboxymethylated phospholipids in the lipid fraction and CML in the protein portion of red cell membranes and also found no increase in these adducts in diabetes (75,76).

Oxidative Stress and Collagen Modification

In all the studies described above measurements were made on products derived from either carbohydrate or lipid precursors. Recently we evaluated oxidation of the collagen backbone itself by measurement of *ortho*-tyrosine (*o*-tyr) and methionine sulfoxide (MetSO) (73). These two oxidized amino acids produced by free radical reactions, and do not require carbohydrate or lipid precursors. Figure 5 compares the changes in these oxidized amino acids as a function of donor age.

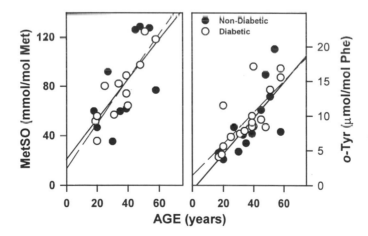

Figure 5. Age-dependent increase in MetSO (left) and o-Tyr (right) in human skin collagen from diabetic and non-diabetic subjects. Reproduced from the Journal of Clinical Investigation (1997) 100: 839-846 by copyright permission of the American Society for Clinical Investigation.

The data for the age-dependent accumulation of each oxidation product was readily approximated by a linear regression, suggesting a constant rate of accumulation of the modified amino acids with age. Based on these studies, we conclude there is no evidence for increased oxidative stress in diabetes, at least in the extracellular milieu. The correlation of *o*-tyr or MetSO with age, for either diabetic or non-diabetic subjects was ~ 0.8. There was also a strong correlation, r = 0.86, between *o*-tyr and MetSO as a function of age. These results indicate that there is a relatively **constant** rate of oxidative damage in skin collagen, and that there is no statistical difference in the rate of accumulation of either *o*-tyr or MetSO in skin collagen of diabetic subjects, compared to non-diabetic donors. At the same time glycoxidation products accumulated at an accelerated rate in these same skin samples. Our interpretation is that at least in the extracellular milieu, diabetic tissues are exposed to increased substrate stress as opposed to oxidative stress.

This conclusion does not imply that oxidative stress is unimportant in the development of diabetic complications. Like concomitant hypertension, higher than average oxidative stress may confer an added risk for complications in the presence of hyperglycemia/ or dyslipidemia. In non-diabetic control subjects, there was a two-fold variation in the rate of accumulation of glycoxidation products with age (6). Since these subjects are euglycemic, we conclude that there is wide variation in oxidative stress within the general population. People with inherently poor antioxidant defenses (or increased oxidative stress) and who develop diabetes may therefore be particularly vulnerable to vascular damage mediated by hyperglycemia or hyperlipidemia.

Carbonyl Stress

The studies summarized above illustrate that glycation and AGE modifications derived from both oxidative and non-oxidative chemistry are increased during hyperglycemia. Similar observations have been noted in non-diabetic uremic subjects. There is a strong correlation between levels of pentosidine in skin collagen and renal function (44), and the highest plasma levels of pentosidine are associated with end stage renal disease, independent of the presence of diabetes. In a recent study Miyata *et al*. (77) measured glycoxidation and lipoxidation products in plasma proteins obtained from uremic subjects with and without diabetes. Pentosidine served as a marker for modification by glycoxidation, malondialdehyde (MDA)-lysine for lipid peroxidation, and CML as a general marker for oxidation reactions. The analyses revealed that concentrations of pentosidine, MDA-lysine and CML in plasma proteins were elevated to similar extents in both groups of uremic subjects. The increases were marked compared to values for non-uremic, non-diabetic individuals, but not significantly different between the diabetic and non-diabetic uremic subjects. The authors suggest that either increased oxidative stress and/or impaired detoxification of carbonyl compounds, independent of glycemia, may explain the parallel elevations in protein modification by carbonyls derived from both carbohydrates and lipid in the non-diabetic subjects. (77,78). The increase in modified protein results from an increase in various carbonyl compounds so that carbonyl stress has been proposed as a more general term for substrate stress (77,78). Carbonyl stress may be distinguished from oxidative stress because it includes compounds that are formed by both oxidative and non-oxidative reactions, including 3-deoxyglucosone and methylglyoxal. The increase in both circulating and protein-bound carbonyl compounds in diabetes and uremia suggests that the elevation may result from both increased production and/ or decreased renal elimination and detoxification of dicarbonyl compounds.

Detoxification of Carbonyl Compounds

There are several enzymatic pathways for detoxification of carbonyl compounds that convert them to less reactive alcohols or acids. The glyoxylase system forms D-lactate following glutathione (GSH)-catalyzed rearrangements of methylglyoxal. Aldose reductase converts glucose to sorbitol, and methylglyoxal to hydroxyacetone in NADPH dependent reactions. NADPH- dependent aldehyde reductases convert 3-deoxyglucosone to 3-deoxyfructose, and NAD^+-dependent aldehyde dehydrogenases form carboxylic acid *e.g.*, 2-keto,3-deoxygluconate from 3-deoxyglucosone.

The end product of glyoxylase reduction of methylglyoxal is D-lactate, and increased concentrations of both methylglyoxal and D-lactate have been measured in blood of IDDM and NIDDM patients, documenting an increased flux of methylglyoxal through the glyoxylase pathway (23,24). Beisswenger *et al.* (80) also provided evidence for decreased methylglyoxal metabolism via the glyoxylase system with progression of retinopathy in IDDM patients. The first of the enzymes of the glyoxylase system catalyzes the formation of S-D-lactoylglutathione from the stoichiometric conjugation of methylglyoxal and GSH (22). The increased flux of methylglyoxal in cells such as erythrocytes, which are insulin-independent for glucose uptake, may contribute to decreased intracellular concentrations of reduced GSH. Treatment with precursors of GSH and lipoic acid have had beneficial effects in retarding cataract development in animal models and diabetic neuropathy in human and animal diabetes (81,82). The extent to which the benefit derives from the antioxidant versus the detoxification function of these compounds is uncertain. However, the generalized increase in carbonyl compounds derived from both carbohydrates and lipids by oxidative and non-oxidative pathways suggests that both overproduction and impaired detoxification of carbonyls contribute to the increased chemical modification of proteins in diabetes and uremia. Oxidative stress may occur secondarily to the demands on GSH and redox nucleotides for carbonyl detoxification.

Impaired intracellular detoxification of carbonyl compounds may also result from the alteration of NADH/NAD+ and NADPH/NADP+ ratios because of increased flux of glucose through glycolysis and the polyol (sorbitol) pathway, and of lipids through β-oxidation in various tissues. Based on measurements of 3-deoxyglucosone and its reduction product, 3-deoxyfructose, in diabetic plasma and urine, Beisswenger, Brown and colleagues (83,84) concluded that there is impaired detoxification of 3-deoxyglucosone in both type I and type II diabetes. Their preliminary data suggest there may be a relationship between impaired detoxification of 3-deoxyglucosone and presence of early nephropathy, based on the association between plasma 3-deoxyglucosone and glomerular hyperfiltration and urinary albumin excretion. The beneficial effects of aldose reductase inhibitors, sorbitol dehydrogenase inhibitors and pyruvate on vascular function in diabetic animals suggest that there are pathogenically relevant redox imbalances in diabetic tissue. While there is controversy as to whether true hypoxia (85) or pseudohypoxia (86) is the source of these intracellular redox imbalances in diabetes, the net effect will be an impairment of detoxification of carbonyl compounds.

Shamsi *et al.* (34), have pointed out that the concentrations of dicarbonyl sugars in plasma under hyperglycemic (or uremic) conditions may well exceed those of the open chain form of glucose. The reactivity of dicarbonyl compounds with protein, their formation intracellularly, and permeability to cell membranes all suggest that the inability to detoxify these compounds will leads to enhanced protein damage in diabetes. Further, reactive dicarbonyls themselves are potentially cytotoxic. Thus, 3-deoxyglucosone and methylglyoxal added to some human macrophage-derived cell lines in culture induced apoptotic cell death (87). While the concentrations of dicarbonyls used in these studies were admittedly higher than those measured in plasma in either diabetes or uremia, it is possible that higher levels are achieved intracellularly. Sources and routes to detoxification of reactive carbonyl compounds, as well as the potential consequences of impaired detoxification are summarized in Figure 6.

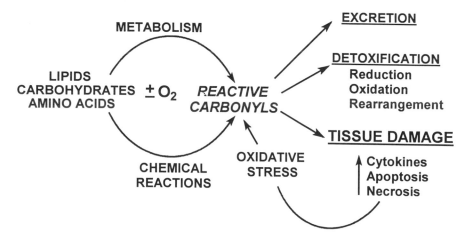

Figure 6. Overview of generation and disposition of reactive carbonyls *in vivo*. Formation of carbonyl compounds from lipids and amino acids requires oxidation chemistry, but carbonyls may be formed from carbohydrates in both oxygen-dependent and independent reactions. Tissue damage results when the elimination by excretion and cellular capacity for detoxification of carbonyls is exceeded by the rate of production.

Implications of Carbonyl Stress for Pharmacological Intervention

If our conclusion is correct, *i.e.* that oxidative stress is not increased in diabetes, then antioxidant intervention may not have a major impact on the progression of complications. Indeed, there is limited support to date for beneficial effects of antioxidant therapy in limiting the progression of diabetic vascular disease. In one prospective study there was an trend for a reduction in nonfatal myocardial infarction in diabetic subjects taking vitamin E (87). However, this may be related to improvement in vascular tone and other metabolic effects of the vitamin, independent of its anti-oxidant activity (88, 89). Our alternative hypothesis, *i.e.* that the deleterious sequelae of chemical modification of protein in diabetes result in part from over production, and/ or impaired detoxification of carbonyl compounds, may provide an alternative target for pharmacological intervention.

Aminoguanidine is one of the most successful agents for improving retinal and renal disease in rat models of diabetes. This nucleophilic hydrazine traps reactive dicarbonyl compounds and has been reported to decrease immunologically detectable AGE formation, including CML, in diabetic rat kidney (90). An additional mechanism of action, however, may be through its activity in limiting the production of carbonyl compounds by enzymatic pathways. As noted above, plasma activity of semicarbizide sensitive amine oxidase is increased in diabetic subjects and reactive carbonyls, including methylglyoxal, formaldchyde, and acrolein, are products of its action (26,28). Aminoguanidine has now been reported to be an inhibitor of semicarbizide sensitive amine oxidase (91), which may be another source of its beneficial effects *in vivo*. Further, aminoguanidine inhibits LDL oxidation and lowers plasma LDL, so that it may also contribute to improvement in diabetic dyslipidemia (92,93). Thus, although aminoguanidine does not affect diabetic hyperglycemia, it may still decrease reactive carbonyl formation from either carbohydrates or lipids.

Hudson and colleagues have shown that pyridoxamine is also effective in preventing AGE formation from both glucose and Amadori compounds (94,95). After 6 months of treatment of diabetic rats with pyridoxamine in the drinking water we have found that pyridoxamine is more effective than aminoguanidine in preserving renal function and normalizing urinary creatinine (unpublished). Pyridoxamine also decreased plasma triglyceride and cholesterol levels in treated compared to untreated diabetic animals. It is not clear whether the preservation of renal function by either aminoguanidine or pyridoxamine retards the development of dyslipidemia, or whether inhibition of dyslipidemia is involved in retarding the development of nephropathy.

GLYCATION/ GLYCOXIDATION OF PLASMA PROTEINS AND DIABETIC VASCULAR DISEASE

The discussion above focused primarily on studies of insoluble skin collagen, a slowly turning over protein that will accumulate chemical modifications and thus serve to integrate protein damage over time. However, even comparatively short-lived plasma proteins can accumulate carbonyl modifications which may have deleterious consequences for vascular cells. Below we briefly discuss studies on albumin and LDL showing how even limited glycation and glycoxidation of these proteins may also contribute to the pathogenesis of diabetic vascular disease. It is important to point out, however, that many of the cellular responses elicited by AGE-proteins are similar to those resulting from exposure of cells to elevated glucose (10-25 mM). For example, hyperglycemia itself, through multiple enzymatic pathways, stimulates increased production of diacylglycerol which in turn activates protein kinase C. Increased protein kinase C activity is linked to the pathogenesis of many vascular changes associated with diabetic complications, including capillary basement membrane thickening, increased vascular permeability, decreased vascular tone and neovascularization (96). As noted below, however, glycated and AGE-proteins also stimulate diacylglycerol production and protein kinase C activity and induce expression of cytokines and growth factors. Thus, the relative contribution of chronic hyperglycemia versus increased glycated or AGEd protein in the biochemical derangements associated with diabetes is not known. It is clear, however, that each has the potential to contribute to pathology.

Proteins modified by glucose, methylglyoxal and AGEs, can have dramatic effects on cell proliferation and viability, as well as gene expression, in cultured cells under euglycemic conditions. The following discussion will highlight results of some studies using proteins chemically characterized with respect to the nature and extent of glycation or glycoxidation, rather than on studies using proteins highly modified by AGEs. There is much evidence that AGE-protein prepared *in vitro* can have profound effects on cellular metabolism *in vitro*, including induction of oxidative stress, and cause pathology *in vivo* when administered to euglycemic animals (40,41,97). There are reasons for caution in interpreting results of such studies, however.

AGE-proteins are frequently prepared by incubation with 100-500 mM glucose or glucose-6-phosphate, in 0.1-0.2 M phosphate buffer, for 1-8 weeks at 37°C. We recently showed that incubation of collagen under similar conditions resulted both in increased concentrations of fructose-lysine and CML, and in increased concentrations of oxidized amino acids in the protein backbone (98). Among others, the redox active amino acids dihydroxy-phenylalanine and valine and leucine hydroperoxides were formed in concert with glycoxidation products. The presence of amino acids such as dihydroxy-phenylalanine and aliphatic hydroperoxides in artificial AGE-proteins makes for possible confusion in interpretation of experiments since observed effects may be the result of either carbohydrate dependent- and/ or independent formation of reactive oxygen species. A recent report by Yamauchi *et al.* (99) illustrates this point. Their results showed that albumin modified with CML in the range found for albumin isolated from *in vivo* sources, had no effect on either diacylglycerol production or stimulating protein kinase C activity in rat aortic smooth muscle cells. In contrast, albumin highly modified with glucose or glucose-6-phosphate markedly increased both diacylglycerol formation and protein kinase C activity; these effects were quenched by pre-incubation of the AGE-albumin with the hydrogen peroxide scavenger catalase. The result of the catalase treatment suggests that oxidant generation by AGE-albumin was important in eliciting the biological responses, since oxidants are well known to stimulate diacylglycerol production and protein kinase C activity (96). What is unclear is whether the oxidants were derived from AGEs or *e.g.*, peroxidized amino acids. Clarification of this issue will require identification of the AGE structure(s) on protein that may be responsible for their biological effects, independent of other modifications.

Protein Glycation and Nephropathy

Work by Cohen and co-workers suggests that minimally glycated albumin may contribute significantly to diabetic nephropathy. Thus, mildly glycated albumin (28 mM glucose, incubated 4-5 days at 37°C) inhibited proliferation of renal mesangial cells in culture (67,68). This effect was blocked by antibodies directed against albumin containing the Amadori product, but unreactive with either unmodified or AGE-albumin. Further, glycated albumin elicited an increase in TGF-β mRNA expression in renal mesangial cells, a growth factor considered to have a major role in renal pathology in diabetes, in part through its effect on increasing extracellular collagen production (100). Collagen mRNA and protein expression were also increased in mesangial cells *in vitro* by glycated albumin, and were inhibited by the anti-glycated albumin antibody (67,68). *In vivo*, weekly injections of the anti-glycated albumin antibody reduced proteinuria, inhibited mesangial expansion, and attenuated overexpression of mRNAs for fibronectin and collagen type IV in *db/db* mice, a model of type II diabetes (69). One possible limitation in the interpretation of these effects of minimally glycated albumin is that it is unclear if the glycated protein remains intact or undergoes either rearrangement or oxidation reactions during further incubations *in vitro*. However, Cohen and co-workers argue that the time frame is too short. Overall, their results show how even a limited increase in glycation of albumin may affect cellular metabolism, in the absence of hyperglycemia *in vitro*, and may contribute to nephropathy *in vivo*.

In recent studies we have found that LDL glycated or glycoxidized under mild conditions (50 mM glucose, 3 days, 0.27 mM EDTA, 37°C, ± nitrogen atmosphere) also increased TGF-β mRNA expression in renal mesangial cells (101). Further, glycated LDL stimulated production of mitogen activated protein kinase in these cells, which was blocked by inhibitors of protein kinase C and mitogen activated protein kinase. The modified LDLs also stimulated mRNA expression of the redox sensitive enzyme heme oxygenase in renal mesangial and proximal tubule cells (unpublished). These results suggest that glycation of LDL, at levels consistent with those found in diabetes, has the potential to elicit cytokine expression and alter intracellular redox status in renal cells, thus contributing to the induction or propagation of diabetic renal disease.

Glycated/Glycoxidized LDL and Retinopathy

We have reported that LDL glycated or glycoxidized under the conditions described above, to extents similar to those found *in vivo*, have cytotoxic effects on retinal pericytes and endothelial cells (102). This result points to a potential mechanism for modified LDL in contributing to retinal disease in diabetes. Thus, the increased permeability of the retinal vasculature in diabetes may expose endothelial cells and pericytes to glycated and glycoxidized LDL leading to vascular damage and pericyte loss. Of interest, when even low levels of aminoguanidine (1 µM) were present in the medium during the glycation or glycoxidation incubations, LDL toxicity was largely prevented. The mechanism of action of aminoguanidine in these experiments is unclear because the low glucose concentration and presence of metal chelator would appear to limit either autoxidation of glucose or the Amadori product in producing dicarbonyl compounds. Further, we detected only minimal lipid oxidation in the LDL preparations. It is possible, however, that even limited oxidation of the lipid component of the lipoprotein, undetected by our assays, may have been inhibited by aminoguanidine, since oxidized lipids are thought to be the source of cellular toxicity in minimally oxidized LDL.

Glycated LDL and Macrovascular Disease

Glycation has been implicated as a catalyst of LDL oxidation, and oxidation of LDL is believed to be an important contributing factor to atherosclerotic disease (103). Thus, evidence that glycation increases susceptibility of LDL to oxidation could provide an important link between hyperglycemia and macrovascular disease. Several *in vitro* studies have shown that glycation increased the generation of oxidized lipid in LDL, based on measurements of conjugated dienes or thiobarbituric acid reactive substances (64,92,93,104). Although AGE-LDL has been implicated in atherogenesis, neither CML-LDL nor methylglyoxal-LDL caused increased cholesterol esterification in macrophages *in vitro* (105,106), considered an important first step in the initiation of atherosclerotic disease (103). In contrast, the glycated subfraction of LDL, whether from diabetic or non-diabetic individuals, did promote increased cholesterol esterification in human macrophages (107, suggesting that chronic elevation in LDL glycation may contribute to foam cell formation, the early hallmark of atherosclerosis (103).

As noted above, increased concentrations of methylglyoxal-modified protein have been measured in plasma proteins and tissues in diabetes. No data are presently available on methylglyoxal modification of LDL *in vivo*. However, *in vitro,* minimally modified methylglyoxal-albumin causes expression of inflammatory cytokines, including TNF-α, IL-1-β and monocyte-macrophage colony stimulating factor in macrophages and monocytic cells (108,109). All of these cytokines have been implicated in the progression of macrovascular disease, so that extravasated protein modified by methylglyoxal could further exacerbate the cycle of reactive carbonyl production, macrophage recruitment and differentiation in the vascular wall. Of interest, strong co-localization of antibody reactivity to methylglyoxal-protein and CML has recently been reported in the cytoplasm of foam cells in atherosclerotic plaque of a non-diabetic individual (110). The results emphasize that chronic elevations in levels of reactive carbonyls, and proteins modified by these compounds, whether from hyperglycemia in diabetes or dyslipidemia in atherosclerotic disease, all have the potential to contribute to pathology in vascular cells.

SUMMARY

Glycation of protein remains a reasonable chemical link between hyperglycemia and the development of complications in diabetes, particularly those involving long-lived structural proteins that are likely to accumulate chemical damage with time. During the past several years it has become clear that carbohydrates other than glucose have important roles to play in this process, and that oxidation reactions are additional chemical sources of protein damage. Chemical modifications of protein are enhanced during diabetic hyperglycemia both because of the increase in blood glucose itself and because of alterations in cellular metabolism leading to elevated concentrations of carbohydrate- and lipid-derived carbonyl compounds. In turn, chemically modified proteins may interact with cells in the vascular wall, inducing expression of cytokines and growth factors that contribute to the pathophysiology of diabetic vascular disease. Hyperglycemia itself, leading to increases in carbohydrate and lipid substrates, appears to account for the increase in chemically modified protein, without the necessity of invoking increased oxidative stress. However, shifts in intracellular redox balances and decreases in cofactors needed for removal of reactive carbonyls may also contribute to the increase in precursors of protein modification. Although oxidative stress in diabetes may play less of a role in the early stages of vascular complications, it may become more important during the later stages of disease in tissues with established complications. As an alternative to increased oxidative stress in diabetic vascular disease, increased carbonyl stress, whether from increased generation and/ or decreased elimination or detoxification of carbonyl compounds may be responsible for the increase in chemical modification of protein contributing to vascular pathology. It may be useful to focus on pharmacological interventions that enhance detoxification of carbonyl compounds as a useful approach for retarding early vascular changes in diabetes.

REFERENCES

1. Van Dam PS, Van Asbeck BS, Erkelens BW, Marx JJM, Gispen W-H, Bravenboer B: The role of oxidative stress in neuropathy and other diabetic complications: *Diabetes/Metabolism Reviews.* 1995;11:181.

2. Giugliano D, Ceriello A, Paolisso G: Oxidative stress and diabetic vascular complications. *Diabetes Care.* 1996:19:257.

3. Baynes JW. "Reactive oxygen in the aetiology and complications of diabetes" In *Drugs, Diet and Disease, Vol2: Mechanistic approaches to diabetes,* Ioannides, C, ed. Pergamon Press: London, UK pp 203.

4. Baynes JW, Thorpe SR: The role of oxidative stress in diabetic complications. *Cur Opin Endocrin.* 1997;3:277.

5.   Garlick RL, Bunn, HF, Spiro, RG: Non-enzymatic glycosylation of basement membranes from human glomeruli and bovine sources. *Diabetes.* 1988;37:1144.
6.   Dyer DG, Dunn JA, Thorpe SR, Bailie KE, Lyons TJ, McCance DR, Baynes JW: Accumulation of Maillard reaction products in skin collagen in diabetes and aging. *J Clin Invest.* 1993;91:2463.
7.   Lyons TJ, Silvestri G, Dunn JA, Dyer DG, Baynes JW: Role of glycation in modification of lens crystallins in diabetic and non-diabetic senile cataracts. *Diabetes.* 1991;40:1010.
8.   Zyzak DV, Richardson JM, Thorpe SR, Baynes JW: Formation of reactive intermediates from Amadori compounds under physiological conditions. *Arch Biochem Biophysics.* 1995;316:547.
9.   Yamada H, Miyata S, Igaki N, Yatabe H, Miyauchi Y, Ohara T, Sakai M, Shoda H, Oimomi M, Kasuga M: Increase in 3-deoxyglucosone levels in diabetic rat plasma. *J Biol Chem.* 1995;269:20275.
10.   Hamada Y, Nakamura J, Fujisawa H, Yago H, Nakashima E, Koh N, Hotta N: Effects of glycemic control on plasma 3-deoxyglucosone levels in NIDDM patients. *Diabetes Care.* 1997;20:1466.
11.   Niwa T, Takeda N, Yoshizumi H, Tatematsu A, Ohara M, Tomiyama S, Niimura K: Presence of 3-deoxyglucosone, a potent protein crosslinking intermediate of Maillard Reaction, in diabetic serum. *Biochem Biophysic Res Comm.* 1993;196:837.
12.   Niwa T, Takeda N, Miyazaki T, Yoshizumi H, Tatematsu A, Maeda M, Ohara S, Tomiyama S, Kiimura K: Elevated serum levels of 3-deoxyglucosone, a potent crosslinking intermediate of the Maillard reaction, in uremic serum. *Nephron.* 1995;69:438.
13.   Wells-Knecht KJ, Lyons TJ, McCance DR, Thorpe SR, Feather MS, Baynes JW: 3-Deoxyfructose concentrations are increased in human plasma and urine in diabetes. *Diabetes.* 1994;43:1152.
14.   Lal, S, Szwergold BS, Taylor AH, Randall WC, Kappler F, Wells-Knecht KJ, Baynes JW, Brown TR: Metabolism of fructose-3-phosphate in the diabetic rat lens. *Arch Biochem Biophysics.* 1995;318:191.
15.   Petersen A, Kappler F, Szwergold BS, Brown TR: Fructose metabolism in the human erythrocyte: Phosphorylation to fructose-3-phosphate. *Biochem J.* 1991;284:363.
16.   Dyer DG, Blackledge JA, Thorpe SR, Baynes JW: Formation of pentosidine during nonenzymatic browning of proteins by glucose. Identification of glucose and other carbohydrates as possible precursors of pentosidine *in vivo. J Biol Chem.* 1991;266:11654.
17.   Niwa T, Katsuzaki T, Miyazaki S, Miyazaki t, Ishizaki Y, Hayase F, Tatemichi N, Takei Y: Immunohistochemical detection of imidazolone, a novel advanced glycation end product, in kidneys and aortas of diabetic patients. *J Clin Invest.* 1997;99:1272.
18.   Portero-Otin M, Nagaraj RH, Monnier VM: Chromatographic evidence for pyrraline formation during protein glycation *in vitro* and *in vivo. Biochimica Biophysica Acta.* 1995;1247:74.
19.   Horie K, Miyata T, Maeda K, Miyata S, Sugiyama S, Sakai H, van Ypersele de Strihou C, Monnier VM, Witztum JL, Kurokawa K. Immunohistochemical colocalization of glycoxidaton products and lipid peroxidation products in diabetic renal glomerular lesions. *J Clin Invest.* 1997;100:2995.
20.   Portero-Otin M, Pamplona R, Bellmut MJ, Bergua M, RH, Prat J: Glycaemic control and *in vivo* non-oxidative Maillard reaction: urinary excretion of pyrraline in diabetes patients. *Eur J Clin Invest.* 1997;27:763.
21.   Richard JP: Kinetic parameters for the elimination reaction catalyzed by triosephosphate isomerase and an estimation of the reaction's physiological significance. *Biochemistry.* 1991;39:4581.
22.   Thornalley PJ: Pharmacology of methylglyoxal. *Gen Pharmacol.* 1996;27:565.
23.   Thornalley PJ, Hooper NI, Jennings PE, Florkowski CM, Jones AF, Lunec J, Barnett AH: The human red blood glyoxalase system in diabetes mellitus. *Diabetes Research and Clinical Practice.* 1989;7:115.
24.   McLellan AC, Thornalley PJ, Benn J, Soenksen, PH: Glyoxylase system in clinical diabetes mellitus and correlation with diabetic complications. *Clin Sci.* 1994;87:21.
25.   Lyles GA, Chalmers J: The metabolism of aminoacetone to methylglyoxal by semicarbizide-sensitive amine oxidase in human umbilical artery. *Biochem Pharm.* 1992;43:1409.

26. Boomsma F, Derkx FHM, van den Meiracker AH, in't Veld AJM, Schalekamp MADH: Plasma semicarbizide-sensitive amine oxidase activity is elevated in diabetes mellitus and correlates with glycosylated hemoglobin. *Clin Sci.* 1995;88:675.

27. Boomsma F, van Veldhuisen DJ, de Kam PJ, in't Veld AJM, Lie, KI, Schalekamp MADH: Plasma semicarbizide-sensitive amine oxidase is elevated in patients with congestive heart failure. *Cardiovascular Research.* 1997;33:387.

28. Yu PH, Zuo D-M: Oxidative deamination of methylamine by semicarbizide-sensitive amine oxidase leads to cytotoxic damage in endothelial cells. *Diabetes.* 1993;42:594.

29. Hayashi T, Namiki, M: Role of sugar fragmentation in the Maillard reaction. *Developments in Food Science.* 1986;13:29.

30. Niyati-Shirkhodaee F, Shibamoto T: Gas chromatographyic analysis of glyoxal and methylglyoxal formed from lipids and related compounds upon ultraviolet irradiation. *J Agricul Food Chem.* 1993;41:227.

31. Ahmed MU, Brinkmann-Frye E, Degenhardt TP, Thorpe SR, Baynes JW: Nε(Carboxy)ethyllsyine, a product of the chemical modification of proteins by methylglyoxal, increases with age in human lens protein. *Biochem J.* 1997;324:565.

32. Lo TWC, Westwood ME, McLellan AC, Selwood T, Thornally PJ: Binding and modification of proteins by methylglyoxal under physiological conditions. *J Biol Chem.* 1994;269: 32299.

33. Shipanova IN Glomb M, Nagaraj RH: Protein modification by methylglyoxal: chemical nature and synthetic mechanism of a major fluorescent adduct. *Arch Biochem Biophysics.* 1997;344:29.

34. Shamsi FA, Partal A, Sady C, Glomb M and Nagaraj RH: Immunological evidence for methylglyoxal-derived modifications *in vivo. J Biol Chem.* 1998;273:6928.

35. Nagaraj RH, Shipanova IN, Faust, FM: Protein cross-linking by the Maillard reaction. *J Biol Chem.* 1996;271:19338.

36. Brinkmann-Frye E, Degenhardt TP, Thorpe SR, Baynes JW. Role of the Maillard reaction in aging of tissue proteins. *J Biol Chem.* 1998;273:18714.

37. Odani H, Shinzato T, Matsumoto Y, Brinkmann-Frye E, Baynes JW, Maeda K: Imidazolium crosslinks derived from reaction of lysine with glyoxal and methylglyoxal are increased in serum proteins of uremic patients: evidence for increased oxidative stress in uremia. *FEBS Let.* 1998;427:381.

38. Yim HS, Kang SO, Hah YC, Chock PB, Yim MB: Free radicals generated during the glycation reaction of amino acids by methylglyoxal. A model study of protein-cross-linked free radicals. *J Biol Chem.* 1995:270:28228.

39. Fu M-X, Knecht KJ, Lyons TJ, Thorpe SR, Baynes JW: Role of oxygen in the cross-linking and chemical modification of collagen by glucose. *Diabetes.* 1994;43:676.

40. Brownlee M: Advanced protein glycosylation in diabetes and aging. *Ann Rev Med.* 1996;46:223.

41. Vlassara H: Recent progress in advanced glycation end-products and diabetic complications. *Diabetes.* 1997;46 (Suppl 2):S19.

42. Ahmed MU, Thorpe SR, Baynes JW: Identification of carboxymethyllysine as a degradation product of fructose-lysine in glycosylated protein. *J Biol Chem.* 1986;261:4889.

43. Sell DR, Monnier VM. Structure elucidation of a senescence cross-link from human extracellular matrix: Implication of pentoses in the aging process. *J Biol Chem.* 1989;264:21597.

44. Sell DR, Monnier VM: End-stage renal disease and diabetes catalyze the formation of a pentose-derived crosslink from aging human collagen. *J Clin Invest.* 1990;85:380.

45. Reddy S, Bichler J, Wells-Knecht KJ, Thorpe SR, Baynes JW: Nε(carboxymethyl)lysine is a dominant advanced glycation end-product (AGE) antigen in tissue proteins. *Biochemistry.* 1995;34:10872.

46. Baynes, JW: The role of oxidative stress in the development of complications in diabetes. *Diabetes.* 1991;40:405.

47. Wells-Knecht KJ, Zyzak DV, Litchfield JE, Thorpe SR, Baynes JW: Mechanism of autoxidative glycosylation: identification of glyoxal and arabinose as intermediates in the autoxidative modification of proteins by glucose. *Biochemistry.* 1995;34:3702.

48. Glomb MA, Monnier VM: Mechanism of protein modification by glyoxal and glycoaldehyde, reactive intermediates of the Maillard reaction. *J Biol Chem.* 1995;270:10017.

49.   Anderson MM, Hazen SL, Hsu FF, Heinecke JH: Human neutrophils employ the myeloperoxidase-hydrogen peroxide-chloride system to convert hydroxy-amino acids into glycolaldehyde, 2-hydroxypropanol, and acrolein. *J Clin Invest.* 1997;99:424.

50.   Fu M-X, Requena JR, Jenkins AJ, Lyons TJ, Baynes JW, Thorpe SR: The advanced glycation end-product, Nε(carboxymethyl)lysine, is a product of both lipid peroxidation and glycoxidation reactions. *J Biol Chem.* 1996;271:9982.

51.   Kume S, Takeya M, Mori T, Araki N, Suzuki H, Horiuchi S, Kodama T, Miyauchi T, Takahashi K: Immunohistochemical and ultrastructural detection of advanced glycation end products in atherosclerotic lesions of human aorta with a novel specific monoclonal antibody. *Amer J Path.* 1995;147:654.

52.   Wolff SP, Dean RT: Glucose autoxidation and protein modification: the potential role of autoxidative glycosylation in diabetes. *Biochem J.* 1987;245:243.

53.   Wells-Knecht MC, Thorpe SR, Baynes JW: Pathways of formation of glycoxidation products during glycation of collagen. *Biochemistry.* 1995;34:15134.

54.   Elgawish A, Glomb M, Friedlander M, Monnier VM: Involvement of hydrogen peroxide in collagen cross-linking by high glucose *in vitro* and *in vivo. J Biol Chem.* 1996;271;12964.

55.   Hamlin CR, Kohn RR: Evidence for progressive, age-related structural changes in post-mature human collagen. *Biochimica Biophysica Acta.* 1971;236:458.

56.   Eble AS, Thorpe SR, Baynes JW: Non-enzymatic glucosylation and glucose-dependent crosslinking of protein. *J Biol Chem.* 1983;258:9406.

57.   Oxlund H, Rasmussen LM, Andreassen TT, Heickendorff L: Increased aortic stiffness in patients with type 1 (insulin-dependent) diabetes mellitus. *Diabetologia.* 1989;32:748.

58.   Monnier VM, Vishwanath V, Frank KE, Elmets CA, Dauchot P, Kohn RR: Relations between complications to Type I diabetes mellitus and collagen-linked fluorescence. *N Engl J of Med.* 1986;314:403.

59.   Monnier VM, Sell DR, Abdul-Karim FW, Emancipator SN: Collagen browning and cross-linking are increased in chronic experimental hyperglycemia. Relevance to diabetes and aging. *Diabetes.* 1988;37:867.

60.   Sell DR, Lapolla A, Odetti P, Fogarty J, Monnier VM: Pentosidine formation in skin correlates with severity of complications in individuals with long-standing IDDM. *Diabetes.* 1992;41:1286.

61.   McCance DR, Dyer DG, Dunn JA, Bailie KE, Thorpe SR, Baynes JW, Lyons TJ: Maillard reaction products and their relation to complications in insulin dependent diabetes mellitus. *J Clin Invest.* 1993;91:2470.

62.   Bucala R, Tracey KJ, Cerami A: Advanced glycosylation products quench nitric oxide and mediate defective endothelium-dependent vasodilatation in experimental diabetes. *J Clin Invest.* 1991;87:432.

63.   Brownlee M, Vlassara H, Cerami A: Nonenzymatic glycosylation products on collagen covalently trap low-density lipoprotein. *Diabetes.* 1985;34:938.

64.   Hicks M, Delbridge L, Yue, DK, Reeve TS: Increase in crosslinking of nonenzymatically glycosylated collagen induced by products of lipid peroxidation. *Arch Biochem Biophysics.* 1989;268:249.

65.   Lyons TJ, Kennedy L: Non-enzymatic glycosylation of skin collagen in patients with limited joint mobility. *Diabetologia.* 1985;28:2.

66.   Vishwanath V, Frank KE, Elmets CA, Dauchot PJ, Monnier VM: Glycosylation of skin collagen in Type I diabetes mellitus: correlations with long-term complications. *Diabetes/* 1986;35:916.

67.   Ziyadeh FN, Cohen MP: Effects of glycated albumin on mesangial cells: evidence for a role in diabetic nephropathy. *Mol Cell Biochem.* 1993;125:19.

68.   Cohen MP, Ziyadeh FN: Amadori glucose adducts modulate mesangial cell growth and collagen gene expression. *Kidney Internl.* 1994;45:475.

69.   Cohen MP, Sharma K, Jin Y, Hud E, Wu V-Y, Tomaszewski J, Ziyadeh FN: Prevention of diabetic nephropathy in *db/db* mice with glycated albumin antagonists. *J Clin Invest.* 1995;95:2338.

70.   Lyons TJ: Oxidized low density lipoproteins: a role in the pathogenesis of atherosclerosis in diabetes? *Diabetic Medicine.* 1991;8:411.

71. Tsai EC, Hirsch IB, Brunzell JD, Chait A: Reduced plasma peroxyl radical trapping capacity and increased susceptibility of LDL to oxidation in poorly controlled IDDM. *Diabetes.* 1994;43:1010.

72. Stringer MD, Gorog PG, Freeman A, Kakkar VV. Lipid peroxides and atherosclerosis. *Brit Med J.* 1989;298:281.

73. Wells-Knecht MC, Lyons TJ, McCance, DR, Thorpe SR, Baynes JW: Age-dependent increase in *ortho*-tyrosine and methionine sulfoxide in human skin collagen is not accelerated in diabetes. *J Clin Invest.* 1997;839.

74. Knecht KJ, Dunn JA, McFarland KF, McCance DR, Lyons TJ, Thorpe SR, Baynes JW: Effect of diabetes and aging on carboxymethyllysine levels in human urine. *Diabetes.* 1991;41:190.

75. Requena JR, Ahmed MU, Fountain CW, Degenhardt TP, Reddy S, Perez C, Lyons TJ, Jenkin AJ, Baynes JW, Thorpe, SR: Carboxymethylethanolamine, a biomarker of phospholipid modification during the Maillard reaction *in vivo. J Biol Chem.* 1997;272:17473.

76. Jenkins AJ, Lyons TJ, Smyth B, Requena JR, Fountain CW, Degenhardt TP, Hermayer K, Phillips, K, King L, Baynes JW, Thorpe S: Glycoxidation and lipoxidation products in red cell membranes in IDDM- Relationship to glycemic control and microvascular complications. *Diabetes.* 1998; 47(supplement 1) :A127.

77. Miyata T, Fu M-X, Kurokawa K, van Ypersele de Strihou C, Thorpe SR, Baynes JW: Products of both carbohydrates and lipids are increased in uremic plasma. *Kidney International.* 1998; in press

78. Miyata T, van Ypersele de Strihou C, Kurokawa K, Baynes JW: Alterations in non-enzymatic biochemistry in uremia. Origin and significance of "carbonyl stress" in long-term uremic complications. *Kidney International.* 1998; in press

79. Lyons TJ, Jenkins AJJ: Glycation, oxidation and lipoxidation in the development of the complications of diabetes: a carbonyl stress hypothesis. *Diabetes Reviews.* 1997;5:365.

80. Beisswenger PJ, Howell S., Stevens RA, Cavender JC, Lal S, Randall W, Szwergold BS, Kappler F,Brown T: The role of glycation products, α dicarbonyls and their degradative pathways in diabetic retinopathy. *Invest Ophthalmol Visual Sci.* 1996,38 (supplement).765.

81. Packer L: Antioxidant properties of lipoic acid and its therapeutic effects in prevention of diabetes complications and cataracts. *Ann NY Acad Sci.* 1994;38:257.

82. Packer L, Tritschler HJ, Wessel K: Nueroprotection by the metabolic antioxidant alpha-lipoic acid. *Free Rad Biol Med.* 1997;22:359.

83. Lal S, Szwergold BS, Walker M, Randall W, Kappler F, Besisswenger PJ, Brown T. "Production and metabolism of 3-deoxyglucosone in humans". In *The Maillard reaction in foods and Medicine*, O'Brien J, Nursten HE, Crabbe JC, Ames JM, eds. Royal Society of Chemistry: London, UK 1998 pp. 291.

84. Beisswenger, PJ, Howell S, Stevens R, Siegal A, Lal S, Randall W, Szwergold BS, Kappler F, Brown T. "The role of 3-deoxyglucosone and the activity of its degradative pathways in the etiology of diabetic microvascular disease". In *The Maillard reaction in foods and Medicine*, O'Brien J, Nursten HE, Crabbe JC, Ames JM, eds. Royal Society of Chemistry: London, UK 1998 pp.298.

85. Cameron NE, Cotter MA: Metabolic and vascular factors in the pathogenesis of diabetic neuropathy. *Diabetes.* 1997;46 (Supplement 2): S31.

86. Williamson JR, Chang K, Khalid MF, Hasan KS, Ido Y, Kawamura T, Nyengaard JR, Van den Enden M, Kilo C, Tilton RG: Hyperglycemic pseudohypoxia and diabetic complications. *Diabetes.* 1993;42: 801.

87. Okado A, Kawasaki Y, Hasuke Y, Takahashi M, Teshima T, Fujii J, Taniguchi N: Induction of apoptotic cell death by methyglyoxal and 3-deoxyglucosone in Macrophage-derived cell lines. *Biochem Biophysic Res Comm.* 1996; 225:219.

88. Stephens NG, Parsons A, Schofield PM, Kelly F, Cheeseman K, Mitchinson MJ: Randomised controlled trial of vitamin E in patients with coronary disease: Cambridge Heart Antioxidant Study (CHAOS). *Lancet.* 1996;347:781.

89. Diaz, MD, Frei B, Vita JA, Keaney JF: Antioxidants and atherosclerotic heart disease. *N Engl J Med.* 1997;337:408.

90. Rumble, JR, Cooper ME, Soulis T, Cox A, Wu L, Youssef S, Jasik M, Jerums G, Gilbert RE: Vascular hypertrophy in experimental diabetes. Role of advanced glycation end products. *J Clin Invest.* 1997;99:1016.

91.   Yu PH, Zuo DM: Aminoguanidine inhibits semicarbizide-sensitive amine oxidase activity: implications for advanced glycation and diabetic complications. *Diabetologia.* 1997;40:1243.

92.   Bucala R, Makita Z, Koschinsky T, Cerami A, Vlassara H: Lipid advanced glycosylation: Pathway for lipid oxidation *in vivo. Proc Natl Acad Sci USA.* 1993;90:6434.

93.   Bucala R, Makita Z, Vega G, Grundy S, Koschinsky T, Cerami A, Vlassara H: Modification of low density lipoprotein by advanced glycation end products contributes to the dyslipidemia of diabetes and renal insufficiency. *Proc Natl Acad Sci USA.* 1994;91:9441.

94.   Booth, AA, Khalifah RG, Hudson BG: Thiamine pyrophosphate and pyridoxamine inhibit the formation of antigenic advanced glycation end-products: comparison with aminoguanidine. *Biochem Biophysic Res Comm.* 1996;220:113.

95.   Booth, AA, Khalifah RG, Todd P, Hudson BG: In vitro kinetic studies of formation of antigenic advanced glycation end products (AGEs). Novel inhibition of post-Amadori glycation pathways. *J Biol Chem.* 1997;272:5430.

96.   Ishi H, Daisuke K, King GL: Protein kinase C activation and its role in the development of vascular complicatinos in diabetes mellitus. *J Mol Med.* 1998;76:21.

97.   Bierhaus A, Hofmann MA, Ziegler R, Nawroth PP: AGEs and their interaction with AGE-receptors in vascular disease and diabetes mellitus. I. The AGE concept. *Cardiovascular Research.* 199;37:586.

98.   Fu S, Fu M-X, Baynes JW, Thorpe SR, Dean RT: Presence of DOPA and amino acid hydroperoxides in proteins modified with advanced glycation end products (AGEs): amino acid oxidation products as a possible source of oxidative stress induced by AGE-proteins. *Biochem J.* 1998;330:233.

99.   Yamauchi, T, Igarashi M, Brownlee M, Thorpe S, King G: Activation of diacylglyercol and protein kinase C in aortic smooth muscle cells by oxidants and advanced glycation products. *Diabetes.* 1998;47 (supplement 1) :A372.

100.   Ziyadeh FN, Cheol D, Cohen JA, Guo J, Cohen MP: Glycated albumin stimulates fibronectin expression in glomerular mesangial cells: Involvement of the transforming growth factor-β system. *Kidney International.* 1998;53:631.

101.   Verlade V, Jenkins A, Christopher J, Lyons T, Mayfield R, Jaffa A: Modified lipoproteins induce mitogen activated protein kinase (MAPK) and TGF-β expression in mesangial cells. *Diabetes.* 1998;47(supplment 1):A127.

102.   Lyons TJ, Li W, Wells-Knecht M, Jokl R: Toxicity of mildly modified low density lipoproteins to cultured retinal capillary endothelial cells and pericytes. *Diabetes.* 1994;43:1090.

103.   Witztum JL, Steinberg D: Role of oxidized low density lipoprotein in atherogenesis. *J Clin Invest.* 1991;88:1785.

104.   Mullarkey CJ, Edelstien D, Brownlee M: Free radical generation by early glycation products: a mechanism for accelerated atherogenesis in diabetes. *Biochem Biophysicl Res Comm.* 1990;177:932.

105.   Sakurai T, Yamamoto Y, Shimoyama M, Nakano M. "Low density lipoprotein carboxymethylated in vitro does not accelerate cholesterylester synthesis in mouse peritoneal macrophages: In *The Maillard reaction in foods and Medicine,* O'Brien J, Nursten HE, Crabbe JC, Ames JM, eds. Royal Society of Chemistry: London, UK 1998 pp. 351.

106.   Schalkwijk, CG, Vermeer MA, Verzijl N, Stehouwer CDA, te Koppele J, Prncen HMG, van Hinsbergh VWM. "Modification of low-density lipoproteins by methylglyoxal alters its physio-chemical and biological properties". In *The Maillard reaction in foods and Medicine,* O'Brien J, Nursten HE, Crabbe JC, Ames JM, eds. Royal Society of Chemistry: London, UK 1998 pp. 285.

107.   Klein RL, Laimins M, Lopes-Virella MF: Isolation, characterization and metabolism of the glycated and non-glycated subfractions of low density lipoproteins isolated from type I diabetic patients and non-diabetic subjects. *Diabetes.* 1995;44:109.

108.   Westwood ME, Thornalley PJ: Induction of synthesis and secretion of interleukin 1 beta in the human monocytic THP-1 cells by human serum albumins modified with methylgloxal and advanced glycation endproducts *Immunol Lett.* 1996;50:17.

109.   Abordo EA, Westwood ME, Thornalley PJ: Synthesis and secretion of macrophage colony stimulating factor by mature human monocytes and human monocytic THP-1 cells induced by human serum albumin derivatives modified with methylglyoxal and glucose-derived advanced glycation end-products. *Immun Lett.* 1996;53:7.

110.   Uchida K, Khor OT, Oya T, Osawa T, Yasuda Y, Miyata T: Protein modification by a Maillard reaction intermediate methylglyoxal.   Immunochemical detection of a fluorescent 5-methyimidazolone derivatives in vivo. *FEBS Lett.* 1997;410:313.

15 ADVANCED GLYCOSYLATION ENDPRODUCTS AND DIABETIC VASCULAR DISEASE

Richard Bucala

INTRODUCTION

Long-term, persistent hyperglycemia has become well-accepted as an underlying cause of diabetic complications, which can become manifest over time as retinopathy, nephropathy, neuropathy, and atherosclerotic vascular disease (1). Since diabetes mellitus afflicts at least 12 million individuals in the United States alone, the contribution of these complications to the overall morbidity and mortality of this disease is considerable (1,2). An important contributing factor for the development of diabetic sequelae is a progressive vasculopathy that has been traditionally characterized into two anatomic types: a microvascular disease affecting capillary beds, and a macrovascular type affecting arteries and arterioles (2,3). Emerging data obtained both from basic laboratory and clinical pharmacological studies indicate that one fundamental biochemical abnormality, increased non-enzymatic glycosylation (glycation), may play a critical, etiologic role in the development of diabetic vascular disease.

GLYCATION CHEMISTRY

Glycation, or nonenzymatic glycosylation, describes the covalent attachment of sugars such as glucose to free amino groups. Although proteins have been the most studied substrate for glycation, the free amino groups of phospholipids and DNA nucleotides can also participate in this process (4,5). In the first step of this pathway, the carbonyl group of the sugar attaches to a primary amino group to form a reversible Schiff base (Fig 1). The Schiff base then slowly undergoes an Amadori rearrangement (or Heyns rearrangement in the case of a ketose sugar reactant) to produce a more stable, but still slowly reversible adduct. An Amadori rearrangement product attached to the N-terminal valine of the hemoglobin-β chain produces the minor hemoglobin species, HbA1c. Thirty years ago, investigation into the physiological basis of HbA1c formation provided the first indication that nonenzymatic glycosylation could occur *in vivo* (6). HbA1c was found to circulate in increased amounts in the red cells of diabetic

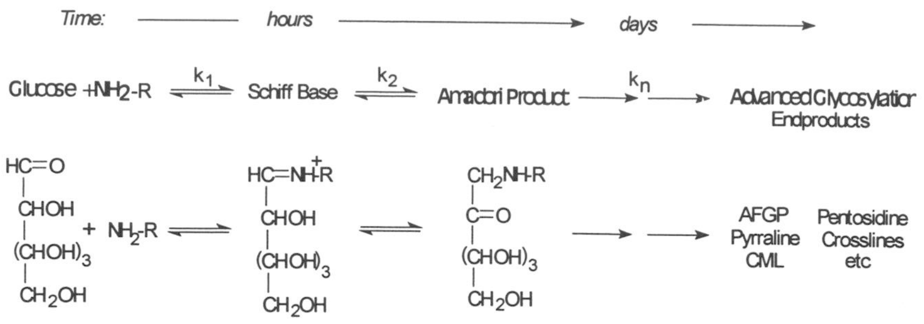

Figure 1. General scheme for the formation of advanced glycation endproducts (AGEs). Equilibrium levels of the reversible Schiff base and Amadori products are reached within hours and days respectively. AGEs form over a longer time period by remain irreversibly bound to amino groups. R=amino acid or lipid backbone.

patients. Since the Amadori product forms over the entire 120 day lifespan of the red cell, it was soon realized that HbA_{1c} measurements could provide a clinically useful index of ambient glucose levels over a period of several weeks (7,8).

Amadori rearrangement products are not the final product of protein glycation however, and over a time period of days to weeks, further chemical reactions can occur. These involve dehydration, rearrangement, and oxidation steps that lead ultimately to a heterogeneous group of adducts that remain irreversibly bound to the protein. This stage of glycation remains only partially characterized, but is known to proceed through the formation of reactive intermediates that have the capacity to crosslink proximate amino groups (9,10). It was realized early on that at least some of these advanced products, which have come to be termed advanced glycation endproducts or AGEs, exhibit characteristic absorbance and fluorescence properties. This in turn provided a useful, albeit relatively insensitive means to begin to assess AGE formation *in vivo*. It was then determined that the glycation process contributes to much of the structural damage associated with "aged" proteins *in vivo*. Thus, long-lived proteins such as connective tissue and basement membrane collagen accumulate the products of advanced glycation and become increasingly fluorescent, crosslinked, and rigid with age. As expected, this process is accelerated under the hyperglycemic environment of diabetes mellitus (9-11).

Recent studies have led to the elucidation of several defined AGE structures, and there is evidence that certain of these products form *in vivo*, as assessed by immunochemical and chromatographic criteria (Fig 2) (12-29). Many AGEs appear to arise from Amadori product-derived dicarbonyl intermediates such as 1- and 3-deoxyglucosones, protein-bound dideoxyosones, and fragmentation products such as glyoxal and methylglyoxal (9-11). Nevertheless, there remains evidence to suggest that the pathologically important, crosslinking adducts are not fluorescent and that the presently known glycation adducts may only represent biomarkers of the more "toxic" AGEs that form *in vivo*.

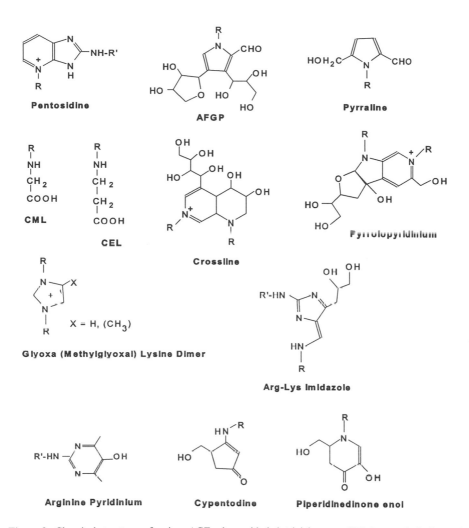

Figure 2. Chemical structures of various AGEs along with their trivial names. "R" denotes the lysine and "R'" signifies the arginine carbon backbone. Direct chemical or immunochemical evidence for the *in vivo* formation of pyrraline, pentosidine, carboxymethyllysine (CML), crossline, arg-lys imadazole, and cypentodine has been obtained (23 – 29).

In addition to long-lived connective tissue and basement membrane protein components, AGEs have been shown to form *in situ* on a variety of blood proteins such as albumin (25), hemoglobin (30), immunoglobulins (31), low-density lipoprotein (LDL) (4), and β_2-microglobin (32). AGE formation on proteins such as LDL or β_2-microglobulin may be directly toxic - delaying plasma clearance and inducing LDL oxidation for instance (4,33), or promoting tissue deposition and amyloidosis in the case of β_2-microglobulin (32). Alternatively, such modification may serve as a useful diagnostic maker of AGE "burden" in the host, as in the case of circulating AGE-modified hemoglobin (Hb-AGE) (34).

While plasma protein AGEs can form by the direct attachment of glucose (or other reducing sugars) to proteins, experimental studies indicate that the AGEs in blood also arise from the entry into the plasma compartment of reactive, AGE-peptides produced by the normal catabolism of AGE-modified tissue proteins. High concentrations of circulating AGE-peptides therefore can occur even under non-hyperglycemic conditions if plasma filtration is impaired by renal disease. The reactive nature of AGE-peptides together with their normal clearance by the kidneys has led to the concept that circulating AGE-peptides comprise a component of the so-called uremic toxins or "middle molecules" which accumulate during renal insufficiency and which may contribute to the morbidity and mortality of chronic renal failure (35,36). Importantly, dyslipidemia and severe atherosclerosis occurs in patients with renal insufficiency irrespective of diabetes. Diabetic patients with end-stage renal disease for example, suffer from a particularly poor long-term prognosis. Their two year survival rate is $\leq 50\%$ and cardiovascular complications account for the single most common cause of pre-mature death (37).

CELLULAR RESPONSES AND AGE TURNOVER

Several years ago, quantitative considerations suggested that net AGE formation occurred faster *in vitro* than *in vivo*. While differences in the oxidative environment of *in vitro* versus *in vivo* conditions have since been found to play a role in this discrepancy (38), it was proposed several years ago that significant AGE-specific turnover mechanisms may exist in the body to limit the net accumulation and tissue toxicity of AGE-modified proteins (39). Experimental studies have since established the existence and functions of several cellular-based AGE uptake systems. Monocyte/macrophages are prominent components of this system, however AGE binding and uptake also have been described in numerous other cell types. The potential importance of the AGE-receptor system to diabetic (and age-related) pathologies is underscored by the profound biological response of many cell and tissue types to AGE exposure. In the case of endothelium for instance, it has been proposed that these AGE-binding proteins mediate several of the toxic effects of glucose on blood vessel wall function (40-44).

Two cell surface binding proteins specific for AGEs that have been described include a 35 kDa member of the immunoglobulin superfamily called RAGE (receptor for AGE), and a 32 kDa protein named Galectin-3, Mac-2, or carbohydrate binding protein-35 (CBP-35) (45,46). Each of these diverse binding proteins has been implicated in the cellular responses to AGEs. RAGE in particular has been functionally linked to AGE-related increases in NF-κB activation, which may serve to greatly amplify the subcellular response to AGE contact (47).

Recent studies with gene-knockout mice also have provided support for a role for the macrophage scavenger receptor in the clearance of AGE-modified proteins. Model calculations suggest that as much as 60% of the macrophage endocytic uptake of AGE-proteins may be mediated by this cell surface protein, which also is responsible for the uptake and degradation of a variety of other modified proteins, and that are generally of a polyanionic character (48,49).

AGEs are chemotactic for monocyte/macrophages, and have been shown to induce monocyte recruitment from the circulation across normal endothelium (42). Occupancy of macrophage receptors by AGEs induces the release of TNFα, IL-1, PDGF, and IGF-1 (50, 51). These mediators act in turn to recruit nearby connective tissue cells, induce their proliferation, and promote extracellular matrix production (52). Variability in the constitutive or inducible expression of these AGE-receptor or binding proteins may underlie differences in the susceptibility of patients to various tissue-specific diabetic sequelae, and perhaps account for the long-standing observation that while some diabetics develop few complications despite a long-history of poor glucose control, others suffer severe and debilitating complications despite relatively good control.

Vascular Dynamics and Hypertension

Long-standing diabetes is associated with abnormalities in vascular tone and regional blood flow that contribute significantly to tissue hypoperfusion, end-organ hypoxia, and cardiovascular compromise (54,55). Recent biochemical studies have provided evidence for a potentially important activity for AGEs *in vivo*: the capacity to chemically inactivate nitric oxide (NO), *i.e.* endothelium-derived relaxing factor (56). In experimentally-induced diabetes, defective vasodilatory responses develop in a pattern, and over a time frame (weeks to months) which are consistent with the quenching of nitric oxide by accumulated, subendothelial AGEs. A similar loss of vascular reactivity that correlates with subendothelial AGE accumulation has been demonstrated to occur in normal, non-diabetic animals which have been intravenously administered autologous, AGE-modified proteins (57). In both of these experimental systems, the loss of vasodilatory function occurs more slowly after treatment with the advanced glycosylation inhibitor aminoguanidine. Inactivation of nitric oxide by vascular wall AGEs may explain in large part the progressive impairment in nitric oxide-mediated responses that occurs in the renal, coronary, and systemic circulation of diabetic patients (54,55). Of note, this dynamic effect is distinct from the AGE-mediated crosslinking that occurs at an accelerated rate within the vascular wall of diabetics. Such covalent crosslinking has been shown recently to contribute importantly to the structural rigidity of diabetic vessels, with significant effects on large vessel hemodynamics (58).

Epidemiological studies have established that the prevalence of hypertension is more than two-fold higher in the diabetic than in the non-diabetic population (59,60). Furthermore, the occurrence of high blood pressure in patients with established diabetes increases markedly their risk for developing a rapidly progressive course of atherosclerosis, retinopathy, and nephropathy. Precisely what factors account for the increased susceptibility of diabetics to hypertensive disease is unclear. Endothelium-derived nitric oxide plays an important role in maintaining normal vascular tone and blood pressure (61) and the progressive accumulation of subendothelial AGEs may be an important mechanism for inactivating nitric oxide and contributing to hypertensive pathology.

Nitric oxide also exerts potent homeostatic and anti-proliferative effects on different cell types and has been proposed to be responsible for maintaining the mitogenic quiescence of subendothelial vascular smooth muscle cells (62). Experimental damage or removal of endothelium is associated with a proliferation of underlying smooth muscle cells that contributes importantly to luminal occlusion (63). Recent studies utilizing model cell culture systems have confirmed that nitric oxide displays potent cytostatic effects on different mesenchymal cell types. AGE-modified matrix proteins specifically block the anti-proliferative effect of nitric oxide on vascular smooth muscle cells and kidney mesangial cells (64). These data implicate tissue AGEs as important modulators of nitric oxide-mediated cytostasis and suggest a common, biochemical pathway for the evolution of the proliferative glomerular and vascular lesions present in diabetes mellitus.

Vascular Wall Homeostasis

Numerous epidemiological studies over the years have established that patients with diabetes suffer at least a 3-4 fold increased risk of heart attack or stroke when compared to the general population (3,65,66). These complications arise from an accelerated atherosclerosis which occurs at a younger age and affects the vasculature more extensively in diabetic than in non-diabetic persons. Atherosclerotic plaque formation is the hallmark of the disease process, and results from a complex interaction between vascular wall endothelial, macrophage, and smooth muscle cell types, blood-borne lipoproteins, and secreted growth factors (63). Histologically, the atheromatous lesions in diabetics are indistinguishable from those in non-diabetics (3).

The interaction of diverse AGE-modified proteins with endothelial cells has been shown to initiate a cascade of deleterious effects on vascular wall homeostasis. Occupancy of endothelial cell AGE-receptors increases vascular permeability, one of the earliest abnormalities which occurs in vessels exposed to high glucose concentrations. AGEs also act to down-regulate endothelial cell expression of the surface anticoagulant thrombomodulin and to increase the synthesis of the procoagulant tissue factor (42). These effects promote thrombosis, a long-noted feature of diabetic vasculature, and suggest that endothelial cell toxicity may be a primary and important consequence of high, circulating AGE levels. A significant pro-atherogenic effect of protein glycation was observed in a study of AGE-infusion in rabbits, which also noted an increase in VCAM-1 and ICAM-1 expression on the aortic endothelium *in vivo*. These AGE-mediated changes were accelerated in rabbits placed briefly on a cholesterol-rich diet, which manifested multifocal atheroma formation in less than 2 weeks (67). Significantly, the AGE-R1 and AGE-R2 molecules have been found to be expressed in several cellular components of human atherosclerotic plaque, where they co-localize with intracellular AGEs (53).

Lipoprotein Metabolism

Prominent among the factors which exacerbate atherosclerosis in diabetes is a dyslipidemia due in part to an elevation in the circulating levels of the apolipoprotein B (apo B)-containing particles VLDL, LDL, and IDL (68,69). LDL is the major lipoprotein component responsible for transferring exogenously-absorbed and endogenously-synthesized lipids to peripheral tissues, and persistent elevation of either LDL or its metabolic precursor, VLDL, has been shown repeatedly to be an important risk factor in both diabetic and non-diabetic populations for the development of atherosclerosis (70, 71). Lipoproteins isolated from diabetic plasma exhibit important qualitative abnormalities, such as an impaired capacity to be taken up by fibroblast or tissue LDL receptors (72,73). Acquired biochemical modifications of LDL are believed to play an important role in atherogenesis and the precise molecular basis for this uptake abnormality has been of considerable interest.

One chemical modification pathway which has received much attention for its capacity to increase the atherogenicity of the LDL particle is "oxidative modification" (see Chapter 4). When LDL is exposed *in vitro* to divalent transition metals or other sources of free radical generation, it undergoes a variety of changes such as oxidative degradation of unsaturated fatty acids, an increase in electrophoretic mobility, and chemical modification of apolipoprotein amino groups (74). As a consequence, oxidized LDL exhibits diminished recognition by cellular LDL receptors and preferential uptake by macrophage scavenger receptors. Vascular wall macrophages then may become transformed into the lipid-laden "foam" cells which appear to prestage the development of fatty streaks and the complex, proliferative lesions of atherosclerotic plaque (70, 74).

Unsaturated fatty acids (*i.e.* fatty acids bearing one or more double bonds in their carbon backbone) readily undergo oxidative modification, a process that begins when an unspecified oxidant abstracts the relatively labile *bis*-allylic hydrogen atom from the fatty acid side chain (75). The addition of molecular oxygen then generates a lipid peroxyl radical. This serves to propagate oxidative modification by initiating hydrogen atom abstraction at additional unsaturated bonds. Fatty acid peroxidation and breakdown then ensues, producing a variety of shorter chain, α,β-unsaturated aldehydes such as the hydroxyalkenals that in turn can react with nucleophilic sites on proteins to form Michael addition products and resonance-stabilized Schiff bases. Although transition metal-catalyzed lipid peroxidation occurs readily *in vitro* and continues to be studied as a model for the "propagative" phase of oxidative degradation, it should be noted that the identity of the oxidant(s) responsible for initiating lipid peroxidation *in vivo* has yet to be established (75). This situation has led to certain conceptual difficulties in assessing the prevalence and the pathological significance of lipid peroxidation, particularly with respect to atherogenesis. *In vivo*, low trace metal concentrations , the high availability of ligands that form tight coordination complexes with metals, and the abundant anti-oxidant capacity of plasma provide strong arguments against the possibility that metal-catalyzed oxidation plays a significant role in mediating lipid peroxidation *in vivo* (75,76).

The possibility that lipids and lipoproteins might undergo advanced glycation *in vivo* was first proposed a number of years ago as a result of studies showing that amine-containing phospholipids could react with glucose to form AGEs in much the same way that polypeptide amines form AGEs (4). It then was hypothesized that intramolecular oxidation-reduction reactions, which are known to occur during advanced glycosylation, might act within the hydrophobic microenvironment of phospholipids to promote, and possibly even initiate fatty acid oxidation. Further links between glycation and oxidation chemistry were provided by observations regarding the mechanism of formation of certain AGEs that form *in vivo*. Pentosidine for instance, which is the first structurally-defined AGE crosslink to be identified in human tissue, undergoes an obligate oxidation step in pathway of formation (12,77,78). Similarly, the product carboxymethyllysine (CML) may arise in part by the oxidative cleavage of Amadori product (15). While CML has since been shown form by other pathways as well (79,80), these initial observations provided impetus for the view that advanced glycation chemistry may involve certain oxidative steps *in vivo*, perhaps via intramolecular oxidation-reduction or by interaction with other redox-sensitive biomolecules. Accordingly, it was proposed that an AGE-mediated oxidative pathway might proceed independently of added transition metals or exogenous free-radical generating systems, and could serve potentially as one mechanism for initiating lipid oxidation *in vivo*.

When purified human LDL was incubated with glucose (in the presence of metal chelators) oxidative modification was found to occur in an AGE-dependent manner. Phospholipid-linked AGEs formed more rapidly than apolipoprotein B-linked AGEs (apoB-AGEs), and reached a specific activity 100-fold greater than that of apoB-linked AGEs. These results suggested that the rate of advanced glycosylation is much faster in lipid phases than in aqueous (apolipoprotein) phases, presumably because non-polar microenvironments favor the dehydration and subsequent rearrangement reactions that characterize the advanced glycosylation process. Measurements of oxidative modification further showed that LDL was oxidized concomitantly with AGE formation (4).

In more recent studies, gas chromatography - electron impact mass spectrometry analyses of AGE-modified LDL have identified specific oxidation products which form during either phospholipid- or LDL-advanced glycosylation (81). One product produced mass ions consistent with 4-hydoxynonenal, and a second product was identified as 4-hydroxyhexenal. These data provide direct chemical support for the concept that lipid-advanced glycosylation reactions lead to the oxidation of unsaturated fatty acids and the formation of reactive lipid species.

Once attached to phospholipid head groups, reactive AGE products may interact with fatty acid side chains to promote redox cycling directly within the hydrophobic, lipid microenvironment. In fact, there has long been evidence that advanced glycation reactions proceed via a succession of oxidation-reduction reactions that are accompanied by the formation of transient free radicals and species bearing unpaired electrons (82,83). Recent support for this concept has been provided by model electron spin resonance studies of the 3-carbon, Maillard decomposition product methylglyoxal (84). These data show evidence for the formation of both crosslinked radical cations and dicarbonyl-based radical anions which arise by a pathway that is independent of oxygen or metal ions.

Whether AGE-derived radicals actually possess sufficient reactivity to abstract hydrogen atoms from the *bis*-allylic position of unsaturated bonds remains to be established. This mechanism would provide an important unifying link between glycation chemistry, which occurs ubiquitously *in vivo*, and oxidative modification, and offer new insight into the origin of atherogenic forms of LDL. Experimental resolution of the precise biochemical basis of lipid and lipoprotein modification together with the identification of important oxidation initiators *in vivo* should lead ultimately to the more rational development of pharmacological agents aimed at protecting lipid and lipoprotein integrity *in vivo*.

Lipoprotein (LDL) Glycation *In Vivo*

To better define the relationship between advanced glycation and LDL metabolism, we recently analyzed LDL from patients with diabetes or renal insufficiency for the presence of phospholipid-AGEs and apoB-AGEs (33). As discussed earlier, it had been determined that reactive AGEs circulate in high concentrations during renal insufficiency and that these AGEs can attach readily to plasma components such as LDL. There was a significant elevation in the levels of apoB-AGE and lipid-AGE in LDL when each of the patient groups was compared to the control (non-diabetic/normal renal function) group. The highest levels of AGE-modification were observed in patients with renal insufficiency, pointing to the important role of circulating, reactive AGE-peptides in producing AGE-modified LDL.

Chemical modification of basic residues within the LDL-receptor binding domain of apolipoprotein B has been shown in the past to interfere with the ability of LDL to undergo receptor-mediated uptake and degradation (85,86). Because AGEs form on the lysine and arginine residues of proteins, it was reasoned that AGE-modified LDL might exhibit delayed clearance kinetics *in vivo*. When the plasma clearance of AGE-LDL was examined in transgenic mice expressing the human LDL-receptor, markedly delayed clearance kinetics were observed. Of note, the level of AGE-modification utilized in these studies was comparable to that observed in diabetic/end-stage renal disease patients *in vivo*, and there was a significant relationship between the extent of apoB-advanced glycosylation and impaired plasma clearance of LDL *in vivo* (33).

Initial studies established that a major site for the AGE modification of apo B is within a 67 amino acid domain located between residues 1388 and 1454 of the apo B primary sequence (87). This domain lies 1791 residues N-terminal to the putative LDL-receptor binding domain, and an important question posed by these findings was the mechanism by which the modification of lysine residue(s) remote from the receptor-binding domain of apo B can have such a profound effect on LDL-receptor binding. Of note, the 67 amino acid AGE-reactive domain has been mapped to a lipid-associating region of the apolipoprotein B sequence, and advanced glycosylation at this site may be favored by the fact that anhydrous, lipophilic environments can enhance the dehydration and rearrangement reactions leading to AGE formation (88). More recent studies employing a well characterized panel of 29 different anti-apo B monoclonal antibodies showed that glycation decreased the immunoreactivity of six distinct apoB epitopes, including two that closely flank the apoB-LDL receptor binding domain. Nevertheless, residues that are known to be within the apoB-LDLr-binding site are not apparently modified (89). AGE modification presumably induces a conformational change within the LDL particle which is sufficient to perturb ligand-receptor interaction. This may result from an alteration of charge or conformation of the affected lysine, or possibly by the formation of metastable, AGE-crosslinks. These studies provide the first structural basis for beginning to assess how advanced glycosylation can exert such profound impact on LDL clearance. Interestingly, low but detectable levels of AGE-immunoreactivity were found to be present in LDL obtained from non-diabetic individuals, verifying prior observations that measurable quantities of AGE-modified LDL also exist in the circulation of normal, non-diabetic subjects (87).

Lowering of Plasma LDL in Human Subjects By Aminoguanidine

The potential contribution of advanced glycosylation to altered LDL clearance kinetics has been assessed recently in a cohort of diabetic patients who were enrolled in a 28 day, double-blind placebo-controlled trial of the advanced glycosylation inhibitor aminoguanidine. Eighteen patients received aminoguanidine at an average daily dose of 1200 mg and 8 patients received placebo. Blood samples were obtained at the initiation and at the termination of treatment and analyzed for total cholesterol, triglycerides, VLDL-cholesterol, LDL-cholesterol, HDL-cholesterol, Hb-AGE, and HbA_{1c}. The efficacy of aminoguanidine as an inhibitor of advanced glycosylation in these subjects was verified by the observation that circulating Hb-AGE levels decreased by almost 28% in the aminoguanidine-treated group (30). Of significance, amino-guanidine therapy also was associated with a 19% decrease in total cholesterol, a 19% decrease in triglycerides, and a 28% decrease in LDL-cholesterol (33).

A recent clinical trial of aminoguanidine in diabetic dyslipidemia (Type II disease) also has afforded an opportunity to directly examine the AGE-modification of LDL *in vivo*. In this study, 90 diabetic patients were randomized to receive placebo or aminoguanidine for 3 months. Statistical significance was achieved in the lowering of LDL, VLDL, total cholesterol, triglycerides, and apoB-AGE (Table 1) (90). This study provides the most direct evidence to date that AGE modification impairs lipoprotein clearance in human subjects, an important factor in promoting atherogenesis. Further Phase II/III clinical studies of aminoguanidine are presently underway as part of the large, multicenter ACTION I trial that is examining the role of AGE modification in diabetic renal disease and other complications.

Table 1.

Component	Aminoguanidine Treatment	
VLDL	↓ 26%	P = 0.03
LDL	↓ 7.2%	P = 0.04
LDL >160	↓ 16%	P = 0.003
Total Cholesterol	↓ 8.2%	P = 0.001
Total Cholesterol >240	↓ 11%	P = 0.001
HDL	↑ 0.03%	P = 0.16
Triglycerides	↓ 12.7%	P = 0.075
Triglycerides >165	↓ 20%	P = 0.011
ApoB-AGE	↓ 15%	P = 0.045

Average % change in plasma lipid values at 3 months in an aminoguanidine-treated group of diabetics (Type II) versus a placebo (control) group. Dara are from 90 randomized patients and are expressed as a percentage change from baseline (90).

In studies of diabetic, end-stage renal disease patients, high levels of AGE-modified protein breakdown products, *i.e* AGE-peptides, have been found to circulate in blood and this has been attributed to poor clearance by conventional hemodialysis methods (36). "High-flux" hemodialysis membranes are more efficacious in this respect and recent work has shown that diabetic patients treated by high-flux hemodialysis have significantly lower levels of AGE-peptides levels than those treated by conventional dialysis (35% versus 16%). Moreover, high-flux dialysis was found to reduce circulating LDL levels much better than conventional dialysis (27% versus 6%) (91). This study also helps establish the causal link between AGE clearance and dyslipidemia in diabetic patients with end-stage renal failure, and suggests that dialysis methods that favor the removal of circulating AGEs could significantly benefit clinical outcome with regard to vascular disease, the major cause of mortality in this patient group.

Using an immunohistochemical method to quantitate AGEs in atherosclerotic vessels, arterial AGE levels and lesion severity correlate with circulating apoB-AGE levels in non-diabetic patients undergoing endarterectomy, further suggesting a relationship between AGE modification of lipoprotein and clinical vascular disease (92). Circulating levels of AGE-modified LDL (AGE-ApoB) may prove ultimately to be an important marker for atherosclerosis risk, in non-diabetic as well as in diabetic subjects. The elevated circulating level of AGE-ApoB in diabetic patients together with the impaired plasma clearance kinetics of AGE-modified LDL in human LDL-receptor transgenic mice point to the important role of advanced glycation in diabetic atherogenesis. Impairment in the normal, receptor-mediated clearance of LDL is likely to act in concert with abnormalities in lipoprotein production, increases in lipoprotein oxidation and vascular wall lipoprotein trapping, and alterations in endothelial cell function to produce the rapidly progressive vasculopathy of diabetes or renal insufficiency. Lower levels of AGE-modified LDL occur in non-diabetic/non-renal impaired individuals, and it is important to consider that over a time period of many years, advanced glycation also may contribute to the age-related development of atherosclerosis in the general population.

Tobacco Smoke as a Source of AGEs

Smoking has been identified to be the single greatest preventable cause of morbidity and mortality in the United States. The principle cause of death related to smoking is myocardial infarction, but smoking also increases the risk of death from peripheral vascular disease and stroke, as well as pulmonary diseases and cancer (93-95). While assaying AGE levels in certain series of patient plasma, it was noticed that the content of immunoreactive AGEs was significantly higher in the blood of patients who had a history of smoking, irrespective of diabetes or renal disease. The AGE fractions were localized on total serum proteins and on fractions of apo B. Because the curing of tobacco takes place under conditions that favor Maillard chemistry - the process responsible for AGE formation - we embarked on an examination of whether tobacco and tobacco smoke could generate AGEs that might react with plasma and tissue proteins *in vivo*. We found that immunoreactive AGEs with chemical crosslinking potential were present within the aqueous extracts of tobacco, as well as in tobacco smoke that was collected as an aqueous condensate. Smoke-derived AGEs also induced AGE-like fluorescence changes in target proteins, and both crosslinking and fluorescence could be inhibited by aminoguanidine. Of interest, these smoke-derived AGEs were mutagenic and, given their prevalence in aqueous condensate, it likely that they account for a significant portion of the mutagenic potential of tobacco (96).

To ascertain whether AGEs also accumulate in tissues as a consequence of smoking, we next examined specimens of coronary arteries obtained from smokers. Significantly greater levels of immunoreactive AGEs were identified in these arteries, providing the first etiologic link between tobacco smoke-derived glycation products and coronary

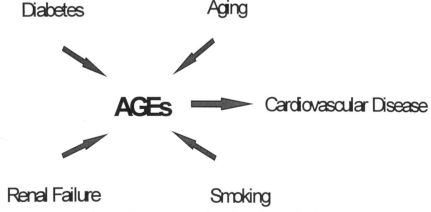

Figure 3. AGEs can be regarded as a common denominator in several pathological processes. It is worth noting that diabetics who smoke are at a significantly increased risk of developing vascular complications compared to their nonsmoking counterparts (98).

artery disease (97). This recently emerging concept has important ramifications for the understanding of discases associated with tobacco usage, points to a new and significant source of AGEs in the human environment, and significantly broadens the role of advanced glycation in pathological processes (Fig 3).

CONCLUSIONS

There is now conclusive evidence that hyperglycemia is associated with the formation of AGEs that have important implications for vascular homeostasis and perhaps, the clinical manifestations of diabetic vascular disease. Large-scale clinical trials will be required to determine if reducing the burden of AGEs translates into demonstrable benefit for patients with diabetes mellitus.

REFERENCES

1.   The Diabetes Control and Complications Trial Research Group. The effect of intensive treatment of diabetes on the development and progression of long-term complications in insulin-dependent diabetes mellitus. *N Engl J of Med.* 1993;329:977.
2.   Donahue RP, Orchard TJ. Diabetes mellitus and microvascular complications. An epidemiological perspective. *Diabetes Care.* 1992;15:1141.
3.   Ruderman NB, and Haudenschild C. Diabetes as an atherogenic factor. *Prog Cardiovasc Dis.* 1981;26:373.
4.   Bucala R, Makita Z, Koschinsky T, Cerami A, Vlassara H. Lipid advanced glycosylation: Pathway for lipid oxidation *in vivo. Proc Natl Acad of Sci USA.* 1993;90:6434.
5.   Bucala R and Cerami A (1996) DNA-advanced glycosylation. In: *Maillard Reactions in Chemistry, Food, and Health.* Labuza T P, Reineccius GA, Monnier V, O'Brien J, and Baynes J (eds), Royal Society of Chemistry, Cambridge UK, pp. 161.
6.   Rahbar S. An abnormal hemoglobin in red cells of diabetics. *Clin Chim Acta.* 1968;22:296.
7.   Koenig RJ, Peterson CM, Jones RL, Saudek C, Lehrman M, Cerami A. Correlation of glucose regulation and hemoglobin A_{1c} in diabetes mellitus. *N Eng J Med.* 1976;295:417.
8.   Larsen ML, Horder M, Mogensen EF. Effect of long-term monitoring of glycosylated hemoglobin levels in insulin-dependent diabetes mellitus. *N Eng J Med.* 1990;323:1021.
9.   Njoroge FG, Monnier VM. The chemistry of the Maillard reaction under physiological conditions. A Review. *Prog Clin Biol Res.* 1989;304:85.
10. Ledl F, Schliecher E. New aspects of the Maillard reaction in foods and in the human body. *Angewandte Chemie.* 1990;29:565.
11. Bucala R, Cerami A. Advanced glycosylation: chemistry, biology, and implications for diabetes and aging. *Adv Pharmacol.* 1992;23:1.
12. Sell DR, Monnier VM. Structure elucidation of a senescence cross-link from humanextracellular matrix. *J Biol Chem.* 1989;264:21597.
13. Farmer J, Ulrich P, Cerami A. Novel pyrroles from sulfite-inhibited Maillard reactions: insight into the mechanism of inhibition. *J Org Chem.* 1988;53:2346.
14. Njoroge FG, Sayre LM, Monnier V. Detection of D-glucose-derived pyrrole compounds during Maillard reaction under physiological conditions. *Carbohydrate Res.* 1987;167:211.
15. Ahmed MU, Thorpe SR, Baynes JW. Identification of N-epsilon-carboxymethyllysine as a degradation product of fructoselysine in glycated protein. *J Biol Chem.* 1986;261:4889
16. Nakamura K., Hasegawa T, Fukunaga Y, Ienaga K. Crosslines A and B as candidates for the fluorophores in age- and diabetes-related cross-linked proteins, and their diacetates produced by Maillard reaction of α-N-acetyl-L-lysine with D-glucose. *J Chem Soc Chem Commun.* 1992; 14:992.
17. Hayase F, Hinuma H, Asano M, Akto H, Arai S. Identification of novel fluorescent pyrrolopyridinium compound formed from Maillard reaction of 3-deoxyglucosone and butylamine. *Bioscience Biotech Biochem.* 1994;58:1936.
18. Wells-Knecht KJ, Brinkmann E, Baynes JW. Characterization of an imidazolium salt formed from glyoxal anfd N^α-hippuryllysine: A model for Maillard reaction crosslinks in proteins. *J Org*

Chem. 1995;60:6246.

19.   Al-Abed Y, Mitsuhashi T, Ulrich P, Bucala R. Novel modifications of N^α-Boc-Arginine and N^α-CBZ-lysine by methylglyoxal. *Bioorg & Med Chem Letts.* 1996;6:1577.

20.   Al-Abed Y, Bucala R. A novel AGE-crosslink exhibiting immunological crossreactivity with *in vivo*-formed AGEs. *Maillard Reactions in Chemistry, Food, and Health.* 1998 (in press).

21.   Zhang X, Ulrich P. Directed approaches to reactiveMaillard intermediates: Formation of a novel 3-alkylamino-2-hydroxy-4-hydroxymethyl-2-cyclopenten-1-one ("cypentodine"). *Tet Letts.* 1996;37:4667.

22.   Schoetter C, Piscetsrieder M, Lerche H, Severin T. Formation of aminoreductones from maltose. *Tet Letts.* 1994;35:7369.

23.   Makita Z, Vlassara H, Cerami A, Bucala R. Immunochemical Detection of Advanced Glycosylation End Products *In Vivo*. *J Biol Chem.* 1992;267:5133.

24.   Nakamura Y, Horii Y, Nishino T, Shiiki H, Sakaguchi Y, Kagoshima T, Dohi K,Makita Z, Vlassara H, Bucala R. Immunohistochemical Localization of Advanced Glycosylation Endproducts (AGEs) in Coronary Atheroma and Cardiac Tissue in Diabetes Mellitus. *Am J Pathol.* 1993;143:1649.

25.   Hayase F, Nagaraj RH, Miyata S, Njoroge FG, Monnier VM. Aging of proteins: immunological detection of a glucose-derived pyrrole formed during Maillard reaction *in vivo*. *J Biol Chem.* 1989;264:3758.

26.   Odetti P, Fogarty J, Sell DR, Monnier VM. Chromatographic quantitation of plasma and erythrocyte pentosidine in diabetic and uremic subjects. *Diabetes.* 1992;41:153.

27.   Beisswenger PJ, Moore LL, Brinck-Johnnsen T, Curphey TJ. Increased collagen-linked pentosidine levels and advanced glycosylattion endproducts in early diabetic nephropathy. *J Clin Invest.* 1993;92:212.

28.   Dyer DG, Dunn JA, Thorpe SR, Bailie KE, Lyons TJ, McCance DR, Baynes JW. Accumulation of Maillard reaction products in skin collagen in diabetes and aging. *J Clin Invest.* 1993;91:2463.

29.   Ienaga K, Nakamura K, Hocji T, Nakazawa Y, Fukunaga Y, Kakita H, Nakano K. Crosslines, fluorophores in the AGE-related cross-linked proteins. In: Diabetes-related amyloidosis, Maeda K, Shinzato T (eds). Contrib Nephrol Basel. Karger 1995; vol 112 pp 42.

30.   Makita Z, Vlassara H, Rayfield E, Cartwright K, Friedman E, Rodby R, Cerami A, Bucala R. Hemoglobin-AGE: A Circulating Marker of Advanced Glycosylation. *Science.* 1992;258:1.

31.   Vasan S, Zhang X, Zhang X, Kapurniotu A, Bernhagen J, Teichberg S, Basgen J, Wagle D, Shih D,   Terlecky I, Bucala R, Cerami A, Egan J, Ulrich P. An agent cleaving glucose-derived protein crosslinks *in vitro* and *in vivo*. *Nature.* 1996;382:275.

32.   Miyata T, Oda O, Inagi R, Iida Y, Araki N, Yamada N, Horiuchi S, Taniguchi N, Maeda K, Kinoshita T. β_2-Microglobulin modified with advanced glycation end products is a major component of hemodialysis-associated amyloidosis. *J Clin Invest.* 1993;92:1243.

33.   Bucala R, Makita Z, Vega G, Grundy S, Koschinsky T, Cerami A, Vlassara H. Modification of LDL by advanced glycosylation endproducts contributes to the dyslipidemia of diabetes and renal insufficiency. *Proc Natl Acad Sci USA.* 1994;91:9441.

34.   Wolffenbuttel BHR, Giordano D, Founds H W, and Bucala R. Long-term assessment of glucose control by haemoglobin-AGE measurement. *The Lancet.* 1996;347:513.

35.   Makita Z, Radoff S, Rayfield EJ, Yang Z, Skolnik E, Delaney V, Friedman EA, Cerami A, Vlassara H. Advanced glycosylation end products in patients with diabetic nephropathy. *N Engl J Med.* 1991;325:836.

36.   Makita Z, Bucala R, Rayfield EJ, Friedman EA, Kaufman AM, Korbet SM, Barth RH, Winston JA, Fuh H, Manogue K, Cerami A, Vlassara H. Diabetic-uremic serum advanced glycosylation endproducts are chemically reactive and resistant to dialysis therapy: Role in mortality of uremia. *Lancet.* 1994;343:1519.

37.   Friedman EA. Treatment options for diabetic nephropathy. *Diabetes Spectrum* 1992; 5 :6.

38.   Fu MX, Knecht KJ, Thorpe SR, Baynes JW. Role of oxygen in cross-linking and chemical modification of collagen by glucose. *Diabetes.* 1992;41 (Suppl 2):42.

39.   Vlassara H, Brownlee M, Cerami A. High-affinity receptor-mediated uptake and degradation of glucose-modified proteins: a potential mechanism for the removal of senescent macromolecules. *Proc Natl Acad Sci USA.* 1985;82:5588.

40.   Vlassara H and Bucala R. Recent progress in advanced glycation and diabetic vascular disease: Role of advanced glycation end product receptors. *Diabetes.* 1996; Suppl.30:S65.

41.   Yang Z, Makita Z, Horii Y, Brunelle S, Cerami A, Sehajpal P, Vlassara H. Two novel rat liver membrane proteins that bind advanced glycosylation endproducts: relationship to macrophage receptor for glucose-modified proteins. *J Exp Med.* 1991;174:515.

42.   Esposito C, Gerlach H, Brett J, Stern D, Vlassara H. Endothelial receptor-mediated binding of glucose-modified albumin is associated with increased monolayer permeability and modulation of cell surface coagulant properties. *J Exp Med.* 1989;170:1387.

43.   Imani F, Horii Y, Suthanthiran M, Skolnik EY, Makita Z, Sharma V, Sehajpal P, Vlassara H. Advanced glycosylation endproduct-specific receptors on human and rat T-lymphocytes mediate synthesis of interferon-γ: role in tissue remodeling. *J Exp Med.* 1993;178:2165.

44.   Skolnik EY, Yang Z, Makita Z, Radoff S, Kirstein M, Vlassara H: Human and rat mesangial cell receptors for glucose-modified proteins: Potential role in kidney tissue remodelling and diabetic nephropathy. *J Exp Med.* 1991;174:931.

45.   Schmidt AM, Vianna M, Gelach M, Brett J, Ryan J, Kao J, Esposito C, Hegarty H, Hurley W, Clauss M, Wang F, Pan Y-CE, Tsang TC, Stern D. Isolation and characterization of two binding proteins for advanced glycosylation endproducts from bovine lung which are present on the endothelial cell surface. *J Biol Chem.* 1992;267:14987.

46.   Vlassara H, Li YM, Imani F, Wojciechoiwicz D, Yang Z, Liu F, Cerami A. Identification of Galectin-3 as a high affinity binding protein of advanced glycation endproducts (AGE): a new member of the AGE-receptor complex. *Mol Med.* 1995;1:634.

47.   Yan SD, Schmidt AM, Anderson GM, Zhang J, Brett J, Zou YS, Pinsky D, Stern D. Enhanced cellular oxidant stress by the interaction of advanced glycation end products with their receptors/binding proteins. *J Biol Chem.* 1994;269:9889.

48.   Araki N, Higashi T, Mori T, Shibayama R, Kawabe Y, Kodama T, Takahashi K, Shichiri M, Horiuchi S. Macrophage scavenger receptor mediates the endocytic uptake and degradation of advanced glycation end products of the Maillard reaction. *Eur J Biochem.* 1995;230:408.

49.   Suzuki H, Kurihara Y, Wada Y, *et al.* Establishment and analysis of scavenger receptor knockout mice. *Circulation.* (suppl) 92;I-428.

50.   Vlassara H, Brownlee M, Manogue K, Dinarello C, Cerami A. Cachectin/TNF and IL-1 induced by glucose-modified proteins: role in normal tissue remodeling. *Science.* 1988;240:1546.

51.   Doi T, Vlassara H, Kirstein M, Yamada Y, Striker GE, Striker LJ. Receptor-specific increase in extracellular matrix production in mouse mesangial cells by advanced glycosylation end products is mediated via platelet-derived growth factor. *Proc Natl Acad Sci USA.* 1992;89: 2873.

52.   Haitoglou CS, Tsilibary EC, Brownlee M, Charonis AS. Altered cellular interactions between cells and nonenzymatically glucosylated laminin-Type IV collagen. *J Biol Chem.* 1992;267: 12404.

53.   Stitt A, Li YM, Gardiner TA, Bucala R, Archer D, and Vlassara H. Advanced glycation end products (AGEs) co-localize with AGE receptors in the retinal vasculature of diabetic and of AGE-infused rats. *Am J Pathol.* 1997;150:523.

54.   de Tejada IS, Goldstein I, Azadzoi K, Krane RJ, Cohen RJA: Impaired neurogenic and endothelium-mediated relaxation of penile smooth muscle in diabetic men with impotence. *N Engl J Med.* 1989;320:1025.

55.   McVeigh GE, Brennan GM, Johnston GD, McDermott BJ, McGrath LT, Henry WR, Andrews JW, Hayes JR. Impaired endothelium-dependent and independent vasodilation in patients with type 2 (non-insulin-dependent) diabetes mellitus. *Diabetologia.* 1992;35:771.

56.   Bucala R, Tracey KJ, Cerami A. Advanced glycosylation products quench nitric oxide and mediate defective endothelium-dependent vasodilatation in experimental diabetes. *J Clin Invest.* 1991;87:432.

57.   Vlassara H, Fuh H, Makita Z, Krungkrai S, Cerami A, Bucala R: Exogenous advanced glycosylation endproducts induce complex vascular dysfunction in normal animals: a model for diabetic and aging complications. *Proc Natl Acad Sci USA.* 1992;89:12043.

58.   Huijberts MS, Wolffenbuttel BH, Boudier HA, Crijns FR, Kruseman AC, Poitevin P, Levy BI. Aminoguanidine treatment increases elasticity and decreases fluid filtration of large arteries from diabetic rats. *J Clin Invest.* 1993;92:1407.

59.   Barnett AH. Diabetes and hypertension. *Brit Med Bull.* 1994;50:397.

60.   Teuscher A, Egger M, Hermann JB: Diabetes and nephropathy: blood pressure in clinical diabetic patients and control population. *Arch Int Med.* 1989;149:1942.

61.   Vallance P, Collier J, Moncada S: Effects of endothelium-derived nitric oxide on peripheral

arteriolar tone in man. *Lancet.* 1989;2:997.

62.   Garg UC, Hassid A. Nitric oxide-generating vasodilators and 8-bromo-cyclic guanosine monophosphate inhibit mitogenesis and proliferation of cultured rat vascular smooth muscle cells. *J Clin Invest.* 1989;83:1774.

63.   Ross R. The pathogenesis of atherosclerosis. An update. *N Eng J Med.* 1989;314:488.

64.   Hogan M, Cerami A, Bucala R. Advanced glycosylation endproducts block the antiproliferative effect of nitric oxide. *J Clin Invest.* 1992;90:1110.

65.   Pyorala K. Diabetes and coronary artery disease: what a coincidence? *J Cardiovascular Pharm.* 1990;16:S8.

66.   Lithner F, Asplund K, Eriksson S, Hagg E, Strand T, Wester PO. Clinical characteristics of in diabetic stroke patients. *Diabetes Metab.* 1988;44:15.

67.   Vlassara H, Fuh H, Donnelly T, and Cybulsky M. Advanced glycation endproducts promote adhesion molecule (VCAM-1, ICAM-1) expression and atheroma formation in normal rabbits. *Mol Medicine.* 1995;1:447.

68.   Jensen T, Stender S, Deckert T. Abnormalities in plasma concentrations of lipoproteins and fibrinogen in Type I diabetic patients with increased urinary albumin excretion. *Diabetologia.* 1988;31:142.

69.   Brown WV, Lipoprotein disorders in diabetes mellitus. *Med Clin N Am.* 1994;78:143.

70.   Ross R. The pathogenesis of atherosclerosis: a perspective for the 1990s. *Nature.* 1993;362: 801.

71.   Goldstein JL, Brown MS. The low-density lipoprotein pathway and its relation to athero-sclerosis. *Annu Rev Biochem.* 1977;46:897.

72.   Lopes-Virella MF, Sherer GK, Lees AM, Wohltmann H, Mayfield R, Sagel J, LeRoy EC, Colwell JA: Surface binding, internalization and degradation by cultured human fibroblasts of low density lipoproteins isolated from type 1 (insulin-dependent) diabetic patients: changes with metabolic control. *Diabetologia.* 1982;22:430.

73.   Hiramatsu K, Bierman EL, Chait A. Metabolism of low-density lipoprotein from patients   with diabetic hypertriglyceridemia by cultured human skin fibroblasts. *Diabetes.* 1985;34:8.

74.   Steinberg D, Parthasarathy S, Carew TE, Khoo JC, Witztum JL: Modifications of low-density lipoprotein that increases its atherogenicity. *New Eng J Med.* 1989;320:915.

75.   Dix TA, Aikens J. Mechanisms and biological relevance of lipid peroxidation initiation. *Chem Res Toxicol.* 1992;6:2.

76.   Bucala R. Lipid and lipoprotein oxidation: Basic mechanisms and unresolved questions *in vivo.* *Redox Report.* 1996;2:291.

77.   Grandhee SK Monnier VM. Mechanism of formation of the Maillard protein cross-link pentosidine. Glucose, fructose, and ascorbate as pentosidine precursors. *J Biol Chem.* 1991; 266:11649.

78.   Dyer DG, Blackledge JA, Thorpe SR, Baynes JW. Formation of pentosidine during nonenzymatic browning of proteins by glucose. Identification of glucose and other carbohydrates as possible precursors of pentosidine *in vivo. J Biol Chem.* 1991;266:11654.

79.   Fu MX, Requena JR, Jenkins AJ, Lyons TJ, Baynes JW, Thorpe SR. The advanced glycation end product, N-epsilon-(carboxymethyl)lysine, is a product of both lipid peroxidation and glycoxidation reactions. *J Biol Chem.* 1996;271:9982.

80.   Al-Abed Y, Bucala R. *N*-Carboxymethyllysine formation by direct addition of glyoxal to lysine during the Maillard reaction. *Biorg Med Chem Lett.* 1995;5:2161.

81.   Al-Abed Y, Liebich H, Voelter W, Bucala R. Hydroxyalkenal formation induced by advanced glycosylation of low density lipoprotein. *J BiolChem.* 1996;271:2892.

82.   Mitsuda H, Yasumoto K, Yokoyama K. Studies of Free Radicals in Amino-carbonyl Reaction. *J Agric Biol Chem.* 1965;29:751.

83.   Hayashi T, Ohta Y, Namiki M. Electron Spin Resonance Spectral Study on the Structure of the Novel Free Radical Products Formed by the Reactions of Sugars with Amino Acids or Amines. *J Agric Fd Chem.* 1977;25:1282.

84.   Yim H-S, Kang S-O, Hah Y-C, Chock PB, Yim MB. Free radicals generated during the glycation reaction of amino acids and methylglyoxal. *J Biol Chem.* 1995;270:28228.

85.   Mahley RW, Innerarity TL, Pitas RE, Weisgraber KH, Brown JH, Gross E. Inhibition of lipoprotein binding to cell surface receptors of fibroblasts following selective modification of arginyl residues in apoprotein B. *J Biol Chem.* 1987;252:7279.

86.   Mahley RW, Innerarity TL, Weisgraber KH, Oh SY. Altered metabolism (*in vivo* and *in vitro*) of plasma lipoproteins after selective chemical modification of lysine residues of the apoprotein B.

J Clin Invest. 1979;64:743.

87.   Bucala R, Mitchell R, Arnold K, Innerarity T, Vlassara H, Cerami A. Identification of the major site of apolipoprotein-B modification by advanced glycosylation endproducts (AGEs) blocking uptake by the LDL receptor. *J Biol Chem.* 1995;270:10820.

88.   Chen GC, Hardman DA, Hamilton RL, Mendel CM, Schilling JW, Zhu S, Lau K, Wong JS, Kane JP. Distribution of lipid-binding regions in human apolipoprotein B-100. *Biochemistry.* 1989;28:2477.

89.   Wang X, Bucala R, Milne R. Epitopes close to the apolipoprotein B low density lipoprotein binding site are modified by advanced glycation end products. *Proc Natl Acad Sci USA.* 95:7643.

90.   Alteon, Inc. Press release. Reuters News Service 09:55 AM ET, 4/17/97.

91.   Fishbane S, Bucala R, Pereira BJG, Founds H, Vlassara H. Reduction of plasma apolipoprotein-B by effective removal of circulating glycation derivatives in uremia. *Kidney Int.* 1997;52:1645.

92.   Stitt A, He C, Freidman S, Scher L, Rosssi P, Ong L, Founds F, Li Y, Bucala R, Vlassara H. Elevated AGE-modified ApoB in sera of euglycemic, normolipidemic patients with atherosclerosis: Relationship to tissue AGEs. *Mol Med.* 1997;3:617.

93.   Bartecchi CE, MacKenzie TD, Schrier RW. The human costs of tobacco use. *N Engl J Med.* 1994;330:907.

94.   Shah PK, Helfant RH. Smoking and coronary artery disease. *Chest.* 1988;94:449.

95.   Sherman CB. Health affects of cigarette smoking. *Clin Chest Med.* 1991;12:643.

96.   Cerami C, Founds H, Nicholl ID, Mitsuhashi T, Giordano D, Vanpatten S, Lee A, Al-Abed Y, Vlassara H, Bucala R, Cerami A. Tobacco smoke is a source of toxic reactive glycation products. *Proc Natl Acad Sci USAi.* 1997;94:13915.

97.   Nicholl ID, Stitt AW, Moore JE, Ritchie AJ, Archer DB, Bucala R. Increased levels of advanced glycation endproducts in the lenses and blood vessels of cigarette smokers. *Mol Med.* 1998 (in press).

98.   Suarez L, Barrett-Connor E. Interaction between cigarette smoking and diabetes mellitus in the prediction of death attributed to cardiovascular disease. *Am J Epidemiol.* 1984;120:670.

16 HYPERGLYCEMIA AND DIABETES -INDUCED VASCULAR DYSFUNCTION: ROLE OF OXIDATIVE STRESS

Galen M. Pieper

INTRODUCTION

There is substantial indirect evidence that oxidative stress occurs during the course of diabetes mellitus. This is based upon reports of elevation in lipid peroxides (*i.e.*, malondialdehyde) in plasma of experimental diabetic rodents (1-3) and in plasma of human type I and type II diabetes mellitus (2,4-7). More recently, F_2-isoprostancs, nonenzymatic peroxidation products, were shown to be increased in plasma of diabetic patients (8). In addition to elevated concentrations of lipid peroxides, oxidation of LDL, increased formation of glycated proteins, and elevated plasma concentrations of ceruloplasmin (9,10) have supported a role for increased oxidative stress in diabetic patients.

Studies conducted in human diabetic patients show that elevations in plasma lipid peroxide levels were higher in individuals with macro- and microangiopathy (5-7). These observations have led to the hypothesis that oxidative stress is pivotal in the development of vascular disease and complications of diabetes mellitus (11,12). While elevations in lipid peroxides have been reported in vascular tissue of experimental diabetic animals (13), it is not possible to preclude that increases in circulating oxidant products correlate with frank increases in lipid peroxides, or other oxidant end-points in vascular tissue. Indeed, temporal changes in thiobarbituric acid-reactive substances in arteries and myocardium do not parallel changes observed in the plasma (13). The balance between oxidant production and antioxidant defense mechanisms *per se* regulates the net effect of systemic oxidative stress on vascular tissue.

Several reviews have addressed the issue of the role of oxidative stress in diabetic vascular complications, in general (11,12,14-17). In contrast, less attention has been played to the role of oxidative stress in diabetes-induced vascular complications specific to the endothelium. The present paper attempts to provide the current state of knowledge regarding the relationship between endothelial dysfunction and oxidative stress in diabetes mellitus. This discussion will focus on two separate facets of oxidative stress on diabetes-induced endothelial dysfunction. The first is the acute effect of reactive oxygen produced concurrently during the actual evaluation of endothelium-dependent relaxation. The second is the role of reactive oxygen produced chronically during the course of the disease on the actual etiology of endothelial dysfunction.

ENDOTHELIAL DYSFUNCTION IN DIABETES MELLITUS

There is broad consensus that endothelial dysfunction (characterized by impaired endothelium-dependent relaxation) occurs in diabetes mellitus (see reviews; 18-23). This dysfunction occurs in both conduit and resistance arteries of chemically- and genetically-induced diabetic animals and under *in vitro* and *in vivo* conditions. There is general agreement that impaired relaxation is specific to the endothelium as relaxation is normal in response to nitrovasodilators which act directly to activate vascular smooth muscle guanylyl cyclase. Observations made in these experimental models are significant and relevant to human disease as similar observations have been observed in both type I and type II diabetic patients. Although in human disease, there appears to be some additional evidence that a superimposed defect in vascular responsiveness to nitrovasodilators may be present in some diabetic patients (23). This issue of impaired nitrovasodilator responses in human diabetes mellitus may need to be resolved with appropriate patient selection and better screening techniques.

The studies conducted in animal models suggest that the mechanism of diabetes-induced endothelial dysfunction is complex and that a single universal factor may be inadequate to explain impaired endothelium-dependent relaxation under all conditions. This most likely is due to variations in the duration and severity of disease, the contribution of other factors to dilation (*i.e.* hyperpolarizing factors and prostaglandins) vs. nitric oxide (NO) in individual artery types and differences in experimental design and methods of evaluation. Individual factors present at the time of functional evaluation that have been proposed to contribute to defective relaxation include: (a) increased release of an endothelium-derived constricting factor arising from the cyclooxygenase pathway; (b) increase in protein kinase C activity; (c) inhibition of $Na^+K^+ATPase$; (d) a deficiency or inappropriate utilization of substrate or co-factors for NO synthase; (e) increased quenching of NO by advanced glycosylation end products; (f) decreased NO release; (g) increased NO destruction by increased formation of superoxide anion radical ($^.O_2^-$).

This chapter will review the evidence that oxidative stress contributes to endothelial dysfunction. It is important to note that the degree to which this occurs in the acute setting depends on the contribution of NO to relaxation in any given artery type and whether diabetes is associated with specific defects in NO-mediated relaxation. This issue has been addressed in the author's recent review (23).

Indirect Evidence Supporting Enhanced Superoxide Anion Radical Formation During *In Vitro* Analysis of Endothelial Function in Diabetic Arteries

The enzyme, superoxide dismutase (SOD), converts superoxide to hydrogen peroxide (H_2O_2) and O_2. Several studies have shown that addition *in vitro* of SOD restores defective basal NO activity (24,25) and completely or partially restores defective endothelium-dependent relaxation in conduit and resistance arteries of chemical-induced (26-32) and genetically-diabetic animals (33). A few studies have shown that SOD alone had no effect in renal arterioles (34), mesenteric arteries (35) or coronary arteries (36). It is possible that these latter observations reflect variances in the contribution of NO to relaxation versus other factors such as prostanoids and endothelium-derived hyperpolarizing factor (EDHF). In those cases in which the agonist-induced component of relaxation is largely due to prostanoids and/or EDHF, the addition of SOD to quench superoxide and its subsequent interactions with NO would not be expected to be effective. Indeed, bioassay studies conducted in rat aorta which have virtually a complete component related to NO indicate that luminal perfusion with SOD enhanced acetylcholine-stimulated endothelium-derived NO activity arising from diabetic but not control donor arteries (27).

Other reactive oxygen species may also impact on endothelial dysfunction in diabetes. While addition *in vitro* of catalase to detoxify H_2O_2 had no effect on endothelium-dependent relaxation in diabetic aorta (26,32,37), the combination of SOD + catalase improved relaxation (37). Furthermore, intra-arterial infusion of SOD failed but topical application of SOD + catalase improved relaxation in diabetic canine coronary artery (38). This observation suggests that diabetes elicits enhanced production of both superoxide and H_2O_2 but do not prove that diabetic blood vessels produced increased amounts of these reactive oxygen species. Using the ferricytochrome C technique, two laboratories have reported enhanced basal production of superoxide arising from isolated diabetic rat aorta (39,40) while another technique revealed increased release of H_2O_2 (40).

Increased vascular production of superoxide and H_2O_2 has been confirmed in isolated aorta of 2-week diabetic rats (40, Figure 1). Both of these reactive oxygen species are precursor molecules for hydroxyl radical formation via Haber-Weiss or Fenton reactions. A role of hydroxyl radical in diabetes-induced endothelial dysfunction is consistent with the observation of increased detection of hydroxyl radical by salicylic acid trapping in experimental diabetes (41) and in diabetic patients (42). It is also consistent with reports showing that scavengers of hydroxyl radical or hydroxyl radical formation such as dimethylthiourea (29,34) or diethylenetriaminepentaacetic acid (DTPA) (37) improved endothelium-dependent relaxation in experimental diabetic models. An alternative explanation for these findings is that thiols and DTPA bind redox-active iron. Iron may directly interact with endothelium-derived relaxing factor or NO (43). Thus, endothelial function might be improved by removing the ability of iron to destroy NO, thereby increasing NO bioactivity. This action might also explain the restoration of vasodilator response to cold pressor challenges (believed to be indicative of endothelial function) in NIDDM patients infused with the iron chelator, deferoxamine (44).

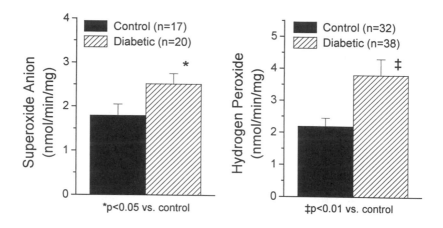

Figure 1. Increased production of superoxide and H_2O_2 from diabetic rat aorta.

The nature of increased reactive oxygen arising from isolated diabetic blood vessels *in vitro* and the mechanism of benefits of the combination of SOD + catalase or hydroxyl radical inhibitors remain in need of further study. This includes detailed investigation of the location (*i.e.* cell specificity) and source (*i.e.* enzymatic or nonenzymatic) of reactive oxygen production by isolated diabetic arteries

Role of Endogenous Antioxidant Enzymes

The increased detection of reactive oxygen may be influenced by the balance between the rate of production and the level of antioxidant defense/enzymes which may vary depending on the severity and stage/duration of disease. Diabetic cerebral microvessels possess a diminished capacity to detoxify peroxides (45). After 4 months of diabetes, diminished activity of glutathione peroxidase but unaltered catalase was observed in diabetic rat aorta (2). In contrast, other authors have noted either no change in SOD activity after 3 days of diabetes (46), or unaltered SOD but augmented catalase after diabetes of 8 weeks duration (47). In yet another study with diabetic rats, SOD, catalase and glutathione peroxidase were reported to be elevated after 1-2 weeks of diabetes (13). It is important to note that some of the increased antioxidant enzyme activity observed in that latter study were followed by a period of normalization and re-induction of activity with length of disease. Increased vascular antioxidant enzyme activities are likely due to a compensatory induction from chronic oxidative stress *in vivo* as pancreatic islet transplantation after 8 weeks of diabetes quickly restores these activities to normal (47).

Observations that antioxidant enzyme activities might increase with diabetes suggests that simple evaluation of intrinsic reactive oxygen production within vascular tissue may underestimate the true oxidative stress. This situation might explain the failure to detect oxidants including lipid peroxide in plasma and various tissues at certain stages of the disease (13,48-50). Indeed, increased vascular production of superoxide and H_2O_2 after 2 weeks of diabetes was not apparent at 8 weeks, a time when tissue catalase activity was increased (40). In contrast, arteries treated with aminotriazole to inhibit endogenous catalase activity demonstrated greater aortic H_2O_2 production in these 8-week diabetic rats.

There is an implicit assumption in all of the above studies that the activities of endogenous antioxidants are uniformly distributed between cell types in the vascular wall. This assumption may be invalid. There is a study showing that endothelial cells isolated from the aorta of rabbits after 17 days of diabetes display decreased catalase, glutathione peroxidase and CuZnSOD activity but unchanged MnSOD activity (51). This suggests that increased production of reactive oxygen by endothelial cells may be due to decreased detoxification by endogenous antioxidant enzymes. There still are important questions to be addressed. There is a need to more clearly identify potential time- and cell-dependent heterogeneity in the expression of antioxidant enzyme activities in diabetic arteries. Furthermore, there is a need to determine the specific location and cell-type that is responsible for the increased production of reactive oxygen in the vascular wall of diabetic arteries.

Sources of Increased Reactive Oxygen Production *In Vitro*

It is also unclear whether the enhanced reactive oxygen production and/or the increased NO destruction by isolated diabetic arteries arises from enzymatic or nonenzymatic pathways. In the *in vitro* assays reported above, the level of glucose in the media for control and diabetic arteries did not vary. Thus, elevations in glucose concentration present at the time of functional evaluation cannot account for this difference. Nonenzymatic sources might arise from glycated proteins located within the vessel wall. Indeed, glycated proteins have been reported to inhibit endothelium-dependent relaxation in isolated rat aorta (52,53) presumably by quenching NO. The impairment of endothelium-dependent, but not endothelium-independent relaxation, by glycated human hemoglobin (Hb) is prevented by SOD (54) but not by catalase, deferoxamine, indomethacin, thromboxane receptor antagonists, endothelin receptor antagonists or L-arginine. This suggests a significant role of superoxide arising from glycated proteins in this defect.

A more recent study has challenged the role of glycated proteins in producing endothelial dysfunction. Using 10-fold higher concentrations of glycated Hb that the study discussed above, Oltman *et al.* failed to observe altered endothelium-dependent relaxation in a variety of blood vessel types including: cardiac ventricular microvessels and coronary, mesenteric, femoral and renal arteries (55). While these findings may point to important regional and species differences in action of glycated proteins, these authors speculated but did not test the hypothesis that previous results showing impaired relaxation to glycated Hb are artifacts due to the high oxygen tensions employed (55). Nevertheless, this conclusion does not exclude the possibility that glycated proteins located within the vascular tissue may be important sources of reactive oxygen in diabetes mellitus.

NADPH/NADH Oxidases as Enzymatic Sources of Reactive Oxygen

An enzymatic pathway for increased reactive oxygen production was suggested by a recent histochemical study conducted in diabetic retinal vessels. In that study, NADH oxidase activity was increased in endothelial cells and basement membrane of diabetic retinal arteries (56). In normal arteries, there is evidence for NADPH/NADH oxidase in both endothelial cells (57,58) and vascular smooth muscle cells (59). This spatial heterogeneity of NADPH/NADH oxidase activity in the vascular wall may give insight into sources of enhanced oxidative stress in diabetic vasculature. It is interesting to note that topical application *in situ* of SOD + catalase improved relaxation in diabetic basilar artery (30) and that topical SOD + catalase (but not luminal perfusion with SOD) improved endothelial function in diabetic coronary arterioles (38). These data suggest that the location of the reactive oxygen production may be highest on the adventitial side of the artery wall. In normal rabbit aorta, immunohistochemical studies reveal highly localized NADPH oxidase activity in the adventitia (60). Furthermore, it is interesting to note that iron deposition is increased in adventitia of diabetic arteries (61). Redox-active iron in this case might enhance hydroxyl radical formation from superoxide and H_2O_2 precursors or quench NO directly. There clearly is a need for more extensive research to clarify the location and enzymatic pathways for increased reactive oxygen production arising from diabetic blood vessels.

Nitric Oxide Synthase: A Putative Source Of Reactive Oxygen

Under normal conditions, NO synthase converts arginine to citrulline and NO. Under limiting conditions of substrate or the cofactor, tetrahydrobiopterin, the purified brain enzyme *in vitro* also produces superoxide and H_2O_2 as by-products (62). Interestingly, while homogenates of diabetic tissue reveal normal or enhanced NO production, endothelium-dependent relaxation is still impaired suggesting that NO synthase activity is diminished in intact cell conditions (63). This might reflect a 'relative deficiency' or inadequate utilization of arginine and/or cofactor. Indeed, plasma and vascular tissue arginine is decreased in diabetes (64). The cofactor, tetrahydrobiopterin, has been shown to be reduced in diabetic rat brain (65) and calmodulin is reduced in diabetic tissue including aorta (66).

The beneficial effects of acute *in vivo* supplementation with arginine (36), or *in vitro* supplementation with tetrahydrobiopterin (67) or arginine (68-71) reverse endothelial dysfunction and improve cGMP generation in diabetic vascular tissue and this could be explained by combined increase in NO production and diminished reactive oxygen production from NO synthase. If this hypothesis proves true, then an aberrant NO synthase may serve as a chronic source of reactive oxygen production within diabetic vascular tissue. While the effects of these interventions to reduce intrinsic rates of reactive oxygen production in diabetic arteries have not yet been documented, dietary arginine has been shown to reduce reactive oxygen production arising from isolated atherosclerotic arteries (72).

ACUTE EFFECTS OF ANTIOXIDANT INTERVENTION TO PREVENT ENDOTHELIAL DYSFUNCTION PRODUCED BY ELEVATED GLUCOSE CONCENTRATION

Incubation with elevated glucose concentration for short periods of time (*i.e.* hours) impaired endothelium-dependent relaxation in normal conduit and resistance arteries in *vitro* (28,73-75). Furthermore, topical application of elevated glucose concentration *in situ* also impaired endothelium-dependent relaxation (76,77). In contrast to these studies, infusion of glucose in humans for 24 hours failed to elicit impaired endothelium-dependent relaxation (78). The nature of this ineffectiveness is not yet known particularly since another report revealed impaired relaxation conducted during a glucose-tolerance protocol (79). As multiple agonists were used in the former study, it is difficult to evaluate these findings due to the potential masking by latent crossover effects between individual agonist challenges.

The detrimental effects of high glucose concentrations in arteries of experimental animals were ameliorated using SOD (28,73,75,76), a protein kinase C (PKC) inhibitor (77) or by indomethacin (28,73,75,76). These findings suggest that reactive oxygen production is enhanced by activation of PKC and cyclooxygenase pathways. It is not yet certain in these experiments whether the reactive oxygen arises from smooth muscle or endothelial cell sources or both. Studies conducted in cultured endothelial and smooth muscle cells reveal that elevated glucose concentration can activate PKC in both cell types (80). Furthermore, thromboxane A_2 synthesis arising from intact arteries exposed to elevated glucose (28) is increased but is not increased in isolated endothelial cells (81).

Endothelial-Specific Effects of High Glucose Concentrations: Role of Oxidants

Impaired agonist-stimulated Ca^{2+} signaling and/or NO production have been observed after exposure of isolated rat, bovine and porcine endothelial cells to elevated glucose concentration (82-86). Intracellular hydroxyl radical scavengers with metal chelation activity such as dimethylthiourea and pyrrolidine dithiocarbamate, but not the extracellular scavenger, mannitol, prevented these defects (82,85).

Few studies have actually quantified reactive oxygen production in endothelial cells following exposure to elevated glucose concentration. Using the ferricytochrome C technique which measures extracellular superoxide release only, increases in the intrinsic rates of basal and agonist-stimulated reactive oxygen production were observed following glucose exposure (87-89). Pretreatment with vitamin E or probucol prevented this increase (88). These studies show that glucose can alter the spontaneous rate of endogenous radical production by endothelial cells but do not address the issue whether reactive oxygen is, in fact, generated within endothelial cells during the period of glucose exposure. Acute increases in reactive oxygen production within endothelial cells during the actual glucose exposure period were demonstrated using the fluorescent probe, dichlorofluorescein (82). Reactive oxygen was not produced by elevated glucose under acellular conditions and the response was specific for D-glucose as L-glucose did not produce this effect (unpublished observations). These studies show that intracellular reactive oxygen is generated within the endothelial cell during the time of elevated glucose exposure.

Acute Effects of Antioxidant Intervention on Endothelial Function *In Vivo*

There are few studies that have examined diabetic endothelial function under ambient diabetic conditions. Studies conducted in cerebral arteries reveal that either topical application of SOD (30) or inhibitors of PKC (90) normalize relaxation in diabetic arteries. This suggests that increased production of superoxide arising from a PKC-dependent pathway may be involved. Similarly, stimulation of superoxide in arteries by lysophosphatidylcholine was shown to be PKC-dependent (91).

In human IDDM or NIDDM, infusion with vitamin C (92,93) or infusion with the iron chelator, deferoxamine, (44) restored endothelial function. Collectively, these studies support a role of concurrent oxidative stress in eliciting diminished endothelial function in human diabetes mellitus. The precise source of this increased oxidative stress *in vivo* is not yet known with certainty. Possible sources include: elevated glucose concentration, glycated proteins or oxidized LDL.

Beneficial Effects of Chronic Antioxidant Intervention *In Vivo* on Endothelial Dysfunction in Experimental Diabetes

There is a need to evaluate the effects of chronic administration of antioxidants on endothelial function in diabetes mellitus. In the streptozotocin-diabetic rat, chronic treatment with vitamin E (94,95), N-acetylcysteine (96,97), butylated hydroxytoluene (96), dimethylthiourea (98,99) or modified deferoxamine (100) prevented endothelial dysfunction in large arteries. Vitamin E also partially prevented ultrastructural changes in the endothelium (101). In resistance arteries, vitamin E (31) prevented endothelial dysfunction in diabetic coronary resistance arteries whereas probucol (102) and vitamin E, vitamin C or a combination of both (103) failed to prevent dysfunction in diabetic mesenteric arteries despite a reduction in plasma lipid peroxides.

It is uncertain whether these findings suggest important regional differences in protection by antioxidants as there is insufficient corroborating information for these findings in mesenteric studies. Again, the contribution of NO versus EDHF and prostanoids to total relaxation may be important in determining the potential efficacy of antioxidant interventions in these arteries. The salient effect of vitamin E on coronary resistance arteries (31) and the flavonoid, delphinidin chloride, on hamster cheek pouch microcirculation (104) would argue against a lack of efficacy of antioxidants to prevent endothelial dysfunction in resistance arteries in general. This is supported by the apparent improvement in deficits in sciatic nutritive endoneurial blood flow in diabetic rats using a variety of antioxidants including: probucol (105), a probucol analog BM15.0639 (106), vitamins E and C (107) and the iron chelators, deferoxamine or trientine (108).

Interestingly, chronic treatment with a 21-aminosteroid, a potent inhibitor of lipid peroxidation, also failed to prevent endothelial dysfunction in diabetic rat aorta despite normalization of plasma lipid peroxides (109). These findings might suggest that lipid peroxides might not be direct mediators of diabetes-induced endothelial dysfunction. Alternatively, it is possible that the specific 21-aminosteroid chosen for these studies may have intercalated at levels in the cell membrane which do not impact on lipid peroxides formed at deeper levels of the lipid bilayer. Taken together with the variant studies using probucol and vitamin E in both conduit and resistant arteries, it is not yet clear whether lipid peroxides *per se* play a significant role in the etiology of diabetes-induced endothelial dysfunction.

It is equally plausible that the failure of probucol and vitamins E and C to prevent dysfunction in diabetic mesenteric arteries is due to the disease duration/severity. For example, the beneficial effects of vitamin E in rat aorta and coronary resistance arteries were conducted in diabetic animals of 2-3 months duration whereas the animals were only diabetic for 4 weeks in the studies lacking antioxidant efficacy in the mesenteric model.

In addition to the classical agents used for antioxidant intervention, it is possible that a variety of other classes of drugs throught to act via different mechanisms may actually provide benefit via an antioxidant pathway. For example, aminoguanidine has shown benefit in preventing diabetic vascular alterations. Aminoguanidine has putative specificity for inhibition of inducible NO synthase (110), but this agent can also inhibit aldose reductase (111) and the formation of advanced glycation endproducts (112) as well as provide antioxidant properties (113,114). There is no clear indication which property of aminoguanidine may be predominate under *in vivo* conditions. Chronic treatment with aldose reductase inhibitors has also been shown to prevent endothelial dysfunction in streptozotocin-diabetic rat and alloxan-diabetic rabbit models (115-117). It is known that at least some aldose reductase inhibitors are potent inhibitors of iron- and copper-catalyzed oxidation (118). Thus, these agents may need to be re-evaluated for their efficacy *in vivo* in preventing diabetes-associated endothelial dysfunction via an alternative mechanism of preventing metal ion-catalyzed reactive oxygen production.

Effects of Chronic Treatment With Antioxidants On Glucose or Glycation

Most studies showing benefits of chronic antioxidant intervention to prevent endothelial dysfunction have shown that plasma glucose levels remain elevated. It has not been routinely evaluated in such functional studies whether this form of therapeutic intervention alters glycated protein levels. Glycated proteins are diminished by iron chelators in response to elevated glucose concentration (119) and by large doses of vitamin E and C in diabetic patients (120,121). In contrast, lower vitamin E intake did not correlate with changes in glycated Hb levels (122).

In diabetic animals, we have shown only marginal or modest effects to reduce glycated Hb levels and no changes in glucose or insulin levels by chronic treatment with a deferoxamine analog (100), dimethylthiourea (98); or N-acetylcysteine (97) despite prevention of endothelial dysfunction. This suggests that chronic antioxidant intervention might act via scavenging of reactive products produced as a result of glucose autoxidation or glycation reactions rather than by changing glucose concentrations or levels of glycated proteins. These conclusions do not exclude the possibility that antioxidants might decrease advanced glycation products in tissue without altering system glycated Hb levels as has been shown in renal tissue following treatment with NO synthase inhibitors (123).

EFFECTS OF ANTIOXIDANTS ON CELL ADHESION MOLECULE EXPRESSION: ROLE OF NF-κB

Most studies have not evaluated the effects of antioxidant intervention on cell adhesion. There is increased expression of E-selectin and vascular cell adhesion molecule-1 (VCAM-1) on aortic endothelium of diabetic rabbits (124) and increased expression of intercellular adhesion molecule-1 (ICAM-1) and P-selectin in diabetic human retina and choroid (125). Circulating levels of soluble adhesion molecules have been proposed as biomarkers that play a significant role in the pathogenesis of macrovascular and microvascular dysfunction and neuropathy of diabetes mellitus (126-128).

Incubation of isolated human umbilical vein endothelial cells with high glucose concentrations also increases ICAM-1 expression (129,130). In contrast, one study failed to detect increased expression of E-selectin, VCAM-1 or ICAM-1 in human aortic endothelial cells exposed to 25 mM glucose for 7-10 days (131). A complicating factor that might explain this discrepancy is that the media in this study contained high concentrations of pyruvate, a known scavenger of H_2O_2.

Antioxidants are known to reduce cell adhesion molecule expression in cultured cells exposed to cytokines (132-136). This occurs via inhibition of transcription regulated by the oxidant-sensitive transcription factor, nuclear factor-κB (NF-κB). Indeed, there are known NF-κB binding domains in the promoter region for genes encoding VCAM-1, ICAM-1 and E-selectin expression. It has now been documented in our laboratory that exposure of isolated endothelial cells to elevated glucose concentrations increases NF-κB binding activity within the nuclear fraction (137). NF-κB activation in these endothelial cells was prevented by incubation with the PKC inhibitor, calphostin C, and subsequently was shown to be prevented by the antioxidants, aspirin or pyrrolidine dithiocarbamate (unpublished observation). Other authors have shown that advanced glycation end-products can activate NF-κB in isolated endothelial cells and this activation can be prevented by the antioxidant N-acetylcysteine (138) or α-lipoic acid (139). Likewise, activation of endothelial cell NF-κB by oxidized LDL is prevented by α-tocopherol (140).

Thus, there are at least 3 candidate stimuli (*i.e.* glucose, advanced glycation products and oxidized LDL) present under diabetic conditions which can potentially activate this important oxidant-sensitive transcription factor and its gene products under *in vivo* conditions. Whether this increased in NF-κB activity occurs in diabetic tissue *in vivo*, remains to be determined. In this regard, we have found a doubling of NF-κB binding activity in the nuclear fraction of rat aortic vascular tissue within 5 days of streptozotocin-diabetes (Figure 2). That oxidative stress may play a role to cell adhesion to the endothelium under *in vivo* diabetic conditions is suggested by an isolated study showing that chronic treatment with a flavonoid reduced leukocyte adherance to diabetic hamster microvessels (104).

Accordingly, it appears important that research be directed to understanding how antioxidant administration plays a role in transcription factor-regulated expression of endothelial gene products such as cell adhesion molecules. Understanding this regulation may provide a better design of therapeutic agents to prevent the development of vascular complications associated with diabetes mellitus.

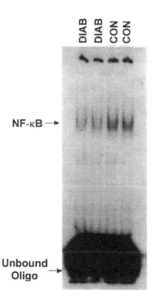

Figure 2. Increased NF-κB binding activity in aorta of 5-day streptozotocin-diabetic rats compared to nondiabetic control rats.

REFERENCES

1.   Matkovics B, Varga SI, Szabó L, Witas H. The effect of diabetes on the activities of the peroxide metabolism enzymes. *Horm Metab Res.* 1982;14:77.

2.   Dohi T, Kawamura K, Morita K, Okamoto H, Tsujimoto A. Alterations of the plasma selenium concentrations and the activities of tissue peroxide metabolism enzymes in streptozotocin-induced diabetic rats. *Horm Metab Res.* 1988;20:671.

3.   Higuchi Y. Lipid peroxides and ⟨-tocopherol in rat streptozotocin-induced diabetes mellitus. *Acta Med Okayama.* 1982;3:165.

4.   Sato Y, Hotta N, Sakamoto N, Matsuoka S, Ohishi N, Yagi K. Lipid peroxide level in plasma of diabetic patients. *Biochem Med.* 1979;21:104.

5.   Gallou G, Ruelland A, Legras B, Maugendre D, Allannic H, Cloarec L.   Plasma malondialdehyde in type 1 and type 2 diabetic patients. *Clin Chim Acta.* 1993;214:227.

6.   Gallou G, Ruelland A, Campion L, Maugendre D, Le Moullec N, Legras B, Allannic H, Cloarec L. Increase in thiobarbituric acid-reactive substances and vascular complications in type 2 diabetes mellitus. *Diabete & Metabolisme (Paris).* 1994;20:258.

7.   Griesmacher A, Kindhauser M, Andert SE, Schreiner W, Toma C, Knoebl P, Pietschmann P, Prager R, Schnack C, Schernthaner G, Mueller MM.   Enhanced serum levels of thiobarbituric-acid-reactive substances in diabetes mellitus. *Am J Med.* 1995;98:469.

8.   Gopaul NK, Änggård, Mallet AI, Betteridge DJ, Wolff SP, Nourooz-Zadeh J. Plasma 8-epi-PGF$_2$ levels are elevated in individuals with non-insulin dependent diabetes mellitus. *FEBS Lett.* 1995;368:225.

9.   Cunningham J, Leffell M, Mearkle P, Harmatz P. Elevated plasma ceruloplasmin in insulin-dependent diabetes mellitus: evidence for increased oxidative stress as a variable complication. *Metabolism.* 1995;44:996.

10.   MacRury SM, Gordon D, Wilson R, Bradley H, Gemmell CG, Paterson JR, Rumley AG, MacCuish AC. A comparison of different methods of assessing free radical activity in type 2 diabetes and peripheral vascular disease. *Diab Med.* 1992;10:331.

11.   Tribe RM, Poston L. Oxidative stress and lipids in diabetes: a role in endothelium vasodilator dysfunction? *Vasc Med.* 1996;1:195.

12.   Giugliano D, Ceriello A, Paolisso G. Oxidative stress and diabetic vascular complications. *Diabetes Care.* 1996;19:257.

13.   Kakkar R, Mantha SV, Kalra J, Prasad K. Time course study of oxidative stress in aorta and heart of diabetic rat. *Clin Sci.* 1997;91:441.

14.   Wolff SP, Jiang ZY, Hunt JV. Protein glycation and oxidative stress in diabetes mellitus and ageing. *Free Radical Biol Med.* 1991;10:339.

15.   Baynes JW. Role of oxidative stress in development of complications of diabetes. *Diabetes.* 1991; 40:405.

16.   Williamson JR, Chang K, Frangos M, Hasan KS, Ido Y, Kawamura T, Nyengaard JR, Van Den Enden M, Kilo C, Tilton RG.   Hyperglycemic pseudohypoxia and diabetic complications. *Diabetes.* 1993;42:801.

17.   Chappey O, Dosquet C, Wautier M-P, Wautier J-L.   Advanced glycation end products, oxidant stress and vascular lesions. *Eur J Clin Invest.* 1997;27:97.

18.   Pieper GM, Gross GJ. "Endothelial Dysfunction in Diabetes" In *Cardiovascular Significance of Endothelium-Derived Vasoactive Factors,* GM Rubanyi, ed. Mount Kisco, NY: Futura Publishing Co., Inc., 1991:223.

19.   Kamata N, Miyata N, Abiru T, Kasuya Y. Functional changes in vascular smooth muscle and endothelium of arteries during diabetes mellitus. *Life Sci.* 1992;50:1379.

20.   Cohen RA.   Dysfunction of vascular endothelium in diabetes mellitus. *Circulation.* 1993;87(suppl. V):V-67.

21.   Poston L, Taylor PD. Endothelium-mediated vascular function in insulin-dependent diabetes mellitus. *Clin Sci.* 1995;88:245.

22.   Sobrevia L, Mann GE. Dysfunction of the endothelilal nitric oxide signalling pathway in diabetes and hyperglycaemia. *Exp Physiol.* 1997;82:423.

23.   Pieper GM.   Review of alterations in endothelial nitric oxide production in diabetes: protective role of arginine on endothelial dysfunction. *Hypertension.* 1998;31:1047.

24.   Langenstroer P, Pieper GM. Regulation of spontaneous EDRF release in diabetic rat aorta by oxygen free radicals. *Am J Physiol.* 1992;263(*Heart Circ Physiol* 32):H257.

25.   Ohishi K, Carmines PK. Superoxide dismutase restores the influence of nitric oxide on renal arterioles in diabetes mellitus. *J Am Soc Nephrol.* 1995;5:1559.

26.   Hattori Y, Kawasakie H, Abe K, Kanno M.   Superoxide dismutase recovers altered endothelium-dependent relaxation in diabetic rat aorta. *Am J Physiol.* 1991;261(*Heart Circ Physiol* 30):H1086.

27.   Pieper GM, Mei DA, Langenstroer P, O'Rourke ST. Bioassay of endothelium-derived relaxing factor in diabetic rat aorta. *Am J Physiol.* 1992:263 (*Heart Circ Physiol* 32):H676.

28.   Tesfamariam B, Cohen RA. Free radicals mediate endothelial cell dysfunction caused by elevated glucose. *Am J Physiol.* 1992;263 (*Heart Circ Physiol* 32):H321.

29.   Diederich D, Skopec J, Diederich A, Dai F-X. Endothelial dysfunction in mesenteric resistance arteries of diabetic rats: role of free radicals. *Am J Physiol.* 1994;266 (*Heart Circ Physiol* 35):H1153.
30.   Mayhan WG. Superoxide dismutase partially restores impaired dilatation of the basilar artery during diabetes mellitus. *Brain Res.* 1997;760:204.
31.   Rösen P, Ballhausen T, Bloch W, Addicks K. Endothelial relaxation is disturbed by oxidative stress in the diabetic rat heart: influence of tocopherol as antioxidant. *Diabetologia.* 1995;38:1157.
32.   Kamata K, Kobayashi T. Changes in superoxide dismutase mRNA expression by streptozotocin-induced diabetes. *Br J Pharmacol.* 1996;119:583.
33.   Pieper GM, Moore-Hilton G, Roza AM. Evaluation of the mechanism of endothelial dysfunction in the genetically-diabetic BB rat. *Life Sci.* 1996;58:147.
34.   Dai F-X, Diederich A, Skopec J, Diederich D. Diabetes-induced endothelial dysfunction in streptozotocin-treated rats: role of prostaglandin endoperoxides and free radicals. *J Am Soc Nephrol.* 1993;4:1327.
35.   Heygate KM, Lawrence IG, Bennett MA, Thurston H. Impaired endothelium-dependent relaxation in isolated resistance arteries of spontaneously diabetic rats. *Br J Pharmacol.* 1995:116:3251.
36.   Matsunaga T, Okumura K, Ishizaka H, Tsunoda R, Tayama S, Tabuchi T, Yasue H. Impairment of coronary blood flow regulation by endothelium-derived nitric oxide in dogs with alloxan-induced diabetes. *J Cardiovasc Pharmacol.* 1996;28:60.
37.   Pieper GM, Langenstroer P, Siebeneich W. Diabetic-induced endothelial dysfunction in rat aorta: role of hydroxyl radicals. *Cardiovasc Res.* 1997;34:145.
38.   Ammar RF Jr, Gutterman DD, Dellsperger KC. Topically applied superoxide dismutase and catalase normalize coronary arteriolar responses to acetylcholine in diabetes mellitus *in vivo.* *Circulation.* 1994;90:I-57 (abstract).
39.   Chang KC, Chung SY, Chong WS, Suh JS, Kim SH, Noh HK, Seong BW, Ko HJ, Chun KW. Possible superoxide radical-induced alteration of vascular reactivity in aortas from streptozotocin-treated rats. *J Pharmacol Exp Thera.* 1993;266:992.
40.   Pieper GM. Oxidative stress in diabetic blood vessels. *FASEB J* 1995;9:A891 (abstract).
41.   Ohkuwa T, Sato Y, Naoi M. Hydroxyl radical formation in diabetic rats induced by streptozotocin. *Life Sci.* 1995;56:1789.
42.   Ghiselli A, Laurenti O, De Mattia G, Maiani G, Ferro-Luzzi A. Salicylate hydroxylation as an early marker of *in vivo* oxidative stress in diabetic patients. *Free Radical Biol Med.* 1992;13:621.
43.   Gryglewski RJ, Palmer RMJ, Moncada S. Superoxide anion is involved in the breakdown of endothelium-derived relaxing factor. *Nature.* 1986;320:454.
44.   Nitenberg A, Paycha F, Ledoux S, Sachs R, Attali J-R, Valensi P. Coronary artery responses to physiological stimuli are improved by deferoxamine but not by L-arginine in non-insulin-dependent diabetic patients with angiographically normal coronary arteries and no other risk factors. *Circulation.* 1998;97:736.
45.   Mooradian AD. The antioxidant potential of cerebral microvessels in experimental diabetes mellitus. *Brain Res.* 1995;671:164.
46.   Crouch R, Kimsey G, Priest DG, Sarda A, Buse MG. Effect of streptozotocin on erythrocyte and retinal superoxide dismutase. *Diabetologia.* 1978;15:53.
47.   Pieper GM, Jordan M, Dondlinger LA, Adams MB, Roza AM. Peroxidative stress in diabetic blood vessels: reversal by pancreatic islet transplantation. *Diabetes.* 1995;44:884.
48.   Armstrong D, Al-Awadi F. Lipid peroxidation and retinopathy in streptozotocin-induced diabetes. *Free Radical Biol Med.* 1991;11:433.
49.   Low PA, Nickander KK. Oxygen free radical effects in sciatic nerve in experimental diabetes. *Diabetes.* 1991;40:873.
50.   Tatsuki R, Satoh K, Yamamoto A, Hoshi K, Ichihara K. Lipid peroxidation in the pancreas and other organs in streptozotocin diabetic rats. *Jap J Pharmacol.* 1997;75:267.
51.   Tagami S, Kondo T, Yoshida K, Hirokawa J, Ohtsuka Y, Kawakami Y. Effect of insulin on impaired antioxidant activities in aortic endothelial cells from diabetic rabbits. *Metabolism.* 1992;41:1053.
52.   Bucala R, Tracey KJ, Cerami A. Advanced glycosylation products quench nitric oxide and mediate defective endothelium-dependent vasodilatation in experimental diabetes. *J Clin Invest.* 1991;87:432.

53.   Rodríguez-Mañas L, Arribas S, Girón C, Villamor J, Sánchez-Ferrer CF, Marín J. Interference of glycosylated human hemoglobin with endothelium-dependent responses. *Circulation.* 1993;88[part 1]:2111.

54.   Angulo J, Sánchez-Ferrer CF, Peiró C, Marín J, Rodríguez-Mañas L. Impairment of endothelium-dependent relaxation by increasing percentages of glycosylated human hemoglobin: possible mechanisms involved. *Hypertension.* 1996;28:583.

55.   Oltman CL, Gutterman DD, Scott EC, Bocker JM, Dellsperger KC. Effects of glycosylated hemoglobin on vascular responses *in vitro*. *Cardiovasc Res.* 1997;34:179.

56.   Ellis EA, Grant MB, Murray FT, Wachowski MB, Guberski DL, Kubilis PS, Lutty GA. Increased NADH oxidase activity in the retina of the BBZ/Wor diabetic rat. *Free Radical Biol Med.* 1998;24:111.

57.   Mohazzab-H KM, Kaminski PM, Wolin MS. NADH oxidoreductase is a major source of superoxide anion in bovine coronary artery endothelium. *Am J Physiol.* 1994;266 (*Heart Circ Physiol* 35):H2568.

58.   Jones SA, O'Donnell VB, Wood JD, Broughton JP, Hughes EJ, Jones OTG. Expression of phagocyte NADPH oxidase components in human endothelial cells. *Am J Physiol.* 1996;271 (*Heart Circ Physiol* 40):H1626.

59.   Ushio-Fukai M, Zafari AM, Fukui T, Ishizaka N, Griendling KK. P22^{phox} is a critical component of the superoxide-generating NADH/NADPH oxidase system and regulates angiotensin II-induced hypertrophy in vascular smooth muscle cells. *J Biol Chemi.* 1996;271:23317.

60.   Pagano PJ, Clark JK, Cifuentes-Pagano ME, Clark SM, Callis GM, Quinn MT. Localization of a constitutively active, phagocyte-like NADPH oxidase in rabbit aortic adventitia: enhancement by angiotensin II. *Proc Natl Acad Sci USA.* 1997;94:14483.

61.   Quian M, Brunk UT, Pieper GM, Eaton JW. Diabetic peripheral neuropathy: a possible involvement of iron bound to glycated basement membrane proteins. *Ped Res.* 1998;43:83A (abstract).

62.   Heinzel B, John M, Klatt P, Böhme E, Mayer B. Ca^{2+}/calmodulin-dependent formation of hydrogen peroxide by brain nitric oxide synthase. *Biochem J.* 1992;281:627.

63.   Rösen P, Ballhausen T, Stockklauser K. Impairment of endothelium dependent relaxation in the diabetic rat heart: mechanisms and implications. *Diabetes Res Clin Pract.* 1996;31(suppl.):S143.

64.   Pieper GM, Dondlinger LA. Plasma and vascular tissue arginine are decreased in diabetes: acute arginine supplementation restores endothelium-dependent relaxation by augmenting cGMP production. *J Pharmacol Exp Thera.* 1997;283:684.

65.   Hamon CG, Cutler P, Blair JA. Tetrahydrobiopterin metabolism in the streptozotocin induced diabetic state in rats. *Clin Chim Acta.* 1989;181:249.

66.   Öztürk Y, Aydin S, Altan VM, Yildizoglu-Ari N, Özçelikay AT. Effect of short and long term streptozotocin diabetes on smooth muscle calmodulin levels in the rat. *Cell Calcium.* 1994;16:81.

67.   Pieper GM. Acute amelioration of diabetic endothelial dysfunction with a derivative of the nitric oxide synthase cofactor, tetrahydrobiopterin. *J Cardiovasc Pharmacol.* 1997;29:8.

68.   Pieper GM, Peltier BA. Amelioration by L-arginine of a dysfunctional arginine/nitric oxide pathway in diabetic endothelium. *J Cardiovasc Pharmacol.* 1995;25:397.

69.   Pieper GM, Jordan M, Adams MB, Roza AM. Syngeneic pancreatic islet transplantation reverses endothelial dysfunction in experimental diabetes. *Diabetes.* 1995;44:1106.

70.   Pieper GM, Siebeneich W, Moore-Hilton G, Roza AM. Reversal by L-arginine of a dysfunctional arginine/nitric oxide pathway in the endothelium of the genetic diabetic BB rat. *Diabetologia.* 1997;40:910.

71.   Pieper GM, Siebeneich W, Dondlinger LA. Short-term oral administration of L-arginine reverses defective endothelium-dependent relaxation and cGMP generation in diabetes. *Eur J Pharmacol.* 1996;317:317.

72.   Böger RH, Bode-Böger SM, Brandes RP, Phivthong-ngam L, Böhme M, Nafe R, Mügge A, Frölich JC. Dietary L-arginine redues the progression of atherosclerosis in cholesterol-fed rabbits: comparison with lovastatin. *Circulation.* 1997;96:1282.

73.   Taylor PD, Poston L. The effect of hyperglycaemia on function of rat isolated mesenteric resistance artery. *Br J Pharmacol.* 1994;113:801.

74.   Félétou M, Rasetti C, Duhault J. Magnesium modulates endothelial dysfunction produced by elevated glucose incubation. *J Cardiovasc Pharmacol.* 1994;24:470.

75. Dorigo P, Fraccarollo D, Santostasi G, Maragno I. Impairment of endothelium-dependent but not endothelium-independent dilatation in guinea pig aorta rings incubated in the presence of elevated glucose. *Br J Pharmacol.* 1997;121:972.

76. Bohlen HG, Lash JM. Topical hyperglycemia rapidly suppresses EDRF-mediated vasodilation of normal rat arterioles. *Am J Physiol.* 1993;265*(Heart Circ Physiol* 34):H219.

77. Mayhan WG, Patel KP. Acute effects of glucose on reactivity of cerebral microcirculation: role of activation of protein kinase C. *Am J Physiol.* 1995;269(*Heart Circ Physiol* 38):H1297.

78. Houben AJHM, Schaper NC, DeHaan HA, Huvers FC, Slaaf DW, DeLeeuw PW, Nieuwenhuijzen-Kruseman AC. Local 24-h hyperglycemia does not affect endothelium-dependent or –independent vasoreactivity in humans. *Am J Physiol.* 1996;270 (*Heart Circ Physiol* 39):H2014.

79. Akbari C, Saouaf R, Barnhill D, Newman P, Logerfo F. Endothelium-dependent vasodilatation is impaired during acute hyperglycemia. *Diabetes.* 1997;46 (supp. 1):114A (abstract).

80. Lee T-S, Saltsman KA, Ohashi H, King GL. Activation of protein kinase C by elevation of glucose concentration: proposal for a mechanism in the development of diabetic vascular complications. *Proc Natl Acad Sci USA.* 1989;86:5141.

81. Weisbrod RM, Brown ML, Cohen RA. Effect of elevated glucose on cyclic GMP and eicosanoids produced by porcine aortic endothelium. *Arterterioscler Thromb.* 1993;13:915.

82. Pieper GM, Dondlinger L. Glucose elevations alter bradykinin-stimulated intracellular calcium accumulation in cultured endothelial cells. *Cardiovasc Res.* 1997;34:169.

83. Magill SB, Danaberg J. "Effects of hyperglycemia on vascular endothelium nitric oxide metabolism" In *Contemporary Endocrinology: Endocrinology of the Vasculature,* JR Sowers, ed,. Totowa, NJ: Humana Press Inc.; 1996:145.

84. Salameh A, Dhein S. Influence of chronic exposure to high concentrations of D-glucose and long-term ®-blocker treatment on intracellular calcium concentrations of porcine aortic endothelial cells. *Diabetes.* 1998,47:407.

85. Pieper GM, Dondlinger LA. The antioxidant, pyrrolidine dithiocarbamate, prevents defective bradykinin-stimulated calcium accumulation and nitric oxide activity following exposure of endothelial cells to elevated glucose concentration. *Diabetologia.* 1998;41:806.

86. Kimura C, Oike M, Kashiwagi S, Ito Y. Effects of glucose overload on histamine H_2 receptor-mediated Ca^{2+} mobilization in bovine cerebral endothelial cells. *Diabetes.* 1998;47:104.

87 Mazière C, Auclari M, Rose-Robert F, Leflon P, Mezière JC. Glucose-enriched medium enhances cell-mediated low density lipoprotein peroxidation. *Febs Lett.* 1995;363:277.

88. Graier WF, Simecck S, Hoebel BG, Wascher TC, Dittrich P, Kostner GM. Antioxidants prevent high D-glucose-enhanced endothelial Ca^{2+}/cGMP response by scavenging superoxide anions. *Eur J Pharmacol.* 1997;322:113.

89 Cosentino F, Hishikawa K, Katusic ZS, Lüscher TF. High glucose increases nitric oxide synthase expression and superoxide anion generation in human aortic endothelial cells. *Circulation.* 1997;96:25.

90. Pellligrino DA, Koenig HM, Wang Q, Albrecht RF. Protein kinase C suppresses receptor-mediated pial arteriolar relaxation in the diabetic rat. *NeuroReport.* 1994;5:417.

91. Ohara Y, Peterson TE, Zheng B, Kuo JF, Harrison DG. Lysophosphatidylcholine increases vascular superoxide anion production via protein kinase C activation. *Arterioscler Thromb.* 1994;14:1007.

92. Ting HH, Timimi FK, Boles KS, Creager SJ, Ganz P, Creager MA. Vitamin C improves endothelium-dependent vasodilation in patients with non-insulin-dependent diabetes mellitus. *J Clin Invest.* 1996;97:22.

93. Timimi FK, Ting HH, Haley EA, Roddy M-A, Ganz P, Creager MA. Vitamin C improves endothelium-dependent vasodilation in patients with insulin-dependent diabetes mellitus. *J Am Coll Cardiol.* 1998;31:552.

94. Keegan A, Walbank H, Cotter MA, Cameron NE. Chronic vitamin E treatment prevents defective endothelium-dependent relaxation in diabetic rat aorta. *Diabetologia.* 1995;38:1475.

95. Karasu Ç, Ozansoy G, Bozkurt O, Erdogan D, Ömeroglu S. Isoprenaline-induced endothelium-dependent and –independent relaxations of aorta in long-term STZ-diabetic rats: reversal effect of dietary vitamin E. *Gen Pharmacol.* 1997;29:561.

96. Archibald V, Cotter MA, Keegan A, Cameron NE. Contraction and relaxation of aortas from diabetic rats: effects of chronic anti-oxidant and aminoguanidine treatments. *Naunyn-Schmiedeberg's Arch Pharmacol.* 1996;353:584.

Diabetic Vascular Dysfunction

97.   Pieper GM, Siebeneich W. Oral administration of the antioxidant, N-acetylcysteine, abrogates diabetes-induced endothelial dysfunction. *J Cardiovasc Pharmacol.* 1998; 41:101.

98.   Pieper GM, Siebeneich W, Roza AM, Jordan M, Adams MB. Chronic treatment *in vivo* with dimethylthiourea, a hydroxyl radical scavenger, prevents diabetes-induced endothelial dysfunction. *J Cardiovasc Pharmacol.* 1996;28:741.

99.   Mayhan WG, Patel KK. Treatment with dimethylthiourea prevents impaired dilatation of the basilar artery during diabetes mellitus. *Am J Physiol.* 1998;274(*Heart Circ Physiol.* 43):H1895.

100.   Pieper GM, Siebeneich W. Diabetes-induce endothelial dysfunction is prevented by long-term treatment with the modified iron chelator, hydroxyethyl starch conjugated-deferoxamine. *J Cardiovasc Pharmacol.* 1997;30:734.

101.   Karasu Ç, Ozansoy G, Bozhurt D, Ömeroglu S. Antioxidant and triglyceride-lowering effect of vitamin E associated with the prevention of abnormalities in the reactivity and morphology of aorta from streptozotocin-diabetic rats. *Metabolism.* 1997;46:872.

102.   Palmer AM, Gopaul N, Dhir S, Thomas CR, Poston L, Tribe RM. Endothelial dysfunction in streptozotocin-diabetic rats is not reversed by dietary probucol or simvastatin supplementation. *Diabetologia.* 1998;41:157.

103.   Palmer AM, Thomas CR, Gopaul N, Dhir S, Änggård EE, Poston L, Tribe RM. Dietary antioxidant supplementation reduces lipid peroxidation but impairs vascular function in small mesenteric arteries of the streptozotocin-diabetic rat. *Diabetologia.* 1998;41:148.

104.   Bertuglia S, Malandrino S, Colantuoni A. Effects of the natural flavonoid delphinidin on diabetic microangiopathy. *Arzn-Forschung/Drug Res.* 1995;45:481.

105.   Cameron NE, Cotter MA, Archibald V, Dines KC, Maxfield EK. Anti-oxidant and pro-oxidant effects on nerve conduction velocity, endoneurial blood flow and oxygen tension in non-diabetic and streptozotocin-diabetic rats. *Diabetologia.* 1994;37:449.

106.   Cameron NE, Cotter MA. Reversal of peripheral nerve conduction and perfusion deficits by the free radical scavenger, BM15.0639, in diabetic rats. *Naunyn-Schmiedeberg's Arch Pharmacol.* 1995;352:685.

107.   Cotter MA, Love A, Watt MJ, Cameron NE, Dines KC. Effects of natural free radical scavengers on peripheral nerve and neurovascular function in diabetic rats. *Diabetologia.* 1995;38:1285.

108.   Cameron NE, Cotter MA. Neurovascular dysfunction in diabetic rats. Potential contribution of autoxidation and free radicals examined using transition metal chelating agents. *J Clin Invest.* 1995;96:1159.

109.   Pieper GM, Jordan M, Roza AM. Chronic treatment with the 21-aminosteroid U74389F an inhibitor of lipid peroxidation, does not prevent diabetic endothelial dysfunction. *Cardiovasc Drugs Therapy.* 1997;11:435.

110.   Tilton RG, Chang K, Hasan KS, Smith SR, Petrash JM, Misko TP, Moore WM, Currie WG, Corbett JA, McDaniel ML, Williamson JR. Prevention of diabetic vascular dyfsunction by guanidines. Inhibition of nitric oxide synthase versus advanced glycation end-product formation. *Diabetes.* 1993;42:221.

111.   Kumari K, Umar S, Bansal V, Sahib MK. Inhibition of diabetes-associated complications by nucleophilic compounds. *Diabetes.* 1991;1079.

112.   Brownlee M, Vlassara H, Kooney A, Ulrich P, Cerami A. Aminoguanidine prevents diabetes-induced arterial wall protein cross-linking. *Science.* 1986;232:1629.

113.   Picard S, Parthasrathy S, Fruebis J, Witztum JL. Aminoguanidine inhibits oxidative modification of low density lipoprotein protein and the subsequent increase in uptake by the macrophage scavenger receptor. *Proc Natl Acad Sci USA.* 1992;89:6876.

114.   Philis-Tsimikas A, Parthasarathy S, Picard S, Palinski W, Witztum J. Aminoguanidine has both pro-oxidant and antioxidant activity toward LDL. *Arterioscler Thromb Vasc Biol.* 1994;15:367.

115.   Cameron NE, Cotter MA. Impaired contraction and relaxation in aorta from streptozotocin-diabetic rats: role of polyol pathway. *Diabetelogia.* 1992;35:1011.

116.   Tesfamariam B, Palacino JJ, Weisbrod RM, Cohen RA. Aldose reductase inhibition restores endothelial cell function in diabetic rabbit aorta. *J Cardiovasc Pharmacol.* 1993;21:205.

117.   Otter DJ, Chess-Williams R. The effects of aldose reductase inhibition with ponalrestat on changes in vascular function in streptozotocin diabetic rats. *Br J Pharmacol.* 1994;113:576.

118.   Jian ZY, Zhou Q-L, Eaton JW, Koppenol WH, Hunt JV, Wolff SP. Spirohydantoin inhibitors of aldose reductase inhibit iron- and copper-catalyzed ascorbate oxidation *in vitro*. *Biochem Pharmacol.* 1991;42:1273.

119. Hunt JV, Dean RT, Wolff SP. Hydroxyl radical production and autoxidative glycosylation. Glucose autoxidation as the cause of protein damage in the experimental glycation model of diabetes mellitus and ageing. *Biochem J.* 1988;256:205.
120. Ceriello A, Giugliano D, Quatraro A, Donzella C, Cipalo G, Lefebvre PJ. Vitamin E reduction of protein glycosylation in diabetes. New prospect for prevention of diabetic complications. *Diabetes Care.* 1991;14:68.
121. Davies SJ, Gould BJ, Yudkin JS. Effect of vitamin C on glycosylation of proteins. *Diabetes.* 1992;41:167.
122. Shoff SM, Mares-Perlman JA, Cruickshanks KJ, Klein R, Klein BEK, Ritter LL. Glycosylated hemoglobin concentrations and vitamin E, vitamin C, and ®-carotene intake in diabetic and nondiabetic older aldults. *Am J Clin Nutr.* 1993;58:412.
123. Soulis T, Cooper ME, Sastra S, Thallas V, Panagiotopoulos S, Bjerrum OJ, Jerums G. Relative contributions of advanced glycation and nitric oxide synthase inhibition to aminoguanidine-mediated renoprotection in diabetic rats. *Diabetologia.* 1997;40:1141.
124. Richardson M, Hadcock SJ, DeReske M, Cybulsky MI. Increase expression *in vivo* of VCAM-1 and E-selectin by the aortic endothelium of normolipemic and hyperlipemic diabetic rabbits. *Arterioscler Thromb.* 1994;14:760.
125. McLeod DS, Lefer DJ, Merges C, Lutty GA. Enhanced expression of intracellular adhesion molecule-1 and P-selectin in the diabetic human retina and choroid. *Am J Pathol.* 1995;147:642.
126. Schmidt AM, Crandall J, Hori O, Cao R, Lakatta E. Elevated plasma levels of vascular cell adhesion molecule-1 (VCAM-1) in diabetic patients with microalbuminuria: a marker of vascular dysfunction and progressive vascular disease. *Br J Haematol.* 1996;92:747.
127. Fasching P, Veitl M, Rohac M, Streli C, Schneider B, Waldhäusl W, Wagner OF. Elevated concentrations of circulating adhesion molecules and their association with microvascular complications in insulin-dependent diabetes mellitus. *J Clin Invest.* 1996;81:4313.
128. Jude EB, Abbott CA, Young MJ, Anderson SG, Douglas JT, Boulton AJM. The potential role of cell adhesion molecules in the pathogenesis of diabetic neuropathy. *Diabetologia.* 1998;41:330.
129. Baumgartner-Parzer SM, Wagner L, Pettermann M, Gessl A, Waldhäsl W. Modulation by high glucose of adhesion molecule expression in cultured endothelial cells. *Diabetologia.* 1995;38:1367.
130. Taki H, Kashiwagi A, Tanaka Y, Horiike K. Expression of intercellular adhesion molecules (ICAM-1) via an osmotic effect in human umbilical vein endothelial cells exposed to high glucose medium. *Life Sci.* 1996;58:1713.
131. Kim JA, Berliner JA, Natarajan RD, Nadler JL. Evidence that glucose increases monocyte binding to human aortic endothelial cells. *Diabetes.* 1994;43:1103.
132. Weber C, Erl W, Pietsch A, Sröbel M, Ziegler-Heitbrock HWL, Weber PC. Antioxidants inhibit monocyte adhesion by suppressing nuclear factor-κB moblilization and induction of vascular cell adhesion molecule-1 in endothelial cells stimulated to generate radicals. *Arterioscler Thromb.* 1994;14:1665.
133. Weber C, Erl W, Pietsch A, Weber PC. Aspirin inhibits nuclear factor--κB mobilization and monocyte adhesion in stimulated human endothelial cells. *Circulation.* 1995;91:1914.
134. Ferrans C, Millan MT, Csizmadia V, Cooper JT, Brostjan C, Bach FH, Winkler H. Inhibition of NF-κB by pyrrolidine dithiocarbamate blocks endothelial cell activation. *Biochem Biophys Res Comm.* 1995;214:212.
135. Mauri N, Offerman Mk, Swerlick R, Kunsch C, Rosen CA, Ahmad M, Alexander RW, Medford RM. Vascular cell adhesion molecule-1 (VCAM-1) gene transcription and expression are regulated through an antioxidant-sensitive mechanism in vascular endothelial cells. *J Clin Invest.* 1993;92:1866.
136. Gerritsen ME, Carley WW, Ranges GE, Shen C-P, Phan SA, Ligon CF, Perry CA. Flavonoids inhibit cytokine-induced endothelial cell adhesion protein gene expression. *Am J Pathol.* 1995;147:278.
137. Pieper GM, ul-Haq R. Activation of nuclear factor-κB in cultured endothelial cells by increased glucose concentration: prevention by calphostin C. *J Cardiovasc Pharmacol.* 1997;30:528.
138. Schmidt AM, Hori O, Chen JX, Li JF, Crandall J, Zhang J, Cao R, Yan SD, Brett J, Stern D. Advanced glycation endproducts interacting with their endothelial receptor induce expression of vascular cell adhesion molecule-1 (VCAM-1) in cultured human endothelial cells and in mice.

A potential mechanism for the accelerated vasculopathy of diabetes. *J Clin Invest.* 1995;96:1395.

139.   Bierhaus A, Chevion S, Chevion M, Hofmann M, Quehenberger P, Illmer T, Luther T, Berentshtein E, Tritscher H, Müller M, Wahl P, Ziegler R, Nawroth PP. Advanced glycation end produt-induced activation of NF-κB is suppressed by 〈-lipoic acid in cultured endothelial cells. *Diabetes.* 1997;46:1481.

140.   Mazière C, Auclair M, Djavaheri-Mergny M, Packer L, Mazière J-C. Oxidized low density lipoprotein induces activation of the transcription factor NF-κB in fibroblasts, endothelial and smooth muscle cells. *Biochem Mol Biol Int.* 1996;39:1201.

17 THE ROLE OF OXIDATIVE STRESS IN HYPERTENSION

Mark J. Somers, Kathy K. Griendling, and
David G. Harrison

INTRODUCTION

In the past decade, substantial attention has been directed toward understanding how reactive oxygen species contribute to the pathophysiology of vascular disease. Increasing evidence suggests that increases in vascular production of oxygen-derived radicals represent a common pathway whereby many pathological conditions can promote vascular disease and lesion formation. In particular, it has become clear that reactive oxygen species play a critical role in the pathology of hypertension. Likewise, many of the neurohumoral alterations that accompany hypertension accelerate vascular production of reactive oxygen species. In this review, we will discuss this evidence and examine the potential consequences of "oxidative stress" as it pertains to hypertension and its vascular consequences.

OXIDATIVE STRESS – THE BALANCE BETWEEN REACTIVE OXYGEN SPECIES AND ANTIOXIDANT DEFENSES

In the process of normal cellular metabolism, oxygen undergoes a series of reductions leading sequentially to the production of superoxide anion ($O_2^{\cdot-}$), hydrogen peroxide (H_2O_2) and subsequently H_2O. Superoxide and hydrogen peroxide can participate in a variety of subsequent redox reactions and may serve as precursors to other reactive oxygen species, including hydroxyl anion, peroxynitrite anion, lipid radicals, hypochlorous acid, and others. Not all of these are oxygen radicals, in that they lack an unpaired electron in their outer atomic orbital, and thus they are collectively referred to as reactive oxygen species. Under normal physiological conditions, mammalian cells tightly regulate the ambient levels of such reactive oxygen species, limiting their toxic potential. This is accomplished by not only keeping their production in check, but also by using a variety of antioxidant defense mechanisms. As discussed in Chapter 3, these include small molecule antioxidants (thiol groups, uric acid, nitric oxide, and antioxidant vitamins) and antioxidant enzymes (superoxide dismutases, catalase and glutathione peroxidase) (1). It has become clear that under certain conditions, the balance between the production of reactive oxygen species and their inactivation is altered, leading to a condition generally referred to as "oxidative stress" (Chapter 1).

PRODUCTION OF REACTIVE OXYGEN SPECIES IN VASCULAR CELLS

Traditionally, production of reactive oxygen species was considered a unique property of phagocytic cells such as neutrophils and macrophages. In these cells, production of reactive oxygen species plays critical immune and inflammatory roles. In the last several years, considerable evidence has been accumulated to suggest that numerous mammalian cells produce reactive oxygen species, albeit in lower steady state levels. In these cells, reactive oxygen species have important functions in both physiological and pathophysiological states.

In the blood vessel, there is evidence that endothelial, vascular smooth muscle, and adventitial cells produce reactive oxygen species (2-6). While there are numerous potential sources of radical formation in these cells, the predominant enzymatic sources seem to be enzyme systems recently identified as NADH/NADPH-driven, membrane bound oxidases (4,7,8). The molecular structure of these enzymes may differ among endothelial, vascular smooth muscle, and adventitial cells; however, they seem to share several similarities. Functionally, several characteristics of the neutrophil NADPH oxidase are shared by the vascular smooth muscle cell enzyme system. Both can be stimulated by phosphatidic and arachidonic acid, both are associated with the membrane, and both are sensitive to the flavin-containing enzyme inhibitor diphenylene iodonium (8). However, the vascular smooth muscle cell oxidase differs from that of the neutrophil oxidase in at least two respects. The time course of stimulation of the oxidase differs dramatically in the two cell types. Superoxide generation by the neutrophil NADPH oxidase is massive and occurs in bursts when the neutrophils are activated (9). In contrast, superoxide production by the vascular oxidase is about one-tenth the amount of phagocytes and is constant in output (4,8). Secondly, the vascular smooth muscle cell enzyme appears to utilize NADH in preference to NADPH, which is exactly the opposite of the situation in neutrophils.

On a molecular level, the vascular oxidase may share only limited homology to the neutrophil enzyme. At least one neutrophil component, the large subunit of the membrane cytochrome b558, gp91phox, seems to be absent in smooth muscle cells (10). One component, p22phox, has been cloned in vascular smooth muscle cells and is relatively abundant at the mRNA level (11). Functionally, it appears that p22phox is critical for function of the oxidase, since antisense inhibition of p22phox expression in VSMC decreases superoxide and hydrogen peroxide production by these cells, as discussed in the following sections (10).

Recent evidence suggests that the NADH/NADPH oxidase in endothelial cells may have more molecular similarity to the neutrophil oxidase than does the vascular smooth muscle cell. Using RT-PCR, gp91phox, p22phox, p67phox, and p47phox have been identified in cultured human endothelial cells that have NADH/NADPH oxidase activity (12). Despite the presence of mRNA for gp91phox and p22phox, spectrophotometric evidence of cytochrome b558 could not be demonstrated, suggesting that these proteins may not be expressed or do not function in a manner similar to the neutrophil cytochrome.

Regulation of Oxidase Activity in Vascular Cells

A particularly important aspect of the vascular NADH/NADPH oxidase systems is that physical forces, angiotensin II and certain cytokines regulate their activity. Two important physical forces exerted on vascular cells are forces parallel to flow (shear) and pressure perpendicular to flow (strain). These two forces exert very different effects on production of reactive oxygen species. For example, Howard *et al.* showed that cyclic strain caused an early (2 hour) transient increase in NADH/NADPH oxidase activity and a sustained increase in H_2O_2 in cultured porcine aortic endothelial cells (13). It has also been shown that pulsatile stretch causes NADH/NADPH oxidase-dependent increases in superoxide production in human coronary smooth muscle cells which is inhibitable by the NADH/NADPH oxidase inhibitor diphenylene iodonium (14). Shear stress also alters the oxidative state of vascular cells (Figure 1). Shear increases expression of both the endothelial cell NO synthase and the endothelial Cu/Zn SOD, both of which impact on superoxide levels in the endothelium (15,16). In contrast to this antioxidant effect of laminar shear, De Keulanaer *et al.* have also shown oscillatory shear causes a

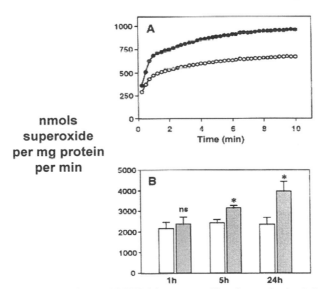

nmols superoxide per mg protein per min

Figure 1. Effect of oscillatory shear on NADH-driven superoxide anion production in human umbilical vein endothelial cells. Upper Panel: Human umbilical vein endothelial cells were exposed for 5 hours to static conditions (O) or oscillatory shear (●, ±5 dyne/cm2, 1 Hz), then washed, homogenized, and assayed for NADH (100 μmol/L)–driven O_2^{-} production using lucigenin chemiluminescence. B, Human umbilical vein endothelial cells were exposed for 1, 5, or 24 hours to static conditions (open bars) or oscillatory shear (±5 dyne/cm2, 1 Hz, shaded bars), then washed and homogenized. NADH (100 μmol/L)–driven O_2^{-} production was then examined using lucigenin chemiluminescence. Values are mean ± SEM of O_2^{-} (*P<0.05). From reference 15, with permission from the American Heart Association.

sustained significant increase in NADH oxidase activity in cultured human endothelial cells (17). The effect of laminar shear on NADH oxidase activity was a transient upregulation (Figure 1). Together, these findings suggest that while laminar flow predisposes to an antioxidant state, oscillatory flow and strain create a significant increase in oxidative stress.

In addition to physical forces, humoral factors play a role in mediating the oxidative environment. In vascular smooth muscle cells, the inflammatory cytokine TNF-α caused a concentration-dependent increase in p22phox mRNA and NADH oxidase activity which was inhibited by transfection with antisense to p22phox (18). Likewise, treatment of cultured vascular smooth muscle cells with nanomolar levels of angiotensin II markedly increases NADH and NADPH oxidase activity (Figure 2), resulting in an increased production of both superoxide and hydrogen peroxide.

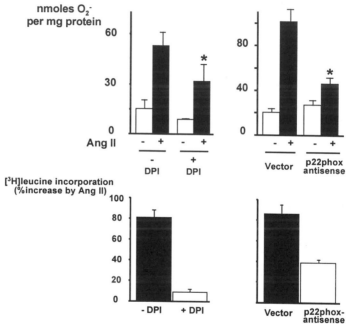

Figure 2: **Upper panels:** Effect of angiotensin II on rat aortic vascular smooth muscle cell superoxide production. Cells either were not treated (open bars) or treated with angiotensin II (filled bars) for 4 hours. In some cases, cells were treated with diphenylene iodonium (DPI), which inhibits flavin-containing enzymes. In other experiments, cells were stably transfected with either vector alone or a vector containing the full-length antisense against p22phox. Assays of NADH oxidase activity were performed on homogenates of cells using lucigenin-enhanced chemiluminescence following addition of 100 μM NADH. Angiotensin II markedly increased NADH oxidase activity, and this was inhibited both by DPI and in cells stably transfected with the p22phox antisense. **Lower Panels:** Effect of angiotensin II on leucine incorporation as a marker of cell hypertrophy. Cells were treated as described above and exposed to ^{3}H-labeled leucine. Leucine incorporation was markedly enhanced by angiotensin II. Cells were also exposed to DPI or transfected with vector alone or vector containing p22phox antisense as described above. Angiotensin II markedly stimulated leucine incorporation; this was prevented by both DPI and the antisense against p22phox. From reference 12, with permission from the American Chemical Society.

This increase in production of reactive oxygen species seems essential for the hypertrophy of vascular smooth muscles induced by angiotensin II. Cells in which the NADH oxidase expression has been diminished by stable transfection of the full-length p22phox antisense or in which NADH oxidase activity is inhibited with diphenylene iodonium exhibit markedly diminished growth in response to angiotensin II (8, 10). These findings emphasize the importance of p22phox as a component of this oxidase system.

Nitric Oxide/Superoxide Interactions

Because superoxide and nitric oxide are both radicals and contain an unpaired electron in their outer orbital, they undergo an extremely rapid, diffusion-limited radical/radical reaction, occurring at a rate of 1.9×10^{10} $M^{-1} \cdot sec^{-1}$ (19). This reaction rate is ten times faster than the rate of reaction between superoxide and the superoxide dismutases and >10,000 times faster than reactions between superoxide and the common antioxidant enzymes such as vitamin A, E, and C. Importantly, this reaction with superoxide markedly alters the biological activity of nitric oxide. A major product of this reaction is the peroxynitrite anion ($ONOO^-$). Peroxynitrite is a weak vasodilator compared to nitric oxide and thus this reaction markedly impairs the vasodilatory capacity of nitric oxide. Likewise, many of the favorable biological actions of nitric oxide, such as inhibition of platelet aggregation and smooth muscle growth and inhibition of VCAM-1 expression are not shared by peroxynitrite. Peroxynitrite is a strong oxidant and is has been implicated t in numerous pathophysiological processes including lipid peroxidation and membrane damage.

Because of this radical-radical chemistry, it appears that superoxide plays a critical role in modulating ambient levels of nitric oxide. Normally, the balance between nitric oxide and superoxide favors the net production of nitric oxide, and permits a state of basal vasodilation and maintenance of normal blood pressure. Of note, this balance is altered in several pathological states, including atherosclerosis (20), diabetes (21), heart failure and cigarette smoking (22). In hypercholesterolemia, vessels produce excess quantities of superoxide, leading to destruction of nitric oxide, and impaired endothelium-dependent vascular relaxation (20). In hypercholesterolemia, treatment of vessels or animals with membrane-targeted forms of SOD markedly improves endothelium-dependent vascular relaxations (23). Likewise, infusions of antioxidant vitamins improve endothelium-dependent vasodilation of forearm vessels in human subjects with diabetes (21) and cigarette smokers (22).

HYPERTENSION, ANGIOTENSIN, AND SUPEROXIDE

As discussed in the paragraph above, increased vascular oxidant stress seems to be a common phenomenon in numerous conditions known to be "risk factors" for atherosclerosis. In each of these conditions, elevated superoxide levels seem to reduce the biological activity of nitric oxide. One of the most common and important of these is hypertension.

The first suggestion that superoxide might contribute to hypertension came from work by Nakazono and his co-workers (24). These investigators showed that a form of superoxide dismutase, modified to bind to heparan sulfates in the vessel extracellular matrix, would acutely lower blood pressure in spontaneously hypertensive rats (SHR) while having no effect on blood pressure in normal rats.

As discussed above, angiotensin II potently modulates activity of the NADH/NADPH oxidase in cultured vascular smooth muscle cells. Recently, these findings have been extended to an *in vivo* model of angiotensin II-induced hypertension (4, 25). Osmotic mini-pumps were used to infuse angiotensin II subcutaneously (0.7mg/kg/day) into Sprague-Dawley rats. To study hypertension independent of angiotensin, rats were treated with a subcutaneous infusion of norepinephrine for a similar period of time. At the end of five days the animals were sacrificed and their aortas removed for studies of superoxide production using lucigenin-enhanced chemiluminescence. Angiotensin II infusion significantly increased superoxide production in the vessel wall. In experiments in which the endothelium was intentionally removed, the increase in superoxide production between vessels from angiotensin II-treated and sham-operated animals persisted, suggesting that the source of the increase in superoxide was likely the vascular smooth muscle. Subsequent studies indicated the oxidase involved in the increase in superoxide production was indeed the membrane-associated NADH-oxidase.

Interestingly, in these experiments infusion of angiotensin II (0.7 mg/kg/day) did not produce hypertension until the third day. In subsequent studies, it became clear that the time course of induction of vascular NADH oxidase activity and the onset of hypertension were similar, both beginning about day 3 following onset of exposure to angiotensin II. Of note, aortas from angiotensin II-treated rats demonstrated markedly increased expression of p22phox mRNA, beginning approximately 3 days following onset of angiotensin II infusion. Thus, the time course of p22phox expression, oxidase activity, and the onset of hypertension roughly parallel one another during chronic angiotensin II infusion, suggesting that they are closely related (Figure 3).

The increase in vascular smooth muscle production of superoxide caused by angiotensin II treatment was associated with a marked impairment in endothelium-dependent vascular relaxation (4) (Figure 4, left panel). This was not observed in vessels from rats treated with norepinephrine. In vessels not exposed to increased levels of oxygen free radicals, the balance between nitric oxide and superoxide favors the net production of nitric oxide, permitting a state of basal vasodilation and maintenance of normal blood pressure. An increase in superoxide in the resistance circulation might contribute to the hypertension caused by angiotensin II infusion through scavenging of nitric oxide by superoxide. To address this possibility, endogenous steady state levels of vascular superoxide were lowered by treatment of rats with daily injections of liposome-entrapped SOD (26). This treatment had no effect on blood pressure in either control or norepinephrine-infused rats, but lowered blood pressure by 60 mg Hg in rats with angiotensin II-induced hypertension. (Figure 4, right panel).

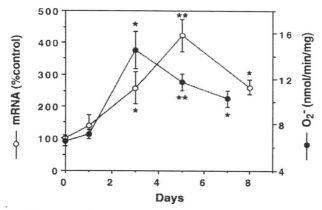

Figure 3. p22phox mRNA expression and NADPH oxidase activity in aortas after Ang II infusion. Rats were infused with Ang II for the indicated times and were killed, their aortas were removed for measurement of p22phox mRNA (left ordinate) or NADPH oxidase activity (right ordinate). Each point represents the mean +/- SE of 3 to10 determinations. *P<.05 vs. sham-operated rats, **P<.01 vs. sham-operated rats. Angiotensin II infusion causes a significant increase in both p22phox mRNA expression and NADPH oxidase activity beginning at 3 days after the start of infusion. From reference 25, with permission from the Journal of Clinical Investigation and the American Heart Association

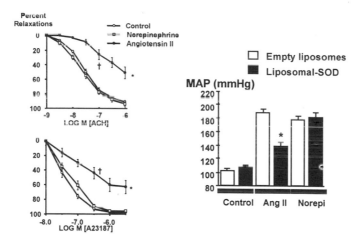

Figure 4. **Left Panel**: Effects of Norepinephrine and Angiotensin II induced hypertension on endothelium-dependent vascular relaxation. Rats were infused with angiotensin II (0.7 mg/kg/d), norepinephrine (2.8 mg/kg/d) or vehicle for 5 days. The rats were then sacrificed and relaxation of preconstricted aortic rings was measured in response to acetylcholine (upper left) or the calcium ionophore A23187 (lower left). Rings from angiotensin II-treated rats (●) showed marked impairment in endothelium dependent vascular relaxation compared to rings from norepinephrine-treated (□) or vehicle-treated rats (O). **Right Panel**: Effect of superoxide dismutase on norepinephrine and angiotensin-II induced hypertension. Rats were injected with empty liposomes (open bars) or liposome-entrapped superoxide dismutase (1000 U/d, filled bars) before and during angiotensin II, norepinephrine, or vehicle infusion, and blood pressure measured before sacrifice. Superoxide dismutase caused a significant attenuation in the hypertension induced by angiotensin II but not norepinephrine. From references 4 and 26, with permission from the Journal of Clinical Investigation and the American Heart Association.

These data suggest that a portion of the hypertension in physiologic conditions where angiotensin II is elevated is associated with an increase in vascular superoxide production. These findings may provide some insight into why forms of hypertension associated with elevated plasma renin activity are linked with increased cardiovascular event rates. It is of interest that hypertension induced by norepinephrine infusion was not associated with an increase in vascular superoxide production and did not alter endothelial regulation of vasomotion (4). Of note, infusion of lower doses of angiotensin II, which had minimal effects on blood pressure, also increased (by about 2-fold) NADH oxidase activity. This suggested that conditions in which circulating or local levels of angiotensin II are elevated might have unique effects on the vessel wall independent of elevating blood pressure. Furthermore, hypertension not associated with increases in angiotensin II, and not associated with activation of vascular oxidases, may be less prone to produce vascular disease. However, it is still possible that hypertension alone may cause a significant degree of oxidative stress. In preliminary studies, we have examined the effect of prolonged, low renin hypertension on vascular redox state. In uni-nephrectomized rats treated for 21 days with desoxycorticosterone acetate (DOCA) and high salt (DOCA-salt hypertension), aortic superoxide production was increased and endothelium-dependent vascular relaxation was impaired. This DOCA-salt model is associated with a suppressed renin-angiotensin system, and indeed treatment with an angiotensin receptor antagonist did not lower vascular superoxide levels (unpublished data). Thus, prolonged hypertension in the absence of elevated angiotensin II can also increase vascular $O_2^{-\bullet}$ production. This is likely related to increased stretch of vascular cells exposed to hypertension as observed previously in cell culture.

These studies have examined how superoxide may modulate nitric oxide's biological activity. It is important to point out that superoxide and other reactive oxygen species can have effects on vascular reactivity potentially independent of nitric oxide. In vascular smooth muscle, intracellular calcium levels may be increased by reactive oxygen species by interfering with calcium uptake by the sarcoplasmic reticulum (27). It has recently been shown that reactive oxygen species may react with fatty acids in the membrane to produce isoprostanoids. These can be detected in the blood of humans with several conditions thought associated with increased oxidative stress such as hypercholesterolemia, diabetes, and cigarette smoking (28, 29). Such oxidatively modified fatty acids act on prostaglandin H/thromboxane receptors to enhance vasoconstriction, potentially increasing systemic vascular resistance. Ultimately, this could predispose to hypertension.

Another mechanism involved in hypertension caused by angiotensin II relates to endothelin production by the vascular smooth muscle cell. It is now clear angiotensin II can enhance endothelin-1 (ET-1) gene expression in the vessel wall (30, 31). Two separate groups have shown that ET-1 antagonists can prevent hypertension caused by angiotensin II infusion (32, 33). We have also observed that the expression of ET-1 protein is markedly increased in vessels from rats that have been exposed to 5 days of angiotensin II infusion (32). The manner in which angiotensin II, oxidative stress, loss of nitric oxide bioactivity, and increased ET-1 protein production interact *in vivo* is unclear. It is likely that these work in concert to produce hypertension and its numerous effects on the vessel wall.

SUMMARY AND FUTURE DIRECTIONS

The mechanisms whereby vascular cells produce reactive oxygen species and the functional consequences of their production are only now coming to light. It is clear, however, that numerous vascular diseases involve perturbations of the balance between production of vascular reactive oxygen species and antioxidant defense mechanisms. A growing body of literature strongly suggests that the vascular NADH/NADPH oxidase plays a crucial role in these conditions. In the case of hypertension, the mechanical forces and humoral factors to which the vessel is exposed activate the NADH/NADPH oxidase. As shown in Figure 5, this has multiple consequences and it is likely that this increase in vascular oxidant stress contributes to hypertension's role as a risk factor for atherosclerosis. In this fashion, hypertension shares similarities with other conditions identified as risk factors, including hypercholesterolemia, diabetes, cigarette smoking and aging, all of which are associated with increased vascular oxidant stress. In the future, it may be possible to specifically alter activity of the vascular NADH/NADPH oxidase, thereby providing novel therapeutic approaches to these diseases.

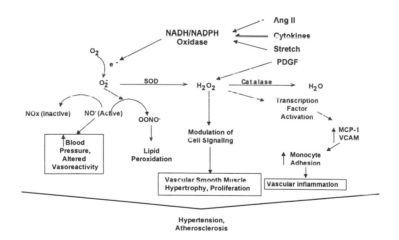

Figure 5. Paradigm for interactions between physiologic stimuli, reactive oxygen species, and hypertension. Oxygen free radicals are generated in response to angiotensin II, stretch, and cytokines. These contribute to hypertension, altered vasomotor reactivity and vessel wall inflammation both directly by scavenging nitric oxide and indirectly through modulation of signaling and gene expression.

REFERENCES

1.   Lu D, Maiulik N, Moraru II, Kreutzer DL, Das DK. Molecular adaptation of vascular endothelial cells to oxidative stress. *Am J Physiol.* 1993;264:C715.

2.   Pagano PJ, Tornheim K, Cohen RA. Superoxide anion production by rabbit thoracic aorta: effect of endothlium-derived nitric oxide. *Am J Physiol.* 1993:265:H707.

3.   Panus PC, Radi R, Chumley PH, Lillard RH, Freeman BA. Detection of H_2O_2 release from vascular endothelial cells. *Free Rad Biol Med.* 1993;14:217.

4.   Rajagopalan S, Kurz S, Munzel T, Tarpey M, Freeman B, Griendling K, Harrison D. Angiotensin II-mediated hypertension in the rat increases vascular superoxide production via membrane NADH/NADPH oxidase activation: contribution to alterations of vasomotor tone. *J Clin Invest.* 1996;97:1916.

5.   Friedl HP, Till GO, Ryan US, Ward PA. Mediator-induced activation of xanthine oxidase in endothelial cells. *FASEB J.* 1989;3:2512.

6.   Mohazzab KM, Wolin MS. Sites of superoxide anion production detected by lucigenin in calf pulmonary artery smooth muscle. *Am J Physiol.* 1994;267:L815.

7.   Mohazzah KM, Kaminski PM, Wolin MS. NADH oxidoreductase is a major source of superoxide anion in bovine coronary artery endothelium. *Am J Physiol.* 1994;266:H2568.

8.   Griendling K, Ollerenshaw JD, Minieri CA, Alexander RW. Angiotensin II stimulated NADH activity in cultured vascular smooth muscle cells. *Circ Res.* 1994;74:1141.

9.   Watson F, Robinson J, Edwards SW. Protein kinase C-dependent and –independent activation of the NADPH oxidase of human neutrophils. *J Biol Chem.* 1991;266:7432

10.   Ushio-Fukai M, Zafari AM, Fukui T, Ishizaka N, Griendling KK. P22phox is a critical component of the superoxide-generating NADH/NADPH oxidase system and regulated angiotensin II-induced hypertrophy in vascular smooth muscle cells. *J Biol Chem.* 1996;271:23317.

11.   Fukui T, Lassegue B, Kai H, Alexander RW, Griendling KK. Cytochrome b558 a-subunit cloning and expression in rat aortic smooth muscle cells. *Biochim Biophys Acta.* 1995;1231:215.

12.   Jones SA, O'Donnell VB, Wood JD, Broughton JP, Hughes EJ, Jones OT. Expression of phagocyte NADPH oxidase components in human endothelial cells. *Am J Physiol.* 1996;271:H1626.

13.   Howard AB, Alexander RW, Nerem RM, Griendling KK, Taylor WR. Cyclic strain induces and oxidative stress in endothelial cells. *Am J Physiol.* 1997;272:C421.

14.   Hishikawa K, Luscher TF. Pulsatile stretch stimulates superoxide production in human aortic endothelial cells. *Circulation.* 1997;96:3610.

15.   Inoue N, Ramasamy S, Fukai T, Nerem RM, Harrison DG. Shear stress modulates expression of Cu/Zn superoxide dismutase in human aortic endothelial cells. *Circ Res.* 1996;79:32.

16.   Nishida K, Harrison DG, Navas JP, Fisher AA, Dockery SP, Uematsu M, Nerem RM, Alexander RW, Murphy TJ. Molecular cloning and characterization of the constitutive bovine aortic endothelial cell nitric oxide synthase. *J Clin Invest.* 1993;90:2092.

17.   De Keulenaer GW, Chappell DC, Ishizaka N, Nerem RM, Alexander RW, Griendling KK. Oscillatory and steady laminar shear stress differentially affect human endothelial redox state: role of a suerpoxde-producing NADH oxidase. *Circ Res.* 1998;82:1094.

18.   De Keulenaer GW, Alexander RW, Ushio-Fukai M, Ishizaka N, Griendling KK. Tumor necrosis factor alpha activates a pssphox-based NADH oxidase in vascular smooth muscle. *Biochem J.* 1998;329:653.

19.   Kissner R, Nauser T, Bugnon P, Lye PG, Koppenol WH. Formation and properties of peroxynitrite as studied by laser flash photolysis, high-pressure stopped flow technique, and pulse radiolysis. *Chem Res Toxicol* 1997;10:1285

20.   Ohara Y, Peterson TE, Harrision DG. Hypercholesterolemia increases endothelial superoxide anion production. *J Clin Invest.* 1993;91:2546.

21.   Ting HH, Timimi FK, Boles K, Creager S, Ganz P, Creager MA. Vitamin C acutely improves endothelim-dependent vasodilation in patients with non-insulin-dependent diabetes mellitus. *Circulation.* 1995;92:1747.

22. Heitzer T, Just H, Munzel T. Antioxidant vitamin C improves endothelial dysfunction in chronic smokers. *Circulation.* 1996;94:6.
23. Mugge A, Elwell JH, Peterson TE, Hofmeyer TG, Heistad DD, Harrision DG. Chronic treatment with polyethylene-glycolated superoxide dismutase partially restores endothelim-dependent vascular relaxation in cholesterol-fed rabbits. *Circ Res.* 1991;69:1293.
24. Nakazono I, Watanabe N, Matsuno K, Sasaki J, Sato T, Inoue M. Does superoxide underlie the pathogenesis of hypertension? *Proc Natl Acad Sci USA.* 1991;88:10045.
25. Fukui T, Ishizaka N, Rajagopalan S, Laursen JB, Capers QT, Taylor WR, Harrison DG, de Leon H, Wilcox JN, Griendling KK. p22phox mRNA expression and NADPH oxidase activity are increased in aortas from hypertensive rats. *Circ Res.* 1997:80:45.
26. Laursen JB, Rajagopalan S, Tarpey M, Freeman B, Harrison DG. A role of superoxide in angiotensin II - but not catecholamine-induced hypertension. *Circulation* 1997;95:588.
27. Kwan CY, Beazley JS. Mechanisms of inhibition of alloxan of ATP-driven calcium transport by vascular smooth muscle microsomes. *J Bioenerg Biomembr.* 1988;20:517.
28. Reilly M, Delanty N, Lawson JA, FitzGerald GA. Modulation of oxidants stress *in vivo* in chroinc cigarette smokers. *Circulation* 1996;94:19.
29. Bachi A, Zuccato E, Baraldi M, Fanelli R, Chiabrando C. Measurement of urinary 8-epi-prostaglandin F_2-α, a novel index of lipid peroxidation *in vivo*, by immunoaffinity extraction/gas chromatography-mass spectrometry: Basal levels in smokers and nonsmokers. *Free Rad Biol Med.* 1996;20:619.
30. Chua BH, Chua CC, Diglio CA, Siu BB. Regulation of endothelin-1 mRNA by angiotensin II in rat heart endothelial cells. *Biochim Biophys Acta.* 1993;1178:201.
31. Imai T, Hirata Y, Emori T, Yanagisawa M, Masaki T, Marumo F. Induction of endothelin-1 gene by angiotensin and vasopressin in endothlial cells. *Hypertension.* 1992;19:753.
32. Rajagopalan S, Bech Laursen J, Borthayre A, Kurz S, Keiser J, Haleen S, Giaid A, Harrision DG. A role for endothelin-1 in angiotensin II mediated hypertension. *Hypertension.* 1997;30:29.
33. d'Uscio LV, Moreau P, Shaw S, Takase H, Barton M, Luscher TF. Effects of chronic ETA-receptor blockade in angiotensin II-induced hypertension. *Hypertension.* 1997;29:435.

18 PROTEIN KINASES THAT MEDIATE REDOX-SENSITIVE SIGNAL TRANSDUCTION

Bradford C. Berk

INTRODUCTION

Reduction-oxidation (redox) reactions that generate reactive oxygen species (ROS) have been identified as important chemical processes that regulate signal transduction. In this chapter ROS will refer to hydrogen peroxide (H_2O_2), superoxide ($O_2^{\cdot-}$) and $OH^{\bullet}$. Because increased ROS may be a risk factor for cardiovascular events such as unstable angina, myocardial infarction and sudden death, understanding the biological processes that generate ROS and the intracellular signals elicited by ROS will be important to gain insight into the pathogenesis of these diseases. In this review, the role of the mitogen-activated protein (MAP) kinase pathway in redox-sensitive signal transduction, and the nature of the tyrosine kinases that act as proximate "sensors" for redox-mediated signal events are presented. Four major points will be discussed as they relate to the nature of redox sensitive signal events. 1) Signal transduction will differ when ROS generation is intracellular versus extracellular. Also extracellular generation is usually acute and related to ischemia/reperfusion settings, while intracellular generation is usually chronic and related to stimulation of cell metabolism. 2) There are species specific differences in generation and response to ROS. 3) Because of different reactions, the three primary ROS species will exert different effects on intracellular signals. 4) Signal pathways that are redox sensitive may be defined by specific activation of upstream mediators which include phospholipases, small G proteins and tyrosine kinases. The mechanisms by which these mediators regulate gene transcription are then discussed to provide insight into the pathogenic roles of ROS in hypertension, atherosclerosis and vascular remodeling.

REDOX-SENSITIVE KINASES PROVIDE INSIGHT INTO MECHANISMS OF GENE REGULATION IN THE VASCULATURE

Initial studies in our lab showed that exposure of vascular smooth muscle cells to extracellular ROS altered vascular smooth muscle cells growth (1), MAP kinase activity (2), and proto-oncogene expression (3). Recently it has become clear that intracellular ROS generated in response to hormonal stimuli may act as second messengers. Three lines of evidence support this concept. 1) Stimulation of vascular smooth muscle cells with PDGF or angiotensin II increases ROS production (4, 5). 2) Most of the superoxide generated in vascular smooth muscle cells appears to be produced intracellularly (5), in contrast to phagocytes which generate extracellular superoxide. 3) Inhibiting superoxide production with transduced SOD, catalase or antioxidants blocks signal transduction by PDGF (4). In cultured vascular smooth muscle cells, the predominant source of agonist-stimulated superoxide formation is a plasma membrane NADH oxidase (5) which accounts for >90% of superoxide formation in vessels (6). Dr. Griendling's lab showed that angiotensin II caused a sustained increase in vascular smooth muscle cells superoxide. Importantly, angiotensin II hypertrophy was inhibited by transfection with antisense p22phox cDNA, a component of NADH oxidase. These findings indicate that intracellular ROS in vascular smooth muscle cells activate signal transduction analogous to calcium.

Recent data suggest that ROS may also serve as second messengers in endothelial cells, and that flow modulates endothelial cell redox state. Based on findings discussed below, a general concept may be proposed that steady laminar flow activates "antioxidant mechanisms" while oscillatory (and turbulent) flow stimulates "pro-oxidant mechanisms." For example, laminar flow inhibits induction of vascular cell adhesion molecule-1 by interleukin-1, a transcriptional event that is mediated by NF-κB in a redox-sensitive manner (7, 8). Similarly, monocyte chemotactic protein-1 expression (which is redox-sensitive), is initially stimulated by flow, but expression is then markedly inhibited (9) suggesting that flow exerts an initial pro-oxidant followed by an antioxidant effect. Both Harrison's and Gimbrone's labs recently demonstrated that steady laminar flow induced expression of SOD, the predominant intracellular antioxidant enzyme (10, 11). In contrast, oscillatory flow failed to induce SOD. As discussed above, there is a predilection for atherosclerosis at sites of oscillatory flow (12). Our published data show that oscillatory flow fails to increase intracellular calcium in contrast to steady flow (13), which should result in decreased NO production (since endothelial nitric oxide synthase [eNOS] is calcium-dependent). Thus the flow pattern may modulate endothelial cell redox state.

REMODELING IS IMPORTANT IN THE PATHO-GENESIS OF ATHEROSCLEROSIS, HYPERTENSION, AND RESTENOSIS AND IS REGULATED BY VASCULAR REDOX STATE

Vascular remodeling is a well-described response of blood vessels to both physiological and pathological stimuli. My laboratory and others have promoted the concept that the nature of vascular remodeling is a function of the balance between NO and ROS in the vessel. As discussed above, the redox state and level of eNOS expression are also regulated, in part, by the nature of the flow pattern. Vascular remodeling was first described in response to flow and/or pressure in rabbits (14,

15) and rats (16), in fetal development (17), and clinically following graft placement (18). Increased pressure and wall tension are associated with a thickened vascular wall (19), whereas increased flow and shear stress are associated with enlarged lumen diameter (20, 21) . Shear stress and its effects on endothelial cells have been proposed to be primary mediators for remodeling because endothelial denudation limits the ability to remodel (14). Shear stress alters the gene expression and protein function of several important mediators including eNOS (22-24), platelet-derived growth factor (PDGF) A- and B-chains (25-27), and extracellular signal regulated kinases (ERK) forms 1 and 2 (28, 29). Inhibiting eNOS function with the L-arginine analog N^G-nitro-L-arginine-methyl ester (L-NAME) prevents flow-induced remodeling (20) consistent with the impaired remodeling observed in eNOS knockout mice (30).

An important role for vessel redox state as a determinant of remodeling was initially suggested by our study of balloon-injured pig coronary arteries treated with vitamins C and E or placebo. Compared to placebo, vitamin C and E treatment produced a significant increase in total vessel area and lumen diameter without a change in intimal area (31). Vitamin C and E concentrations determined in plasma and lymphocytes (as an index for tissue levels) from treated animals showed 2 - 3 fold increases compared to controls. Superoxide production from the injured left anterior descending artery was 2.5-fold greater than superoxide production from the uninjured left anterior descending or right coronary arteries. In both the right and left anterior descending arteries, superoxide production was significantly inhibited by treatment with vitamins C and E, with decreases of ~45% relative to untreated vessels. There was a significant correlation between vessel superoxide production and lymphocyte vitamin E levels. These results were the first to show increased superoxide production in injured vessels and to demonstrate that antioxidant vitamins reduce superoxide production (31, 32). More recently, the antioxidant probucol was shown to limit restenosis following PTCA in a manner consistent with a positive effect on remodeling (33). Alterations in remodeling must therefore be considered as one mechanism by which ROS contribute to the pathogenesis of restenosis and atherosclerosis.

REDOX-SENSITIVE SIGNAL TRANSDUCTION

General Concepts And Overall Model

Signal transduction proceeds from cell surface through the plasma membrane to generate second messengers which then transmit the signal to intracellular mediators in both cytoplasm and nucleus. ROS participate in signal transduction by both generating classic second messengers (calcium and lipid mediators) and by themselves acting as second messengers. Classic second messengers will be discussed first, followed by more recent studies which show that generation of ROS by growth factors is an important component of growth factor-mediated responses. Both aspects will be presented based on the concept that kinases act to coordinate intracellular signal transduction through the integration of multiple extracellular stimuli via shared, convergent kinases. In addition, there is amplification of signal transduction events by kinase cascades in which activation of multiple downstream kinases occurs from the action of a single upstream kinases. There is important positive and negative crosstalk between kinase cascades. Also, translocation and subcellular localization of enzymes determines access to substrates and regulators. Finally, induction and activation of phosphatases that inhibit kinases is a prominent mechanism for turning off signal transduction. These general concepts are discussed in greater detail for ROS mediated signal events below using the MAP kinases as a specific model.

Stimulation of Calcium-Dependent Signal Transduction

Both endothelial cells and vascular smooth muscle cells are highly dependent on changes in intracellular calcium for normal biological function. For example NO production from endothelial cells is controlled by eNOS, a calcium/calmodulin-dependent enzyme, and activation of myosin light chain kinase is required for smooth muscle cell contraction and this event is dependent on a rise in calcium. ROS have been shown to stimulate increases in calcium via at least three pathways (Fig. 1). In the first of these, ROS produce intracellular calcium release from endoplasmic reticulum through generation of IP_3 (see below) which binds to an IP_3-sensitive calcium channel. In addition, ROS may directly increase the open probability of calcium release channels. It has been proposed that ROS stimulate formation of mixed disulfides with GSSG or other oxidized thiols that interact with the IP_3 receptor/channel to stimulate calcium release (34). In addition, a calcium-ATPase is required to maintain calcium within the inositol triphosphate (IP_3)-sensitive pool and inhibiting this ATPase would increase intracellular calcium (35). A second target for ROS-mediated changes in intracellular calcium involves calcium channels. Extracellular calcium concentrations are 1000 to 10,000 times greater than intracellular concentrations so that changes in the permeability of calcium channels and exchangers dramatically alters intracellular calcium. In several cell types, ROS have been shown to stimulate extracellular calcium entry by effects on

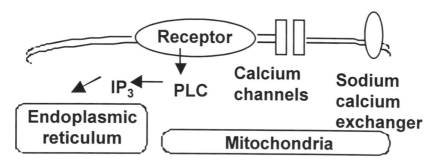

Figure 1. Mechanisms by which ROS increase intracellular calcium concentrations.

channels (36) and the sodium-calcium exchanger (37). The third and final mechanism of altered calcium homeostasis with ROS involves the mitochondrion. Mitochondria also store intracellular calcium, and significant oxidative stress inhibits this ability resulting in release of calcium, especially in response to oxidized pyridine nucleotides (38,39). The importance of mitochondrial calcium release in response to physiological levels of ROS remains unclear.

Stimulation of Phospholipid-Dependent Signal Transduction

The finding that ROS increased intracellular calcium indicated that phospholipases were activated by ROS, since generation of IP$_3$ from phosphatidylinositol bis-phosphate (PIP$_2$) is a well-established mechanism in vascular cells for the release of calcium from intracellular stores. At least three important phospholipases have been shown to be activated by ROS (Fig. 2): phospholipase A$_2$ (PLA$_2$), phospholipase C (PLC) and phospholipase D (PLD).

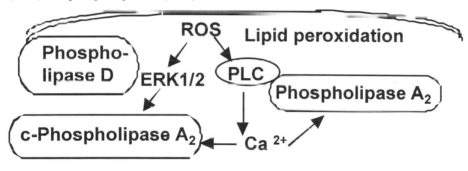

Figure 2. Mechanisms by which ROS activate phospholipase

Two mechanisms appear to account for activation of PLA$_2$ enzymes. First, because these phospholipases are calcium-dependent, increased calcium augments their activity. This may occur by a reduced calcium dependence stemming from alterations in enzyme/substrate calcium binding (40), substrate availability, or substrate replenishment (41). In addition, type IV PLA$_2$ (also termed cPLA$_2$) is regulated by translocation to the plasma membrane in a phosphorylation-dependent manner. ERK1/2 appear to be required for this activation suggesting that cPLA2 is a mediator of later signaling events. Phospholipase C is a calcium-dependent enzyme that hydrolyses PIP$_2$ to generate IP$_3$ and diacylglycerol. There are no published data to suggest that ROS directly activate PLC. However, as discussed below, generation of ROS may be an early event in growth factor-dependent signaling and hence, activation of PLC. Phospholipase D has been shown to be stimulated by H$_2$O$_2$, fatty acid hydroperoxides (42), and 4-hydroxynonenal in endothelial cells. Regulation of PLD is presently unclear, but may require tyrosine phosphorylation (43), although it appears to be calcium-independent (42). Future studies will be required to define the mechanisms by which phospholipases are activated.

Table 1. Examples of Agonists that Use Intracellular ROS

Ligands	ROS	Reference
Angiotensin II	H_2O_2, $O_2^{\cdot-}$	(5, 44)
Insulin	H_2O_2	(45)
Interleukin 1β	H_2O_2, $O_2^{\cdot-}$	(4, 46)
Parathyroid hormone	$O_2^{\cdot-}$	(47)
Platelet derived growth factor	H_2O_2	(4, 48)
Transforming growth factor-β	H_2O_2	(49)
Tumor necrosis factor-α	H_2O_2, $OH^{\cdot}$	(4, 46)
Vitamin D3	$O_2^{\cdot-}$	(47)

REACTIVE OXYGEN SPECIES AS SECOND MESSENGERS

The concept that ROS are second messengers similar to calcium or phospholipids is supported by the findings that agonist-receptor binding leads to rapid generation of ROS and that antioxidants block agonist-mediated signaling. Table 1 lists several ligand/receptor interactions that seem to use ROS as second messengers. Data are strong that vascular smooth muscle cells generate ROS in response to several agonists including angiotensin II and PDGF. Our group initially demonstrated that extracellular ROS (via xanthine + xanthine oxidase [1]), or intracellular ROS (via naphthoquinolinediones [2]) were able to stimulate vascular smooth muscle cell growth. More recently, Griendling and colleagues demonstrated that angiotensin II rapidly increased production of ROS. Angiotensin II-mediated cell hypertrophy was dependent on ROS generation as inhibition of ROS generation prevented the angiotensin II-mediated increase in protein synthesis (5, 44). Similar data have been generated for PDGF. Sundaresan *et al.* (4, 46) observed that PDGF transiently increased H_2O_2 that was required for PDGF-induced tyrosine phosphorylation and ERK1/2 activation. In other cell types, agonists have been shown to stimulate gene expression (especially, NF-kB activity) via generation of ROS (46). These findings suggest that intracellular generation of ROS is likely to be important in the actions of many agonists. It should be noted that there are ROS-specific and species-specific determinants of cell responsiveness to ROS. For example, in rat aortic vascular smooth muscle cells, there was a concentration-dependent increase in ERK1/2 activity by a superoxide generating napthoquinolinedione, but not by H_2O_2 which was associated with cell growth (2). In contrast, in human aortic vascular smooth muscle cells, H_2O_2 but not superoxide stimulated ERK1/2 activity, yet neither ROS was able to stimulate cell growth (50). These differences were not explained by alterations in glutathione levels which were the same in both cell types.

REDOX-SENSITIVE SIGNAL TRANSDUCTION: INTEGRATION BY ROS ACTIVATED KINASES

Tyrosine Kinases As Mediators of Redox-Sensitive Pathways

The importance of tyrosine kinases as intracellular mediators is evident by their rapidly activation by many stimuli including ROS. Several tyrosine kinases are readily activated by ROS, the Src-family kinases playing a prominent role in this regard. For example, H_2O_2 and diamide, which oxidize free sulfhydryl groups, both stimulated tyrosine phosphorylation of multiple proteins (especially a 55-kD protein) in cultured T lymphocytes (51). The 55-kD molecule phosphorylated by diamide was identified as p56Lck , a Src-family protein tyrosine kinase. Including this report, at least three members of the Src family (p60Src, p56Lck, and p59Fyn) have demonstrated sensitivity to H_2O_2 and diamide. Two other redox-sensitive tyrosine kinases identified in white blood cells are Syk and ZAP-70 (52). Src appears to be especially important for activation of MAP kinases by ROS as discussed below.

At least three mechanisms have been proposed by which ROS activate tyrosine kinases. First, ROS may directly activate kinases by altering protein-protein interactions depending on sulfhydryl groups and "liberating" kinases from endogenous inhibitors. Second, ROS inhibit phosphotyrosine phosphatases (PTPases) by oxidation of a redox-sensitive cysteine in the active site (53). Oxidation of the sulfhydryl group inactivates the PTPase and, because many tyrosine kinases are inactivated by PTPases, oxidation of PTPases stimulates tyrosine kinases. This mechanism is supported by observations that immunoprecipitated Syk-family kinases were not responsive to oxidants, indicating that these kinases may not be directly regulated by ROS. In addition, similar patterns of protein tyrosine phosphorylation were found in white blood cells in response to ROS and to PTPase inhibition (52). Third, oxidation has been shown to stimulate proteolysis of regulatory proteins that may inhibit tyrosine kinase activity.

Small G Proteins in Redox Sensitive Signal Transduction

Small G proteins are thought to be important mediators of ROS signaling. For example, activation of ERK1/2 by H_2O_2 was prevented in cells in which p21ras activity was blocked either through expression of a dominant negative mutant or by treating with a farnesyltransferase inhibitor. Using recombinant p21ras in vitro it was found that ROS directly promoted guanine nucleotide exchange on p21ras (54). Furthermore, H_2O_2 activation of ERK2 was abolished by expression of dominant negative ras-N-17 (55). These results suggest that ROS may directly activate p21ras and thus trigger downstream events via the MAP kinase pathway. Potential mechanisms for p21ras activation include alterations of the lipid environment and inhibition of post-translational modifications such as palmitoylation that may regulate small G protein activity. It also appears that another small G protein, rac, may regulate ROS production (48,56). Expression of constitutively active V12-rac1 in HeLa cells or stimulation with cytokines resulted in a significant increase in intracellular ROS and activation of NF-kB. Treatment of cells with antioxidants inhibited the rise in ROS that occurred following V12-rac1 expression as well as the ability of V12-rac1 to stimulate NF-kB activity. These results suggest that rac1 also regulates intracellular ROS production.

Mitogen-Activated Protein (MAP) Kinase Pathway in Redox Sensitive Signal Transduction

MAP kinase family members are logical candidates to mediate the many changes in gene expression observed in response to ROS. MAP kinases are serine and threonine protein kinases activated in response to a wide variety of extracellular stimuli and are encoded by a multigene family (Figure 3) (57). MAP kinases are activated by phosphorylation on threonine and tyrosine residues within a T-X-Y phosphorylation motif, where "X" can be Glu (E), Pro (P), or Gly (G). Three classes of dual-specificity MAP kinases may be defined based on their phosphorylation motifs. For example, both ERK1/2 and big MAP kinase-1 (BMK1) are phosphorylated on a TEY motif. In contrast, c-Jun N-terminal protein kinases (JNK), also called stress-activated protein kinases (SAPK), are phosphorylated via a TPY motif (Fig. 3). Finally, p38 kinase (also called ERK6) is activated by phosphorylation on a TGY motif. Activation of the three classes of MAP kinases is characteristic for particular stimuli. For example, growth factors and phorbol myristate acetate (PMA) activate ERK1/2 strongly, but JNK and p38 kinases weakly (58). Hyperosmolar stress and TNF-α are strong stimuli for p38 (59). In vascular smooth muscle cells we have shown that growth factors and angiotensin II are powerful activators of ERK1/2 (60). Arachidonic acid and 15-HETE (a 15-lipoxygenase product of arachidonic acid), have both been shown to activate ERK1/2 in vascular smooth muscle cells (61). The specificity for MAP kinase activation is determined, in part, by members of the MAPK/ERK kinase (MEK) family which exhibit unique pairing with downstream MAP kinases. For example, MEK1 and MEK2 activate ERK1/2, MEK3 activates p38, and MEK4 activates JNK (Figure 3). Thus, cell- and stimulus-specific events regulate MAP kinase activity. The specific activation of MAP kinases by individual stimuli is reiterated by specific substrates for each class (Figure 3). Common substrates for the MAP kinases are transcription factors that, upon phosphorylation, may be activated and induce changes in gene expression. ERK1/2 phosphorylate ternary complex factor (TCF)/Elk-1 on sites essential for transactivation (62). JNK phosphorylates c-Jun, and increases its transcriptional activating potential (63). Activating transcription factor 2 (ATF2) is phosphorylated and activated by both JNK and p38 (64, 65). BMK1 activates myocyte enhancer factor 2 (MEF2) transcription factors (66).

Extracellular signal regulated kinases 1 and 2 (ERK1/2)

Recently we found that ROS activated ERK1/2 when the ROS was superoxide, but not H_2O_2 (2). In other systems, ROS activate JNK strongly (67). Griendling and

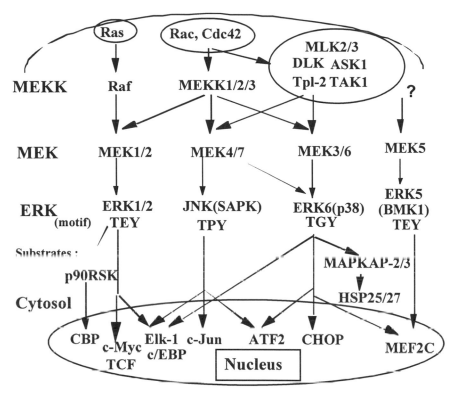

Figure 3. Sheme for ROS-activated MAP kinase cascades.
Abbreviations: ASK, apoptosis signal–regulating kinase; ATF2, activating transcription factor 2; BMK1, big MAP kinase 1; CHOP, C/EBP-homologous protein, DLK, dual leucine zipper bearing kinase; ERK, extracellular signal regulated kinase; HSP, heat-shock protein, JNK, c-Jun N-terminal protein kinase; MAPKAP, MAP kinase-acivated protein; MEF2, myocyte enhancer factor 2; MEK, MAPK/ERK kinase; MEKK, MEK kinase; MLK, mixed lineage kinase; SAPK; stress activated protein kinase; TAK1, transforming growth factor β activated kinase; .

colleagues found that angiotensin II-dependent hypertrophy was dependent on generation of ROS, as angiotensin II rapidly stimulated NADH oxidase and hypertrophy was inhibited by catalase, SOD and inhibition of NADH oxidase. Both ERK1/2 and p38 appear necessary for angiotensin II-mediated hypertrophy as inhibition of these MAP kinases with PD98059 and SB205380, respectively led to additive decreases in cell protein synthesis (2).

Stress Activated Protein Kinases (SAPK): p38 and c-Jun N Terminal Kinase (JNK)

Stimulation of vascular smooth muscle cells with H_2O_2 or superoxide (generated by LY83583) failed to activate p21-activated kinase-1 (PAK1), the upstream regulator of both p38 and JNK. In contrast, angiotensin II rapidly stimulated PAK1, and stimulated p38 and JNK in vascular smooth muscle cells (44, 68). These results suggest that additional signals activated by angiotensin and/or the nature of intracellular ROS generation versus extracellular ROS provide critical differences in signal transduction events.

Big MAP Kinase 1 (BMK1)

A MAP kinase termed Big MAP kinase 1 (BMK1) or ERK5 was recently cloned by two groups (69, 70). Because the primary structure and molecular mass (~110 kD) differ from ERK1/2 (69), the name BMK1 will be used. BMK1 has a TEY sequence in its dual phosphorylation site, like ERK1/2, but has unique C-terminal and loop-12 domains, suggesting that its regulation and function may be different from ERK1/2. The upstream kinase that phosphorylates BMK1 has been identified as MEK5 (69, 70). However, upstream regulators of MEK5 remain unknown. In our laboratory we observed that in response to several different vascular smooth muscle cells agonists, BMK1 was stimulated to the greatest extent by H_2O_2 , with a relative potency of $H_2O_2 >>> PDGF>PMA=TNF\alpha$ (71). It is noteworthy that while ERK1/2 and JNK are activated by ROS, they are activated to a much greater extent by growth factors and cytokines. Thus, these findings suggest that BMK1 is the first MAP kinase which is specifically redox sensitive.

We found that BMK1 was rapidly and specifically activated by H_2O_2, but not by growth factors in vascular smooth muscle cells. Hydrogen peroxide caused a time- and concentration-dependent activation of BMK1, which was calcium-and tyrosine-kinase dependent as shown by inhibition with thapsigargin and herbimycin A, respectively (71). Stimulation of BMK1 by H_2O_2 appeared ubiquitous as shown by increases in BMK1 activity in human skin fibroblasts, human vascular smooth muscle cells and human umbilical vein endothelial cells (71). These findings demonstrate that activation of BMK1 is different from ERK1/2, JNK and p38 and depends on calcium and tyrosine kinases, but not on protein kinase C (PKC). To show that BMK1 activation in vascular smooth muscle cells is regulated by redox state, we used ebselen (a glutathione peroxidase mimic that we have previously shown to enter cultured cells rapidly). Vascular smooth muscle cells were treated with 30 μM ebselen or vehicle for 30 min and then exposed to 200 μM H_2O_2 for 20 min. Ebselen completely inhibited H_2O_2 -mediated increases in BMK1 activity.

An essential role for c-Src in H_2O_2-mediated BMK1 activation in vascular smooth muscle cells is suggested by 4 experiments (72). First, H_2O_2 stimulated c-Src activity rapidly in vascular smooth muscle cells and fibroblasts (peak at 5 min) temporally preceding peak activity of BMK1 (20 min). Second, specific Src-family tyrosine kinase inhibitors (herbimycin A and CP-118,556) blocked BMK1 activation by H_2O_2 in a concentration-dependent manner. Third, BMK1 activation in response to H_2O_2 was completely inhibited in cells derived from mice deficient in c-Src, but not Fyn. Mouse fibroblasts from transgenic animals that lacked Src (Src-/-), Fyn (Fyn-/-) or both (Src-/-&Fyn-/-) were prepared (73, 74). BMK1 activation was decreased only in Src-/- and Src-/-&Fyn-/- cells. Fourth, BMK1 activity was much greater in v-Src transformed NIH-3T3 cells than wild type cells. These results demonstrate an essential role for c-Src in H_2O_2-mediated activation of BMK1 and suggest that redox-sensitive regulation of BMK1 is a new function for c-Src.

SUMMARY

It is clear that multiple enzymes may stimulate ROS production in vascular smooth muscle cells and endothelial cells. These include NADH/NADPH oxidase, xanthine oxidase, lipoxygenases, cyclo-oxygenase, p450 mono-oxygenases and the enzymes of mitochondrial oxidative phosphorylation. In addition to generation of intracellular superoxide by these enzymes, extracellular stimuli including lipophilic substrates, membrane permeant oxidants (*e.g.* H_2O_2), cytokines, and growth factors may modulate cellular redox state. The increased ROS may act as second messengers to activate kinases such as tyrosine kinases of the Src and Syk families, serine-threonine kinases such as the MAP kinase family, and ROS inhibit protein tyrosine phosphatases (PTPases). As discussed above, regulation of the MAP kinases is one example of the complexity of ROS-dependent signal transduction. A further level of complexity that remains to be explored in greater detail are the effects of ROS-dependent signal transduction on the activity of transcription factors resulting in changes in gene expression. While the complexity of ROS-mediated signal transduction is daunting, the diversity offers multiple therapeutic targets for pharmacological intervention.

REFERENCES

1. Rao GN, Berk BC. Active oxygen species stimulate vascular smooth muscle cell growth and proto-oncogene expression. *Circ Res.* 1992;70:593.
2. Baas AS, Berk BC. Differential activation of mitogen-activated protein kinases by H_2O_2 and superoxide in vascular smooth muscle cells. *Circ Res.* 1995;77:29.
3   Rao GN, Lassegue B, Griendling KK, Alexander RW, Berk BC. Hydrogen peroxide-induced c-fos expression is mediated by arachidonic acid release: Role of protein kinase C. *Nucl Acids Res.* 1993;21:1259.
4. Sundaresan M, Yu ZX, Ferrans VJ, Irani K, Finkel T. Requirement for generation of H_2O_2 for platelet-derived growth factor signal transduction. *Science.* 1995;270:296.
5. Griendling KK, Minieri CA, Ollerenshaw JD, Alexander RW. Angiotensin II stimulates NADH and NADPH oxidase activation in cultured vascular smooth muscle cells. *Circ Res.* 1994;74:1141.
6. Mohazzab KM, Kaminski PM, Wolin MS. NADH oxidoreductase is a major source of superoxide anion in bovine coronary artery endothelium. *Am J Physiol.* 1994;266:H2568.
7. Ahmad M, Marui N, Alexander RW, Medford RM. Cell type-specific transactivation of the VCAM-1 promoter through an NF-kappa B enhancer motif. *J Biol Chem.* 1995;270:8976.
8. Medford R, Erickson S, Chappel D, Offermann M, Nerem R, Alexander R. Laminar shear stress and redox sensitive regulation of human vascular endothelial cell VCAM-1 gene expression. *Circulation.* (abstract). 1994;90:I-83.
9. Shyy YJ, Hsieh HJ, Usami S, Chien S. Fluid shear stress induces a biphasic response of human monocyte chemotactic protein 1 gene expression in vascular endothelium. *Proc Natl Acad Sci USA.* 1994;91:4678.
10. Inoue N, Ramasamy S, Fukai T, Nerem RM, Harrison DG. Shear stress modulates expression of Cu/Zn superoxide dismutase in human aortic endothelial cells. *Circ Res.* 1996;79:32.
11. Topper JN, Cai J, Falb D, Gimbrone MA, Jr. Identification of vascular endothelial genes differentially responsive to fluid mechanical stimuli: cyclooxygenase-2, manganese

superoxide dismutase, and endothelial cell nitric oxide synthase are selectively up-regulated by steady laminar shear stress. *Proc Natl Acad Sci USA.* 1996;93:10417.

12.   Ku DN, Giddens DP, Zarins CK, Glagov S. Pulsatile flow and atherosclerosis in the human carotid bifurcation. Positive correlation between plaque location and low oscillating shear stress. *Arteriosclerosis.* 1985;5:293.

13.   Helmlinger G, Berk BC, Nerem RM. The calcium responses of endothelial cell monolayers subjected to pulsatile and steady laminar flow differ. *Am J Physiol (Cell Physiol).* 1995;269:C367.

14.   Langille BL, O'Donnell F. 1986. Reductions in arterial diameter produced by chronic decreases in blood flow are endothelium-dependent. *Science.* 1986;231:405.

15.   Langille BL, Bendeck MP, Keeley FW. Adaptations of carotid arteries of young and mature rabbits to reduced carotid blood flow. *Am J Physiol.* 1989;256:H931.

16.   Guyton JR, Hartley CJ. Flow restriction of one carotid artery in juvenile rats inhibits growth of arterial diameter. *Am J Physiol.* 1985;248:H540.

17.   Langille BL. Remodeling of developing and mature arteries: endothelium, smooth muscle, and matrix. *J Cardiovasc Pharmacol.* 1993;1:S11.

18.   Geary RL, Kohler TR, Vergel S, Kirkman TR, Clowes AW. Time course of flow-induced smooth muscle cell proliferation and intimal thickening in endothelialized baboon vascular grafts. *Circ Res.* 1994;74:14

19.   Folkow B, Grimby G, Thulesius O. Adaptive structural changes of the vascular walls in hypertension and their relation to the control of peripheral resistance. *Acta Phy Scand.* 1958;44:255.

20.   Tronc F, Wassef M, Esposito B, Henrion D, Glagov S, Tedgui A. Role of NO in flow-induced remodeling of the rabbit common carotid artery. *Arterioscler Thromb Vasc Biol.* 1996;16:1256.

21.   Brownlee RD, Langille BL. Arterial adaptations to altered blood flow. *Can J Physiol Pharmacol.* 1991;69:978.

22.   Corson MA, Berk BC, Navas JP, Harrison DG Phosphorylation of endothelial nitric oxide synthase in response to shear stress. *Circulation.* 1993;88:I-183.

23.   Korenaga R, Ando J, Tsuboi H, Yang W, Sakuma I, Toyo OT, Kamiya A. Laminar flow stimulates ATP- and shear stress-dependent nitric oxide production in cultured bovine endothelial cells. *Biochem Biophys Res Comm.* 1994;198:213-9.

24.   Uematsu M, Ohara Y, Navas JP, Nishida K, Murphy TJ, Alexander RW, Nerem RM, Harrison DG. Regulation of endothelial cell nitric oxide synthase mRNA expression by shear stress. *Am J Physiol.* 1995;269:C1371.

25.   Hsieh H-J, Li N-Q, Frangos JA. Shear stress increases endothelial platelet-derived growth factor mRNA levels. *Am J Physiol. (Heart Circ Physiol)*1991;260:H642.

26.   Mitsumata M, Fishel RS, Nerem RN, Alexander RW, Berk BC. Fluid shear stress stimulates platelet-derived growth factor expression in endothelial cells. *Am J Physiol.* 1993;265:H3.

27.   Mondy JS, Lindner V, Miyashiro JK, Berk BC, Dean RH, Geary RL. Platelet-derived growth factor ligand and receptor expression in response to altered blood flow in vivo. *Circ Res.* 1997;81:320.

28.   Tseng H, Peterson TE, Berk BC. Fluid shear stress stimulates mitogen-activated protein kinase in endothelial cells. *Circ Res.* 1995;77:869.

29.   Ishida T, Peterson TE, Kovach NL, Berk BC. MAP kinase activation by flow in endothelial cells. Role of beta 1 integrins and tyrosine kinases. *Circ Res.* 1996; 79:310.

30.   Rudic RD, Shesely EG, Maeda N, Smithies O, Segal SS, Sessa WC. Direct evidence for the importance of endothelium-derived nitric oxide in vascular remodeling. *J Clin Invest.* 1998;101:731.

31.   Nunes GL, Sgoutas DS, Redden RA, Sigman SR, Gravanis MB, King SBr, Berk BC. Combination of vitamins C and E alters the response to coronary balloon injury in the pig. *Arterioscler Thromb Vasc Biol.* 1995;15:156.

32.   Nunes GL, Robinson K, Kalynych A, King III SB, Sgoutas DS, Berk BC. Vitamins C and E inhibit superoxide production in the pig coronary artery. *Circulation.* 1997;96:3593.

33.   Tardif JC, Coté G, Lespérance J, Bourassa M, Lambert J, Doucet S, Bilodeau L, Nattel S, de Guise P. Probucol and multivitamins in the prevention of restenosis after coronary angioplasty. Multivitamins and Probucol Study Group. *N Engl J Med.* 1997;337:365.

34.   Renard DC, Seitz MB, Thomas AP. Oxidized glutathione causes sensitization of calcium release to inositol 1,4,5-trisphosphate in permeabilized hepatocytes. *Biochem J.* 1992;284:507.

35.   Sweetman LL, Zhang NY, Peterson H, Gopalakrishna R, Sevanian A. Effect of linoleic acid hydroperoxide on endothelial cell calcium homeostasis and phospholipid hydrolysis. *Arch Biochem Biophys*. 1995;323:97.

36.   Wang SY, Clague JR, Langer GA. Increase in calcium leak channel activity by metabolic inhibition or hydrogen peroxide in rat ventricular myocytes and its inhibition by polycation. *J Mol Cell Cardiol*. 1995;27:211.

37.   Reeves JP, Bailey CA, Hale CC. Redox modification of sodium-calcium exchange activity in cardiac sarcolemmal vesicles. *J Biol Chem*. 1986;261:4948.

38.   Lehninger AL, Vercesi A, Bababunmi EA. Regulation of Ca^{2+} release from mitochondria by the oxidation-reduction state of pyridine nucleotides. *Proc Natl Acad Sci USA*. 1978;75:1690.

39.   Sies H, Graf P, Estrela JM. Hepatic calcium efflux during cytochrome P-450-dependent drug oxidations at the endoplasmic reticulum in intact liver. *Proc Natl Acad Sci USA*. 1981;78:3358.

40.   Salgo MG, Corongiu FP, Sevanian A. Enhanced interfacial catalysis and hydrolytic specificity of phospholipase A_2 toward peroxidized phosphatidylcholine vesicles. *Arch Biochem Biophys*. 1993;304:123.

41.   Jain MK, Rogers J, Berg O, Gelb MH. Interfacial catalysis by phospholipase A_2: activation by substrate replenishment. *Biochemistry*. 1991;30:7340.

42.   Natarajan V, Taher MM, Roehm B, Parinandi NL, Schmid HH, Kiss Z, Garcia JG. Activation of endothelial cell phospholipase D by hydrogen peroxide and fatty acid hydroperoxide. *J Biol Chem*. 1993;268:930.

43.   Bourgoin S, Grinstein S. Peroxides of vanadate induce activation of phospholipase D in HL-60 cells. Role of tyrosine phosphorylation. *J Biol Chem*. 1992;267:11908.

44.   Ushio-Fukai M, Alexander RW, Akers M, Griendling KK. p38 Mitogen-activated protein kinase is a critical component of the redox-sensitive signaling pathways activated by angiotensin II. Role in vascular smooth muscle cell hypertrophy. *J Biol Chem*. 1998;273:15022.

45.   Krieger-Brauer HI, Kather H. Human fat cells possess a plasma membrane-bound H_2O_2-generating system that is activated by insulin via a mechanism bypassing the receptor kinase. *J Clin Invest*. 1992;89:1006.

46.   Schreck R, Rieber P, Baeuerle PA. Reactive oxygen intermediates as apparently widely used messengers in the activation of the NF-kappa B transcription factor and HIV-1. *Embo J*. 1991;10:2247.

47.   Garrett IR, Boyce BF, Oreffo RO, Bonewald L, Poser J, Mundy GR. Oxygen-derived free radicals stimulate osteoclastic bone resorption in rodent bone in vitro and in vivo. *J Clin Invest*. 1990;85:632.

48.   Sundaresan M, Yu ZX, Ferrans VJ, Sulciner DJ, Gutkind JS, Irani K, Goldschmidt C-PJ, Finkel T. Regulation of reactive-oxygen-species generation in fibroblasts by Rac1. *Biochem J*. 1996;318:379.

49.   Ohba M, Shibanuma M, Kuroki T, Nose K. Production of hydrogen peroxide by transforming growth factor-beta 1 and its involvement in induction of egr-1 in mouse osteoblastic cells. *J Cell Biol*. 1994;126:1079.

50.   Baas AS, Duff JL, Berk BC. Oxidative stress stimulates mitogen-activated protein kinases (ERK1/2) and cell death in human aortic smooth muscle cells. *Circ Res*. 1997;submitted.

51.   Nakamura K, Hori T, Sato N, Sugie K, Kawakami T, Yodoi J. Redox regulation of a src family protein tyrosine kinase p56lck in T cells. *Oncogene*. 1993;8:3133.

52.   Schieven GL, Mittler RS, Nadler SG, Kirihara JM, Bolen JB, Kanner SB, Ledbetter JA. ZAP-70 tyrosine kinase, CD45, and T cell receptor involvement in UV- and H_2O_2-induced T cell signal transduction. *J Biol Chem*. 1994;269:20718.

53.   Brondello JM, McKenzie FR, Sun H, Tonks NK, Pouyss'egur J. Constitutive MAP kinase phosphatase (MKP-1) expression blocks G1 specific gene transcription and S-phase entry in fibroblasts. *Oncogene*. 1995;10:1895.

54.   Lander HM, Ogiste JS, Teng KK, Novogrodsky A. p21ras as a common signaling target of reactive free radicals and cellular redox stress. *J Biol Chem*. 1995;270:21195.

55.   Irani K, Xia Y, Zweier JL, Sollott SJ, Der CJ, Fearon ER, Sundaresan M, Finkel T, Clermont-Goldschmidt PJ. Mitogenic signaling mediated by oxidants in Ras-transformed fibroblasts. *Science*. 1997;275:1649.

56.   Sulciner DJ, Irani K, Yu ZX, Ferrans VJ, Clermont-Goldschmidt P, Finkel T. rac1 regulates a cytokine-stimulated, redox-dependent pathway necessary for NF-kappaB activation. *Mol Cell Biol.* 1996;16:7115.
57.   Blenis J. Signal transduction via the MAP kinases: proceed at your own RSK. *Proc Natl Acad Sci USA.* 1993;90:5889.
58.   Cano E, Hazzalin CA, Mahadevan LC. Anisomycin-activated protein kinases p45 and p55 but not mitogen-activated protein kinases ERK-1 and -2 are implicated in the induction of c-fos and c-jun. *Mol Cell Biol.* 1994;14:7352.
59.   Han J, Lee JD, Bibbs L, Ulevitch RJ. A MAP kinase targeted by endotoxin and hyperosmolarity in mammalian cells. *Science.* 1994;265:808.
60.   Duff JL, Berk BC, Corson MA. Angiotensin II stimulates the pp44 and pp42 mitogen-activated protein kinases in cultured rat aortic smooth muscle cells. *Biochem Biophys Res Comm.* 1992;188:257.
61.   Rao GN, Baas AS, Glasgow WC, Eling TE, Runge MS, Alexander RW. Activation of mitogen-activated protein kinases by arachidonic acid and its metabolites in vascular smooth muscle cells. *J Biol Chem.* 1994;269:32586.
62.   Marais R, Wynne J, Treisman R. The SRF accessory protein Elk-1 contains a growth factor-regulated transcriptional activation domain. *Cell.* 1993;73:381.
63.   Kyriakis JM, Banerjee P, Nikolakaki E, Dai T, Rubie EA, Ahmad MF, Avruch J, Woodgett JR. The stress-activated protein kinase subfamily of c-Jun kinases. *Nature.* 1994;369:156.
64.   Gupta S, Campbell D, D'Erijard B, Davis RJ. Transcription factor ATF2 regulation by the JNK signal transduction pathway. *Science.* 1995;267:389.
65.   Raingeaud J, Gupta S, Rogers JS, Dickens M, Han J, Ulevitch RJ, Davis RJ. Pro-inflammatory cytokines and environmental stress cause p38 mitogen-activated protein kinase activation by dual phosphorylation on tyrosine and threonine. *J Biol Chem.* 1995;270:7420.
66.   Kato Y, Kravchenko VV, Tapping RI, Han J, Ulevitch RJ, Lee JD. BMK1/ERK5 regulates serum-induced early gene expression through transcription factor MEF2C. *Embo J.* 1997;16:7054.
67.   Devary Y, Gottlieb RA, Smeal T, Karin M. The mammalian ultraviolet response is triggered by activation of src tyrosine kinases. *Cell.* 1992;71:1081.
68.   Schmitz U, Ishida T, Ishida M, Surapisitchat J, Hasham MI, Pelech S, Berk BC. Angiotensin II stimulates p21-activated kinase in vascular smooth muscle cells: Role in activation of JNK. *Circ Res.* 1998;82:1272.
69.   Lee JD, Ulevitch RJ, Han J. Primary structure of BMK1: a new mammalian MAP kinase. *Biochem Biophys Res Comm.* 1995;213:715.
70.   Zhou G, Bao ZQ, Dixon JE. Components of a new human protein kinase signal transduction pathway. *J Biol Chem.* 1995;270:12665.
71.   Abe J, Kusuhara M, Ulevitch RJ, Berk BC, Lee JD. Big mitogen-activated protein kinase 1 (BMK1) is a redox-sensitive kinase. *J Biol Chem.* 1996;271:16586.
72.   Abe J, Takahashi M, Ishida M, Lee J-D, Berk BC. c-Src is required for oxidative stress-mediated activation of big mitogen-activated protein kinase (BMK1). *J Biol Chem.* 1997;272:20389.
73.   Thomas SM, Soriano P, Imamoto A. Specific and redundant roles of Src and Fyn in organizing the cytoskeleton. *Nature.* 1995;376:267.
74.   Soriano P, Montgomery C, Geske R, Bradley A. Targeted disruption of the c-src proto-oncogene leads to osteopetrosis in mice. *Cell.* 1991;64:693.

19 ANTIOXIDANTS AND RESTENOSIS: ANIMAL AND CLINICAL STUDIES

John F. Paolini and Elazer R. Edelman

INTRODUCTION

While percutaneous revascularization procedures (*i.e.*, angioplasty) can restore luminal flow in atherosclerotic and occluded vessels, initial high success rates ultimately diminish due to gradual reclosure of the vessel over time. This phenomenon, referred to as restenosis, occurs in up to 40% of patients undergoing angioplasty and is a major health hazard. Angioplasty involves high-pressures balloon inflation in the coronary artery that typically causes significant mechanical injury to the intima, often with concomitant rupture of the internal elastic lamina. Smooth muscle cells subsequently migrate from the media to the intima, then proliferate and secrete extracellular matrix producing neointimal hyperplasia and a fibromuscular lesion that may occlude the vessel lumen.

Endovascular stents extend the benefit of angioplasty procedures but are themselves beset by accelerated forms of restenosis. Though new classes of anticoagulants limit early stent thrombosis, restenosis persists, necessitating either a return to the catheterization laboratory for additional interventions or referral for surgical bypass grafting. It is somewhat counter-intuitive that despite lower clinical restenosis rates observed with stenting, arterial injury during stent implantation is more severe than with simple balloon angioplasty. There is deep penetration of the stent limbs into the vessel wall and laceration of the media, triggering aggressive neointimal formation. However, the mechanical scaffolding properties of the stent limit luminal encroachment and allow a greater extent of neointimal hyperplasia before clinical restenosis occurs. Thus, the scaffolding properties of the stent result in an overall reduction in restenosis.

Oxidative stress is recognized as a potentially important contributor to atherogenesis and restenosis after vascular intervention and injury. Reactive oxygen species and oxidized lipids have profound and wide-ranging effects which can dramatically increase vascular toxicity and initiate a cascade of molecular and cellular responses (see Chapters 4 and 18). As described in chapter 4, oxidized LDL impairs endothelial cell function, activates monocytes/macrophages, and is cytotoxic to vascular smooth muscle cells. Macrophages bind oxidized LDL but not native LDL via the acetyl-LDL ("scavenger") receptor (1). Once internalized, oxidized LDL induces secretion of chemokines by endothelial cells (2) and increases adhesion of monocytes to endothelial cells (3,4), thus promoting the influx of inflammatory cells into the lesion. Subsequently, oxidized LDL promotes differentiation of monocytes into tissue macrophages (5). T cells are then activated in a monocyte-dependent manner (6). Restenosis involves the creation of similar lesions typified by lipid-laden macrophages accumulating in the injured arterial wall, causing the migration of smooth muscle cells from media to the intima and subsequent cell proliferation and secretion of extracellular matrix. Rosenfeld *et al.* demonstrated (7) that isolated macrophage-derived foam cells after balloon injury have an intrinsically high capacity to oxidize LDL.

It is not surprising, therefore, that antioxidants have been proposed as a means to control restenosis in the clinical setting. There is a wealth of epidemiological data linking supplemental dietary intake of antioxidant vitamins (vitamins C and E and β-carotene) with reduction of the clinical manifestations of atherosclerosis (8) and more powerful antioxidants such as probucol have also been heavily tested. However, the clinical experience with antioxidants has been variable, with some studies showing beneficial effects and others showing no net effect. The enthusiasm generated by promising initial clinical trials raised expectations that these agents would significantly reduce atherosclerosis and restenosis,. The resultant trials, however, generated conflicting results. On the one hand, the progression of femoral artery intimal thickening in the Probucol Quantitative Regression Swedish Trial (PQRST) (9) showed no beneficial effect from probucol therapy. In contrast, studies dealing exclusively with restenosis such as the Probucol Angioplasty Restenosis Trial (PART) (10) showed that probucol was more effective than placebo in preventing restenosis. The Multivitamins and Probucol (MVP) trial added to the confusion with the data showing that probucol was more effective than placebo in preventing post-angioplasty restenosis but its combination with multivitamins diminished the probucol effect (11). Questions were raised about dose and duration of therapy as well as an apparent need to pretreat with these agents prior to intervention.

To reconcile apparently conflicting evidence among clinical trials, it will be necessary to first revisit the preclinical and animal studies and glean a basic understanding of the biological mechanisms of antioxidants and restenosis. Methodological details of the clinical studies must be reviewed as well, to determine whether attributes of study design might explain any discrepancies.

BIOCHEMICAL AND *IN VITRO* DATA

Antioxidant vitamins and probucol may interfere with the development of atherosclerosis and restenosis through both direct and indirect mechanisms. Both vitamin E and probucol can directly decrease LDL and total cholesterol as well as protect LDL from oxidation (12), resulting in a decreased uptake of LDL by macrophages (13). Either directly or indirectly, probucol decreases interleukin-1 (IL-1) secretion by macrophages (14) and inhibits the production and release of growth factors like platelet-derived growth factor (PDGF). α–Tocopherol restores NO release from cells inhibited by oxidized LDL (15), eliminates macrophage binding to IL-1β-stimulated endothelium by regulating surface expression of E-selectin (16), increases the resistance of endothelial cells and macrophages to oxidized LDL-mediated cytotoxicity, and decreases platelet activation by arachidonic acid and phorbol ester through a decrease in protein kinase C (PKC) stimulation (17,18). Tanaka and colleagues (19) showed that probucol directly inhibits smooth muscle cell proliferation in a dose-dependent manner as assayed *in vitro* by cell number (25.3% maximum inhibition) and BrdU incorporation (46% maximum inhibition). This was not a toxic effect, probucol appeared to directly inhibit the mitogen-activated protein (MAP) kinase and PKC pathways. Thus, any model to explain the inhibitory effect of probucol on restenosis must include direct drug effects as well as any proposed antioxidant effects.

ANIMAL STUDIES

Among the first animal model tested for an effect of probucol an atherosclerosis was the Watanabe heritable hypercholesterolemic rabbit (WHHL) (20, see also Chapter 11). In one study, 2 month old WHHL rabbits were fed either standard rabbit chow or rabbit chow with 1% wt/wt probucol for 6 months. Despite only modest reductions in serum cholesterol concentration in the probucol group (approximately 20%), there was impressive reduction in visible atherosclerosis compared to controls. Biochemical studies of the LDL from the probucol-treated rabbits demonstrated increased resistance to oxidation and minimal recognition by macrophage scavenger receptors, suggesting that the mechanism for prevention of atherosclerosis was through decreased LDL oxidation and foam cell formation rather than a direct cholesterol lowering effect (20).

Other studies demonstrated that lipid-lowering alone was not sufficient to control atherosclerosis. Carew *et al.* (21) measured the uptake and degradation of LDL in WHHL rabbits which were treated with placebo, probucol, or lovastatin. The investigators found that the rate of LDL degradation in the fatty streak lesions of WHHL rabbits treated with probucol was approximately half that of WHHL rabbits fed placebo. Moreover, treatment with lovastatin sufficient to reduce cholesterol to the same level as the probucol-treated animals did not have the same protective effect. These results might well indicate that the antiatherogenic effect of probucol is independent of its lipid-lowering effect and is likely due to an antioxidant effect. Bjorkhem *et al.* (22) confirmed this hypothesis by administering the pure antioxidant butylated hydroxytoluene (BHT), which has no intrinsic lipid-lowering effect, to cholesterol-fed normal rabbits. Interestingly, although the addition of BHT to a 1% cholesterol diet actually increased total cholesterol (+40%), triglycerides (+250%), LDL and VLDL levels; there was significantly less atherosclerosis in the BHT-treated animals compared to placebo. Serum levels of cholesterol autoxidation products were lower in the BHT-treated animals, supporting the hypothesis that oxidation state rather than quantity is the important determinant.

Antioxidants have been tested in animal models of restenosis as well. Most studies were performed in cholesterol fed animals rather than WHHL rabbits. Ferns and colleagues (23) assigned rabbits to one of three groups: 2% cholesterol, 2% cholesterol and 1% probucol, and control chow. Rabbits were fed diets for one week before balloon denudation of the left carotid artery and maintained or their respective diets until sacrifice at 5 weeks. Total serum cholesterol was 32% lower in probucol-treated animals fed a cholesterol-rich diet compared to those receiving cholesterol alone. Probucol treatment resulted in a 68% decrease in neointimal macrophage accumulation, a 51% decrease in absolute intimal size, and a 51% decrease in the intima/media thickness ratio. There was an inverse relation between serum probucol levels and intimal macrophage content, but no correlation between serum cholesterol levels and intimal hyperplasia in animals treated with probucol. These data suggest the protective effect of probucol against restenosis must be independent of its lipid effects.

Kisunaki *et al.* (24) confirmed these findings and further demonstrated that pretreatment with probucol was unnecessary in the rabbit model. The aortas of forty-eight normal rabbits underwent balloon denudation and were then subsequently divided into four groups, receiving a standard chow or a 0.5% cholesterol diet alone, each or in combination with probucol. The neointima of cholesterol-fed animals was populated with numerous foam cells as well as more abundant smooth muscle cells than in the chow-fed rabbits. Of note, the intimal thickness of the probucol-treated animals was much less than the placebo-fed animals, with that difference being apparent in the normal diet-fed rabbits but more pronounced in the cholesterol-fed animals. There were also fewer infiltrating macrophages in the probucol groups. Total cholesterol and triglycerides were increased in the cholesterol-fed animals but were unchanged by probucol treatment. Probucol did markedly reduce lipid peroxides, and the greatest amount of oxidized LDL detectable by immunohistochemical techniques was found in the cholesterol-fed, placebo-treated group. These data strongly suggest that oxidized LDL is a critical determinant for infiltration of foam cells and neointimal proliferation after vascular injury, a pathway which is interrupted by treatment with probucol.

Protection from restenosis seems to depend more on the oxidation state of LDL than overall serum cholesterol levels. Schneider *et al.* (25) showed that HMG-CoA reductase inhibitors did not protect against restenosis. In this study, 25 pigs fed either a regular diet or a 2% cholesterol diet for 2 weeks subsequently underwent coronary artery balloon injury and were then treated either with placebo or with lovastatin (2 mg/kg/d). Increased total serum cholesterol did not correlate with increased intimal hyperplasia; moreover, the extent of hyperplasia 28 days after injury was not diminished by lovastatin. Freyschuss and colleagues (26) demonstrated that BHT prevented restenosis. Rabbits were fed either 0.25% cholesterol or 0.25% cholesterol with 1% BHT for three weeks, at which time balloon injury of the aorta was performed. After three additional weeks of dietary treatment, rabbits were sacrificed. Intimal thickness in the BHT-treated animals was one-fourth that of the control animals. Additionally, there were half as many intimal smooth muscle cells, fewer intimal macrophages (RAM-11 staining) and no T cells (L11/135 staining) in the BHT-treated animals compared to those fed cholesterol alone. Although there was no difference in serum lipid levels between the two groups, serum levels of cholesterol oxidation products were significantly lower in the BHT-treated animals.

All of the studies noted above examined the effect of antioxidants or restenosis in the setting of cholesterol loading, leaving the effect in normocholesterolemic animals open to question. This issue was addressed by Tanaka *et al.* (19) who demonstrated a reduction in neointima proliferation in denuded carotid artery of Japanese White rabbits fed standard chow supplemented with 1% probucol for one week before injury and continued for two weeks thereafter. Schneider *et al.* (27) confirmed that the effect of probucol in swine coronary arteries was dose-dependent. Probucol at 1 or 2g/d was initiated two days prior to coronary artery balloon injury and continued for 2 weeks. Both doses inhibited intimal thickening but only the high dose reduced total cholesterol, LDL and HDL; low dose probucol actually raised LDL. These data also infer that the effects of probucol on experimental vascular injury is independent of its lipid effects.

The notion of a cholesterol-independent effect of probucol was further supported by Ishizaka *et al* (28) who found that probucol administered locally to the exterior of injured rat arteries at doses that did not provide a systemic anti-cholesterol effect reduced neointima in an equivalent fashion to systemic administration. Rats were divided into four groups: control, treatment with oral probucol (1%), local delivery of 50 mg probucol (in a pluronic gel complex) to the exterior of the carotid artery at the time of injury, and local delivery as well as oral dosing. Diet was continued for 2 weeks following balloon injury and then the animals were sacrificed. Neointimal area and intima/media ratio were significantly reduced by either local or systemic probucol delivery. Dual therapy resulted in a slightly greater effect. As predicted, local delivery did not affect serum cholesterol values. Finally, there is evidence for potentiating effects, of antioxidant combinations. In a study by Nunes and colleagues (29), if vitamins C or E were administered separately one week prior to balloon injury of porcine coronary arteries, no effect was observed on neointima formation two weeks later. When these vitamins were given together, however, both oxidized LDL and the ratio of intimal area to vessel area were significantly reduced.

In summary, available evidence from animal studies demonstrates that probucol reduces atherosclerosis and neointima formation after balloon injury in cholesterol-fed animals. The activity of probucol to diminish neointimal formation after arterial injury is not restricted to hypercholesterolemic animals, and appears independent of its effect to lower cholesterol. Vascular incorporation of probucol, either through pretreating animals or direct vascular application, corresponds to better protection against neointima formation. Current evidence also links the effect of probucol to a reduction in lipid peroxidation as other antioxidant combinations are also effective, albeit less so than probucol. The reason for such a discrepancy may be due to non-antioxidant effects of probucol that may also contribute to the reduction in neointima formation.

HUMAN STUDIES – PTCA AND STENT

Encouraged by the success of preliminary animal studies, investigators hoped that antioxidants would show a similar benefit in the prevention of both clinical atherosclerosis and restenosis. Studies looking at the role of antioxidants in primary and secondary prevention of atherosclerosis have been reviewed elsewhere (see Chapter 13). This section will focus on the effects of antioxidants in preventing restenosis after balloon angioplasty with or without stent implantation. Interestingly, these studies seem to demonstrate a significant reliance on the mode of antioxidant administration to achieve a beneficial effect.

The first clinical studies looking at antioxidants and restenosis were done with vitamins. DeMaio *et al.* (30) randomized 100 patients after successful PTCA to receive 4 months of α-tocopherol (1200 U/d, over 100-fold greater than the average American daily intake) or placebo. Although α-tocopherol treatment reduced both the restenosis rate (35.5% vs 47.5%) and the incidence of abnormal ETT or thallium tests (34.6% vs. 50%), the effects were not statistically significantly because of inadequate sample size. There was no change in plasma lipids, lipoproteins, apolipoproteins, retinol, β-carotene, or even lipid peroxide levels. In light of these findings, it is possible that α-tocopherol, started only at the time of intervention, did not have enough antioxidant potency to demonstrate a statistically significant result.

The experience with probucol in preventing human restenosis have been more robust than that with vitamin E. In a pilot study (31) with 67 patients undergoing elective PTCA, the rate of restenosis was reduced in patients given 750 - 1000 mg probucol (19.4%, 31 patients) compared to those treated with 150 mg dipyridamole (41.7%, 36 patients). Therapy was begun 7 days before PTCA and continued for 3-6 months thereafter. Angiographic follow-up revealed greater lesion progression even in non-restenotic areas in the dipyridamole group. Analysis of serum markers showed that the probucol group had significantly lower total cholesterol at the end of the study. Probucol appeared to show the greatest benefit in patients with higher initial cholesterol values. A slightly larger study of 118 patients with 134 vessels undergoing angioplasty (32) also demonstrated a benefit when probucol (0.5 mg/d) was begun at least 7 days prior to PTCA and continued 3 months thereafter. Restenosis was reduced from 39.7% in placebo-treated patients to 19.7% in the probucol group. Finally, in the PART trial, patients who received probucol (1g/d) that started four weeks prior to angioplasty and continued for 24 weeks had a significantly lower restenosis rate (23%) than placebo-treated patients (57%) as determined by quantitative angiography (10). Both the LDL and HDL levels were also decreased by probucol therapy. Although these three studies demonstrate the effectiveness of probucol in reducing restenosis rates after angioplasty, the required pretreatment period ranging from 7 days to 4 weeks limits the clinical utility of this compound given the urgent nature of many procedures.

Given the limitations of probucol, it is not surprising that some investigators turned to combination therapy with other agents in a search for synergistic effects. Unfortunately, the importance of pretreatment was again supported by combination therapy trials with HMG CoA reductase inhibitors. Given the benefits of cholesterol reduction for primary and secondary prevention of myocardial infarction, it was hoped that HMG CoA reductase inhibitors, either alone or in combination with antioxidants, might also decrease restenosis and decrease the pretreatment interval. Lee *et al.* (33) enrolled 141 patients in a randomized trial in which the active treatment group received probucol (750 mg/d) starting either at least 30 days prior to intervention (34 patients) or less than 14 days prior to intervention (27 patients). The control group received pravastatin at a dose of 10 mg/d for similar periods of time. Patients also received aspirin, dipyridamole, diltiazem, and isosorbide dinitrate. Five months after PTCA or at prior intervening catheterization, total cholesterol levels were similar in all treatment groups with the probucol patients demonstrating the lowest HDL levels and the pravastatin patients the lowest LDL levels. Restenosis rates were influenced by the drug but also by the timing of administration. Restenosis rates were reduced only by long pretreatment with probucol (17.6%) and not with short pretreatment (48.1%), compared to the pravastatin controls (44.7%, long pretreatment and 35.7%, short pretreatment). This study demonstrated that a lipid-lowering effect alone was not sufficient to prevent restenosis and pretreatment with probucol was required. In the Angioplasty Plus Probucol/Lovastatin Evaluation (APPLE) trial (34), investigators attempted to shorten the pretreatment interval using probucol and lovastatin as combination therapy. Probucol (500 mg twice daily) and lovastatin (20 mg twice daily) were started between 48 hrs prior to and 24 hours after PTCA and continued for 6 months. The active therapy resulted in effective reduction in cholesterol: 27% reduction in total cholesterol, 30% reduction in LDL, but no significant difference in angiographic restenosis or secondary endpoints.

The MVP trial (11) looked at probucol in conjunction with antioxidants, specifically vitamins C and E in 317 patients scheduled for elective PTCA. Patients were randomized to one of four treatment groups beginning 30 days prior to PTCA: probucol alone (500 mg twice daily), multivitamins alone (containing 30,000 IU beta carotene, 500 mg vitamin C, and 700 IU alpha-tocopherol), probucol plus multivitamins, or placebo. Twelve hours prior to PTCA, patients received additional medication according to their randomized group: 2000 IU vitamin E, 1000 mg probucol, vitamin E and probucol, or placebo. Additionally, all patients received 325 mg aspirin daily for the entire study period. There was a definite benefit to probucol therapy compared with control: restenosis rates were 38.9% (placebo), 20.7% (probucol), 40.3% (multivitamin), and 28.9% (probucol plus multivitamin). These effects held up in a *post-hoc* subgroup analysis of small vessels (<3.0 mm diameter) as well (35).

Finally, Sekiya *et al.* (36) studied the individual and combined effects of the antioxidant, probucol and the phosphodiesterase inhibitor, cilastazol. Cilostazol inhibits phosphodiesterase type III and thus suppresses platelet aggregation by increasing cAMP levels in the platelet - an activity similar to other PDE inhibitors such as ticlopidine. However, cilostazol has an additional activity not found in ticlopidine, cilostazol also inhibits phosphodiesterase in the blood vessel wall, resulting in increased cAMP in vascular smooth muscle cells causing vasodilation. There are also reports that cilostazol direct suppresses smooth muscle cell proliferation through a cAMP-dependent pathway. These investigators postulated that a treatment regimen combining two independent mechanisms of inhibiting smooth muscle cell proliferation might be more effective in minimizing neointimal proliferation and restenosis. The study enrolled 136 patients with restenosis after stenting or type 3 post-PTCA dissections in vessels >2.5 mm undergoing stenting. The study protocol involved prospective randomization (without double-blinding) to one of four experimental groups: 81 mg/d aspirin; 500 mg/d probucol starting 5 days prior to stenting with 81 mg aspirin; 200 mg/d cilostazol starting 5 days prior to stenting with 81 mg/d aspirin; 500 mg/d probucol and 200 mg/d cilostazol with 81 mg/d aspirin. Heparin and dextran were continuously infused during stenting. Warfarin was given to patients not receiving cilostazol. All therapies were continued for six months, when follow-up angiography was performed on all patients. The vessel restenosis rates were 31.7% (control), 16.7% (probucol alone), 12.5% (cilostazol alone), and 9.5% (cilostazol plus probucol), demonstrating the benefit of combination therapy. In this study, probucol was effective without prolonged pretreatment.

DISCUSSION

There were several important lessons learned from the major clinical probucol trials. First, the effects of the antioxidants appear to be dependent on the mode and timing of drug administration. Early studies by Reaven *et al.* (37) demonstrated that the lipid-soluble antioxidants probucol and α-tocopherol are incorporated into LDL and increase resistance of LDL to oxidative modification; however, several weeks of oral administration are required to achieve steady-state plasma levels (and presumably tissue levels) for sufficient antioxidant protection in humans. β-carotene does not provide the same resistance to oxidation despite accumulation within the lipoprotein, and the water-soluble vitamin C is not incorporated within the LDL particle. Pretreatment appears to be necessary to see a beneficial effect, although the minimum duration of that pretreatment has not been firmly established. The PART and MVP trials began therapy 1 month before angioplasty, whereas other preliminary positive trials provided probucol for as little as 1 week before intervention. In the absence of pretreatment, probucol failed to demonstrate benefit in preventing restenotic lesions. Local delivery might ultimately be comparable to oral administration, as at least one animal study has shown that a controlled-release device can provide adequate tissue levels directly and without the need for pretreatment, suggesting a potential clinical benefit from drug-impregnated stents (28).

Second, probucol appears to decrease restenosis through several potentially independent mechanisms, perhaps explaining why compared to other antioxidants, probucol alone has demonstrated clinical efficacy. It is clear that the beneficial effect of probucol is independent of its effect on serum LDL and total cholesterol. HMG CoA reductase inhibitors are clearly ineffective in preventing restenosis despite their benefit in primary and secondary atherosclerosis. Furthermore, in the APPLE trial, dual therapy with HMG CoA reductase inhibitors and probucol was actually less effective than probucol alone, an unexpected competitive effect. Collectively, these and other studies suggest that the oxidation state, rather than the quantity, of LDL present is most relevant in explaining the beneficial effect of probucol. However, not all antioxidants appear equal in this regard as α-tocopherol also protects LDL from oxidation but does not appear to afford protection against restenosis.

There was an additional expectation that vitamins and probucol would synergize to reduce restenosis; instead, there was again an apparent competition. Some have proposed that the insignificant effect of multivitamins alone on restenosis might reflect a weaker antioxidant effect than that of probucol. However, the diminished effectiveness of probucol and multivitamins in combination compared with probucol alone as seen in the MVP trial, refutes this assertion. The antioxidant vitamins either individually or in combination appear to interfere with the activity of probucol and the mechanism for this observation remains unclear. The MVP investigators speculated that the pre-PTCA bolus of multivitamins may have had a pro-oxidant effect, however there is no evidence to support this contention. Alternatively, one could speculate that the reduced benefit of probucol when administered with vitamins might reflect some interaction between these compounds. It is germane to note that probucol is metabolized into a number of compounds that are biologically active as well. Antioxidant vitamins may interfere with the conversion of probucol to its active metabolites. Alternatively, they may prevent uptake of probucol into the smooth muscle cells or block other direct effect of probucol. The cholesterol-lowering activity of probucol can be excluded as the sole mechanisms of activity as cholesterol-lowering along is ineffective. Ultimately, the beneficial effect of probucol may be related to its diverse influences on inflammatory responses by macrophages as well as direct effects on smooth muscle cell migration and proliferation as described earlier.

Finally, it is difficult to reconcile the experiences in animal models and clinical trials of atherosclerosis using probucol. The fact that probucol unequivocally inhibits atherosclerosis in almost all animal models of atherosclerosis but completely lacks efficacy in human atherosclerosis is discouraging. Although this drug appeared to be effective against both restenosis and native atherosclerosis in animal models, in human clinical trials it is apparently effective only against restenosis, showing no benefit against native atherosclerosis. Ultimately, these observations underscore the complexity of human atherosclerosis and provide considerable impetus for further study.

REFERENCES

1. Steinberg D, Witztum JL. Role of oxidized low density lipoprotein in atherogenesis. *J Clin Invest.* 1991;88:1785.
2. Cushing SD, Berliner JA, Valente AJ, Ternito MC, Navab M, Parhami F, Gerity R, Schwartz CJ, Fogelman AM. Minimally modified low density lipoprotein induces monocyte chemotactic protein I in human endothelial cells and smooth muscle cells. *Proc Nat. Acad Sci USA.* 1990;87:5134.
3. Berliner JA, Territo MC, Sevanian A, Ramin S, Kim JA, Bamshad B, Esterson M, Fogelman AF. Minimally modifed low density lipoprotein stimulates monocyte endothelial interactions. *J Clin Invest.* 1990;85:1260.
4. Frostegard J, Haegerstrand A, Gidlund M, Nilsson J. Biologically modified low density lipoprotein increases the adhesive properties of endothelial cells. *Atherosclerosis.* 1991;90:119.

5. Frostegard J, Nilsson J, Haegerstrand A, Hamstem A, Wigzell H, Gidlund M. Oxidized low density lipoprotein induces differentialtion and adhesion of human monocytes and the monocyte cell line U937. *Proc Natl Acad Sci USA.* 1990;87:904.
6. Frostegard J, Wu R, Giscombe R, Holm G, Lefvert A-K, Nilsson J. Induction of T cell activation by oxidized low density lipoprotein. *Arteriosclerosis and Thrombosis.* 1992;12:461.
7. Rosenfeld ME, Khoo JC, Miller E, Parthasarathy S, Palinski W, Witztum JL. Macrophage-derived foam cells freshly isolated from rabbit atherosclerotic lesions degrade modified lipoproteins, promote oxidation of low-density lipoproteins, and contain oxidation-specific lipid-protein adducts. *J Clin Invest.* 1991;87:90.
8. Diaz MN, Frei B, Vita JA, Keaney JF, Jr. Antioxidants and atherosclerotic heart disease. *N Engl J Med.* 1997;337:408.
9. Walldius G, Erikson U, Olsson AG, Bergstrand L, Hadell K, Johansson J, Kaijser L, Lassvik C, Molgaard J, Nilsson S, Schafer-Elinder L, Stenport G, Holme I. The effect of probucol on femoral atherosclerosis: the probucol quantitative regression swedish trial (PQRST). *Am J Cardiol.* 1994;74:875.
10. Yokoi H, Daida H, Kuwabara Y, Nishikawa H, Takatsu F, Tomihara H, Nakata Y, Kutsumi Y, Ohshima S, Nishimura S, Kanoh T, Yamaguchi H. Effectiveness of an antioxidant in preventing restenosis after percutaneous transluminal coronary angioplasty: the probucol angioplasty restenosis trial (PART). *J Am Coll Cardiol.* 1997;30:855.
11. Tardif J-C, Cote G, Lesperance J, Bourassa M, Lambert J, Doucet S, Bilodeau L, Nattel S, De Guise P. Probucol and multivitamins in the prevention of restenosis after coronary angioplasty. *N Engl J Med.* 1997;337:365.
12. Parthasarathy S, Young SG, Witztum JS, Pittman RC, Steinberg D. Probucol inhibits oxidative modification of low density lipoprotein. *J Clin Invest.* 1986;77:641.
13. Yamamoto A, Takaichi S, Hara H, Nishidawa O, Yokoyama S, Yamamura T. Probucol prevents lipid storage in macrophages. *Atherosclerosis.* 1986;62:209.
14. Ku G, Doherty NS, Wolos JA, Jackson RL. Inhibition by probucol of interleukin-1 secretion and its implication in atherosclerosis. *Am J Cardiol.* 1988;62:77B.
15. Keaney JF, Jr., Xu A, Cunningham D, Jackson T, Frei B, Vita JA. Dietary probucol preserves endothelial function in cholesterol-fed rabbits by limiting vascular oxidative stress and superoxide generation. *J Clin Invest.* 1995;95:2520.
16. Faruqi R, de la Motte C, DeCorletto PE. Alpha-tocopherol inhibits agonist-induced monocytic cell adhesion to cultured human endothelial cells. *J Clin Invest.* 1994;94:592.
17. Kunisaki M, Bursell SE, Umeda F, Nawata H, King GL. Normalization of diacylglycerol-protein kinase C activation by vitamin E in aorta of diabetic rats and cultured rat smooth muscle cells exposed to elevated glucose levels. *Diabetes.* 1994;43:1372.
18. Ozer NK, Sirikci O, Taha S, San T, Moser U, Azzi A. Effect of vitamin E and probucol on dietary cholesterol-induced atherosclerosis in rabbits. *Free Radic Biol Med.* 1998;24:226.
19. Tanaka K, Hayashi K, Shingu T, Kuga Y, Nomura K, Kajiyama G. Probucol inhibits neointimal formation in carotid arteries of normocholesterolemic rabbits and the proliferation of cultured rabbit vascular smooth muscle cells. *Cardiovasc Drugs Ther.* 1998;12:19.
20. Kita T, Nagano Y, Yokode M, Ishii K, Kume N, Ooshima A, Yoshida H, Kawai C. Probucol prevents the progression of atherosclerosis in Watanabe heritable hyperlipidemic rabbit, an animal model for familial hypercholesterolemia. *Proc Natl Acad Sci USA.* 1987;84:5928.
21. Carew TE, Schwenke DC, Steinberg D. Antiatherogenic effect of probucol unrelated to its hypocholesterolemic effect: evidence that antioxidants *in vivo* can selectively inhibit low density lipoprotein degradation in macrophage-rich fatty streaks and slow the progression of atherosclerosis in the Watanabe heritable hyperlipidemic rabbit. *Proc Natl Acad Sc. USA.* 1987;84:7725.
22. Bjorkhem I, Henriksson-Freyschuss A, Breuer O, Diczfalusy U, Berglund L, Henriksson P. The antioxidant butylated hydroxytoluene protects against atherosclerosis. *Arteriosclerosis and Thrombosis.* 1991;11:15.
23. Ferns GAA, Forster L, Stewart-Lee A, Konneh M, Nourooz-Zadeh J, Anggard EE. Probucol inhibits neointimal thickening and macrophage accumulation after balloon injury in the cholesterol-fed rabbit. *Proc Natl Acad Sci USA.* 1992;89:11312.
24. Kisunaki A, Asada Y, Hatakeyama K, Hayashi T, Sumiyoshi A. Contribution of the endothelium to intimal thickening in normocholesterolemic and hypercholesterolemic rabbits. *Arteriosclerosis and Thrombosis.* 1992;12:1198.

25. Schneider JE, Santoian EC, Gravanis MB, Cipolla G, Anderberg K, King SB, III. Lovastatin fails to limit smooth muscle cell proliferation in normolipemic and hyperlipemic swine in an overstretch balloon injury model of restenosis. *J Am Coll Cardiol.* 1992;19:163A.

26. Freyschuss A, Stiko-Rahm A, Swedenborg J, Henriksson P, Bjorkhem I, Berglund L, Nilsson J. Antioxidant treatment inhibits the development of intimal thickening after balloon injury of the aorta inn hypercholesterolemic rabbits. *J Clin Invest.* 1992;91:1282.

27. Schneider JE, Berk BC, Gravanis MB, Santoian EC, Cipolla GD, Tarazona N, Lassegue B, King SB, III. Probucol decreases neointimal formation in a swine model of coronary artery balloon injury. *Circulation.* 1993;88:628.

28. Ishizaka N, Kurokawa K, Taguchi J, Miki K, Ohno M. Inhibitory effect of a single local probucol administration on neointimal formation in balloon-injured rat carotid artery. *Atherosclerosis.* 1995;118:53.

29. Nunes G, Sgoutas DS, Redden RA, Sigman SR, Gravanis MB, King SB, III, Berk BC. Combination of vitamins C and E alters the response to coronary balloon injury in the pig. *Arterioscler Thromb Vasc. Biol.* 1995;15:156.

30. DeMaio SJ, King SB, III, Lembo NJ, Roubin G, S,, Hearn JA, Bhagavan HN, Sgoutas DS. Vitamin E supplementation, plasma lipids and incidence of restenosis after percutaneous transluminal coronary angioplasty (PTCA). *J Am Coll Nut.* 1992;11:68.

31. Setsuda M, Inden M, Hiraoka N, Okamoto S, Tanaka H, Okinaka T, Nishimura Y, Okano H, Kouji T, Konishi T, Nakano T. Probucol therapy in the prevention of restenosis after successful percutaneous transluminal coronary angioplasty *Clin Therap.* 1993;15:374.

32. Watanabe K, Sekiya M, Ikeda S, Miyagawa M, Hashidi K. Preventive effects of probucol on restenosis after percutaneous transluminal coronary angioplasty. *Am Heart J.* 1996;132:2329.

33. Lee YJ, Daida H, Yokoi H, Miyano H, Takaya J, Sakura H, Mokuno H, Yamaguchi H. Effectiveness of probucol in preventing restenosis after percutaneous transluminal cornoray angioplasty. *Jpn Heart J.* 1996;37:327.

34. O'Keefe JH, Jr., Stone GW, McCallister BD, Jr., Maddex C, Ligon R, Kacich RL, Kahn J, Cavero PG, Hartzler GO, McCallister BD. Lovastatin plus probucol for prevention of restenosis after percutaneous transluminal coronary angioplasty. *Am J Cardiol.* 1996;77:649.

35. Rodes J, Cote G, Lesperance J, Bourassa MG, Doucet S, Bilodeau L, Bertrand OF, Harel F, Gallo R, Tardif J-C. Prevention of restenosis after angioplasty in small coronary arteries with probucol. *Circulation.* 1998;97:429.

36. Sekiya M, Funada J, Watanabe K, Miyagawa M, Akutsu H. Effects of probucol and cilostazol alone and in combination on frequency of poststenting restenosis. *Am J Cardiol.* 1998;82:144.

37. Reaven PD, Khouw A, Beltz WF, Parthasarathy S, Witztum JL. Effect of dietary antioxidant combinations in humans. *Artheriosclerosis and Thrombosis.* 1993;13:590.

38. Omenn GS, Goodman GE, Thornquist MD, Balmes J, Cullen MR, Glass A, Keogh JP, Meyskens FL, Valanis B, Williams JH, Barnhart S, Hanmar S. Effects of a combination of beta-carotene and vitamin A on lung cancer and cardiovascular disease. *N Engl J Med.* 1996;334:1150.

INDEX